SEVENTH EDITION

Introduction to Audiology

Frederick N. Martin
The University of Texas at Austin

John Greer Clark
Helix Hearing Care of America

Allyn and Bacon

Boston • London • Toronto • Sydney • Tokyo • Singapore

Executive Editor: Stephen D. Dragin
Editorial Assistant: Bridget McSweeney
Senior Editorial-Production Administrator: Joe Sweeney
Editorial-Production Service: Walsh & Associates, Inc.
Composition Buyer: Linda Cox
Manufacturing Buyer: Dave Repetto

Copyright © 2000, 1997, 1994, 1991, 1986, 1981, 1975 by Allyn & Bacon
A Pearson Education Company
Needham Heights, MA 02494

www.abacon.com

Library of Congress Cataloging-in-Publication Data

Martin, Frederick, N.
    Introduction to audiology / Frederick N. Martin, John Greer Clark.
—7th ed.
       p.   cm.
    Includes bibliographical references and indexes.
    ISBN 0-205-29536-3
    1. Hearing disorders. 2. Audiometry. 3. Audiology. 4. Hearing
disorders exercises, etc. 5. Audiometry exercises, etc. I. Clark, John
Greer. II. Title.
    [DNLM: 1. Audiometry. 2. Hearing Disorders. 3. Hearing Tests.
WV 270 M379i 1999]
RF290.M34   1999
617.8—DC21
DNLM/DLC
for Library of Congress   99-21824
                                              CIP

Printed in the United States of America

10 9 8 7 6 5 4 3 2 1   03 02 01 00 99

To our families for their love and support.

CONTENTS

3 Sound and Its Measurement   25

6 Electrophysiological Tests   151

15 Audiological (Re)Habilitation   419

P R E F A C E

Despite their considerable insights, the founders of audiology could not have envisioned the many ways in which this profession would continue to evolve to meet the needs of children and adults with hearing impairments. Breakthroughs continue to come in areas related to the study of audition that include the principles of human hearing and the diagnosis and remediation of hearing loss. The profession is more exciting today than ever before.

Since treatment is our goal, and that is impossible without diagnosis, some people have developed the erroneous opinion that audiology is about doing hearing tests. Surely, testing the hearing function is essential; however, many tests could be performed by technical personnel who lack the education required to be total hearing health-care managers. Historically, the profession has rejected this approach and has developed a model wherein one highly trained, self-supervised audiologist carries the patient and family from history taking through diagnosis and into patient management.

A new degree, the Doctor of Audiology (Au.D.), has emerged that expands the education and training of prospective audiologists and provides a level of prestige not heretofore seen. To date, those practicing audiology with an earned doctorate usually obtained a doctor of philosophy (Ph.D.), which places an emphasis on research in audition, and not on clinical matters. The Au.D. is intended to replace the master's degree as the entry degree of audiological practice and to restore the Ph.D. to the position of a scholarly research degree. Holders of the Au.D. might function as supervisors of individuals who carry out technical duties, leaving them free for patient management. As the Au.D. will become the entry level degree early in the twenty-first century, programs are being developed to provide the opportunity to upgrade to the Au.D. for practicing audiologists or those about to enter the profession with a master's degree.

Through its history of nearly a quarter of a century, this book has been used by students in classes ranging from introductory to advanced. Students have used it who plan to enter the professions of audiology, speech-language pathology, and education of the deaf. All of these individuals are charged with knowing all they can about hearing loss and its ramifications. To know less is to do a disservice to those children and adults who rely on us for assistance. It is difficult to envision a more rewarding or exciting way to spend a professional career.

How to Use This Book

The chapter arrangement in this book differs somewhat from traditional audiology texts in several ways. The usual approach is to present the anatomy and physiology of the ear and then to introduce auditory tests. After an introduction to the profession of audiology, this book first presents a superficial look at how the ear works. With this conceptual beginning, details of auditory tests can be understood as they relate to the basic mechanisms of hearing. Thus, with a grasp of the test principles, the reader is better prepared to benefit from the many examples of theoretical test results that illustrate different disorders in the auditory system. Presentations of anatomy and physiology, designed for greater detail and application, accompany the descriptions of auditory disorders.

The organization of this book has proved useful because it facilitates early comprehension of what is often perceived as difficult material. Readers who wish a more traditional approach may simply rearrange the sequence in which they read the chapters. Chapters 9 through 12, on the anatomy, physiology, disorders, and treatments of different parts of the auditory apparatus, can simply be read before Chapters 4 through 8 on auditory tests. At the completion of the book the same information will have been covered.

The teacher of an introductory audiology course may feel that the depth of coverage of some subjects in this book is greater than desired. If this is the case, the primary and secondary headings allow for easy identification of sections that may be deleted. If greater detail is desired, the suggested reading list can provide more depth. The book may be read in modules, so that only specified materials are covered.

Each chapter in this book begins with an introduction to the subject matter and a statement of instructional objectives. Liberal use is made of headings, subheadings, illustrations, and figures. A summary at the end of each chapter repeats the important portions. Terms that may be new or unusual appear in **boldface** print and are defined in a glossary at the end of each chapter, thus eliminating the reader's need to underscore or highlight important words or concepts. In addition, review tables summarize the high points of each chapter. Readers wishing to test their understanding of different materials may find the questions at the end of each chapter useful to check their grasp of new information.

A separate review manual has been prepared that tracks the materials in this book chapter by chapter. Different question styles are employed, along with problem-solving exercises, labeling, clinical case studies, and so on. Answers to the questions in the review manual are provided at the end of each unit. By using the two books in tandem, serious students can quickly diagnose any deficiencies they may have had in learning the material or satisfy themselves that the content is, in fact, mastered.

The indexes at the back of this book are intended to help readers to find desired materials rapidly. In the Author Index, page numbers in *italics* direct the reader to complete book or journal references by a particular author. Numbers in *italics* in the Subject Index identify the page on which a term is defined in a glossary.

The appendixes contain helpful instructions for taking hearing examinations, as well as lists of test materials and commonly used prefixes, suffixes, and abbreviations. These materials have appeared in the back of the book in preceding editions but may now be found on the accompanying CD ROM, entitled Instructions for Taking the Hearing Examination; Word Lists for Use in Speech Audiometry; and Common Audiological Prefixes, Suffixes, and Abbreviations.

ABOUT THE AUTHORS

Frederick N. Martin (Ph.D., The City University of New York), holds the Lillie Hage Jamail Centennial Professorship in Communication Sciences and Disorders at The University of Texas at Austin. His specialty is clinical audiology, and he has particular interests in the area of patient/parent counseling. Books authored by Dr. Martin include the previous six editions of *Introduction to Audiology*, as well as the first four editions of *Introduction to Audiology: A Study Guide, Exercises in Audiometry, Clinical Audiometry and Masking*, and *Basic Audiometry*. Dr. Martin has also edited *Pediatric Audiology, Medical Audiology, Hearing Disorders in Children*, and the ten-volume series *Remediation of Communication Disorders*. In addition, he has written 19 book chapters, 114 journal articles, and 99 convention or conference papers. During his more than 30 years at The University of Texas he has won the Teaching Excellence Award of the College of Communication, the Graduate Teaching Award, and the Advisor's Award from the Texas Alumni Association. He was the 1997 recipient of the Career Award in Hearing from the American Academy of Audiology. He serves as a reviewer for the most prominent audiology journals, and for years co-edited *Audiology— A Journal for Continuing Education*.

John Greer Clark (Ph.D., University of Cincinnati) is the Director of Clinical Services for Helix Hearing Care of America and has specialty interests in audiological counseling and hearing instrumentation. He is co-editor of *Tinnitus and Its Management: A Clinical Text for Audiologists* and author of the professional guide, *Audiology for the School Speech-Language Clinician*, and the consumer guide, *The ABCs to Better Hearing*. His nearly fifty publications cover a variety of aspects of communication disorders. Dr. Clark has received the Honors of the Ohio Speech and Hearing Association as well as both the Prominent Alumni and Distinguished Alumni Awards from the University of Cincinnati Department of Communication Sciences and Disorders. He served four years on the Boards of Directors for the Ohio Academy of Audiology and the American Academy of Audiology. A co-founder of the Midwest Audiology Conference, he has been an Associate Editor and editorial consultant for several professional journals.

Drs. Martin and Clark are both Fellows of the American Academy of Audiology and the American Speech-Language-Hearing Association. Together they have co-edited two academic texts: *Effective Counseling in Audiology: Perspectives and Practice*, and *Hearing Care for Children*. In addition to their work together on the seventh edition of *Introduction to Audiology* and the accompanying *Review Manual*, they have collaborated on research for the periodical scientific literature.

PART ONE

Elements of Audiology

The first part of this book requires no preknowledge. Chapter 1 presents an overview of the profession of audiology, its history and directions for the future. Chapter 2 is an elementary look at the anatomy of the auditory system, to the extent that basic types of hearing loss and simple hearing tests can be understood. Oversimplifications are clarified in later chapters. Tuning-fork tests are described here for three purposes: first, because they are practiced today by many physicians; second, because they are an important part of the history of the art and science of audiology; and third, because they illustrate some fundamental concepts that are essential to understanding contemporary hearing tests. Chapter 3 discusses the physics of sound and introduces the units of measurement that are important in performing modern audiologic assessments. Readers who have had a course in hearing science may find little new information in Chapter 3 and may wish to use it merely as a review. For those readers for whom this material is new, its comprehension is essential for understanding what follows in this book.

1 The Profession of Audiology

The profession of audiology has grown remarkably since its inception only a little more than fifty years ago. What began as a concentrated effort to assist hearing-injured veterans of World War II in their attempts to reenter civilian life has evolved into a profession serving all population groups and all ages through increasingly sophisticated diagnostic and rehabilitative instrumentation. The current student of audiology can look forward to a future within a dynamic profession, meeting the hearing needs of an expanding patient base.

Chapter Objectives

The purpose of this opening chapter is to introduce the profession of audiology, from its origins, through its course of development, to its present position in the hearing-health-care delivery system. The prevalence of hearing impairment and its impact on the individual and society at large will be reviewed, revealing the growing importance of adequate hearing care and hearing loss intervention. The reader will become familiar with the specialty areas within the profession of audiology and the variety of employment settings within which audiologists may find themselves. Students and professionals from disciplines outside of audiology, primarily from speech-language pathology and education of the deaf, will discover close allies within audiology's varied employment settings as they work together toward the successful (re)habilitation of people with hearing loss. Those from allied professions often become active consumers of audiologic information as they pursue their own careers, similarly dedicated to individuals with communication impairments.

The Evolution of Audiology

Prior to World War II, hearing-care services were provided by physicians and commercial hearing aid dealers. Because the use of hearing protection was not common until the latter part of the war, many service personnel suffered the effects of high-level noise exposure from modern weaponry. It was the influx of these service personnel reentering civilian life that created the impetus for the professions of **otology** and speech pathology to work together to form military-based **aural rehabilitation** centers. These centers met with such success that following the war many of the professionals involved in the programs' development believed that their services should be made available within the civilian sector. While it was primarily through the efforts of the otologists that the first rehabilitative programs for those with hearing loss were established in communities around the country, it was mainly those from speech-language pathology, who had developed the audiometric techniques and rehabilitative procedures of the military clinics, who staffed the emerging community centers (Henoch, 1979).

Audiology developed rapidly as a profession distinct from medicine in the United States. While audiology continues to evolve outside of the United States, most professionals practicing audiology in other countries are physicians, usually otologists. Audiometric technicians in many of these countries attain competency in the administration of hearing tests; however, it is the physician who dictates the tests to be performed, and solely the physician who decides on the management of each patient. Some countries have developed strong academic audiology programs and independent audiologists like those in the United States, but with the exception of geographically isolated areas, most audiologists around the globe look to American audiologists for the model of autonomous practice that they wish to emulate.

In the United States, the educational preparation for audiologists evolved as technology expanded, leading to an increasing variety of diagnostic procedures and a professional scope of practice (American Academy of Audiology, 1997; American Speech-Language-Hearing Association, 1996b) that has enlarged to encompass the identification of hearing loss, the differential diagnosis of hearing impairment, and the nonmedical treatment of hearing impairment and balance disorders. What began as a profession with a bachelor's level preparation quickly transformed to a profession with a required minimum of a master's degree to attain a state license held forth as the mandatory prerequisite for clinical practice in most states. A quarter of a century ago, Raymond Carhart,[1] one of audiology's founders, recognized the limitations imposed by defining the profession at the master's degree level (Carhart, 1975). Yet it was another thirteen years before a conference, sponsored by the Academy of Dispensing Audiologists, set goals for the profession's transformation to a doctoral level (Academy of Dispensing Audiologists, 1988).

Today, state license or registration is required in 49 of the 50 states and educational requirements are moving toward a required doctorate in audiology, with the professional doctorate designated as the Au.D. Although the required course of study to become an audiologist remains somewhat heterogeneous, course work generally includes hearing and speech science, anatomy and physiology, speech and language pathology, counseling techniques, electronics, computer science, and a range of course work in diagnostic and rehabilitative services for those with hearing disorders. It is through this extensive background that university programs continue to produce clinicians capable of making independent decisions for the betterment of those they serve.

The derivation of the word "audiology" is itself unclear. No doubt purists are disturbed that a Latin root, *audire* (to hear), was fused with a Greek suffix, *logos* (the study of), to form the word "audiology." It is often reported that "audiology" was coined as a new word in 1945 simultaneously, yet independently, by Raymond Carhart and Norton Canfield, an otologist active in the establishment of the military aural rehabilitation programs. However, a course established in 1939 by the Auricular Foundation Institute of Audiology entitled "Audiological Problems in Education" and a 1935 instructional film developed under the direction of Mayer Shier simply entitled "Audiology" clearly predate these claims (Skafte, 1990). Regardless of the origin of the word, an audiologist today is defined as an individual who, "by virtue of academic degree, clinical training, and license to practice and/or professional credential, is uniquely qualified to provide a comprehensive array of pro-

---

[1]Dr. Raymond Carhart (1912–1975), largely regarded as the "Father of Audiology."

fessional services related to the assessment and habilitation/rehabilitation of persons with auditory and vestibular impairments, and to the prevention of these impairments" (American Academy of Audiology, 1997).

Prevalence and Impact of Hearing Loss

Although audiology had its birth under the aegis of the military, its growth was rapid within the civilian sector because of the general prevalence of hearing loss and the devastating impact that hearing loss has on the lives of those affected. The reported prevalence of hearing loss varies somewhat depending on the method of estimation (actual evaluation of a population segment or individual response to a survey questionnaire), the criteria used to define hearing loss, and the age of the population sampled. However, it is generally accepted that as the civilized world enters the second millennium, there are more than 25 million Americans with sufficient hearing loss to adversely affect their lives.

The prevalence of hearing loss increases with age (Figure 1.1), and it has been estimated that the number of persons with hearing loss in the United States over the age of 65 years will reach nearly 13 million by the year 2015. The number of children with permanent hearing loss is far fewer than the number of adults. However, the prevalence of hearing loss in children is almost staggering

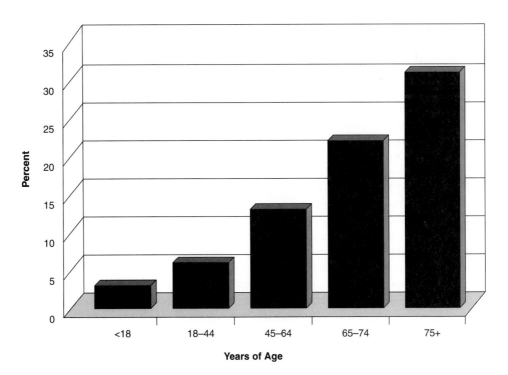

FIGURE 1.1 The percentage of individuals with a hearing loss relative to the general population (Source: National Health Interview Survey, Adams & Marano, 1995).

if we consider those children whose speech and language development and academic performances may be impacted by mild transient ear infections so common among children. While not all children have problems secondary to ear pathologies, 90% of children in the United States will have at least one ear infection before six years of age (National Institute on Deafness and Other Communication Disorders, 1992).

For those children with recurrent or persistent problems with ear infections, the developmental impact may be significant. Studies have shown that children prone to ear pathologies may lag behind their peers in articulatory and phonological development, in the ability to receive and express thoughts through spoken language, in the use of grammar and syntax, in the acquisition of vocabulary, in the development of auditory memory and auditory perception skills, and in social maturation (Clark & Jaindl, 1996). The fact that many children with positive histories of ear infection develop no speech, language, or educational delays suggests that factors additional to fluctuating hearing abilities may also be involved in the learning process (Davis, 1986), but this in no way reduces the need for intervention. The impact of more severe and permanent hearing loss has an even greater effect on a child's developing speech and language and educational performance (Diefendorf, 1996) and also on the psychosocial dynamics within the family and among peer groups (Altman, 1996).

Often, the adult patient's reaction to the diagnosis of permanent hearing loss is as devastating as that of the caregivers of young children with newly diagnosed hearing impairment (Martin, Krall, & O'Neal, 1989). Yet the effects of hearing loss cannot be addressed until diagnosed, and left untreated, hearing loss among adults can seriously erode relationships both within and outside of the family unit. Research has demonstrated that among older adults hearing loss is related to overall poor health, decreased physical activity, and depression. Indeed, Bess, Lichtenstein, Logan, Burger, and Nelson (1989) demonstrated that progressive hearing loss among older adults is associated with progressive physical and psychosocial dysfunction.

In addition to the personal effects of hearing loss on the individual, the financial burden of hearing loss placed upon the individual, and society at large, is remarkable. The total annual costs for the treatment of childhood ear infections alone has been estimated to be as high as $2 billion in the United States (Grundfast & Carney, 1987). When one adds to this figure the costs of educational programs and (re)habilitation services for those with permanent hearing loss and the lost income when hearing impairment truncates one's earning potential, the costs become staggering. Northern and Downs (1991) estimate that for a child of one year of age with severe hearing impairment and an average life expectancy of 71 years, the economic burden of deafness can exceed $1 million.

Audiology Specialties

Most audiology training programs prepare audiologists as generalists, with exposure and preparation in a wide variety of areas. Following graduation, however, many audiologists discover their chosen practice setting leads to a concentration of their time and efforts within one or more specialty areas of audiology. In addition, many practice settings and specialty areas provide audiologists with opportunities to participate in research activities to broaden clinical understanding and application of diagnostic and rehabilitative procedures. When those seeking audiologic care are young, or have concomitant speech or language difficulties, a close working relationship with professionals in speech-language pathology or in the education of those with hearing loss often develops.

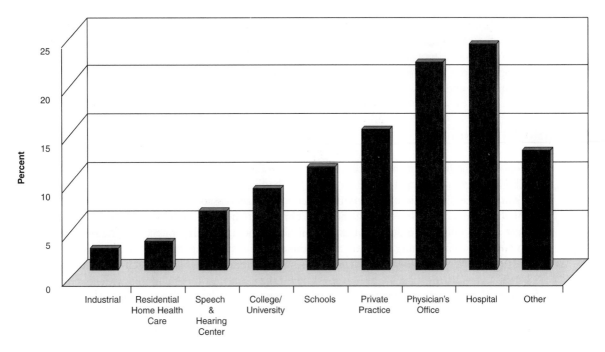

FIGURE 1.2 Audiology practice settings (From demographic profile, American Speech-Language-Hearing Association Research Department, 1996)

It is the varied nature of the practice of audiology that can make an audiology career stimulating and rewarding. Indeed, the fact that audiologists view their careers as both interesting and challenging has been found to result in a high level of job satisfaction within the profession (Martin, Champlin, & Streetman, 1997).

While some audiologists list their primary employment function as a researcher, administrator, or university teacher, nearly 80% consider themselves to be direct clinical service providers (ASHA, 1996a). As noted in Figure 1.2, more audiologists deliver services within a medical environment than any other single employment setting. Private practice constitutes the third largest employment affiliation for audiologists.

Medical Audiology

The largest number of audiologists are currently employed within a medical environment, including community and regional hospitals, physicians' offices, and health maintenance organizations. Audiologists within military-based programs, Veterans Administration medical centers, and departments of public health often work primarily within the specialty of medical audiology. Many of the audiology services provided within this specialty focus on the provision of diagnostic assessments to help establish the location of hearing disorders within the auditory system. The full range of diagnostic procedures detailed in this book may be employed by the medical audiologist with patients of all ages. Results of the final audiologic assessment are combined with the diagnostic findings of other medical and nonmedical professionals to yield a final diagnosis. Medical audiologists may also work within newborn hearing loss identification programs and monitor the hearing levels of patients being treated with medications that can harm hearing. Additional responsibilities may include such nonmedical endeavors as hearing aid dispensing.

Educational Audiology

Following the federal mandates dictated by Public Law 94-142, the Education for All Handicapped Children Act, in 1975 and Public Law 99-457, the Education for the Handicapped Amendments, in 1986, the need for audiologists within the schools has increased. Yet, there remain less than half the number of audiologists to meet the needs of children in the public schools. Educational audiologists bear a wide range of responsibilities in minimizing the devastating impact that hearing loss brings to the education of young children, and in the educational setting they may work closely with professionals in the education of deaf and hearing-impaired children and speech-language pathology. Audiologists in this specialty are responsible for the identification of children with hearing loss and referral for medical and other professional services as needed; the provision of rehabilitative activities including auditory training, speechreading, and speech conservation; the creation of hearing loss prevention programs; counseling and guidance about hearing loss for parents, pupils, and teachers; and the selection and evaluation of individual and group amplification (Blair, 1996).

Pediatric Audiology

Work with children and their families has perhaps more far-reaching effects than any other challenge audiologists undertake. In addition to a honed proficiency in the special considerations involved with the diagnostic evaluation of young children, pediatric audiologists must be prepared to bring to their clinical endeavors an empathy that will help guide parents and families through what is an exceptionally difficult time in their lives. One of the pediatric audiologist's primary roles is the facilitation of parental efforts in meeting the many (re)habilitative challenges the child and family will face.

Nonaudiology professionals who work in the areas of communication and education for children with hearing loss will frequently work closely with pediatric audiologists. Audiologists within a variety of employment settings may work with children and their families. However, those within pediatric hospitals, large rehabilitation centers, and community-based hearing and speech centers will often see a higher percentage of the pediatric population.

Dispensing/Rehabilitative Audiology

More than twenty years ago, the American Speech-Language-Hearing Association rescinded its longstanding ban on the dispensing of hearing aids by audiologists. Since that time, audiologists have become increasingly active in the total hearing rehabilitation of their patients. While many audiologists establish their dispensing/rehabilitative practices within hospitals or physicians' offices, a growing number are attracted to the greater autonomy afforded by an independent practice within their communities. By far the most rapidly growing employment setting for audiologists is that of private practice. Today, private-practice audiology concentrates on the dispensing/rehabilitative efforts of the audiologist, although a number of practices offer a wide array of diagnostic services as well.

Industrial Audiology

As discussed in Chapter 11, exposure to high levels of noise is one of the primary contributors to insidious hearing loss. Many of today's industries produce noise levels of sufficient intensity to permanently damage employees' hearing. According to the National Institute for Occupational Safety and Health (1996), more than 30 million American workers are exposed to hazardous noise levels, resulting in noise-induced occupational hearing loss being the most common occupational disease. Allowable levels and duration of employee noise exposure have been set by the Department of Health. To ensure that adequate hearing protection is both provided by the employer and used effectively by the employee, audiologists who work in industry design hearing conservation programs to identify and measure excessive noise areas, consult in the reduction of noise levels produced by industrial equipment, monitor employee hearing levels, educate employees on the permanent consequences of excessive noise exposure, and fit hearing protection for those employees with excessive exposure (Melnick, 1994). While some audiologists devote their full-time practice exclusively within industrial settings, most who work with industry provide these services as part-time contracted consultants, or as an adjunct to their work within other practice settings. As consultants to industry, audiologists may work in conjunction with attorneys, industrial physicians and nurses, industrial hygienists, safety engineers, and industrial relations and personnel officers within management and unions.

Professional Societies

A number of professional societies for the advancement of the interests of audiologists and those they serve have evolved as the profession itself has grown (see lists on CD-ROM). The American Speech Correction Association (originally founded in 1927 as the American Society for the Study of Disorders of Speech) adopted the new profession of audiology in 1947 when its name was changed to the American Speech and Hearing Association (ASHA). Renamed the American Speech-Language-Hearing Association in 1978 (while retaining its recognized acronym), ASHA was instrumental in setting standards for the practice of audiology and for the accreditation of academic programs for audiologists and speech-language pathologists. ASHA provides continuing education and professional and scientific journals for these two professions, which share a common heritage.

Recognizing the necessity for a strong national association that could represent the unique needs and interests of the audiology profession, the American Academy of Audiology (AAA) was founded in 1988. Rapidly embraced by the profession, AAA became the home of more than 6000 audiologists before the Academy was ten years old. The Academy is committed to the advancement of audiological services through both increased public awareness of hearing disorders and audiological services among the American people, as well as national governmental agencies and congressional representatives. The Academy's journals and continuing education programs are instrumental in audiologists' continuing level of expertise in their chosen profession. AAA, along with ASHA, continues to set and revise practice standards, protocols, and guidelines for the practice of audiology to ensure quality patient care.

In addition to belonging to one or both of the national associations for audiology, as well as their state academy of audiology, many practitioners will belong to organizations that promote their own particular chosen area of expertise. Audiologists may affiliate with other audiologists with similar interests through the Academy of Rehabilitative Audiology, the Academy of Dispensing Audiologists, or the Educational Audiology Association. The American Auditory Society presents a unique opportunity for audiologists to interact with a variety of medical and nonmedical professionals whose endeavors are largely directed toward work with those who have hearing impairment. Finally, some audiologists will find professional growth through affiliation with one or more of the primarily consumer-oriented associations such as Self Help for Hard of Hearing People, Inc. (SHHH) and the Alexander Graham Bell Association for the Deaf.

Summary

Compared to other professions in the health arena, audiology is a relative newcomer, emerging from the combined efforts of otology and speech pathology during World War II. Following the war, this new area of study and practice grew rapidly within the civilian sector because of the high prevalence of hearing loss in the general population and the devastating effects on individuals and families when hearing loss remains untreated. To fully support the needs of those served, especially within the pediatric population, a close working relationship is often maintained with speech-language pathologists and educators of those with hearing impairment. A mutual respect for what each profession brings to the (re)habilitation of those with hearing impairments leads to the highest level of remediation for those served.

Today the profession of audiology supports a variety of specialty areas and is moving toward a professional doctorate as the entry-level degree. Given projected population demographics, students choosing to enter this profession will find themselves well-placed for professional growth and security.

STUDY QUESTIONS

1. List the specialty areas of audiology and the types of employment settings in which they may be practiced.

2. What purpose do professional societies serve for the profession of audiology and its practitioners?

3. Briefly outline the evolution of audiology.

4. Discuss the economic burden hearing loss presents to society.

GLOSSARY

Aural rehabilitation Treatment to improve communication ability of those with hearing loss acquired after the development of spoken language.

Otology Subspecialty of medicine devoted to the diagnosis and treatment of diseases of the ear.

REFERENCES

Academy of Dispensing Audiologists. (1988). *Proceedings, ADA conference on professional education.* October 7–8, Chicago.

Adams, P. F., & Marano, M. A. (1995). *Current estimates from the National Health Interview Survey, 1994.* National Center for Health Statistics. *Vital Health Statistics, 10,* 193.

Altman, E. (1996). Meeting the needs of adolescents with impaired hearing. In F. N. Martin & J. G. Clark (Eds.), *Hearing care for children* (pp. 197–210). Boston: Allyn & Bacon.

American Academy of Audiology. (1997). Audiology: Scope of practice. *Audiology Today, 9*(2), 12–13.

American Speech-Language-Hearing Association (ASHA). (1996a). *Demographic profile.* Speech-Language, Hearing Science and Research Department.

———. (1996b). Scope of practice in audiology. *Asha,* Supplement 16, 12–15.

Bess, F., Lichtenstein, J., Logan, S., Burger, J., & Nelson, E., (1989). Hearing impairment as a determinant of function in the elderly. *Journal of the American Geriatric Society, 37,* 123–128.

Blair, J. C. (1996). Educational audiology. In F. N. Martin & J. G. Clark, (Eds.), *Hearing care for children* (pp. 316–334). Boston: Allyn & Bacon.

Clark, J. G. & Jaindl, M. (1996). Conductive hearing loss in children: Etiology and pathology. In F. N. Martin & J. G. Clark (Eds.), *Hearing care for children* (pp. 45–72). Boston: Allyn & Bacon.

Carhart, R. (1975). Introduction. In M. C. Pollack (Ed.), *Amplification for the hearing-impaired* (pp. xix–xxxvi). New York: Grune & Stratton.

Davis, J. (1986). Remediation of hearing, speech and language deficits resulting from otitis media. In J. F. Kavanagh (Ed.), *Otitis media and child development* (pp. 182–191). Parkton, MD: York Press.

Diefendorf, A. O. (1996). Hearing loss and its effects. In F. N. Martin & J. G. Clark (Eds.), *Hearing care for children* (pp. 3–19). Boston: Allyn & Bacon.

Education For All Handicapped Children Act of 1975. Public Law 94-142. U.S. Congress, 94th Congress, 1st Session. U.S. Code, Section 1041-1456.

Education Of The Handicapped Amendments. (1986). Public Law 99-457, *U.S. Statutes at Large,* 100, 1145-1176. Washington, DC: U.S. Government Printing Office.

Grundfast, K., & Carney, C. J. (1987). *Ear infections in your child.* Hollywood, FL: Compton Books.

Henoch, M. A. (1979). *Aural rehabilitation for the elderly.* New York: Grune & Stratton.

Martin, F. N., Champlin, C. A., & Streetman, P. S. (1997). Audiologists' professional satisfaction. *Journal of the American Academy of Audiology, 8,* 11–17.

Martin, F. N., Krall, L., & O'Neal, J. (1989). The diagnosis of acquired hearing loss: Patient reactions. *Asha, 31,* 47–50.

Melnick, W. (1994). Industrial hearing conservation. In J. Katz (Ed.), *Handbook of clinical audiology* (pp. 534–552). Baltimore: Williams and Wilkins.

National Institute for Occupational Safety and Health (NIOSH). (1996). *National occupational research agenda* (DHHS/NIOSH Pub. No. 96-115). Cincinnati, OH: Author.

National Institute on Deafness and Other Communication Disorders. (1992). *Research in human communication.* (NIH Pub. No. 93- 3562). Bethesda, MD: Author.

Northern, J. L., & Downs, M. P. (1991). *Hearing in children* (4th ed.). Baltimore: Williams and Wilkins.

Skafte, M. D. (1990). Fifty years of hearing health care. *Hearing Instruments,* Commemorative Issue, *41*(9).

SUGGESTED READINGS (Located on Accompanying CD-ROM under Literature)

American Academy of Audiology (1997). Audiology: Scope of practice. *Audiology Today, 9*(2), 12–13.

American Speech-Language-Hearing Association (ASHA). (1996). Scope of practice in audiology. *Asha,* Supplement 16, 12–15.

2 The Human Ear and Simple Tests of Hearing

Anatomy is concerned with how the body is structured, and physiology is concerned with how it functions. To facilitate understanding, the anatomist neatly divides the mechanism of hearing into separate compartments, at the same time realizing that these units actually function as one. Sound impulses pass through the **auditory** tract, where they are converted from acoustical to mechanical to hydraulic to chemical and electrical energy, until finally they are received by the brain, which makes the signal discernible.

We test human hearing by two sound pathways, **air conduction** and **bone conduction.** Tests of hearing utilizing **tuning forks** are by no means modern, but they illustrate hearing via these two pathways. Tuning-fork tests may compare the hearing of the patient to that of a presumably normal-hearing examiner, the relative sensitivity by air conduction and bone conduction, the effects on bone conduction of closing the opening into the ear, and the lateralization of sound to one ear or the other by bone conduction.

Chapter Objectives

The purpose of this chapter is to present a simplified explanation of the mechanism of human hearing and to describe tuning-fork tests that provide information about hearing. The reader will learn a basic vocabulary relative to the ear, acquire a background for study of more sophisticated hearing tests, and gain exposure to the anatomy of hearing. Because of the structure of this chapter, some of the statements have been simplified. These basic concepts are expanded in later chapters in this book.

Anatomy and Physiology of the Ear

A simplified look at a coronal section through the ear (Figure 2.1) illustrates the division of the hearing mechanism into three parts. The **outer ear** comprises a shell-like protrusion from each side of the head, a canal through which sounds travel, and the **eardrum membrane** at the end of the canal. The **middle ear** consists of an air-filled space with a chain of tiny bones, the third of which, the stapes, is the smallest in the human body. The portion of the **inner ear** that is responsible for hearing is called the **cochlea;** it is filled with fluids and many microscopic components, all of which serve to convert waves into a message that travels to the stem (base) of the brain via the **auditory**

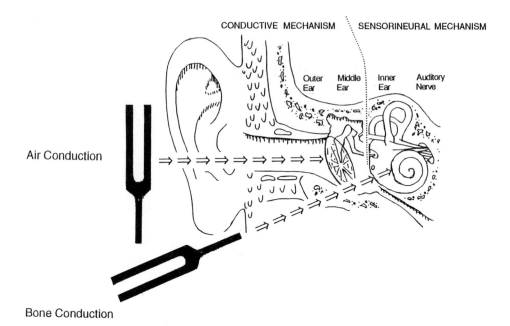

FIGURE 2.1   Cross section of the ear showing the air-conduction pathway and the bone-conduction pathway.

nerve. The brain stem is not coupled to the highest auditory center in the cortex by a simple neural connection. Rather, there is a series of waystations that receive, analyze, and transmit impulses along the auditory pathway.

Pathways of Sound

Those persons whose primary interest is in the measurement of hearing sometimes divide the hearing mechanism differently than anatomists do. Audiologists and physicians separate the ear into the conductive portion—consisting of the outer and middle ears—and the sensorineural portion—consisting of the inner ear and the auditory nerve. This type of breakdown is illustrated in the block diagram in Figure 2.2.

Any sound that courses through the outer ear, middle ear, inner ear, and beyond is heard by air conduction. It is possible to bypass the outer and middle ears by vibrating the skull mechanically and stimulating the inner ear directly. In this way the sound is heard by bone conduction. Therefore, hearing by air conduction depends on the function of the outer, middle, and inner ear and of the neural pathways beyond; hearing by bone conduction depends on the function of the inner ear and beyond.

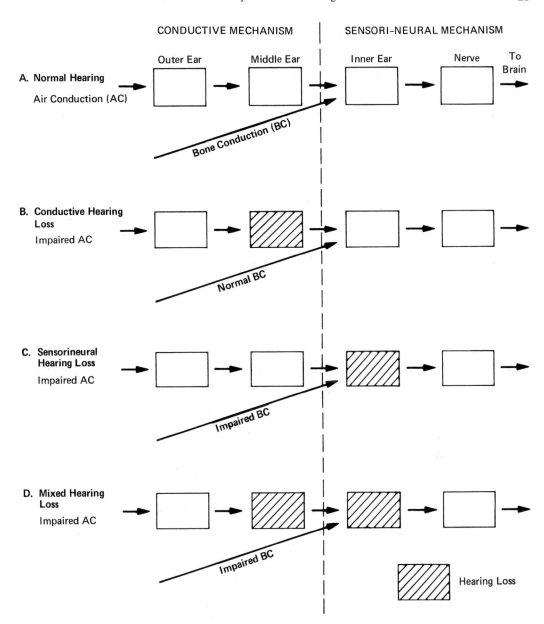

FIGURE 2.2   Block diagram of the ear. A conductive hearing loss is illustrated by damage to the middle ear. Damage to the outer ear would produce the same effect. Similarly, a sensorineural hearing loss could be illustrated by damage to the hearing nerve as well as to the inner ear.

Types of Hearing Loss

Conductive Hearing Loss

A decrease in the strength of a sound is called **attenuation.** Sound attenuation is precisely the result of a conductive hearing loss. Whenever a barrier to sound is present in the outer ear or middle ear, some loss of hearing will result. Individuals will find that their sensitivity to sounds that are introduced by air conduction is impaired by such a blockage. If the sound is introduced by bone conduction, it bypasses the obstacle and goes directly to the sensorineural mechanism. Because the inner ear and the other sensorineural structures are unimpaired, the hearing by bone conduction will be normal. This impaired air conduction with normal bone conduction is called a **conductive hearing loss** and is diagrammed in Figure 2.2B. In this illustration the **hearing loss** is caused by damage to the middle ear. Outer ear abnormalities produce the same relationship between air and bone conduction.

Sensorineural Hearing Loss

If the disturbance producing the hearing loss is situated in some portion of the sensorineural mechanism, such as the inner ear, a hearing loss by air conduction will result. Because the attenuation of the sound occurs along the bone-conduction pathway, the hearing loss by bone conduction will be as great as the hearing loss by air conduction. When a hearing loss exists in which there is the same amount of attenuation for both air conduction and bone conduction, the conductive mechanism is eliminated as a possible cause of the difficulty. A diagnosis of **sensorineural hearing loss** can then be made. In Figure 2.2C the inner ear was selected to illustrate a sensorineural disorder, although the same principle would hold if the auditory nerve were damaged.

Mixed Hearing Loss

Problems can occur simultaneously in both the conductive and sensorineural mechanisms, as illustrated in Figure 2.2D. This results in a loss of hearing sensitivity by bone conduction because of the sensorineural abnormality, but an even greater loss of sensitivity by air conduction. This is true because the loss of hearing by air conduction must include the loss (by bone conduction) in the sensorineural portion plus the attenuation in the conductive portion. In other words, sound traveling on the bone-conduction pathway will be attenuated only by the defect in the inner ear, but sound traveling on the air-conduction pathway will be attenuated by both middle-ear and inner-ear problems. This type of impairment is called a **mixed hearing loss.**

Hearing Tests

Some of the earliest tests of hearing probably consisted merely of producing sounds of some kind, such as clapping the hands or making vocal sounds, to see if an individual could hear them. Asking people if they could hear the ticking of a watch or the clicking of two coins together may have suggested to the examiner that the upper pitch range was being sampled. Obviously, these tests provided little information of either a quantitative or a qualitative nature.

Tuning Fork Tests

The tuning fork (Figure 2.3) is a device, usually made of steel, magnesium, or aluminum, that is used to tune musical instruments, or by singers to obtain certain pitches. A tuning fork emits a tone at a particular pitch and has a clear musical quality. When the tuning fork is vibrating properly, the tines move alternately away from and toward one another (Figure 2.4), and the stem moves with a piston action. The air-conduction tone emitted is relatively pure, meaning that it is free of overtones (more on this subject in Chapter 3).

The tuning fork tests described in this chapter are named for the four German otologists (ear specialists) who described them in the middle nineteenth to early twentieth centuries. They are rarely used by audiologists, who prefer more sophisticated electronic devices. However, tuning-fork tests serve to illustrate the principles involved in certain modern tests.

The tuning fork is set into vibration by holding the stem in the hand and striking one of the tines against a firm but resilient surface. The rubber heel of a shoe does nicely for this purpose, although many physicians prefer the knuckle, knee, or elbow. If the fork is struck against too solid an object, dropped, or otherwise abused, its vibrations may be considerably altered.

The tuning fork was adopted as an instrument for testing hearing over a hundred years ago. It held promise then because it could be quantified, at least in terms of the pitch emitted. Several forks

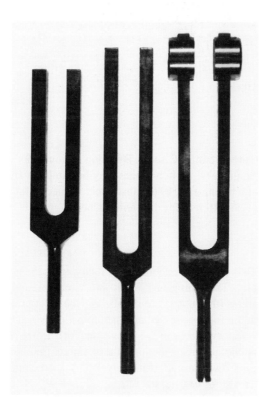

FIGURE 2.3   Several tuning forks. The larger forks vibrate at lower frequencies than the smaller forks.

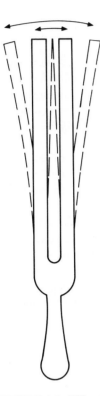

FIGURE 2.4   Vibration pattern of tuning forks.

are available that correspond to notes on the scientific C scale. By using tuning forks with various known properties, hearing sensitivity through several pitch ranges may be sampled. However, any diagnostic statement made on the basis of a tuning-fork test is absolutely limited to the pitch of the fork used because hearing sensitivity is often different for different pitches.

The Schwabach Test

The **Schwabach test,**[1] introduced in 1890, is a bone-conduction test. It compares the hearing sensitivity of a patient with that of an examiner. The tuning fork is set into vibration, and the stem is placed alternately against the **mastoid process** (the bony protrusion behind the ear) of the patient and of the examiner (Figure 2.5A). Each time the fork is pressed against the patient's head, the patient indicates whether the tone is heard. The vibratory energy of the tines of the fork decreases over time, making the tone softer. When the patient no longer hears the tone, the examiner immediately places the stem of the tuning fork behind his or her own ear and, using a watch, notes the number of seconds that the tone is audible after the patient stops hearing it.

---

[1]Named for Dr. Dabobert Schwabach, 1846–1920.

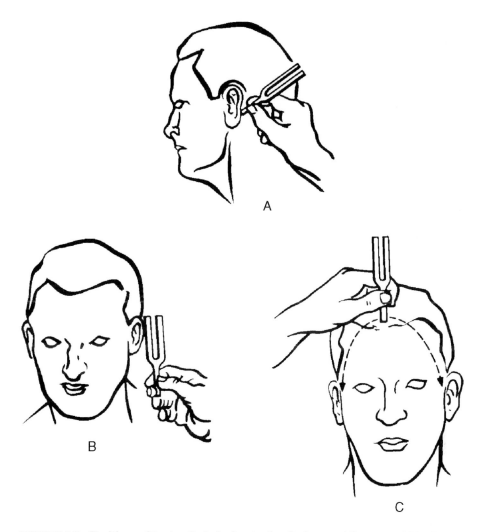

FIGURE 2.5   Positions of tuning fork during tuning-fork tests. (Courtesy of The Ear and Nose-Throat Clinic, P.A., Little Rock, Arkansas)

This test assumes that examiners have normal hearing, and it is less than worthless unless this is true. If both examiners and patients have normal hearing, both will stop hearing the tone emitted by the fork at approximately the same time. This is called a *normal Schwabach*. If patients have sensorineural hearing loss, hearing by bone conduction is impaired, and they will stop hearing the sound much sooner than the examiner. This is called a *diminished Schwabach*. The test can be quantified to some degree by recording the number of seconds an examiner continues to hear the tone after a patient has stopped hearing it. If an examiner hears the tone for 10 seconds longer than a patient, the patient's hearing is "diminished 10 seconds." If patients have a conductive hearing loss, bone conduction is normal and they will hear the tone for at least as long as the examiner, and sometimes longer. In some conductive hearing losses, the patient's hearing in the low-pitch range may appear to be better than normal. When this occurs, the result is called a *prolonged Schwabach.*

Difficulties arise in the administration and interpretation of the Schwabach test. Interpretation of test results in cases of mixed hearing losses is especially difficult. Because both inner ears are very close together and are embedded in the bones of the skull, it is virtually impossible to stimulate one without simultaneously stimulating the other. Therefore, if there is a difference in sensitivity between the two inner ears, a patient will probably respond to sound heard through the better ear, which can cause a *false normal Schwabach.* Thus, the examiner may have difficulty determining which ear is actually being tested.

The Rinne Test

Performance of the **Rinne test**[2] compares patients' hearing sensitivity by bone conduction to their sensitivity by air conduction. This is done by asking them to state whether the tone is louder when the tuning-fork stem is held against the bone behind the ear, as in the Schwabach test (Figure 2.5A), or when the tines of the fork that are generating an air-conducted sound are held next to the opening of the ear (Figure 2.5B). Because air conduction is a more efficient means of sound transmission to the inner ear than bone conduction, people with normal hearing will hear a louder tone when the fork is at the ear than when it is behind the ear. This is called a *positive Rinne.* A positive Rinne also occurs in patients with sensorineural hearing loss. The attenuation produced by a problem in the sensorineural mechanism produces the same degree of loss by air conduction as by bone conduction (Figure 2.2C).

If patients have more than a mild conductive hearing loss, their bone-conduction hearing is normal (Figure 2.2B), and they will hear a louder tone with the stem of the fork behind the ear (bone conduction) than with the tines at the ear (air conduction). This is called a *negative Rinne.* Sometimes patients manifest what has been called the *false negative Rinne,* which occurs when the inner ear not deliberately being tested responds to the tone. As mentioned in the discussion of the Schwabach test, this may happen readily during bone-conduction tests. For example, if the right ear is the one being tested, the loudness of the air-conducted tone in the right ear may inadvertently be compared to the loudness of the bone-conducted tone in the left ear. If the left-ear bone conduction is more sensitive than the right-ear bone conduction, a false negative Rinne may result, giving rise to an improper diagnosis of conductive hearing loss.

The Bing Test

For some time it has been known that when persons with normal hearing close off the opening into the ear canal, the loudness of a tone presented by bone conduction increases. This phenomenon has been called the **occlusion effect,** and it is observed primarily for low-pitched sounds. This effect is also evident in patients with sensorineural hearing loss, but it is absent in patients with conductive hearing loss. This is the premise of the **Bing test.**[3]

---

[2]Named for Dr. Heinrich Rinne, 1819–1868.

[3]Named for Dr. Albert Bing, 1844–1922.

When performing the Bing test, the tuning-fork handle is held to the mastoid process behind the ear (Figure 2.5A) while the examiner alternately closes and opens the ear canal with a finger. For normal hearers and those with sensorineural hearing loss, the result is a pulsating sound, or a sound that seems to get louder and softer (called a *positive Bing*). For patients with conductive hearing losses, no change in the loudness of the sound is noticed (*negative Bing*). The examiner must not suggest to patients what their responses should be. As in the Schwabach and Rinne tests, the danger of a response to the tone by the nontest ear is ever present.

The Weber Test

Since its introduction in 1834, the **Weber test**[4] has been so popular that it has been modified by many audiologists for use with modern electronic testing equipment. It is a test of **lateralization;** that is, patients must state where they hear the tone (left ear, right ear, both ears, or midline).

When performing the Weber test, the tuning fork is set into vibration, and the stem is placed on the midline of the patient's skull. Figure 2.5C shows placement on the forehead, which is probably the most popular location. Other sites are also used, such as the top or the back of the head, the chin, or the upper teeth. In most cases the upper teeth produce the loudest bone-conducted sound. Patients are simply asked in which ear they hear a louder sound. Often the reply is that they hear it in only one ear.

People with normal hearing or with equal amounts of the same type of hearing loss in both ears (conductive, sensorineural, or mixed) will report a midline sensation. They may say that the tone is equally loud in both ears, that they cannot tell any difference, or that they hear the tone as if it originated somewhere in the middle of the head. Patients with sensorineural hearing loss in one ear will hear the tone in their better ear. Patients with conductive hearing loss in one ear will hear the tone in their poorer ear.

The midline sensation is easy to understand. If the ears are equally sensitive and equally stimulated, equal loudness should logically result. One explanation of the Weber effect in sensorineural cases is based on the Stenger effect. The **Stenger principle** states that if two tones that are identical in all ways except loudness are introduced simultaneously into both ears, only the louder tone will be perceived. When the bone-conduction sensitivity is poorer in one ear than in the other, the tone being introduced to both ears with equal energy will be perceived as softer or will not be perceived at all in the poorer ear.

Results on the Weber test are most poorly understood in unilateral conductive hearing losses. The explanation for the tone being louder in the ear with a conductive loss than in the normal ear is probably based on the same phenomenon as prolonged bone conduction, described briefly in the discussion of the Schwabach test.

The Weber test has been known to avert misdiagnosis of unilateral sensorineural hearing loss as conductive when false normal Schwabach or false negative Rinne results are seen but the tone is heard in the poorer-hearing ear rather than the expected better-hearing ear. The Weber test is quick, easy, and often helpful, although like most auditory tests it has some drawbacks. Clinical experience has shown that many patients with a conductive hearing loss in one ear report hearing the tone in their better ear because what they are actually experiencing seems incorrect or even foolish to them.

[4]Named for Dr. Friedrich Weber, 1832–1891.

Again, care must be taken not to lead patients into giving the kind of response they think is "correct." Interpretation of the Weber test is also difficult in mixed hearing losses.

Summary

The mechanisms of hearing may roughly be broken down into conductive and sensorineural portions. Tests by air conduction measure sensitivity through the entire hearing pathway. Tests by bone conduction sample the sensitivity of the structures from the inner ear and beyond, up to the brain. The Schwabach test compares the bone-conduction sensitivity of the patient to that of a presumed normal-hearing person (the examiner); the Rinne tuning-fork test compares patients' own hearing by bone conduction to their hearing by air conduction in order to sample for conductive versus sensorineural loss; the Bing test samples for conductive hearing loss by testing the effect of occluding the ear; and the Weber test checks for lateralization of a bone-conducted tone presented to the midline of the skull to determine if a loss in only one ear is conductive or sensorineural.

STUDY QUESTIONS

1. Sketch a diagram of the ear. Mark the conductive and sensorineural areas.

2. What information is derived from bone conduction that cannot be inferred from air conduction?

3. Why is it a good idea to use more than one tuning fork when doing tuning-fork tests?

4. Why are statements regarding the results of different tuning-fork tests limited to the pitch of the fork used?

5. What are the probable results on the four tuning-fork tests described in this chapter on a person with a conductive hearing loss in the right ear? State results for both ears.

6. What is implied if a person's hearing sensitivity is reduced by air conduction but is normal by bone conduction?

7. What is implied if a person's hearing sensitivity is reduced by air conduction and is reduced the same amount by bone conduction?

8. What are some of the problems with tuning-fork tests?

GLOSSARY

Air conduction The course of sounds that are conducted to the inner ear by way of the outer ear and middle ear.

Attenuation The reduction of energy (e.g., sound).

Auditory Reference to the sense of hearing.

Auditory nerve The VIIIth cranial nerve that connects the inner ear to the brain stem.

Bing test A tuning-fork test that utilizes the occlusion effect to test for the presence or absence of conductive hearing loss.

Bone conduction The course of sounds that are conducted to the inner ear by way of the bones of the skull.

Cochlea That portion of the inner ear responsible for converting sound waves into an electrochemical signal that can be sent to the brain for interpretation.

Conductive hearing loss The loss of sound sensitivity produced by abnormalities of the outer ear and/or middle ear.

Eardrum membrane The vibrating membrane that separates the outer ear from the middle ear. It is more correctly called the *tympanic membrane*.

Hearing loss Any loss of sound sensitivity, partial or complete, produced by an abnormality anywhere in the auditory system.

Inner ear That portion of the hearing mechanism, buried in the bones of the skull, that converts mechanical energy into electrochemical energy for transmission to the brain.

Lateralization The impression that a sound introduced directly to the ears is heard in the right ear or the left ear.

Mastoid process The bony prominence behind the outer ear.

Middle ear An air-filled cavity containing a chain of three tiny bones. Their function is to carry energy from the outer ear to the inner ear.

Mixed hearing loss The sum of the hearing losses produced by abnormalities in both the conductive and sensorineural mechanisms of hearing.

Occlusion effect (OE) The impression of increased loudness of a bone-conducted tone when the outer ear is tightly covered or occluded.

Outer ear The outermost portion of the hearing mechanism, filled with air. Its primary function is to carry sounds to the middle ear.

Rinne test A tuning-fork test that compares hearing by air conduction with hearing by bone conduction.

Schwabach test A tuning-fork test that compares an individual's hearing by bone conduction with the hearing of an examiner (who is presumed to have normal hearing).

Sensorineural hearing loss The loss of sound sensitivity produced by abnormalities of the inner ear or nerve pathways beyond the inner ear to the brain.

Stenger principle When two tones are presented to both ears simultaneously, only the louder one is perceived.

Tuning fork A metal instrument with a stem and two tines. When struck, it vibrates, producing an audible, near-perfect tone.

Weber test A tuning-fork test performed in cases of hearing loss in one ear to determine if the impairment in the poorer ear is conductive or sensorineural.

SUGGESTED READING

Johnson, E. W. (1970). Tuning forks to audiometers and back again. *Laryngoscope, 80,* 49–68.

REVIEW TABLE 2.1   Types of Hearing Loss

Anatomical Area	Purpose	Type of Loss
Outer ear	Conduct sound energy	Conductive
Middle ear	Conduct sound energy Increase sound intensity	Conductive
Inner ear	Convert mechanical to hydraulic to electrochemical energy	Sensorineural
Auditory nerve	Transmit electrochemical (nerve) impulses to brain	Sensorineural

REVIEW TABLE 2.2   Tuning-fork Tests

Test	Purpose	Placement Fork	Normal Hearing	Conductive Loss	Sensorineural Loss
Schwabach	Compare patient's BC to normal	Mastoid process	*Normal Schwabach:* Patient hears tone as long as examiner	*Normal or prolonged Schwabach:* Patient hears tone as long as, or longer than examiner	*Diminished Schwabach:* Patient hears tone for shorter time than examiner
Rinne	Compare patient's AC to BC	Alternately mastoid process and at ear opening	*Positive Rinne:* Louder at ear	*Negative Rinne:* Louder behind ear	*Positive Rinne:* Louder at ear
Bing	Determine presence or absence of occlusion effect	Mastoid process	*Positive Bing:* Tone sounds louder with ear opening occluded	*Negative Bing:* Tone does not sound louder with ear opening occluded	*Positive Bing:* Tone sounds louder with ear opening occluded
Weber	Determine conductive vs. sensorineural loss (in unilateral losses)	Midline of head	Tone equally loud in both ears	Tone louder in poorer ear	Tone louder in better ear

AC = air conduction; BC = bone conduction.

REVIEW TABLE 2.3   Relationship Between Air Conduction and Bone Conduction for Different Hearing Conditions

Finding	Condition
Normal air conduction	Normal hearing
Normal bone conduction	Normal hearing or conductive hearing loss
Poorer hearing for air conduction than for bone conduction	Conductive or mixed hearing loss
Hearing for air conduction the same as hearing for bone conduction	Normal hearing or sensorineural hearing loss

3 Sound and Its Measurement

It is impossible to study abnormalities of human hearing without a basic understanding of the physics of sound, and some of the properties of its measurement and perception. Sound is generated by vibrations and is carried through the air around us in the form of pressure waves. It is only when a sound pressure wave reaches the ear that hearing may take place.

Many factors may affect sound waves during their creation and propagation through the air, and most are specified physically in terms of the frequency and intensity of vibrations. Human reactions to sound are psychological and reflect such subjective experiences as pitch, loudness, sound quality, and the ability to tell the direction of a sound source.

Chapter Objectives

Understanding this chapter requires no special knowledge of mathematics or physics, although a background in either or both of these disciplines is surely helpful. From this chapter, readers should be able to learn about sound waves and their common attributes and express the way these characteristics are measured. They should also come to understand the basic interrelationships among the measurements of sound and be able to do some simple calculations. At this point, however, it is more important to grasp the physical concepts of sound than to gain skill in working equations.

Sound

Sound may be defined in terms of either psychological or physical phenomena. In the psychological sense a sound is an auditory experience—the act of hearing something. In the physical sense, sound is a series of disturbances of molecules within, and propagated through, an elastic medium, such as air.

If a springy object is distorted, it will return to its original shape. The rate at which this occurs is determined by the **elasticity** of the object. Sound may travel through any elastic medium, although our immediate concern is the propagation of sound in air. Every cubic inch of the air that surrounds us is filled with billions and billions of tiny molecules. These particles move about randomly, constantly bouncing off one another. The elasticity, or springiness, of any medium is increased as the distance between the molecules is decreased. Molecules are packed more closely together in a solid than in a liquid and more closely in a liquid than in a gas. Therefore, a solid is more elastic than a liquid, and a liquid is more elastic than a gas.

When water is heated in a kettle, the molecules begin to bounce around, which in turn causes them to move further apart from one another. The energy increases until steam is created, resulting in the familiar teakettle whistle as the molecules are forced through a small opening. As long as there is any heat in the air, there is particle vibration. The rapid and random movement of air particles is called **Brownian motion**[1] and is affected by the heat in the environment. As the heat is increased, the particle velocity is increased.

Waves

Whenever air molecules are disturbed by a body that is set into **vibration,** they move from the point of disturbance, striking and bouncing off adjacent molecules. Because of their elasticity, the original molecules bounce back after having forced their neighbors from their previous positions. When the molecules are pushed close together, they are said to be condensed or compressed. When a space exists between areas of compression, this area is said to be rarefied.

The succession of molecules being shoved together and then pulled apart sets up a motion called **waves.** Waves through the air, therefore, are made up of successive **compressions** and **rarefactions.** Figure 3.1A illustrates such wave motion and shows the different degrees of particle density. Figure 3.1B illustrates the same wave motion as a function of time.

Transverse Waves

The molecular motion in **transverse waves** is perpendicular to the direction of wave motion. The example of water is often useful in understanding transverse wave motion. If a pebble is dropped into a water tank, a hole is made in the area of water through which the pebble falls (Figure 3.2A). Water from the surrounding area flows into the hole to fill it, leaving a circular trough around the original hole (Figure 3.2B). Water from an area surrounding the trough then flows in to fill the first trough (Figure 3.2C). As the circles widen, each trough becomes shallower, until the troughs are barely perceptible. As the water flows in to fill the hole, the waves move out in larger and larger circles. In water, then, a float would illustrate a fixed point of the surface, which could be seen to bob only up and down. In fact, the movement of the float would describe a circle or ellipse on a vertical axis, while the waves move outward in a transverse direction.

Longitudinal Waves

Another kind of wave, more important in the understanding of sound, is the **longitudinal wave.** This wave is illustrated by the motion of wheat blowing in a field, with the tips of the stalks representing the air particles. The air molecules, like the grains of wheat, move along the same axis as the wave itself when a force, such as that provided by the wind, is applied.

Sine Waves

Sound waves pass through the air without being seen. Indeed, they are real, even if there is no one there to hear them. It is useful to depict sound waves in a graphic way to help explain them. Figure 3.3 assists in such a pictorial representation if the reader will concede a bird's-eye view of a bucket

[1]For Robert Brown, British botanist, 1773–1858.

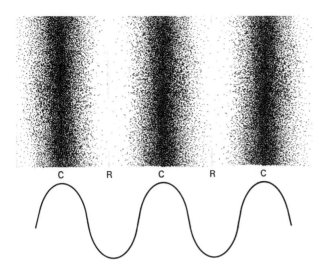

FIGURE 3.1   Simple wave motion in air showing (A) particle displacement (movement of pressure waves through space) and (B) sinusoidal waveform (the pressure wave displayed as a function of time). Note the compressions (C) and rarefactions (R).

of paint suspended by a string above a sheet of paper. If the bucket is pushed forward and backward, a small hole in its bottom allows a thin stream of paint to trace a line on the paper. We assume that forward motions of the bucket stand for compressions of molecules and backward motions for rarefactions. If the bucket continues to swing at the same rate, and if the paper is moved in a leftward direction to represent the passage of time, a smooth wave is painted on the paper; this represents each

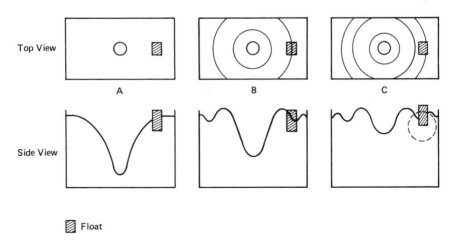

FIGURE 3.2   Wave motion in water as an example of transverse waves. A hole in the water is produced by a pebble (A); the first trough is produced when water flows in to fill the hole (B); the second trough is produced when water flows in to fill the first trough (C). A cork on the surface bobs up and down in a circular fashion.

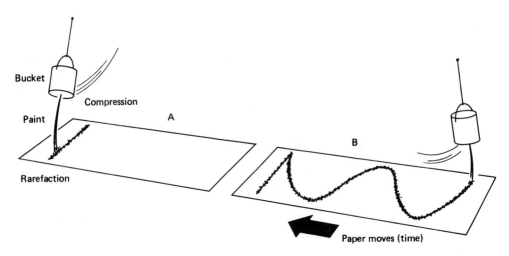

FIGURE 3.3   Sinusoidal motion. Bird's-eye view of a stream of paint from a bucket tracing a line forward (compression) and backward (rarefaction) on a sheet of paper (A). When the paper is moved to the left to represent the passage of time (B), the paint traces a sinusoidal wave.

cycle, consisting of its compression and rarefaction, as a function of time. If the movement of the paper takes one second, during which two complete cycles take place, the **frequency** is 2 cycles per second (cps) and so forth.

A body moving back and forth is said to oscillate. One cycle of vibration, or **oscillation,** begins at any point on the wave and ends at the identical point on the next wave, lending itself to a number of mathematical analyses that are important in the study of acoustics. Such waves are called **sine waves** or **sinusoidal** (sine-like) **waves.** When a body oscillates sinusoidally, showing only one frequency of vibration with no tones superimposed, it is said to be a **pure tone.** The number of complete sine waves that occur in one second constitutes the frequency of that wave. The compression of a sine wave is usually shown by the extension of the curve upward, and rarefaction by the extension of the curve downward. One cycle may be broken down into 360 degrees (Figure 3.4). Look-

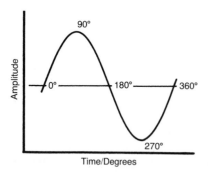

FIGURE 3.4   Denotation of a sine wave into 360 degrees.

ing at a sine wave in terms of degrees is useful, as is seen later in this chapter. When a wave begins at 90 degrees rather than at 0 degrees, it is called a **cosine wave.**

Vibrations

Given the proper amount of energy, a mass can be set into vibration. The properties of its vibration may be influenced by a number of factors.

Effects of Energy on Vibration

Figure 3.5 illustrates the effects of energy on a sine wave. When the oscillating body has swung from point A to point B, it must come to a stop before the onset of the return swing, as the paint bucket in Figure 3.3 must cease its forward swing before it can swing back. At this point there is no **kinetic** (moving) **energy,** but rather all the energy is **potential.** As the vibrating body picks up speed going from B to D, it passes through point C, where there is maximum kinetic energy and no potential energy. As point D is approached, kinetic energy decreases and potential energy increases, as at point B.

Free Vibrations

An object that is allowed to vibrate—for example, a weight suspended at the end of a string (Figure 3.6A)—will encounter a certain amount of opposition to its movement by the molecules in the air. This small amount of friction converts some of the energy involved in the initial movement of the object into heat. Friction has the effect of slowing down the distance of the swing until eventually all swinging will stop. If no outside force is added to perpetuate the swinging, the movement is called

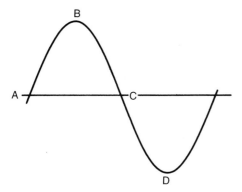

FIGURE 3.5   The effects of energy on a vibrating object. The object is at rest at point A. At point B maximum excursion from the resting position has occurred and all motion stops prior to the return swing. At point B all energy is potential with zero kinetic energy. At point C maximum velocity is reached, so all energy is kinetic and none is potential. Swinging slows down as point D is approached (the same as at point B), and when point D is reached all energy is potential again.

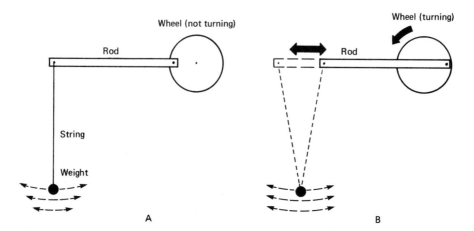

FIGURE 3.6   Free and forced vibrations. If the weight at the end of the string in A is pushed, the swinging back and forth will decrease until it stops. If the rod is caused to move back and forth because of the motion of the wheel (B), the distance of the swing of the weight will remain uniform until the wheel ceases to turn. A illustrates free vibration; B, forced vibration.

a **free vibration.** When the vibrations of a mass decay gradually over time, the system is said to be *lightly damped.* Heavy **damping** causes the oscillations to cease rapidly. When the oscillations cease before a single cycle is completed, the system is said to be *critically damped.*

Forced Vibrations

If an outside force is added to a swinging motion that controls the vibration (Figure 3.6B), swinging will continue unaltered until the outside force is removed. Such movement is called a **forced vibration.** When the external force is removed, the object simply reverts to a condition of free vibration, decreasing the length of its swing until it becomes motionless. In both free and forced vibrations, the number of times the weight moves back and forth (the frequency) is unaltered by the distance of the swing (the amplitude). As the amplitude of particle movement decreases, the velocity of movement also decreases.

Frequency

Nothing may transpire without the passage of time, and it may be questioned how often, or how frequently, an event occurs during some period of time. Occurrences may be rated by using such units as the day or minute; in acoustics, however, when referring to events per unit of time, the duration usually used is the second. Consider the familiar metronome, whose pendulum swings back and forth. Any time the pendulum has moved from any still position to the far right, past the original position to the far left, and then back to the point of origin, one cycle has occurred. Other motions, such as from far left to far right and back again, would also constitute one cycle. If the time required to complete a cycle is one second, it could be said that the frequency is 1 cycle per second (cps). In

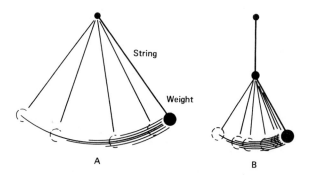

String

Weight

A   B

FIGURE 3.7   Effects of the length of a pendulum on the frequency of the vibration. Given a length of string, the weight at the end will swing back and forth a specific number of times per second. If the string is shortened (B), the weight will swing faster (increase in frequency).

recent years the term **hertz (Hz),**[2] instead of cps, has been adopted as the unit of frequency. The metronome may be adjusted so that the swings of the pendulum occur twice as often. In this way each journey of the pendulum must be made in half the time. This would mean that the time required for each cycle (the **period**) is cut to one-half second. Consequently, the frequency is doubled to 2 Hz. This reciprocal relationship between frequency and period always exists and may be expressed as

period = 1/frequency

Effects of Length on Frequency

With a little imagination, the swinging of an object suspended at the end of a string can be seen to move slowly back and forth (Figure 3.7A). If the length of the string were suddenly shortened by holding it closer to the weight (Figure 3.7B), the number of swings per second would increase, causing the weight to swing back and forth more frequently. Thus, as length decreases, frequency increases. Conversely, as length increases, the number of hertz decreases. The musical harp exemplifies the effects of length on frequency; as the strings get shorter, they are easily seen (and heard) to vibrate at a higher frequency.

Effects of Mass on Frequency

A greater **mass** of an oscillating system results in a decrease in velocity to keep the kinetic energy constant. Simply stated, as the mass is increased, the frequency of vibration is decreased. For example, consider that the increased thickness of the larger strings of a harp produces lower notes.

Effects of Stiffness on Frequency

As a body vibrates, it exhibits a certain amount of compliance (the reciprocal of **stiffness**). As the compliance increases, the frequency at which the body is most easily made to vibrate (the **resonant**

[2]In honor of Dr. Heinrich Hertz, German physicist, 1857–1894.

frequency) decreases. Systems that have more elasticity vibrate better at higher frequencies than at lower frequencies.

Resonance

Almost any mass, regardless of size, may be set into vibration. Because of its inherent properties, each mass has a frequency at which it vibrates most naturally—that is, the frequency at which it is most easily set into vibration and at which the magnitude of vibration is greatest and decays most slowly. The natural rate of vibration of a mass is called its resonant frequency. Although a mass may be set into vibration by a frequency other than its resonant frequency, when the external force is removed, the oscillation will revert to the resonant frequency until it is damped.

Musical notes have been known to shatter a drinking glass. This is accomplished when the resonant frequency of the glass is produced, and the **amplitude** of the sound (the pressure wave) is increased until the glass is set into vibration that is sympathetic to (the same as) the sound source. If the glass is made to vibrate with sufficient amplitude, its shape becomes so distorted that it shatters.

Sound Velocity

The **velocity** of a sound wave is the speed with which it travels from the source to another point. Sound velocity is determined by a number of factors, one of the most important of which is the density of the medium. As stated earlier, molecules are packed closer together in a solid than in a liquid or gas, and more closely in some solids (or liquids or gases) than in others. The closer together the molecules, the shorter the journey each particle makes before striking its neighbor, and the more quickly the adjacent molecules can be set into motion. Therefore, sounds travel faster through a solid than through a liquid and faster through a liquid than through a gas. In audiology our concern is with the movement of sound through air. The velocity of sound in air is approximately 344 meters (1130 feet) per second at standard temperature-pressure conditions (20 degrees Celsius at sea level). When temperature and humidity are increased, the speed of sound increases. At higher altitudes the speed of sound is reduced because the distance between molecules is greater.

The velocity of sound may be determined at a specific moment; this is called the instantaneous velocity. In many cases sound velocity fluctuates as the wave moves through a medium. In such cases the average velocity of the wave may be determined by dividing the distance traveled by the time interval required for passage. Although we often think of velocity in miles per hour (mph), we can shift our thinking to meters per second (m/s) or centimeters per second (cm/s). When velocity is increased, acceleration takes place. When velocity is decreased, deceleration occurs.

As a solid object moves through air, it pushes the air molecules it strikes out of the way, setting up a wave motion. If the object itself exceeds the speed of sound, it causes a great compression ahead of itself, leaving a partial vacuum behind. The compressed molecules rushing in to fill the vacuum result in a sudden overpressure, called the sonic boom. An aircraft flying faster than the speed of sound is first seen to pass by; followed by the boom; followed by the sound of the aircraft approaching, flying overhead, and departing. The loud sound of a gun discharging is made not so much by the explosion of gunpowder, as by the breaking of the sound barrier (exceeding the speed of sound) as the bullet leaves the barrel.

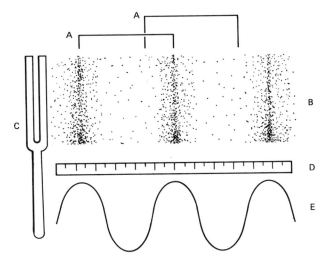

FIGURE 3.8 **Wavelength (A) is measured from any point on the pressure wave to the same point (in degrees) on the next wave. Pressure waves (B) are set up in the air by the vibrating tines of the tuning fork (C). These waves move a given distance as measured by the meter stick (D) and also may be displayed as a function of time (E).**

Wavelength

A characteristic of sound proportionately related to frequency is **wavelength.** The length of a wave is measured from any point on a sinusoid (any degree from 0 to 360) to the same point on the next cycle of the wave (Figure 3.8). The formula for determining wavelength is $w = v/f$, where w = wavelength, v = the velocity of sound, and f = frequency. To solve for velocity, the formula $v = fw$ may be used; to solve for frequency, $f = v/w$ may be used. As frequency goes up, wavelength decreases. For example, the wavelength of a 250 Hz tone is 4.5 feet ($w = 1130/250$), whereas the wavelength of an 8000 Hz tone is 0.14 feet ($w = 1130/8000$). Expressed in the metric system, the wavelength for a 250 Hz tone is 1.4 meters ($w = 344/250$) and for an 8000 Hz tone 0.04 meters ($w = 344/8000$).

Phase

It is convenient to discuss the relationships among corresponding points on different waves in terms of the angular measurements used to describe circular motion. Any point on a sine wave (expressed in degrees) may be compared to a standard. This standard is considered to be zero degrees. If an oscillation has a beginning at 0 (or 360) degrees, it is said to be in **phase** with the standard (Figure 3.9A). Tones presented out of phase (Figure 3.9B, C, and D) are discussed in terms of differences in degrees from the standard function of time (E).

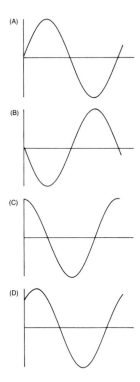

FIGURE 3.9   Relationship of phase on four waves of identical frequency.

Interference

Whenever more than one tone is introduced, there are interactions among sound waves. Such interactions are determined by the frequency, intensity, and phase relationships of the different waves. At any given moment the instantaneous amplitudes of concurrent sound waves are summed. Two tones of the same frequency and phase relationship will reinforce each other, increasing the amplitude. Two tones of identical frequency, but 180 degrees out of phase, will cancel each other, resulting in 0 amplitude at any given moment. Away from laboratory conditions, there are usually more than two concomitant signals, so complete **cancellation** and complete reinforcement rarely occur.

Beats

When two tones of almost identical frequency are presented (e.g., 1000 and 1003 Hz), there will be a noticeable increase and decrease in the resulting sound intensity, which is determined by the separation of the tones in frequency (in this illustration, 3 Hz). These changes in amplitude are perceived as **beats.** When one hears two tones of different frequencies, and the difference between the two frequencies is increased, the number of beats per second increases, changing to a pulsing, then to a roughness, and finally to a series of complex sounds. Depending on the starting frequency, when the difference in frequency between two tones becomes large enough, the ear recognizes number of tones, including the higher one, the lower one, **difference tone,** and summation tone, all of which may be expressed in hertz as multiples of the original two tones.

Intensity

Up to this point we have concerned ourselves with the frequency of vibration and its related functions. It is important that we know not only how fast but also how far a body vibrates—its **intensity.** Figure 3.10A shows two tones of identical frequency; however, there is a difference in the maximum excursions of the two waves. Obviously a greater force has been applied to the wave on the top than to the wave on the bottom to cause this difference to occur. The distance the mass moves from the point of rest is called its amplitude. Because our concern is with particle motion in air, it is assumed that if a greater force is applied to air molecules, they will move further from their points of rest, causing greater compressions and greater rarefactions, increasing the particle displacement and therefore the amplitude. Figure 3.10B shows two tones of identical amplitude and starting phase but of different frequency. Figure 3.10C shows two tones with the same amplitude and frequency but different phase.

Force

When vibrating bodies, such as the tines of a tuning fork, move to and fro, they exert a certain amount of **force** on adjacent air molecules. The greater the force, the greater the displacement of the tines, and therefore the greater the amplitude of the sound wave. Because of the human ear's extreme sensitivity to sound, only very small amounts of force are required to stimulate hearing. The **dyne (d)** is a convenient unit of measurement for quantifying small changes in force.

One dyne is a force sufficient to accelerate a mass of 1 gram at 1 centimeter per second squared. If a mass of 1 gram (one-thirtieth of an ounce) is held at sea level, the force of gravity on this mass is about 1000 dynes. The **Newton (N)**[3] has been used more recently as a force measurement in the United States. One Newton is a force that will accelerate a 1 kg mass at 1 m/s^2.

Pressure

Pressure is generated whenever force is distributed over a surface area. An example is the number of pounds per square inch used in tire-pressure measurements. Normal atmospheric pressure is 14.7 lb/in^2, 1 million dynes/cm^2, or 10^5 **Pascals (Pa).**[4] If a given area remains constant, the pressure increases as the force is increased.

A word might be said here regarding units of measurement. The metric centimeter-gram-second (CGS) system has been popular among scientists in the United States for many years, but is being replaced by the meter-kilogram-second (MKS) system. What might eventually be used exclusively is the International System of Units, abbreviated SI, taken from the French *Le Système International d'Unites.* In the cgs system, pressure is expressed in dynes/cm^2, and in the SI system as Pascals.

Because of the sensitivity of human hearing, micropascals—millionths of a Pascal (μPa)—are used to express sound pressure in the audible range of intensities for humans and most animals. The smallest pressure variation required to produce a just-audible sound to healthy young ears is approximately 0.0002 dyne/cm^2, or 20 μPa. Sound waves that may be damaging to the ear have a pressure of about 2×10^8 μPa.

---

[3]For Sir Isaac Newton, British mathematician, astronomer, and physicist, 1643–1727.

[4]For Blaise Pascal, French mathematician and philosopher, 1623–1662.

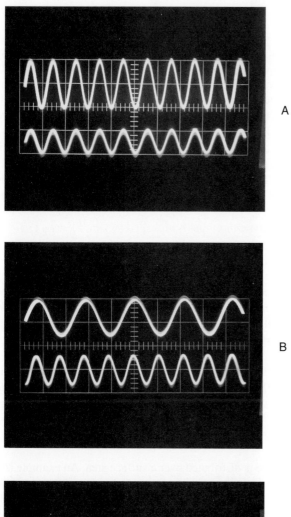

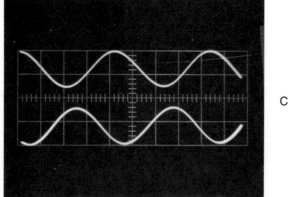

FIGURE 3.10   (A) Two tones of different amplitude (frequency and phase constant), (B) two tones of different frequency (amplitude and phase constant), and (C) two tones differing in phase (amplitude and frequency constant).

Work

When any mass, such as a group of air particles, is moved, a certain amount of work is done as energy is expended. The amount of **work** done may be expressed as the force exerted times the distance the mass is moved. One **erg (e)** is the amount of work done when 1 dyne force displaces an object by 1 cm; one **joule (J)**[5] is 10 million ergs.

Power

Power is the capacity to exert physical force or energy and is expressed as the rate at which energy is expended. Familiar units of power are horsepower and watts.[6] Because human hearing is extremely sensitive, small units of power, such as the erg/second, are used in acoustics. One watt is equal to 1 million ergs/second or 10^{-1} joule/second, and 1 horsepower is equal to 746 watts. Power is a common measure of the magnitude of a sound. As the distance from the source is increased, the sound energy that reaches a given point decreases because the sound's power is spread out over a larger area.

Intensity of a Sound Wave

In any vibration, more air particles are displaced as the distance from the source increases. However, when the intensity of sound is measured, interest is usually centered on a small area at the point of measurement. The intensity of a sound wave is the amount of force per unit of area. Although in any vibration the intensity of the sound decreases proportionately to the square of the distance from the sound source (the **inverse square law**), an intensity of 10^{-12} watt/m^2 (or 10^{-16} watt/cm^2) at 1000 Hz will produce a just-audible sound if that intensity reaches the ear.

Assuming that sound radiates in a spherical pattern from a source, this relationship can be expressed by the following formula:

$$\text{Intensity (watts/cm}^2 \text{ or watts/m}^2) = \frac{\text{power (watts)}}{4\pi \times \text{radius}^2 (\text{cm or m})}$$

Common units of measurement, such as the pound or the mile, are additive in nature. As an example, ten 1-pound weights equal exactly 10 pounds. However, because the range of human hearing is so great, using such units results in very large numbers and becomes cumbersome. It is convenient to discuss one intensity in terms of the number of times it is multiplied by another intensity—that is, in terms of a ratio between the two. The **decibel (dB)** is commonly used for this purpose.

The Decibel

A convenient way of expressing a ratio between two lengthy numbers is to use the logarithm. One unit established in such a way is the **Bel**, named for Alexander Graham Bell.[7] Because a Bel may have a rather large value, the decibel, which is one-tenth of a Bel, is the unit of measurement of intensity used in acoustics and in audiometrics.

[5]For James Prescott Joule, British physicist, 1818–1889.

[6]For James Watt, Scottish inventor, 1736–1819.

[7]American of Scottish descent. Renowned educator of children with hearing loss and inventor of the telephone, 1847–1922.

Five important aspects of the decibel must be remembered: (1) It involves a ratio; (2) it utilizes a logarithm; (3) it is therefore nonlinear; (4) it may be expressed in terms of various reference levels, which must be specified; (5) it is a relative unit of measure.

Logarithms

A **logarithm** (log) is simply a number expressed as an **exponent** that tells how often a number (the base) is multiplied by itself. In the expression 10^2 (ten squared), the log (^{2}) tells us that the base (10) will be multiplied by itself one time ($10 \times 10 = 100$). The exponent is the power, which tells us how many times the base will be used in multiplication (e.g., $10^3 = 10 \times 10 \times 10 = 1000$).

Although any base may be used, in acoustics the base 10 is most common. This is convenient because the log simply tells how many zeros appear after the 1. Table 3.1 (A and B) shows a natural progression of logarithms with the base 10. It is important to note that the log of 1 is zero.

The logarithm is useful in expressing a **ratio** between two numbers. Remember that a ratio is shown when any number is divided by another number. If a number is divided by itself (e.g., 25/25), the ratio is always one to one (1:1), a fact that obtains regardless of the magnitude of the numbers. When numbers with identical bases are used in division, the log of the denominator is subtracted from the log of the numerator (e.g., $10^3/10^2 = 10^1$). These mathematics do not change, regardless of whether the numerator or the denominator is the larger (e.g., $10^2 / 10^3 = 10^{-1}$). When a ratio is expressed as a fraction, the denominator becomes the reference to which the numerator is compared. Ratios expressed without a specific reference are totally meaningless, as in those commercial ads that claim a product is twice as good, three times as bright, or 100 percent faster, and so on, without saying what it is better, brighter, or faster than.

Intensity Level

Under some circumstances it is useful to express the decibel with an intensity reference. A practical unit in such cases is the watt per meter squared (watt/m^2). The intensity reference in a given system may be expressed as I_R (the number of **watts** of the reference intensity). The output (e.g., a loudspeaker) of the system may be expressed as I_O, so that a ratio may be set up between the intensity reference and the intensity output. In solving for the number of decibels using an intensity reference, the formula is

$$dB = 10 \times \log (I_O/I_R)$$

The usual intensity reference (I_R) is 10^{-12} watt/m^2 (or 10^{-16} watt/cm^2), although this may be changed if desired. The exponent tells the number of places the decimal points must be moved to the right or left of the number 1. If the exponent is positive (or unsigned), the number of zeros is added following the 1. If the exponent is negative, the number of zeros placed before the 1 is equal to the exponent minus 1, with a decimal point before the zeros. If the exponent is positive, it suggests a large number; if it is negative, it suggests a small number, less than 1. Therefore, 10^{-12} watt/m^2 is an extremely small quantity (0.000000000001 watt/m^2).

If the intensity reference of a sound system (I_R) is known, the preceding equation may be used to determine the number of decibels of the output above (or below) the reference. As mentioned earlier, it is essential that the reference always be stated. When the reference is 10^{-12} watt/m^2, the term **intensity level (IL)** may be used as shorthand to imply this reference.

TABLE 3.1 Ratios, Logarithms, and Outputs for Determining Number of Decibels with Intensity and Pressure References

A Ratio	B Log	C INTENSITY OUTPUTS (I_O) CGS (watt/cm²)	C INTENSITY OUTPUTS (I_O) SI (watt/m²)	D dB IL*	E Equal Amplitudes	F dB SPL†	G PRESSURE OUTPUTS (P_O) CGS (dyne/cm²)	G PRESSURE OUTPUTS (P_O) SI (μPa)
1:1	0	10^{-16}	10^{-12}	0	Threshold of Audibility	0	.0002	$20.0(2 \times 10^1)$
10:1	1	10^{-15}	10^{-11}	10				
100:1	2	10^{-14}	10^{-10}	20		20	.002	$200.0(2 \times 10^2)$
1,000:1	3	10^{-13}	10^{-9}	30				
10,000:1	4	10^{-12}	10^{-8}	40		40	.02	$2,000.0(2 \times 10^3)$
100,000:1	5	10^{-11}	10^{-7}	50				
1,000,000:1	6	10^{-10}	10^{-6}	60		60	.2	$20,000.0(2 \times 10^4)$
10,000,000:1	7	10^{-9}	10^{-5}	70				
100,000,000:1	8	10^{-8}	10^{-4}	80		80	2.0	$200,000.0(2 \times 10^5)$
1,000,000,000:1	9	10^{-7}	10^{-3}	90				
10,000,000,000:1	10	10^{-6}	10^{-2}	100		100	20.0	$2,000,000.0(2 \times 10^6)$
100,000,000,000:1	11	10^{-5}	10^{-1}	110				
1,000,000,000,000:1	12	10^{-4}	10^{0}	120	Threshold of Pain	120	200.0	$20,000,000.0(2 \times 10^7)$
10,000,000,000,000:1	13	10^{-3}	10^{1}	130				
100,000,000,000,000:1	14	10^{-2}	10^{2}	140		140	2000.0	$200,000,000.0(2 \times 10^8)$

*The number of dB with an intensity reference ($I_R = 10^{-12}$ watt/m²) uses the formula: dB (IL) = $10 \times \log (I_O I_R)$.

†The number of dB with a pressure reference ($P_R = 20$ μPa) uses the formula: dB (SPL) = $20 \times \log (P_O P_R)$.

If the intensity output and the intensity reference are exactly the same ($I_O = I_R$), the ratio is 1:1. Because the log of 1 is 0, use of the formula shows the number of decibels to be 0. Therefore, 0 dB does not mean that sound is absent, but rather that the intensity output is the same as the intensity reference. If I_O were changed to 10^1 watt/m^2, the number of decibels (IL) would be 130. Table 3.1 shows that as the intensity output (C) increases, the ratio (A) increases, raising the power of the log (B) and increasing the number of decibels (D).

It must be remembered that the decibel is a logarithmic expression. When the intensity of a wave is doubled—for example, by adding a second loudspeaker with a sound of identical intensity to the first—the number of decibels is not doubled but is increased by three. This occurs because the intensity outputs of the two signals, and not the number of decibels, are added algebraically according to the principles of wave interference and the rules for working with logs. For example, if loudspeaker A creates a sound of 60 dB IL (10^{-6} watt/m^2) and loudspeaker B also creates a sound of 60 dB IL (10^{-6} watt/m^2) to the same point in space, the result is 63 dB IL (2×10^{-6} watt/m^2).

Sound-pressure Level

Audiologists and acousticians are more accustomed to making measurements of sound in pressure than intensity terms. Such measurements are usually expressed as **sound-pressure level (SPL).** Because pressure ratios are known to be proportional to the square root of intensity ratios (intensity = pressure^2), the conversion from intensity to pressure may be made as follows:

Intensity reference: dB (IL) $= 10 \times \log (I_O/I_R)$
Pressure reference: dB (SPL) $= 10 \times \log (P_O^2/P_R^2)$

Because intensity is proportional to pressure squared, to determine the number of decibels from a pressure reference, I_R may be written as P_R^2 (pressure reference) and I_O may be written as P_O^2 (pressure output). It is a mathematical rule that when a number is squared, its log is multiplied by 2; therefore, the formula for dB SPL may be written

dB (SPL) $= 10 \times \log (P_O^2/P_R^2)$
or
dB (SPL) $= 10 \times 2 \times \log (P_O/P_R)$
or
dB (SPL) $= 20 \times \log (P_O/P_R)$

As in the case of decibels with an intensity reference, when P_O is the same as P_R, the ratio between the two is 1:1 and the number of decibels (SPL) is zero. Just as in the case of intensity, 0 dB SPL does not mean silence; it means only that the output pressure is 0 dB above the reference pressure.

One dyne/cm^2 is equal to 1 **microbar** (one-millionth of normal barometric pressure at sea level), so the two terms are frequently used interchangeably. The pressure of 0.0002 dyne/cm^2 has been the sound-pressure reference in physics and acoustics for some time. It is, however, being replaced by its SI equivalent, 20 micropascals (μPa). This is the reference used for most **sound-level meters** (Figure 3.11), devices designed to measure the sound-pressure levels in various acoustical environments. Therefore, 20 μPa is 0 dB SPL. The threshold of pain at the ear is reached

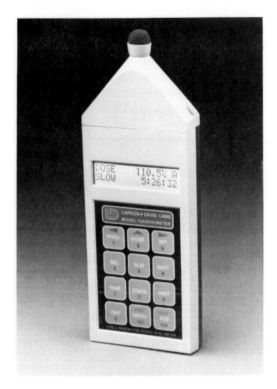

FIGURE 3.11   A commercial sound-level meter. (Courtesy of Larson-Davis Laboratory)

at 140 dB SPL. The term dB SPL implies a pressure reference of 20 μPa. Table 3.1 shows that increases in the number of μPa (or dyne/cm^2) (G) is reflected in the ratio (A), the log (B), and the number of dB SPL (F).

Because the decibel expresses a ratio between two sound intensities or two sound pressures, decibel values cannot be simply added and subtracted. Therefore, 60 dB plus 60 dB does not equal 120 dB. When sound-pressure values are doubled, the number of decibels is increased by six. Therefore, 60 dB (20,000 μPa) plus 60 dB (20,000 μPa) equals 66 dB (40,000 μPa). In actual fact, the SPL will increase by a factor of 3 dB unless the two waves are in perfect correspondence. Also, because of the special relationship between intensity and sound pressure, a 6 dB increase will be shown if the number of loudspeakers is quadrupled, unless they are all in phase.

Note that the amplitude of a wave, whether expressed in decibels with an intensity reference or a pressure reference (Table 3.1, columns C and G), is the same as long as the number of decibels is the same. Intensity and pressure are simply different ways of looking at the same wave. Column E of Table 3.1 is designed to illustrate this point.

Hearing Level

The modern pure-tone audiometer was designed as an instrument to test hearing sensitivity at a number of different frequencies. Originally each audiometer manufacturer determined the SPL required to barely stimulate the hearing of an average normal-hearing individual. Needless to say, there were some differences from manufacturer to manufacturer. Studies were then conducted (e.g., Beasley, 1938) in which the hearing of many young adults was carefully measured. The resulting data culminated in the standard adopted in 1951 by the American Standards Association (ASA). This organization has been renamed the American National Standards Institute (ANSI).

The lowest sound intensity that stimulates normal hearing has been variously called zero hearing loss and zero **hearing level (HL).** Because the ear shows different amounts of sensitivity to different frequencies (being most sensitive in the 1000 to 4000 Hz range), different amounts of pressure are required for 0 dB HL at different frequencies. Even early audiometers were calibrated so that hearing could be tested over a wide range of intensities, up to 110 dB HL (above normal hearing thresholds) at some frequencies. The pressure reference for decibels on an audiometer calibrated to ASA-1951 specifications was therefore different at each frequency, but the hearing-level dial was calibrated with reference to normal hearing (audiometric zero).

Audiometers manufactured in different countries had slightly different SPL values for audiometric zero, until a standard close to what had been used in England was adopted by the International Organization for Standardization (ISO). This revised standard, which was called IS0-1964, showed normal hearing to be more sensitive than the 1951 ASA values, resulting in a lowering of the SPL values averaging approximately 10 dB across frequencies. Differences between the two standards probably occurred because of differences in the studies during which normative data were compiled, in terms of test environment, equipment, and procedure.

Audiologists who had experience testing normal-hearing persons on the ASA standard had noted that many such subjects had hearing better than the zero reference, often in the –10 dB HL range, and welcomed the conversion to the ISO standard. More recently a new American standard has been published by the American National Standards Institute (ANSI, 1996) showing SPL values for normal hearing close to the ISO levels using the usual audiometer earphones (see Table 3.2). These values are termed the reference equivalent threshold sound pressure levels (RETSPLs).

Sensation Level

Another reference for the decibel may be the auditory **threshold** of a given individual. The threshold of a pure tone is usually defined as the level at which the tone is so soft that it can only be perceived 50 percent of the time it is presented, although the 50 percent response criterion is purely arbitrary. The number of decibels of a sound above the threshold of a given individual is that number of decibels **sensation level (SL).**

If a person can barely hear a tone at 5 dB HL at a given frequency, a tone presented at 50 dB HL will be 45 dB above his or her threshold, or stated another way, 45 dB SL. The same 50 dB HL tone presented to a person with a 20 dB threshold will have a sensation level of 30 dB. It is important to recognize that a tone presented at threshold has a sensation level of 0 dB. To state the number of dB SL, the threshold of the individual (the reference) must be known.

Complex Sounds

Pure tones, as described in this chapter, seldom appear in nature. When they are created, it is usually by devices like tuning forks or electronic sine wave generators. Most sounds, therefore, are

TABLE 3.2   Reference Equivalent Threshold Sound Pressure Levels (RETSPLs) (dB re 20 μPa) for Supra-aural Earphones

	Supra-aural Earphone		
Frequency	TDH Type[a]	TDH 39	TDH 49/50
Hz	IEC318	NBS9A	NBS9A
125	45.0	45.0	47.5
160	38.5		
200	32.5		
250	27.0	25.5	26.5
315	22.0		
400	17.0		
500	13.5	11.5	13.5
630	10.5		
750	9.0	8.0	8.5
800	8.5		
1000	7.5	7.0	7.5
1250	7.5		
1500	7.5	6.5	7.5
1600	8.0		
2000	9.0	9.0	11.0
2500	10.5		
3000	11.5	10.0	9.5
3150	11.5		
4000	12.0	9.5	10.5
5000	11.0		
6000	16.0	15.5	13.5
6300	21.0		
8000	15.5	13.0	13.0
Speech	20.0	19.5	20.0

[a]TDH Type or any supra-aural earphone having the characteristics described in clause 9.1.1 or ISO-389 Part 1.

ANSI, 1996

characterized as containing energy at a number of different frequencies, amplitudes, and phase relationships. Fourier[8] first showed that any complex wave can be analyzed in terms of its sinusoidal **components.**

[8]Jean Baptiste Joseph Fourier, French mathematician and physicist, 1768–1830.

Fundamental Frequency

Some complex sounds repeat over time, as do many of the sounds of speech and music. Such sounds are called **periodic.** When a number of pure tones are presented, one of them will naturally have a frequency lower than the others. The lowest rate of a sound's vibration is called the **fundamental frequency,** which is determined by the physical properties of the vibrating body. **Aperiodic** sounds vary randomly over time, do not have fundamental frequencies, and are usually perceived as noise.

Harmonics

In a periodic complex sound, all frequencies are whole-number multiples of the fundamental. These tones, which occur over the fundamental, are called **harmonics** or **overtones.** The spectrum of a sound with a 100 Hz fundamental would therefore contain only higher frequencies of 200, 300, 400 Hz, and so on. With respect to periodic signals, the only difference between overtones and harmonics is the way in which they are numbered: The first harmonic is the fundamental frequency, the second harmonic is twice the fundamental, and so on. The first overtone is equal to the second harmonic, and further overtones are numbered consecutively.

Spectrum of a Complex Sound

When two or more pure tones of different frequencies are generated simultaneously, their combined amplitudes must be summed at each instant in time. This is illustrated in Figure 3.12, which shows that a new and slightly different waveform appears. Adding a fourth and fifth tone would further alter the waveform. **Complex waves** of this nature can be synthesized in the laboratory and constitute, in essence, the opposite of a **Fourier analysis.**

Although the fundamental frequency determines all the harmonic frequencies, the harmonics do not all have equal amplitude (Figure 3.13A). In any wind instrument the fundamental frequency is determined by a vibrating body: in a clarinet, the reed; in a trombone, the lips within the mouthpiece; and in that peculiar wind instrument called the human vocal tract, the vocal folds in the larynx. The length and cross-sectional areas of any of these wind instruments may be varied: in the trombone, by moving the slide; in the clarinet, by depressing keys; and in the vocal tract, by raising or lowering the tongue and moving it forward or back. In this way, even though the fundamental and harmonic frequencies may be the same, the amplitudes of different harmonics vary from instrument to instrument, resulting in the different harmonic **spectrum** (Figure 3.13B and C) and characteristic **qualities** of each.

During speech, altering the size and shape of the vocal tract, mostly by moving the tongue, results in frequency and intensity changes that emphasize some harmonics and suppress others. The resulting waveform has a series of peaks and valleys. Each of the peaks is called a **formant,** and it is manipulation of formant frequencies that facilitates the recognition of different vowel sounds. The peaks are numbered consecutively and are expressed as the lowest, or first, formant (F1); the second formant (F2); and so on. The spectrum of a musical wind instrument may be similar to that of a vowel and is also determined by the resonances of the acoustic systems.

Once the harmonic structure of a wave has been determined by the fundamental, the fundamental is no longer critical for the clear perception of a sound for persons with normal hearing. This is exemplified by the telephone, which does not allow frequencies below about 300 Hz to pass

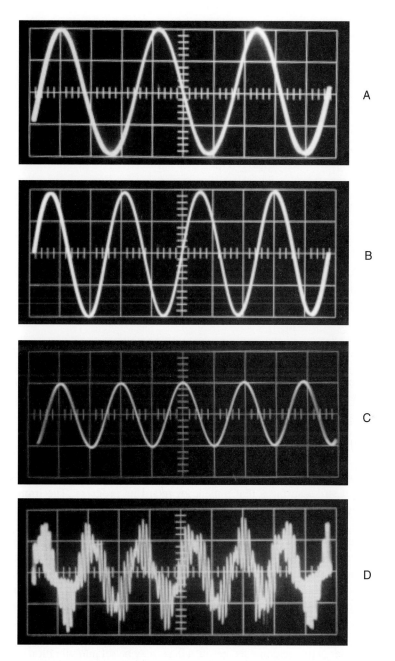

FIGURE 3.12   Synthesis of a complex waveform (D) from three sine waves (A, B, C) of different frequency and/or amplitude. Note that the amplitudes are summed at each moment in time, resulting in a new waveform.

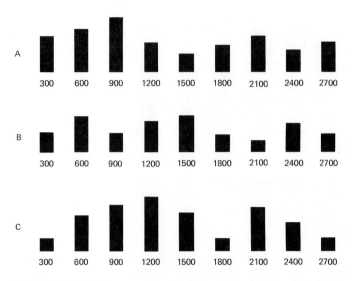

FIGURE 3.13   Histograms showing the spectra of three wind instruments. The fundamental frequency is the same in each (300 Hz), but the amplitudes of the harmonics differ.

through. Although a man's fundamental vocal frequency averages about 85 to 150 Hz and a woman's about 175 to 250 Hz (both the consequences of laryngeal size, shape, and subglottal pressure), the sex of the speakers, as well as their identities, is evident over a telephone even though the fundamental frequency is filtered out.

Impedance

Any moving object must overcome a certain amount of **resistance** to its movement. A sound wave moving through air will strike surfaces that impede or retard its progress. The **impedance** of a medium is the opposition it offers to the transmission of acoustic energy.

As a general rule, as a surface that is placed in the path of a sound wave is made more dense, it offers greater impedance to the wave. For example, when a sound strikes a closed door, some of the energy will be reflected because the door is so much more dense than the air on either side of it. If the sound is to be carried to the adjacent room, the door itself must be set into vibration, whereupon the opposite side of the door, moving against the air molecules in the next room, generates new sound waves. The amount of impedance of the door will determine the amplitude of the waves in the next room. The greater the impedance of the door, the smaller the amplitude of the waves transmitted to the adjacent room.

Given sufficient energy to overcome its inertia, a mass may be set into vibration. The resonant characteristics of a body or medium determine the frequencies of most efficient and least efficient vibration. **Resonance** is determined by the mass, elasticity, and frictional characteristics of an object (or medium). Therefore, resonance characteristics are defined by impedance. In the case of sound moving past an object, like a door, there will be more impedance to some frequencies than to others. As a rule, the mass of the door will attenuate high-frequency sounds more than low-frequency sounds, which is what makes the sound on the opposite side of the door appear "muffled."

Total impedance (Z) is determined by two factors. The first is simple resistance (R)—that is, resistance that is not influenced by frequency of vibration. This simple resistance is analogous to electrical resistance in a direct-current system, such as a battery, in which electrons move in a single direction from a negative to a positive pole. The second factor is complex resistance, or **reactance.** Reactance is influenced by frequency, so that the opposition to energy transfer varies with frequency. Reactance is seen in alternating-current electrical systems, such as household current, in which the flow of electrons is periodically reversed (60 Hz in the United States).

Total reactance is determined by two subsidiary factors called **mass reactance** and **stiffness reactance.** As either the physical mass (M) of an object or the frequency (f) at which the object vibrates is increased, so does the mass reactance. In other words, mass reactance is directly related to both mass and frequency. Stiffness (S) reactance behaves in an opposite manner. As the physical stiffness of an object increases, so does stiffness reactance. However, as frequency increases, stiffness reactance decreases (an inverse relationship).

Together, simple resistance, mass reactance, and stiffness reactance all contribute to the determination of total impedance. All four terms are given the same unit of measurement, the **ohm (Ω).**[9] In the formula for computing impedance Z is the total impedance, R is the simple resistance, $2\pi fM$ is the mass reactance, and $S/2\pi f$ is the stiffness reactance. This equation shows that mass reactance and stiffness reactance combine algebraically.

$$Z = \sqrt{R^2 + \left(2\pi fM - \frac{S}{2\pi f}\right)^2}$$

Sound Measurement

Audiologists are generally interested in making two kinds of measurements: those of the hearing ability of patients with possible disorders of the auditory system, and those of sound-pressure levels in the environment. The first modern step toward quantifying the amount of a patient's hearing loss came with the development of the pure-tone **audiometer.** This device allows for a comparison of any person's hearing threshold to that of an established norm. Hearing threshold is usually defined as the intensity at which a tone is barely audible. Hearing sensitivity is expressed as the number of decibels above (or below) the average normal-hearing person's thresholds for different pure tones. Speech audiometers were designed, in part, to measure thresholds for the spoken word.

The Pure-tone Audiometer

A pure-tone audiometer is diagrammed in Figure 3.14. It consists of an audio oscillator, which generates pure tones of different frequencies, usually at discrete steps of 125, 250, 500, 750, 1000, 1500, 2000, 3000, 4000, 6000, and 8000 Hz. Each tone is amplified to a maximum of about 110 dB HL in the frequency range of 500 to 4000 Hz, with less output above and below those frequencies.

The tones are attenuated with the use of a manual dial or electronic attenuator, which is numbered (contrary to attenuation) in decibels above the normal threshold for each frequency. As the number of decibels is increased, the attenuation is decreased. The audiometer is provided with a

[9]For Georg Simon Ohm, German mathematician and physicist, 1787–1854.

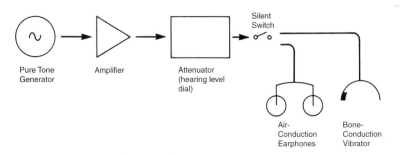

FIGURE 3.14   Block diagram of a pure-tone audiometer.

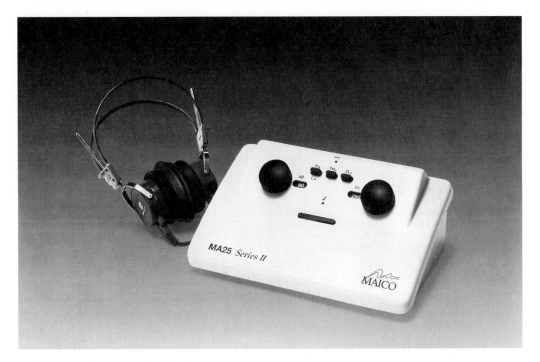

FIGURE 3.15   A pure-tone audiometer. (Courtesy of MAICO)

silent switch that can introduce or interrupt a tone. The signal is routed, via an output selection control, to a right or left earphone or to a bone-conduction vibrator. A photograph of a pure-tone audiometer is shown in Figure 3.15.

Air Conduction.   Earphones are held in place by a steel headband that fits across the top of the head. The phones themselves are connected to the headband by two small metal yokes. The earphone consists of a magnetic device that transduces the electrical translations supplied by the audiometer to a small diaphragm that vibrates according to the acoustic equivalents of frequency and intensity. Around the earphone is a rubber cushion that may fit around the ear (circumaural) or, more usually, over the ear (supra-aural). The movement of the earphone diaphragm generates the sound, which

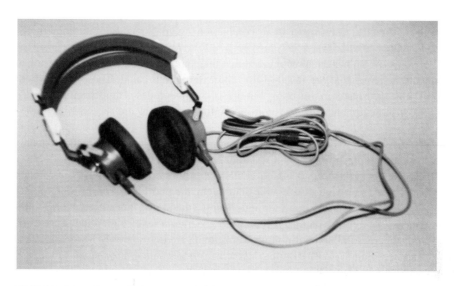

FIGURE 3.16   A set of supra-aural air-conduction receivers. (Courtesy of Starkey Labs)

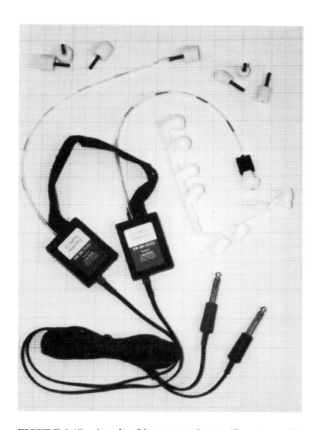

FIGURE 3.17   A pair of insert receivers. (Courtesy of Etymotic Research)

enters the ear directly, resulting in an air conduction signal. Supra-aural audiometric earphones are shown in Figure 3.16.

For some time it has been recognized that there are distinct advantages to using earphones for air-conduction testing that are inserted into the external ear canal. These advantages will be discussed in some detail later in this book, but one of them includes a significant increase in comfort to the patient. Insert earphones that are appropriate for audiometry are shown in Figure 3.17.

Bone Conduction.   Selection of the bone-conduction output of the audiometer causes the signal to terminate in a small plastic device with a slight concavity on one side for comfortable fit against the skull. The principle of the bone-conduction vibrator is the same as that of the air-conduction receiver except that instead of moving a wafer-like diaphragm, the plastic shell of the vibrator must be set into motion. Because they must vibrate a greater mass (the skull), bone conduction vibrators require greater energy than air-conduction receivers to generate a level high enough to stimulate normal hearing. For this reason the maximum power outputs are considerably lower for bone conduction, usually not exceeding 50 to 80 dB HL, depending on frequency. Frequencies of 250 through 4000 Hz are usually available for bone-conduction testing.

The bone-conduction vibrator is held against the skull at either the forehead or the mastoid process. When the forehead is the placement site, a plastic strap is used that circles the head. When the bone behind the ear is the desired place for testing, a spring-steel headband that goes across the top of the skull is employed. A bone-conduction vibrator is shown in Figure 3.18.

The Speech Audiometer

As will be discussed later in this book, measurements made with speech stimuli are very helpful in the diagnosis of auditory disorders. A speech audiometer is required for such measurements. The speech audiometer is usually part of a clinical audiometer (Figure 3.19) that can also perform pure-tone tests.

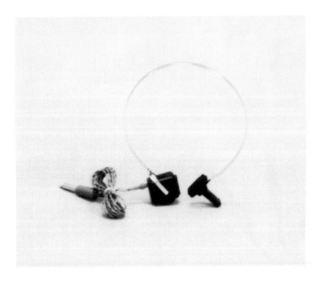

FIGURE 3.18   A bone-conduction vibrator. (Courtesy of Starkey Labs)

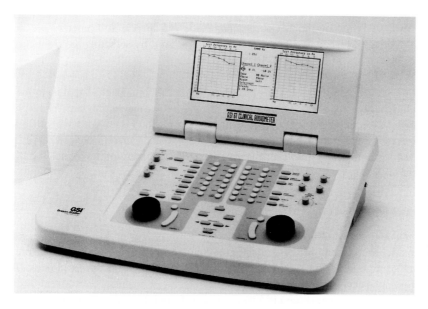

FIGURE 3.19 A diagnostic audiometer. (Courtesy of GSI)

The diagram in Figure 3.20 shows that the speech circuit of an audiometer can have an input signal provided by a microphone, a compact disc (CD) player, or a tape recorder. The input level of the speech signal is monitored by an averaging voltmeter called a VU (volume units) meter. Such a meter reads in dB VU, implying an electrical reference in watts. The signal is amplified and attenuated as in a pure-tone audiometer, with the hearing-level dial calibrated in decibels with reference to audiometric zero for speech (20 dB SPL and the ANSI-1996 standard for a TDH-49 earphone). Some audiometers use light-emitting diodes in lieu of a VU meter.

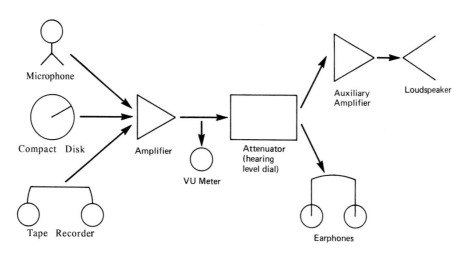

FIGURE 3.20 Block diagram of the speech circuit of a diagnostic audiometer.

Air Conduction.   Most of the measurements made on speech audiometers are accomplished through air-conduction receivers. Testing may be carried out by selecting the right ear, the left ear, or both ears. The usual range is from –10 to 110 dB HL.

Sound Field.   It is often desirable to test with speech in the sound field—that is, to feed the speech signal into the room by using one or more loudspeakers, rather than earphones. The signal generated by the audiometer is designed for air conduction earphones and does not have sufficient power to drive a larger loudspeaker. When the speaker output of the audiometer is selected, the speech signal is usually fed to an auxiliary amplifier that augments the intensity of the signal, creating the additional power necessary to drive the loudspeaker.

Sound-level Meters

As mentioned earlier, airborne sounds are measured by devices called sound-level meters. These consist of a microphone, amplifier, attenuator, and meter that pick up and transduce pressure waves in the air, measure them electrically, and read out the sound pressure levels in decibels. The usual reference for sound-level meters is 20 µPa.

Because the human ear responds differently to different frequencies, many sound-level meters contain systems called weighting networks, which are filters to alter the response of the instrument, much as the ear does at different levels. The phon lines (Figure 3.21) show that the ear is not very sensitive to low frequencies at low SPLs, and that as the sound increases in intensity, the ear is capable of better and better low-frequency response. The three usual weighting networks of sound-level meters are shown in Figure 3.22, which illustrates how the meters respond.

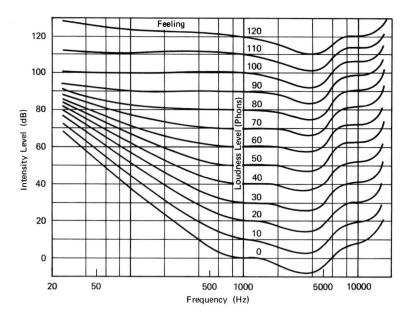

FIGURE 3.21   Equal loudness contours showing the relationship between loudness level (in phons) and intensity (in dB) as a function of frequency.

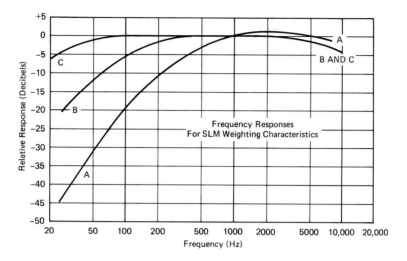

FIGURE 3.22   Weighting networks for sound-level meters. (Courtesy of General Radio Corporation)

Sound-level meters are useful in the study of acoustics and are common tools in industry as concern over noise pollution grows. Background noise levels can play a major role in the testing of hearing because, if they are sufficiently high, they may interfere with accurate measurement by **masking** the test stimuli. Whenever hearing testing is undertaken, especially with persons who have normal or near normal hearing, the background noise levels should be known.

Acceptable Noise Levels for Audiometry

Table 3.3 shows the maximum room noise allowable for air- and bone-conduction testing on the ANSI-1991 scale. To determine the allowable levels for bone-conduction testing, the attenuation

TABLE 3.3   Maximum Permissible Ambient Noise Sound Pressure Levels in Octave Bands for the Audiometric Conditions Ears Covered and Ears Not Covered and Test Frequency Ranges 125 to 8000, 250 to 8000, and 500 to 8000 Hz. Tabled Values Are in dB re: 20 μPa Rounded to the Nearest 0.5 dB

Octave band intervals	Ears Covered			Ears Not Covered		
	125 to 8000 Hz	*250 to 8000 Hz*	*500 to 8000 Hz*	*125 to 8000 Hz*	*250 to 8000 Hz*	*500 to 8000 Hz*
125	34.0	36.5	47.5	28.0	32.5	42.5
250	22.5	22.5	33.5	18.5	18.5	28.5
500	19.5	19.5	19.5	14.5	14.5	14.5
1000	26.5	26.5	26.5	14.0	14.0	14.0
2000	28.0	28.0	28.0	8.5	8.5	8.5
4000	34.5	34.5	34.5	9.0	9.0	9.0
8000	43.5	43.5	43.5	20.5	20.5	20.5

ANSI, 1991

provided by the usual audiometer earphone and cushion must be subtracted from the maximum allowable levels for air conduction because the ear remains uncovered during bone-conduction audiometry.

Calibration of Audiometers

Although periodic factory checks on audiometer calibration are desirable, many audiologists also perform frequent checks on the operation of their equipment on site in the clinic. In the early days of audiometers, checks on the reliability of the hearing level were conducted by testing a group of subjects with known normal hearing—the "psychoacoustic method." This is done by taking the median of the threshold findings and posting a correction chart on the audiometer to remind the audiologist to correct any readings obtained on a patient by the number of decibels the audiometer had drifted out of calibration.

Many audiology clinics today are equipped with meters and couplers, so that the task of level checking may be accomplished electroacoustically. The earphone is placed over a carefully machined coupler, usually containing a cavity of precisely 6 cm^3 to simulate the average volume of air between the earphone and the eardrum membrane. A weight of 500 grams, or a spring with equivalent tension, holds the receiver in place. Sounds emanating from the diaphragm of the receiver are picked up by a sensitive microphone at the bottom of the coupler (the coupler is often called the **artificial ear**), amplified, and read in dB SPL on a sound-level meter. To be certain that the meter is reading the level of the tone (or other signal) from the receiver, and not from the ambient room noise, the level of the signal is usually high enough to avoid this possibility. Hearing levels of 70 dB are convenient for this purpose, and the readout should correspond to the number of decibels required for threshold of the particular signal (see Table 3.2), plus 70 dB. A form designed for level checking with an artificial ear is shown in Figure 3.23, and a commercial testing unit is shown in Figure 3.24.

Because of differences in size and design, insert earphones cannot be calibrated with a standard 6 cm^3 coupler. Rather, a smaller coupler, which has a volume of 2 cm^3, is used with the calibration device described earlier. Reference equivalent sound-pressure levels for calibrating insert earphones are shown in Table 3.4.

When calibrating the speech circuit of an audiometer, a signal must be fed through one of the inputs. A pure tone, a noise containing approximately equal intensity at all frequencies, or a sustained vowel sound, may be used. The signal is adjusted so that the VU or equivalent meter reads zero. With the hearing-level dial set at 70 dB, and with the earphone on the coupler, the signal should read 90 dB SPL on the meter (70 dB HL plus 20 dB SPL required for audiometric zero for speech on the ANSI-1996 standard) for the most commonly used earphone.

Calibration of the bone-conduction systems of audiometers may be accomplished in several ways. One method of field calibration involves the use of several patients with known sensorineural losses. Their air- and bone-conduction thresholds are compared and median values for the differences taken at each frequency. The amounts by which the bone-conduction thresholds differ from the (calibrated) air-conduction thresholds are averaged and corrections are posted on the audiometer. Persons with normal hearing cannot be used because of the danger of masking their uncovered ears by ambient room noise.

The **artificial mastoid** (Figure 3.25) is a device that allows for electronic calibration of the bone-conduction system of an audiometer. The procedure is similar to that for testing air-conduction

For TDH-49 Earphone

University of Texas Speech and Hearing Center
AUDIOMETER CALIBRATION

Calibrated By _____   Audiometer _____   Serial No. _____   Date _____

Attn. HL Obs.	Attn. HL Err.	Frequency Count	Dial	HL	Right Air Output* Obs.	Cor.	Err.	≉Left Air Output* Obs.	Cor.	Err.	HL	Mastoid Output # Obs.	Cor.	Err.	Forehead Output # Obs.	Cor.	Err.
110			125	70		117.5			117.5		—						
105																	
100			250	70		96.5			96.5		25		66.4			79.9	
95	ᵇ																
90			500	70		83.5			83.5		40		70.7			85.7	
85																	
80			750	70		78.5			78.5		40		59.3			71.8	
75																	
70			1000	70		77.5			77.5		40		56.9			66.9	
65																	
60			1500	70		77.5			77.5		40		55.4			66.4	
55																	
50			2000	70		81.0			81.0		40		48.1			56.6	
45																	
40			3000	70		79.5			79.5		40		46.6			54.1	
35																	
30			4000	70		80.5			80.5		40		51.2			57.7	
25																	
20			6000	70		83.5			83.5		—						
15																	
10			8000	70		83.0			83.0		—						
5																	
0			Speech	70		90.0			90.0		40		( )			( )	
Ttl Err.																	

FUNCTIONAL CHECKS WITH TOLERANCES:
Rise Time (20 – 100 milliseconds) _____ .
Fall Time (5 – 100 milliseconds) _____ .

Overshoot and ringing (± 1dB) _____ .

Total Harmonic Distortion (max. —30dB) _____ .

Comments:

*Figures in this column are dB re 20 μPa for proposed ANSI standards for use with TDH-49 receivers mounted in MX-41/AR cushions.
#These figures include corrections for the B&K Model 4930 artificial mastoid for a B—70A bone-conduction vibrator.

FNM/80

FIGURE 3.23   Sample of form for field check of audiometer air-conduction level and frequency.

55

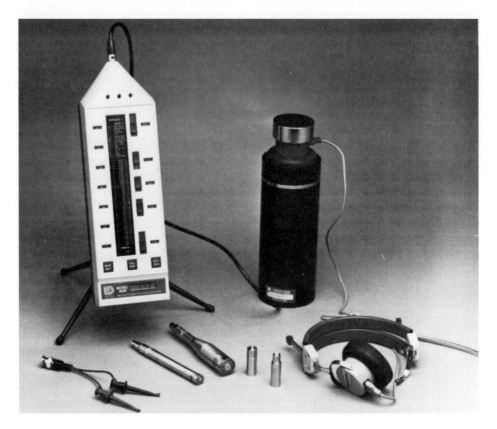

FIGURE 3.24   A commercial audiometer calibration device. (Courtesy Larson-Davis Laboratory)

calibration. The bone-conduction vibrator is placed on the artificial mastoid, which has properties similar to the human skull, scalp, and skin. Vibrations are transduced into electrical currents, which are then converted to decibels for direct readout. The form shown in Figure 3.23 allows for calibration to the ANSI standard for bone conduction testing on either the forehead or the mastoid. The reference equivalent threshold force levels (RETFLs) are shown in Table 3.5.

Calibration of a loudspeaker system with an audiometer requires either the testing of a number of normal-hearing subjects or the use of a sound-level meter. A heavy chair that is difficult to move should be placed before the speaker at a distance of about three times the diameter of the loudspeaker, plus 1 foot, or often just at one meter. This allows the subject to be placed in the "far field." The sound-level meter should be placed in the same position as the head of a patient seated in that same chair.

ANSI (1996) recommends that the loudspeaker output for 0 dB HL in the sound field, when listening with both ears, should be 14.5 dB SPL for speech. If the hearing-level dial is set to 70 dB, the sound-level meter should read 70 dB, plus 20 dB for audiometric zero for speech, minus 5.5 dB (84.5 dB SPL). Five and one-half decibels are subtracted because thresholds for pure tones determined under earphones, called the minimum audible pressure (MAP) (Sivian & White, 1933), are slightly higher (require greater intensity) than thresholds determined in a free sound field, the mini-

TABLE 3.4   Reference Equivalent Threshold Sound Pressure Levels (RETSPLs) (dB re 20 µPa) for Calibration of Insert Earphones to the ANSI (1996) Standard

Coupler Type (Hz)	Frequency Simulator	Occluded Ear Rigid Tube	HA-2 with HA-1
125	28.0	26.0	26.5
160	24.5	22.0	22.0
200	21.5	18.0	19.5
250	17.5	14.0	14.5
315	15.5	12.0	15.0
400	13.0	9.0	10.5
500	9.5	5.5	6.0
630	7.5	4.0	4.5
750	6.0	2.0	2.0
800	5.5	1.5	1.5
1000	5.5	0.0	0.0
1250	8.5	2.0	1.0
1500	9.5	2.0	0.0
1600	9.5	2.0	1.5
2000	11.5	3.0	2.5
2500	13.5	5.0	4.5
3000	13.0	3.5	2.5
3150	13.0	4.0	2.5
4000	15.0	5.5	0.0
5000	18.5	5.0	1.5
6000	16.0	2.0	−2.5
6300	16.0	2.0	−2.0
8000	15.5	0.0	−3.5
Speech	18.0	12.5	12.5

mum audible field (MAF) (Fletcher & Munson, 1933). Because an auxiliary amplifier is usually required to power the loudspeaker, its volume control may often be adjusted to produce the proper level. Reference equivalent sound pressure levels for sound field testing are shown in Table 3.6.

Whenever the audiometer differs from the required level at any frequency by more than 2.5 dB, a correction should be added to the hearing-level dial setting during audiometric testing. Corrections are rounded out to the nearest multiple of 5 dB. Although this may superficially seem illogical, if the calibration procedure reveals that the system is putting out too low a level, the number of decibels of deviation must be *subtracted* from the hearing-level dial setting during any given test. If the intensity is too high, the correction is *added* during testing. Whenever level calibration reveals marked differences from specification, the audiometer should be seen for recalibration. Audiologists should never assume that their audiometers are in proper calibration, even new units, unless they have verified this for themselves.

In addition to level checking, on pure-tone audiometers it is important to check for changes in frequency, to be sure that the ANSI frequency limitations (the nominal frequency ± 3 percent) have not been exceeded. This may be done with a frequency counter.

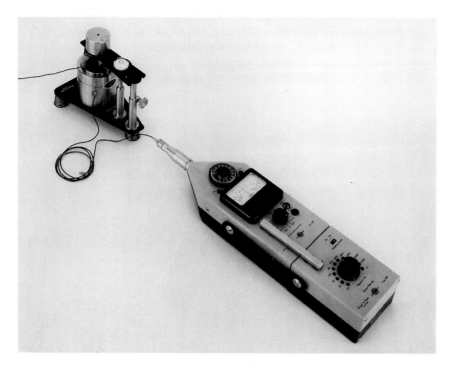

FIGURE 3.25   An artificial mastoid assembly. (Courtesy of B & K Instruments)

The linearity of the attenuator dial is most easily tested electronically with a voltmeter. Checks should be made through the entire intensity range to be certain that when the hearing-level dial is moved a given number of decibels, the level actually changes by this precise amount ± 1.5 dB per 5 dB step, the tolerance allowed by the ANSI 1996 standard. In addition, the total error in the hearing-level dial linearity cannot exceed ± 3 to 5 dB, depending on frequency. The form shown in Figure 3.23 provides space for checking attenuator linearity.

Even though the audiometer generates a pure tone, it is likely that distortion in the system (often the earphone) will result in the emission of the second harmonic of the tone; that is, if a 1000 Hz tone is generated, some energy at 2000 Hz will be present. ANSI standards state that the second harmonic must be at least 30 dB below the fundamental (the nominal frequency). This can be checked with special equipment, such as frequency counters.

Environmental Sounds

Earlier we saw that the range of sound intensities, from threshold of audibility to pain, is extremely wide. All of the sounds that normal-hearing persons may hear without discomfort must be found within this range. Table 3.7 gives examples of some ordinary environmental sounds and their approximate intensities. This table may help the reader to develop a framework from which to approximate the intensities of other sounds.

TABLE 3.5 Reference Equivalent Threshold Force Levels (RETFLs) for Bone Vibrators

Frequency Hz	Mastoid (dB re 1 μN)	Forehead (dB re 1 μN)	Forehead Minus Mastoid
250	67.0	79.0	12.0
315	64.0	76.5	12.5
400	61.0	74.5	13.5
500	58.0	72.0	14.0
630	52.5	66.0	13.5
750	48.5	61.5	13.0
800	47.0	59.0	12.0
1000	42.5	51.0	8.5
1250	39.0	49.0	10.0
1500	36.5	47.5	11.0
1600	35.5	46.5	11.0
2000	31.0	42.5	11.5
2500	29.5	41.5	12.0
3000	30.0	42.0	12.0
3150	31.0	42.5	11.5
4000	35.5	43.5	8.0
5000	40.0	51.0	11.0
6000	40.0	51.0	11.0
6300	40.0	50.0	10.0
8000	40.0	50.0	10.0
Speech	55.0	63.5	8.5

ANSI, 1996

Psychoacoustics

Thus far in this chapter, attention has been focused on physical acoustics. These factors are the same with or without human perception. It is also important that consideration be allocated to psychoacoustics, the study of the relationship between physical stimuli and the psychological responses to which they give rise.

Pitch

Pitch is a term used to describe the subjective impressions of the "highness" or "lowness" of a sound. Pitch relates to frequency; in general, pitch rises as the frequency of vibration increases, at least within the range of human hearing (20 to 20,000 Hz). The Western world uses the **octave** scale in its music. When frequency is doubled, it is raised 1 octave, but raising (or lowering) a sound 1 octave does not double (or halve) its pitch. Intensity also contributes to the perception of pitch, although to a lesser extent than does frequency.

TABLE 3.6   Reference Equivalent Threshold Sound Pressure Levels (RETSPLs) (dB re 20 μPa) for Sound-field Testing

Frequency (Hz)	Binaural Listening[a] In Free Field	Monaural Listening In Sound Field		
	0 Degree Incidence	0 Degree Incidence	45 Degree Incidence	90 Degree Incidence
125	22.0	24.0	23.5	23.0
160	18.0	20.0	19.0	18.5
200	14.5	16.5	15.5	15.0
250	11.0	13.0	12.0	11.0
315	8.5	10.5	9.0	8.0
400	6.0	8.0	5.5	4.5
500	4.0	6.0	3.0	1.5
630	2.5	4.5	1.0	−0.5
750	2.0	4.0	0.5	−1.0
800	2.0	4.0	0.5	−1.0
1000	2.0	4.0	0.0	−1.5
1250	1.5	3.5	−0.5	−2.5
1500	0.5	2.5	−1.0	−2.5
1600	0.0	2.0	−1.5	−2.5
2000	−1.5	0.5	−2.5	−1.5
2500	−4.0	−2.0	−5.5	−4.0
3000	−6.0	−4.0	−9.0	−6.5
3150	−6.5	−4.5	−9.5	−6.5
4000	−6.5	−4.5	−8.5	−4.0
5000	−3.0	−1.0	−7.0	−5.0
6000	2.5	4.5	−3.0	−5.0
6300	4.0	6.0	−1.5	−4.0
8000	11.5	13.5	8.0	5.5
9000	13.5	15.5	10.5	8.5
10000	13.5	15.5	11.0	9.5
11200	12.0	14.0	10.0	7.0
12500	11.0	13.0	11.5	5.0
14000	16.0	18.0		
16000	43.5	44.5		
Speech	14.5	16.5	12.5	11.0

[a]ISO 389-7 Reference Threshold of Hearing Under Free Field and Diffuse Field Conditions.

ANSI, 1996

TABLE 3.7   Scale of Intensities for Ordinary Environmental Sounds*

0 dB	Just audible sound
10 dB	Soft rustle of leaves
20 dB	A whisper at 4 feet
30 dB	A quiet street in the evening with no traffic
40 dB	Night noises in the city
50 dB	A quiet automobile 10 feet away
60 dB	Department store
70 dB	Busy traffic
60–70 dB	Normal conversation at 3 feet
80 dB	Heavy traffic
80–90 dB	Niagara Falls
90 dB	A pneumatic drill 10 feet away
100 dB	A rivet gun 35 feet away
110 dB	Hi-fidelity phonograph with a 10-watt amplifier, 10 feet away
115 dB	Hammering on a steel plate 2 feet away

*The reference is 10^{-16} watt/cm^2 (Van Bergeijk, Pierce, & David, 1960).

The subjective aspect of pitch can be measured by using a unit called the **mel.** One thousand mels is the pitch of a 1000 Hz tone at 40 dB SL. Frequencies can be adjusted so that they sound twice as high (2000 mels), half as high (500 mels), and so on. Except for the fact that the number of mels increases and decreases with frequency, apart from 1000 Hz, the numbers do not correspond. Although the task sounds formidable, pitch scaling can be accomplished on cooperative, normal-hearing subjects with great accuracy after a period of training. The mel scale is illustrated in Figure 3.26.

Loudness

Loudness is a subjective experience, as contrasted with the purely physical force of intensity. The thinking reader has realized, to be sure, that a relationship exists between increased intensity and increased loudness. The decibel, however, is not a unit of loudness measurement, and thus such statements as "The noise in this room is 60 dB loud" are erroneous. The duration and frequency of sounds contribute to the sensation of loudness.

As stated earlier, the ear is not equally sensitive at all frequencies. It is also true that the subjective experience of loudness changes differently at different frequencies. Comparing the loudness of different frequencies to the loudness of a 1000 Hz tone at a number of intensity levels determines the **loudness level** of the different frequencies. Figure 3.21 shows that loudness grows faster for low-frequency tones and certain high-frequency tones than for mid-frequencies. The unit of loudness level is the **phon.**

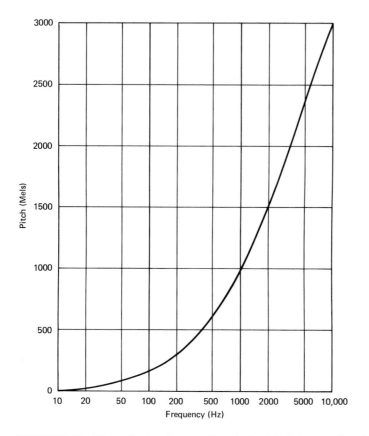

FIGURE 3.26   The mel scale, showing the relationship between pitch (in mels) and frequency (in hertz).

The term **sone** refers to the comparison of the loudness of a 1000 Hz tone at different intensities. One sone is the loudness of 1000 Hz at 40 dB SL. The intensity required for subjects to perceive half the loudness of 1 sone is 0.5 sones, the intensity for twice the loudness is 2 sones, and so forth. Loudness level (in phons) can be related to loudness (in sones), but as Figure 3.27 shows, the measurements do not correspond precisely.

Localization

Hearing is a distance sense, unaffected by many barriers that interfere with sight, touch, and smell. Sound can bend around corners with little distortion, although as frequencies get higher, they become more unidirectional. Under many conditions it is possible, even without seeing the source of a sound, to tell the direction from which it comes. This ability, called **localization,** is a complex phenomenon resulting from the interaction of both ears. The localization of sound, which warned our ancestors of possible danger, was probably a major contributor to the early survival of our species.

Localization is possible because of the relative intensities of sounds and their times of arrival at the two ears (i.e., phase). The greatest single contributors to our ability to localize are interaural

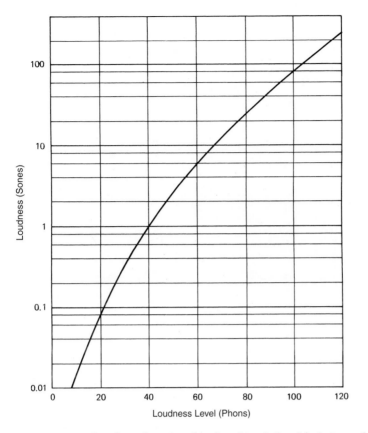

FIGURE 3.27 **Loudness function showing the relationship between loudness (in sones) and loudness level (in phons).**

phase differences in the low frequencies (below 1500 Hz) and intensity differences in the higher frequencies. Naturally, in an acoustical environment with hard surfaces, the sound may **reverberate** and be heard to come from a direction other than its source. An area in which there are no hard surfaces to cause reverberation is called a **free field.** Free fields actually exist only in such exotic areas as mountain tops and specially built **anechoic chambers** (Figure 3.28).

Masking

When two sounds are heard simultaneously, the intensity of one sound may be sufficient to cause the other to be inaudible. This change in the threshold of a sound caused by a second sound with which it coexists is called masking. There is surely no one who has not experienced masking in noisy situations in the form of speech interference. The noise that causes the interference is called the masker. Because masking plays an important role in some aspects of clinical audiology, it is discussed in detail in subsequent chapters of this book.

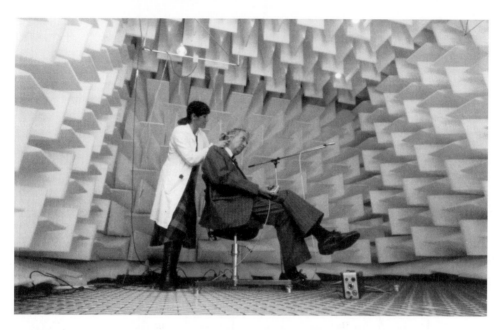

FIGURE 3.28   Photograph of a commercial anechoic chamber. (Courtesy of Industrial Acoustics Company, Inc.)

Summary

Sound may be regarded objectively if we consider its waves in terms of their frequency, intensity, phase, and spectrum. Sounds may also be studied subjectively, in terms of pitch, loudness, or the interactions of signals producing masking or localization. In discussing sound energy it is always important to specify precisely the various aspects and appropriate measurement references, such as hertz, decibels (IL, SPL, HL, or SL), mels, sones, or phons.

STUDY QUESTIONS

1. What is wrong with the statement "The signal has a loudness of 40 dB."?

2. Why may two complex waves with components of identical frequency have different waveforms?

3. What determines the frequency of vibration of a mass?

4. List ten units of sound measurement. Describe what they measure and their references when applicable.

5. Give examples of periodic and aperiodic sounds.

6. Explain why two sounds with SPLs of 60 dB each do not total 120 dB when presented simultaneously. What is the total SPL and why?

7. How is audiometer-level calibration accomplished for air conduction, bone conduction, speech, and sound field?

8. Define the threshold of a sound.

9. What is the number of dB IL with a power output of 10^{-1} watt/m^2? What is the number of dB SPL with a pressure output of 2×10^4 μPa? Check your answers in Table 3.1 and generate more problems if you did not answer these correctly.

10. List the factors that contribute to acoustic impedance.

GLOSSARY

Amplitude The extent of the vibratory movement of a mass from its position of rest to that point furthest from the position of rest.

Anechoic chamber A specially built room with large wedges of sound-absorbing material on all walls, floor, and ceiling. The purpose of the room is to provide maximum sound absorption and to keep reverberation to an absolute minimum.

Aperiodic wave A waveform that does not repeat over time.

Artificial ear A device for calibrating air-conduction earphones. It consists of a 6 cm^3 coupler to connect an earphone to a condenser microphone with cathode follower and a meter that reads in dB SPL. When calibrating insert earphones, a 2 cm^3 coupler must be used.

Artificial mastoid A device for calibrating bone-conduction vibrators. It consists of a resilient surface that simulates the vibrating properties of the mastoid process of the skull and an accelerometer. It is connected to a meter that reads in either decibels or units of force.

Audiometer A device designed for measuring hearing sensitivity for pure tones or for speech.

Beats Periodic variations of the amplitude of a tone when a second tone of slightly different frequency is produced simultaneously.

Bel A unit for expressing ratios of sound pressures in base-10 logarithms.

Brownian motion The constant random colliding movement of molecules in a medium.

Cancellation The reduction of the amplitude of a sound wave to zero. This results when two tones of the same frequency and amplitude are introduced 180 degrees out of phase.

Complex wave A sound wave made up of a number of different sinusoids, each with a different frequency.

Component A pure-tone constituent of a complex wave.

Compression That portion of a sound wave where the molecules of the medium are compressed together. Also called *condensation*.

Cosine wave A sound wave representing simple harmonic motion that begins at 90 degrees.

Cycle The complete sequence of events of a single sine wave through 360 degrees.

Damping Progressive diminution in the amplitude of a vibrating body. Systems are said to be heavily damped when the amplitude decays rapidly, lightly damped when the amplitude decays slowly, and critically damped if all vibration ceases before the completion of one cycle.

Decibel (dB) A unit for expressing the ratio between two sound pressures or two sound powers; one-tenth of a Bel.

Difference tone The perceived pitch of a tone resulting from the simultaneous presentation of two tones of different frequencies. The tone perceived has a frequency equal to the difference in hertz between the other two tones.

Dyne (d) A unit of force just sufficient to accelerate a mass of 1 gram at 1 cm/sec^2.

Elasticity The ability of a mass to return to its natural shape.

Erg (e) A unit of work. One erg results when 1 dyne force displaces an object by 1 centimeter.

Exponent A logarithm or power to which a number may be raised.

Force The impetus required to institute or alter the velocity of a body.

Forced vibration The vibration of a mass controlled and maintained by an external impetus.

Formant A peak of energy in the spectrum of a vowel sound.

Fourier analysis The mathematical breakdown of any complex wave into its component parts, consisting of simple sinusoids of different frequencies.

Free field An acoustic environment with no reverberating surfaces.

Free vibration The vibration of a mass independent of any external force.

Frequency The number of complete oscillations of a vibrating body per unit of time. In acoustics the unit of measurements is *cycles per second* (cps) or *hertz* (Hz).

Fundamental frequency The lowest frequency of vibration in a complex wave.

Harmonic Any whole-number multiple of the fundamental frequency of a complex wave. The fundamental frequency equals the first harmonic.

Hearing level (HL) The number of decibels above an average normal threshold for a given signal. The hearing-level dial of an audiometer is calibrated in dB HL.

Hertz (Hz) Cycles per second (cps).

Impedance The opposition to sound-wave transmission. It comprises frictional resistance, mass, and stiffness and is influenced by frequency.

Intensity The amount of sound energy per unit of area.

Intensity level (IL) An expression of the power of a sound per unit of area. The reference level in decibels is 10^{-12} watt/m^2, or 10^{-16} watt/cm^2.

Inverse square law The intensity of a sound decreases as a function of the square of the distance from the source.

Joule (J) The work obtained when a force of one Newton displaces an object one meter (one J is equal to 10 million ergs).

Kinetic energy The energy of a mass that results from its motion.

Localization The ability of an animal to determine the specific location of a sound source.

Logarithm The exponent that tells the power to which a number is raised; the number of times that a number (the base) is multiplied by itself.

Longitudinal wave A wave in which the particles of the medium move along the same axis as the wave.

Loudness The subjective impression of the power of a sound. The unit of measurement is the *sone*.

Loudness level The intensity above the reference level for a 1000 Hz tone that is subjectively equal in loudness. The unit of measurement is the *phon*.

Masking The process by which the threshold of a sound is elevated by the simultaneous introduction of another sound.

Mass The quantity of a body as measured in terms of its relationship to inertia The weight of a body divided by its acceleration due to gravity.

Mass reactance The quantity that results from the formula $2\pi fM$ (two times pi times frequency times mass).

Mel A unit of pitch measurement. One thousand mels is the pitch of a 1000 Hz tone at 40 dB SL, 2000 mels is the subjective pitch exactly double 1000 mels, and so on.

Microbar (μbar) A pressure equal to one-millionth of standard atmospheric pressure (1 μbar equals 1 dyne/cm^2).

Newton (N) The force required to give a 1 kg mass an acceleration of 1 m/sec^2 (1 N equals 100,000 d).

Octave The difference between two tones separated by a frequency ratio of 2:1.

Ohm (Ω) One acoustic ohm of impedance is the opposition to a sound when a pressure of 1 μbar produces a volume velocity of 1 cm^3/sec.

Oscillation The back-and-forth movement of a vibrating body.

Overtone Any whole-number multiple of the fundamental frequency of a complex wave. It differs from the harmonic only in the numbering used (e.g., the first overtone is equal to the second harmonic).

Pascal (Pa) A unit of pressure equal to 1 N/m^2.

Period The duration (in seconds) of one cycle of vibration. The period is the reciprocal of frequency (e.g., the period of a 1000 Hz tone is 1/1000 second).

Periodic wave A waveform that repeats over time.

Phase The relationship in time between two or more waves.

Phon The unit of loudness level. It corresponds to the loudness of a signal at other frequencies equal to the intensity at numbers of intensity of a 1000 Hz tone.

Pitch The subjective impression of the highness or lowness of a sound. The psychological correlate of frequency.

Potential energy Energy resulting from a fixed and relative position, as a coiled spring.

Power The rate at which work is done. Units of measurement are *watts* or *ergs/second*.

Pressure Force over an area of surface.

Pure tone A tone of only 1 frequency (i.e., no harmonics).

Quality The sharpness of resonance of a sound system; the vividness or identifying characteristics of a sound; the subjective counterpart of spectrum (synonym: *timbre*).

Rarefaction That portion of a sound wave where the molecules become less densely packed per unit of space.

Ratio The mathematical result of a quantity divided by another quantity of the same kind, often expressed as a fraction.

Reactance The contributions of mass, stiffness, and frequency to impedance.

Resistance The opposition to a force.

Resonance The ability of a mass to vibrate at a particular frequency with a minimum application of external force.

Resonant frequency The frequency at which a mass vibrates with the least amount of external force; the natural frequency of vibration of a mass.

Reverberation A short-term echo, or the continuation of a sound in a closed area after the source has stopped vibrating. This results from reflection and refraction of sound waves.

Sensation level (SL) The number of decibels above the hearing threshold of a given subject for a given signal.

Sinusoidal or sine waves The waveform of a pure tone showing simple harmonic motion.

Sone The unit of loudness measurement. One sone equals the loudness of a 1000 Hz tone at 40 dB SPL.

Sound-level meter A device designed for measurement of the intensity of sound waves in air. It consists of a microphone, an amplifier, a frequency weighting circuit, and a meter calibrated in decibels with a reference of 20 μPa.

Sound-pressure level (SPL) An expression of the pressure of a sound. The reference level in decibels is 20 μPa.

Spectrum The sum of the components of a complex wave.

Stiffness The flexibility or pliancy of a mass. The inverse of compliance.

Stiffness reactance The quantity that results when the stiffness of a body is divided by $2\pi f$ (two times pi times frequency).

Threshold In audiology, the least audible sound-pressure level; often defined operationally as the level of a sound at which it can be heard by an individual 50 percent of the time.

Transverse wave A wave in which the motion of the molecules of the medium is perpendicular to the direction of the wave.

Velocity The speed of a sound wave in a given direction.

Vibration The to-and-fro movements of a mass. In a free vibration the mass is displaced from its position of rest and allowed to oscillate without outside influence. In a forced vibration the mass is moved back and forth by applying an external force.

Watt A unit of power.

Wave A series of moving impulses set up by a vibration.

Wavelength The distance between the exact same point (in degrees) on two successive cycles of a tone.

Work Energy expended by displacement of a mass. The unit of measurement is the *erg* or *joule*.

REFERENCES

American National Standards Institute (ANSI). (1991). *Maximum permissible ambient noise levels for audiometric test rooms*. ANSI S3.1-1991. New York: Author.

———. (1996). *American National Standard Specification for Audiometers*. ANSI S3.6-1996. New York: Author.

Beasley, W. C. (1938). *National Health Survey (1935-1936), preliminary reports*. Hearing Study Series Bulletin, 1-7. Washington, DC: U.S. Public Health Service.

Fletcher, H., & Munson, W. A. (1933). Loudness, its definition, measurement, and calculation. *Journal of the Acoustical Society of America, 5,* 82–107.

Sivian, L. J., & White, S. D. (1933). On minimum audible sound fields. *Journal of the Acoustical Society of America, 4,* 288–321.

Van Bergeijk, W. A., Pierce, J. R., & David, E. E. (1960). *Waves and the ear*. New York: Doubleday.

SUGGESTED READINGS

Speaks, C. E. (1993). *Introduction to sound*. San Diego: Singular Publishing Group.

Wilber, L. A. (1994). Calibration, puretone, speech and noise signals. In J. Katz (Ed.), *Handbook of clinical audiology* (pp. 73–94). Baltimore: Williams & Wilkins.

Yost, W. A. (1994). *Fundamentals of hearing: An introduction* (3rd ed.). New York: Holt, Rinehart & Winston.

REVIEW TABLE 3.1   Common Units of Measurement in Acoustics

Measurement	CGS	Unit SI	CGS	Abbreviation	Equivalents
Length	Centimeter	Meter	cm	m	1 cm = 0.01 m I m = 100 cm
Mass	Gram	Kilogram	g	kg	1 g = 0.001 kg 1 kg = 1000 g
Area	Square centimeter	Square meter	cm^2	m^2	1 cm^2 = 0.0001 m^2 1 m = 10,000 cm^2
Work	Erg	Joule	e	J	1 e = 0.0000001 1 J = 10,000,000 e
Power	Ergs per second	Joules per second	e/sec	J/sec	1 e/sec = 0.0000001 J/sec 1 J/sec = 10,000,000 e/sec
	Watts	Watts	w	w	1 w = 1 J/sec 1 w = 10,000,000 e/sec
Force	Dyne	Newton	d	N	1 d = 0.00001 N 1 N 100,000 d
Intensity	Watts per square cm	Watts per square meter	w/cm^2	w/m^2	1 w/cm^2 = 10,000 w/m^2 1 w/m^2 = 0.0001 w/cm^2
Pressure	Dynes per square centimeter	*Newtons per square meter Pascal	d/cm^2	N/m^2	1 d/cm^2 = 0.1 Pa 1 Pa = 10 d/cm^2 1 Pa = 1 N/m^2
Speed (velocity)	Centimeters per second	Meters per second	cm/sec/sec	m/sec	1 cm/sec = 0.01 m/sec 1 m/sec = 100 cm/sec
Acceleration	Centimeters per square second	Meters per second squared	cm/sec^2	m/sec^2	1 cm/sec^2 = 0.01 m/sec^2 1 m/sec^2 = 100 cm/sec^2

*Related to but not strictly on the SI scale.

REVIEW TABLE 3.2   Factors Contributing to Psychological Perceptions of Sound

Percept	Prime Determinant	Other Determinants
Pitch	Frequency	Intensity
Loudness	Intensity	Frequency, duration
Quality	Spectrum	
Protensity	Duration	Intensity

REVIEW TABLE 3.3   Psychological Measurements of Sound

Measurement	Unit	Reference	Physical Correlate
Pitch	Mel	1000 mels (1000 Hz at 40 dB SL)	Frequency
Loudness	Sone	1 sone (1000 Hz at 40 dB SL)	Intensity
Loudness level	Phon	0 phons (corresponding to threshold at 1000 Hz)	Intensity
Quality			Spectrum

REVIEW TABLE 3.4   Physical Measurements of Sound

Measurement	Unit	Reference	Formula	Psychological Correlate
Frequency	cps (Hz)			Pitch
Intensity level	dB IL	10^{-16} watt/cm (CGS) 10^{-12} watt/m^2 (SI)	$NdB = 10 \log I_O/I_R$	Loudness
Sound-pressure level	dB SPL	0.0002 dyne/cm^2 (CGS) 20 µPa (SI)	$NdB = 20 \log$	Loudness
Hearing level	dB HL	ANSI-1996	$NdB = 20 \log P_O/P_R$	Loudness
Sensation level	dB SL	Hearing threshold of subject	$NdB = 20 \log P_O/P_R$	Loudness
Impedance	ohm (Z)		$Z = \sqrt{R^2 + (2\pi f M - S/2\pi f)^2}$	

PART TWO

Hearing Assessment

There is evidence that even seasoned clinicians do not carry out some hearing tests in precise and scientific ways. Often it is the basic tests that do not get the care and attention they deserve. Part II of this book covers the tests that are performed as part of a complete audiologic evaluation. Chapter 4 is concerned with pure-tone tests, which are, in some ways, quantifications of the results found on the tuning-fork tests described in Chapter 2. Chapter 5 presents different forms of speech audiometry and describes ways in which tests carried out with speech stimuli assist in diagnosis and treatment. Tests for determining the site in the auditory system that produce different kinds of auditory disorders are described in Chapters 6 and 7. These tests include both electrophysiological procedures, wherein relatively objective determinations can be made of a lesion site, and behavioral measures, in which the patient plays an active role. In many cases, step-by-step procedures are outlined, along with test interpretation. Special diagnostic procedures for testing children are described in Chapter 8. The importance of using an entire battery of tests in making a diagnosis is stressed.

4 Pure-Tone Audiometry

Pure-tone tests of hearing, performed with an audiometer, are electronic extensions of the same concepts developed in such tuning-fork tests as the Schwabach and Rinne. When such tests are carried out, the procedure is called *audiometry*. The main disadvantage of the tuning-fork tests is that they are difficult to quantify. That is, although the Schwabach might suggest sensorineural sensitivity that is poorer than normal, it does not tell how much poorer; although the Rinne might suggest the presence of a conductive component, it does not tell how large that component is.

The purpose of testing hearing is to aid in the process of making decisions regarding the type and extent of a patient's hearing loss. Because some of these decisions may have profound effects on the patient's medical, social, educational, and psychological status, accurate performance and careful interpretation of hearing tests are mandatory. The reliability of any test is based on interrelationships among such factors as calibration of equipment, test environment, patient performance, and examiner sophistication. In the final analysis, it is not *hearing* that we measure but, rather, *responses* to a set of acoustic signals that we interpret as representing hearing.

Chapter Objectives

Upon completion of this chapter, the reader should have a fundamental understanding of pure-tone audiometry, the basic ingredients of a reliable audiogram, and how different pure-tone tests are performed. The vocabularies in Chapters 2 and 3 are relied on extensively here, and the reader is exposed to new concepts and problems. Some of these problems can be solved; others can only be compensated for and understood. A basic understanding of this chapter should enable the reader to perform and interpret several pure-tone tests, assuming access to an audiometer in good working condition and the opportunity for supervised experience are provided.

The Pure-tone Audiometer

Pure-tone **audiometers** have been in use for nearly a hundred years as devices for determining hearing thresholds, which are then compared to established norms at various frequencies. The original audiometers were electrically driven tuning forks that generated a number of pure tones of different frequencies. In later designs the tones were generated electrically. With the advent of the electronic era, audiometers incorporated vacuum tubes, then transistors, and then the integrated circuits of today. Like other commercial items, audiometers vary considerably in cost. Specifications of the

American National Standards Institute (ANSI, 1996) are imposed on all audiometers so that price differences should not reflect differences in quality of manufacture.

A common type of audiometer, which is sometimes portable, tests hearing sensitivity by *air conduction* and *bone conduction*. A switch allows for easy selection of pure tones. The testable frequencies for these audiometers usually include 125, 250, 500, 750, 1000, 1500, 2000, 3000, 4000, 6000, and 8000 Hz. The range of intensities begins at –10 dB and goes to 110 dB HL at frequencies between 500 and 6000 Hz, with slightly lower maxima at 125, 250, and 8000 Hz. Some special devices, called extended high-frequency audiometers, have been devised that test from 8000 to 20,000 Hz and have specific diagnostic value (Stelmachowicz, Beauchaine, Kalberer, Kelly, & Jesteadt, 1989).

A matched pair of earphones is provided and an output switch directs the tone to either earphone. Usually only the range from 250 through 4000 Hz may be tested by bone conduction. The maximum testable hearing level for bone conduction is considerably lower than for air conduction, not exceeding 50 dB at 250 Hz and 70 or 80 dB at 500 Hz and above. Maximum outputs for bone conduction are lower than for air conduction for several reasons. The power required to drive a bone-conduction vibrator is greater than for an air-conduction earphone. In addition, when the bone-conduction vibrator is driven at high intensities, harmonic distortion takes place, especially in the low frequencies.

In addition to air- and bone-conduction capability, a *masking* control is often provided that allows for introduction of a noise to the nontest ear as needed during audiometry. Often the masking noise is not of a specific spectrum and is not well calibrated for practical clinical purposes. Persons who rely solely on portable air- and bone-conduction audiometers are often unsophisticated about the need for and proper use of masking. Some pure-tone audiometers, however, contain excellent masking-noise generators and can be used for a variety of pure-tone audiometric procedures (Figure 4.1).

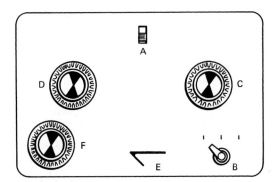

FIGURE 4.1   Typical face of a pure-tone audiometer (A) On-off power switch. (B) Output selector switch. Selects right ear, left ear; or bone conduction. Masking delivered to nontest earphone for air conduction and to left earphone for bone conduction. (C) Frequency selector dial. Air conduction selects 125, 250, 500, 750, 1000, 1500, 2000, 3000, 4000, 6000, or 8000 Hz. Bone conduction selects 250, 500, 750, 1000, 1500, 2000, 3000, or 4000 Hz. (D) Hearing-level dial. Air-conduction range: –10 to 110 dB HL (500 to 6000 Hz), –10 to 90 dB HL (250 to 8000 Hz), and –10 to 80 dB HL (125 Hz). Bone conduction range: –10 to 50 dB HL (250 Hz), –10 to 70 dB HL (500 Hz), and –10 to 80 dB HL (750 to 4000 Hz). (E) Tone-presentation bar. Introduces tone with prescribed rise and fall time and no audible sound from the switch. (F) Masking level dial. Controls intensity of masking noise in the nontest ear: Spectrum and intensity range vary with manufacturer.

Test Environment

Table 3.4 shows the maximum ambient sound-pressure levels allowable for air-conduction and bone-conduction testing. Rooms in which such standards can be met are not readily available. This is true in the case of hearing-test sites in industry or in the public schools. Regardless of the practical limitations imposed by a given situation, the person responsible for audiometric results must realize that background noise may affect audiometric results by elevating auditory thresholds. There are three major ways in which ambient room noise may be attenuated: by using specially designed earphone enclosures, by testing through receivers that insert into the ear, and by using sound-treated chambers.

Earphone Attenuation Devices

Audiometer earphone and cushion combinations do not provide sufficient attenuation of most background noises to allow determination of threshold down to 0 dB HL for people with normal hearing. Several devices are available that allow the supra-aural audiometer earphone and cushion to be mounted within a larger cup, which assists in the attenuation of background noise (see Figure 4.2). Most use a fluid-filled cushion to achieve a tight seal against the head. Such enclosures may be effective but differences exist in the efficiency of different devices (Franks, Engel, & Themann, 1992).

Problems with regard to **calibration** are encountered in the use of some earphone enclosures. The phones cannot be placed on the usual 6 cm³ coupler of an artificial ear. If the earphone is checked and found to be in proper calibration before it is mounted, mounting may alter the calibration slightly, especially in the low frequencies. Because bone-conduction testing is done with the

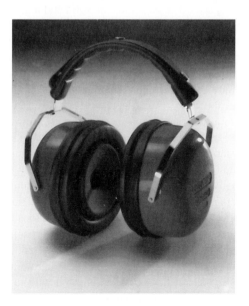

FIGURE 4.2   Commercial earphone enclosure device used to attenuate room noise during threshold audiometry. (Audiocups courtesy of American Overseas Trading Corporation)

ears uncovered, the masking effects of room noise may affect these test results without affecting the air-conduction results, possibly causing a misdiagnosis. Children often find these earphone devices heavy and uncomfortable.

Insert Earphones

Testing hearing with receivers that insert directly into the ear (Figure 4.8) has a number of advantages audiometrically. Clark and Roeser (1988) have shown that when the foam tips are placed into the ears, attenuation of background noise is increased compared to the supra-aural earphone-cushion arrangement. If the foam is inserted deep into the ear, just short of causing discomfort, even more attenuation is obtained. It is desirable to have patients open and close their mouths three or four times to ensure proper seating of the cushion. Insert earphones can be used for testing children as well as adults. Problems with room noise masking remain unsolved for bone-conduction testing, even if insert earphones are used for air conduction.

Sound-isolated Chambers

The term *soundproof room* is often used erroneously. Totally soundproofing a room is a formidable task indeed. All that is necessary in clinical audiometry is to keep the noise in the room below the level of masking that would cause a threshold shift in persons with normal hearing. Sound-isolated rooms may be specially constructed or purchased commercially.

The primary objective in sound-treating a room is to isolate it acoustically from the rest of the building in which it is housed. This usually involves the use of mass (such as cinder block), insulating materials (such as Fiberglas), and dead air spaces. The door must be solid and must close with a tight acoustic seal. Sometimes two doors are used, one opening into the room and the other opening out. The inside walls are covered with soft materials, such as acoustic tile, to help absorb sound and limit reverberation. Some such chambers contain large wedge-shaped pieces of soft material such as Fiberglas on all walls, the ceiling, and the floor, with a catwalk provided for the subject. Rooms in which reverberation is markedly diminished are called anechoic chambers; an example of such a room is shown in Figure 3.28.

Audiometric suites may be designed for either one-room or two-room use. In the one-room arrangement, examiners, their equipment, and the patient are all together in the same room, or the patient is within the room and the clinician just outside. In the two-room arrangement, the examiner and audiometer are in the equipment room and the patient is in the examining room. Windows provide visual communication between the rooms. As a rule there are several panes of glass to attenuate the sounds that emanate from the equipment room. Moisture-absorbing materials must be placed between the panes of glass to keep the windows from fogging. Electrical connections between the rooms are necessary so that signals can be directed from the audiometer to the earphones. In addition, a talkback device, consisting of a microphone, amplifier, and speaker and/or earphone, enables the examiner to hear patients when they speak.

In customizing sound-isolated rooms, a great deal of attention is often paid to attenuating sound from adjoining spaces outside the walls of the room, but insufficient care is given to building-borne vibrations that may enter the room from floor or ceiling. It does little good to have four-foot walls of solid concrete when footsteps can be heard from the floor above.

When sufficient space, money, and architectural know-how are available, custom sound rooms may be the proper choice. Contemporary audiology centers, however, seem to be leaning more toward the commercially prefabricated sound room, which is made of steel panels and can be more easily installed, with wiring included for two-room operation (Figure 4.3). The manufacturer does not guarantee the noise level within the sound room after installation, but only the amount of attenuation the room will provide under specific laboratory conditions, a fact often not fully understood by many purchasers. It is therefore necessary to prepare the room that will enclose the prefabricated booth by making this area as quiet and nonreverberant as possible.

Prefabricated sound booths are available in one- and two-room suites. Windows with several panes of glass are installed to enable the examiner to observe the patient. The inside walls of the booth are constructed of perforated steel and filled with sound-absorbing materials. Some booths are double-walled; that is, there is one booth inside another, larger one. Prefabricated booths are free-

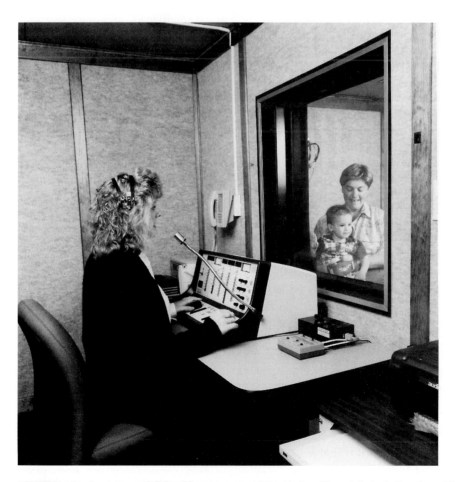

FIGURE 4.3   A commercial double-room sound-treated audiometric test chamber. (Courtesy of Industrial Acoustics Co., Inc.)

standing, touching none of the walls of the room in which they stand, and are isolated from the ceiling by air and from the floor by specially constructed sound rails.

One of the great weaknesses of audiometric rooms, whether custom or commercial, is their ventilation systems. Rooms that are to be tightly closed must have adequate air circulation, requiring the use of fans and motors. Sometimes the air-intake system is coupled directly with the heating and air-conditioning ducts of the building. In such cases care must be taken to minimize the introduction of noise through the ventilation system.

Lighting for both kinds of rooms should be incandescent, but if the use of fluorescent lighting cannot be avoided, the starters must be remotely mounted. Starters for fluorescent tubes often put out an annoying hum that can be heard by the patient or picked up by the audiometer.

The Patient's Role in Manual Pure-tone Audiometry

Patients seeking hearing tests vary a great deal in age, intelligence, education, motivation, and willingness to cooperate. The approach to testing will be very different for an adult than for a child, or for an interested person than for one who is frightened, shy, or even hostile. Procedures also vary depending on the degree of the patient's spoken language. Test results are most easily obtained when a set of instructions can be given orally to a patient, who then complies. As any experienced audiologist will testify, things do not go equally well with all patients.

In pure-tone audiometry, regardless of how the message is conveyed, patients must learn to accept their responsibility in the test if results are to be valid. Spoken instructions, written instructions, gestures, and/or demonstrations may be required. In any case, patients must become aware that they are to indicate when they hear a tone, even when that tone is very soft. The level at which tones are perceived as barely audible is the **threshold** of hearing sensitivity. Auditory thresholds at different frequencies form the basis for pure-tone audiometry.

Patient Response

After patients understand the instructions and know what they are listening for, they must be given some way of indicating that they have heard. Some audiologists request that patients raise one hand when a tone is heard. They then lower the hand when they no longer hear the tone. Sometimes patients are asked to raise their right hands when they hear the tone in the right ear and their left hands when they hear the tone in the left ear. The hand signal is probably the most popular response system used in pure-tone audiometry. Many audiologists like this method because they can observe both how the patient responds and the hearing level that produces the response. Often, when the tone is close to threshold, patients will raise their hands more hesitatingly than when it is clearly audible. Problems occur with this response system when patients either forget to lower their hands or keep them partially elevated.

As with the hand signal, the patient may simply raise one index finger when the tone is heard and lower it when it is not heard. This system has the same advantages and disadvantages as the hand-signal system. It is sometimes difficult to see from an adjacent control room when the patient raises only a finger.

The patient may be given a signal button with instructions to press it when the tone is heard and release it when the tone goes off. Pressing the button illuminates a light on the control panel of the audiometer and/or makes a sound. The use of signal buttons limits the kind of subjective information the audiologist may glean from observing hand or finger signals because the push button is an all-or-none type of response. Use of the push-button technique does have the advantage of training the patient in this response method, which is mandatory in some of the special tests described in Chapter 7. Reaction time is sometimes another important drawback to push-button signaling, as some people may be slow in pushing and releasing the button. Often, if the button is tapped very lightly, the panel light may only flicker, and the response may be missed. Push buttons are usually not a good idea for children or the physically disabled, although they are standard equipment on many audiometers.

Some audiologists prefer vocal responses like "now," "yes," or "I hear it," whenever the tone is heard. This procedure is often useful with children, although some patients have complained that their own voices "ring" in the earphones after each utterance, making tones close to threshold difficult to hear. Play and other motivational techniques are often necessary when testing children or other difficult-to-test persons. Some of these methods are discussed in the chapter on pediatric audiology (Chapter 8).

False Responses

False responses are common during behavioral audiometry, and the alert clinician is always on guard for them because they can be misleading and can cause serious errors in the interpretation of test results.

A common kind of false response occurs when patients fail to indicate that they have heard a tone. Some patients may have misunderstood, or forgotten their roles in the test. Such **false negative responses,** which tend to suggest that hearing is worse than it actually is, are also seen in patients who deliberately feign or exaggerate a hearing loss (see Chapter 13).

False positive responses, where the patient responds when no tone has been presented, are often more irritating to the clinician than are false negatives. Most patients will respond with some false positives if long silent periods occur in the test, especially if they are highly motivated to respond. When false positive responses obscure accurate test results, the clinician must slow down the test to watch for them, which encourages even more false positives. Sometimes even reinstruction to the patient fails to alleviate this vexing situation.

The Clinician's Role in Manual Pure-tone Audiometry

As implied earlier, the first step in manual pure-tone testing is to make patients aware of their task in the procedure. If verbal instructions are given, they may be something like this:

> *You are going to hear a series of tones, first in one ear and then in the other. When you hear a tone, no matter how high or low in pitch, and no matter how loud or soft, please signal that you have heard it. Raise your hand when you first hear the tone, and keep it up as long as you hear it. Put your hand down quickly when the tone goes away. Remember to signal every time you hear a tone. Are there any questions?*

If a different response system is preferred, it may be substituted. There is an advantage to asking the patient to signal quickly to both the onset and the offset of the tone. This permits two responses to each presentation of the tone to be observed. If the patient responds to both the intro-duction and the discontinuation of the tone, the acceptance of false responses may be avoided.

There are some distinct advantages to providing written instructions to patients before they undergo a hearing evaluation. These instructions can be mailed so that they can be read at home before patients arrive at the audiology clinic, or they can be provided when the patients check in with the receptionist, to be read while waiting to be seen by the audiologist. In addition to augmenting verbal instructions, printed instructions can be retained for reference after the patient leaves the clinic, to help clarify what the different tests were intended to measure. Printed instructions should never be used to replace verbal instructions. A sample of patient instructions for the basic test battery may be found on the accompanying CD-ROM under literature.

Patient's Position during Testing

It is of paramount importance that the patient never be in a position to observe the clinician during pure-tone testing. Even small eye, hand, or arm movements by the clinician may cause patients to signal that they have heard a tone when they have not. In one-room situations, patients should be seated so that they are at right angles to the audiometer (Figure 4.4). Some audiologists prefer to have the patient's back to the audiometer to eliminate any possibility of visual cues; however, this is disconcerting to some patients and eliminates observation of the patient's facial expression, which is often helpful to the audiologist in interpreting responses.

Even if the audiologist and patient are in different rooms, care must be taken to ensure that the patient cannot observe the clinician's movements. Figure 4.5 illustrates one satisfactory arrange-ment. Of course, the patient must always be clearly observable by the audiologist.

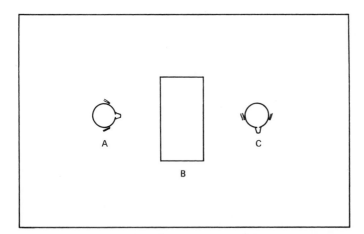

FIGURE 4.4   Proper positioning during pure-tone audiometry for (A) examiner, (B) audiometer, (C) patient.

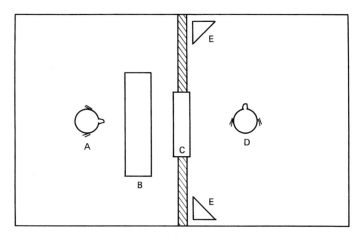

FIGURE 4.5   Proper positioning during pure-tone audiometry conducted in a two-room suite for (A) examiner, (B) audiometer, (C) window separating rooms, (D) patient, and (E) loudspeakers.

Air-conduction Audiometry

The purpose of air-conduction audiometry is to specify the amount of a patient's hearing sensitivity at various frequencies. If there is a loss of hearing, air-conduction test results can specify the degree of loss but not whether the deficit is produced by abnormality in the conductive mechanism, the sensorineural mechanism, or both.

Proper placement of earphones is shown in Figure 4.6. The headband should be placed directly over the top of the head. All interfering hair should be pushed out of the way and earrings should be

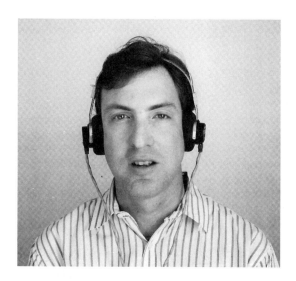

FIGURE 4.6   Properly placed air-conduction earphones.

removed, when possible. Eyeglasses should also be removed as they sometimes lift the cushion of the earphone away from the ear and may become uncomfortable as the earphone cushion presses on the temple bar of the eyeglasses. Some patients are reluctant to remove their eyeglasses as they feel more relaxed when they can see clearly. This is another advantage to insert receivers, which do not interfere at all with the wearing of eyeglasses during testing.

Most earphone cushions are the hard rubber, supra-aural type, fitting tightly against the external ear. The phones should be positioned so that their diaphragms are aimed directly at the opening into the ear canal. The yokes that hold the phones may be pulled down so that the headset is in its most extended position. While the clinician is holding the phones against the ears, the size of the headset can be readjusted for a tight fit.

Some patients' outer ears collapse because of the pressure of the earphones. This creates an artificial conductive hearing loss, which usually shows poorer sensitivity in the higher frequencies, which can be misleading in diagnosis. A useful measure to check for an ear canal that might collapse is to press the rubber cushion from an earphone against the ear and look through the hole to see if the canal appears to collapse (see Figure 4.7). When this occurs, or when the clinician suspects that it may occur because the ear seems particularly supple, certain steps can be taken to overcome the difficulty. One easy solution is to place a small piece of foam rubber (cut in the shape of a behind-the-ear hearing aid) under the pinna (the protrusion of the ear at the side of the head). It is useful to have on hand a number of these foam pieces precut in different sizes for use when they are needed.

Additionally, insert receivers may be used for air-conduction testing when collapsing ear canals are a potential problem. The foam insert must be compressed with the fingers and can be slipped into a small plastic sleeve to maintain this compression until insertion is made into the ear canal. After the insert is in place, the foam quickly expands. The transducer itself is mounted at the end of a 250 mm plastic tube and may be clipped to a blouse or shirt. As with supra-aural phones, insert receivers are colored red and blue for testing the right and left ears, respectively. Properly placed insert earphones are shown in Figure 4.8.

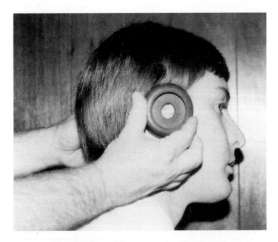

FIGURE 4.7   An empty earphone cushion held against the ear to determine whether it will collapse during air-conduction testing.

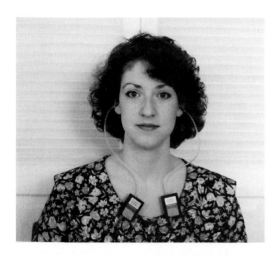

FIGURE 4.8   Properly placed insert earphones.

Procedure for Air-conduction Audiometry

The selection of which ear to test first is purely arbitrary. Although the American Speech-Language-Hearing Association (ASHA) recommends testing the better ear first, it cannot be proved that this has any real effect on test results. Likewise, frequency order probably does not affect results, although most audiologists prefer to test at 1000 Hz initially, test higher frequencies in ascending order, retest 1000 Hz, and then test lower frequencies in descending order (1000, 2000, 4000, 8000, 1000, 500, 250 Hz, etc.). Some audiologists feel that useful information is gained from the 125 Hz threshold; others believe that thresholds at this frequency can be predicted from the 250 Hz results. Some clinicians also prefer to test 6000 rather than 8000 Hz because of the calibration difficulties sometimes encountered at the higher frequency.

Many audiologists only sample hearing at octave points, whereas still others prefer the detail resulting from testing the mid-octave frequencies (750, 1500, 3000, and 6000 Hz). In its guidelines for manual pure-tone audiometry, ASHA (1978) sensibly recommends that mid-octave points be tested when a difference of 20 dB or more is seen in the thresholds at adjacent octaves.

Over the years, a number of different procedures have been devised for determining pure-tone thresholds. Some audiologists have used automatically pulsing tones and some have used manually pulsed tones. Some have used a descending technique, whereby the tone is presented above threshold and lowered in intensity until patients signal that they can no longer hear it. Others have used an ascending approach, increasing the level of the tone from below threshold until a response is given. Still others have used a bracketing procedure to find the threshold of a tone.

Carhart and Jerger (1959) investigated several pure-tone test procedures and found that there were no real differences in test results obtained with different methods. Nevertheless, they recommended that a particular procedure be followed, and this procedure appears to have been widely accepted.

The procedure recommended here, based on Carhart's and Jerger's suggestion, is to begin testing at 1000 Hz because this frequency is easily heard by most people and has been said to have high test-retest reliability. In practice, it may be advisable in some cases to begin testing at other frequencies, perhaps lower ones, in cases of severe hearing loss in which no measurable hearing may be found at 1000 Hz and above.

Following the ASHA (1978) guidelines, a pure tone is presented initially at 30 dB HL. If a response is obtained, it suggests that the 30 dB tone is above the patient's threshold. If no response is seen, the level is raised to 50 dB HL, introduced, and then raised in 10 dB steps until a response is obtained or the limit of the audiometer is reached for the test frequency.

After a response is obtained, the level is lowered in 10 dB steps. Each time a tone is introduced, it is maintained for one or two seconds. The hearing-level dial is never moved while the tone is in the *on* position, as a scratching sound may occur in the earphone, causing the patient to respond as if to a tone. All ascending movements of the hearing-level dial from this point are made in steps of 5 dB. When the tone is lowered below the patient's response level, it is then raised in 5 dB steps until it is audible again, then lowered in 10 dB steps and raised in 5 dB steps until the 50 percent threshold response criterion has been met. The threshold is the lowest level at which the patient can correctly identify three out of a theoretical six tones. This usually, but not always, implies that a point 5 dB above this level will evoke more than a 50 percent response. Levels accepted as threshold are often in the 75 percent to 100 percent response range.

As thresholds are obtained at each frequency, they must be recorded on a data sheet. Some audiologists prefer to record the results directly onto a graph called an **audiogram,** using symbols to depict the threshold of each ear as a function of frequency and intensity (with reference to normal threshold). Others prefer to record their results numerically on a specially prepared score sheet. The form shown in Figure 4.9 has proved to be very useful, especially in the training of new clinicians. This form allows for recording the audiometric data numerically before plotting the graph; for a retest of 1000 Hz; and, if necessary, for retest of all frequencies. Accuracy criteria must be satisfied before the graph is drawn.

Any audiometric worksheet should have some minimal identifying information—the patient's name, age, and sex as well as the date of examination, equipment used, and examiner's name. Some estimate of the test reliability should also be noted. After the air-conduction thresholds have been recorded, the average threshold levels for each ear at 500, 1000, and 2000 Hz should be recorded. This is called the **pure-tone average (PTA),** and it is useful for predicting the threshold for speech as well as for establishing the degree of disability imposed by a hearing loss. Table 4.1 shows the degree of hearing disability created by various degrees of sensitivity loss. Even though this table is based in part on the recommendations made by Stewart and Downs (1984) for children, it has applications for adults as well. The two-frequency pure-tone average (lowest two thresholds at 500, 1000, and 2000 Hz) may be recorded as well and is often a better predictor of hearing for speech than the three-frequency average.

Many laypersons are accustomed to expressing the degree of a hearing impairment in percentage, because they are unfamiliar with such concepts as frequency and intensity. Many physicians also calculate the percentage of hearing impairment, probably because it is easier for their patients to understand. Although percentage of hearing impairment is an outmoded concept, its continued use mandates mention here; however, for practical application in the counseling of patients it is considered inappropriate and even misleading in many cases.

One weakness in the concept of percentage of hearing impairment is that it ignores audiometric configuration, and looks only at the *average* hearing loss. The addition of 3000 Hz to the formula by the American Academy of Ophthalmology and Otolaryngology (AAOO) (1979) improves the situation somewhat. The formula, as modified slightly by Sataloff, Sataloff, and Vassallo (1980), works as follows:

TABLE 4.1 Scale of Hearing Impairment Based on the Pure-tone Average at 500, 1000 and 2000 Hz*

PTA (dB)	Degree of Disability	Consider Hearing Aid	Consider Communication Training
−10 to 15	None	No	No
16 to 25	Slight	Possibly	Possibly
26 to 40	Mild	Probably	Probably
41 to 55	Moderate	Definitely	Definitely
56 to 70	Moderately Severe	Definitely	Definitely
71 to 90	Severe	Definitely	Definitely
>91	Profound	Definitely	Definitely

*Hearing levels refer to the ANSI-1996 scale.

1. Compute the average hearing loss (in decibels) from the threshold responses at 500, 1000, 2000, and 3000 Hz for each ear.
2. Subtract 25 dB—considered to be the lower limit of normal hearing by the AAOO.
3. Multiply the remaining number by 1.5 percent for each ear. This gives the percentage of hearing impairment for each ear.
4. Multiply the percentage of hearing impairment in the better ear by 5, add this figure to the percentage of hearing impairment in the poorer ear, and divide this total by 6. This gives the binaural (both ears) hearing impairment in percentage form.

Obviously, in addition to being somewhat misleading, the computation of percentage of hearing impairment is time-consuming. It is likely that patients are frequently confused by what they have been told about their hearing losses. For example, Table 4.1 indicates that a 25 dB pure-tone average constitutes a slight hearing impairment, but such a loss would prove to be 0 percent by using the AAOO method, which would suggest to patients that their hearing is normal. Likewise, it can be seen that a 92 dB pure-tone average would be shown as 100 percent impairment, which would suggest total deafness to many laypersons. A patient with a 92 dB hearing level often proves to have considerable residual hearing.

When an audiogram is used, the graph should conform to specific dimensions. As Figure 4.9 illustrates, frequency (in hertz) is shown on the abscissa and intensity (in dB HL) on the ordinate. The space horizontally for 1 octave should be the same as the space vertically for 20 dB, forming a perfect square (20 dB by 1 octave). Unlike most graphs, the audiogram is drawn with 0 at the top rather than the bottom. This is done so that as hearing thresholds get poorer, they are shown as lower on the audiogram.

After a hearing threshold is obtained, a symbol is placed under the test frequency at a number corresponding to the hearing-level dial setting (in decibels) that represents threshold. The usual symbols for air conduction are a red circle representing the right ear and a blue X representing the left ear. After all the results are plotted on the audiogram, the symbols are usually connected with a

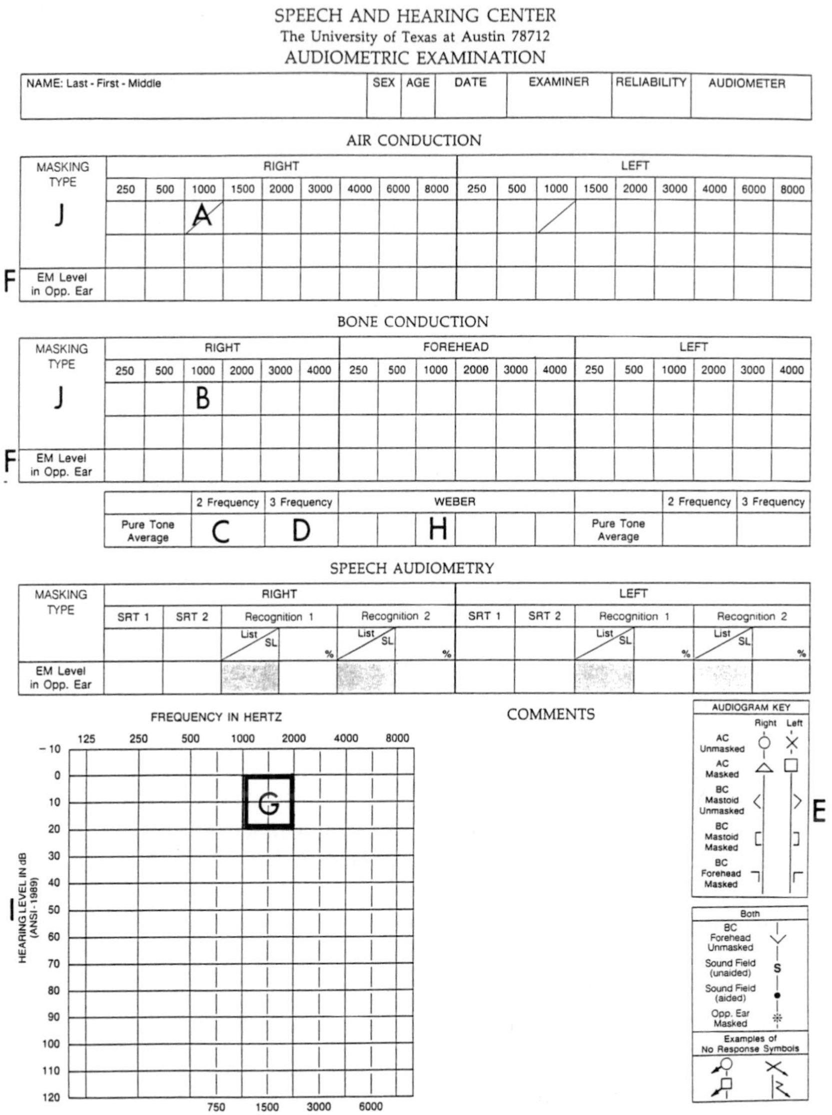

SPEECH AND HEARING CENTER
The University of Texas at Austin 78712
AUDIOMETRIC EXAMINATION

NAME: Last - First - Middle	SEX	AGE	DATE	EXAMINER	RELIABILITY	AUDIOMETER

AIR CONDUCTION

MASKING TYPE	RIGHT									LEFT								
	250	500	1000	1500	2000	3000	4000	6000	8000	250	500	1000	1500	2000	3000	4000	6000	8000
J			A															
F EM Level in Opp. Ear																		

BONE CONDUCTION

MASKING TYPE	RIGHT						FOREHEAD						LEFT					
	250	500	1000	2000	3000	4000	250	500	1000	2000	3000	4000	250	500	1000	2000	3000	4000
J			B															
F EM Level in Opp. Ear																		

		2 Frequency	3 Frequency		WEBER				2 Frequency	3 Frequency
Pure Tone Average		C	D		H		Pure Tone Average			

SPEECH AUDIOMETRY

MASKING TYPE	RIGHT				LEFT			
	SRT 1	SRT 2	Recognition 1	Recognition 2	SRT 1	SRT 2	Recognition 1	Recognition 2
			List / SL %	List / SL %			List / SL %	List / SL %
EM Level in Opp. Ear								

FREQUENCY IN HERTZ

COMMENTS

AUDIOGRAM KEY

	Right	Left
AC Unmasked	O	X
AC Masked	△	□
BC Mastoid Unmasked	<	>
BC Mastoid Masked	[	]
BC Forehead Masked	⌐	⌐

Both
BC Forehead Unmasked
Sound Field (unaided) S
Sound Field (aided)
Opp. Ear Masked
Examples of No Response Symbols

HEARING LEVEL IN dB (ANSI - 1989)

G

FIGURE 4.9   Example of an audiometric worksheet. Note the identifying information regarding the patient's name, sex, and age; examiner's name; date of examination; and description of the audiometer used. The following information is included on the worksheet: (A) air-conduction thresholds (recorded numerically); (B) bone-conduction thresholds (recorded numerically) for either the forehead or the right and left mastoid; a second set of boxes is provided for repeated measurements of air-conduction or bone-conduction tests with opposite-ear masking, if that is necessary; (C) two-frequency pure-tone average (lowest two thresholds at 500, 1000, and 2000 Hz); (D) three-frequency pure-tone average (500, 1000, and 2000 Hz); (E) symbols used for plotting the audiogram; (F) effective masking levels in the nontest ear used, when necessary, during air-conduction or bone-conduction tests; (G) a square to illustrate that the distance of 1 octave (across) is the same as 20 dB (down); (H) audiometric Weber results; (I) indication that the hearing levels refer to ANSI-1996 values; (J) type of noise used in masking for pure-tone tests.

solid red line for the right ear and a solid blue line for the left ear. When masking is used in the non-test ear, the symbol Δ (in red) is substituted for the right ear and the symbol □ (in blue) is used for the left ear. When no response (NR) is obtained at the highest output for the frequency being tested, the appropriate symbol is placed at the point on the intersection of the maximum testable level for the test frequency; an arrow pointing down indicates no response. ASHA (1990) has recommended a set of symbols that has been widely adopted. The currently used symbols are shown in Figure 4.10. The obvious reason for using standardized symbols is to improve communication and minimize confusion when audiograms are exchanged among different clinics.

Figure 4.11 shows an audiogram that illustrates normal hearing for both ears. Note that the normal audiometric contour is flat, because the normal threshold curve, with a sound-pressure level

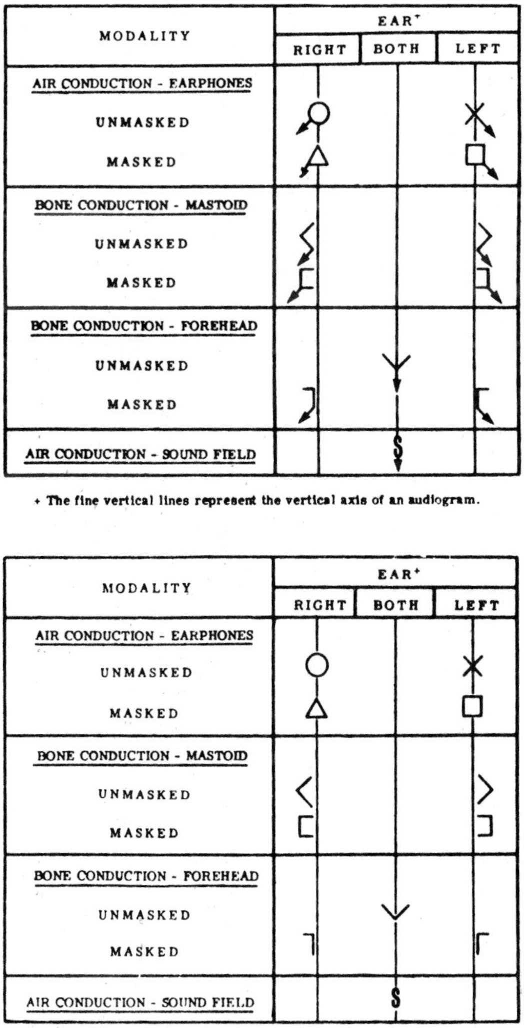

+ The fine vertical lines represent the vertical axis of an audiogram.

FIGURE 4.10   Symbols recommended by the American Speech-Language-Hearing Association (1990) for use in pure-tone audiometry.

SPEECH AND HEARING CENTER
The University of Texas at Austin 78712
AUDIOMETRIC EXAMINATION

NAME: Last - First - Middle	SEX	AGE	DATE	EXAMINER	RELIABILITY	AUDIOMETER

AIR CONDUCTION

MASKING TYPE	RIGHT									LEFT								
	250	500	1000	1500	2000	3000	4000	6000	8000	250	500	1000	1500	2000	3000	4000	6000	8000
	5	10	5/5	5	5	0	10	10	15	10	5	5/5	10	10	5	15	10	10
EM Level in Opp. Ear																		

BONE CONDUCTION

MASKING TYPE	RIGHT						FOREHEAD						LEFT					
	250	500	1000	2000	3000	4000	250	500	1000	2000	3000	4000	250	500	1000	2000	3000	4000
							5	5	5	10	10	10						
EM Level in Opp. Ear																		

	2 Frequency	3 Frequency	WEBER							2 Frequency	3 Frequency
Pure Tone Average	5	7	M	M	M	M	M		Pure Tone Average	5	7

SPEECH AUDIOMETRY

MASKING TYPE	RIGHT						LEFT					
	SRT 1	SRT 2	Recognition 1		Recognition 2		SRT 1	SRT 2	Recognition 1		Recognition 2	
			List / SL	%	List / SL	%			List / SL	%	List / SL	%
EM Level in Opp. Ear												

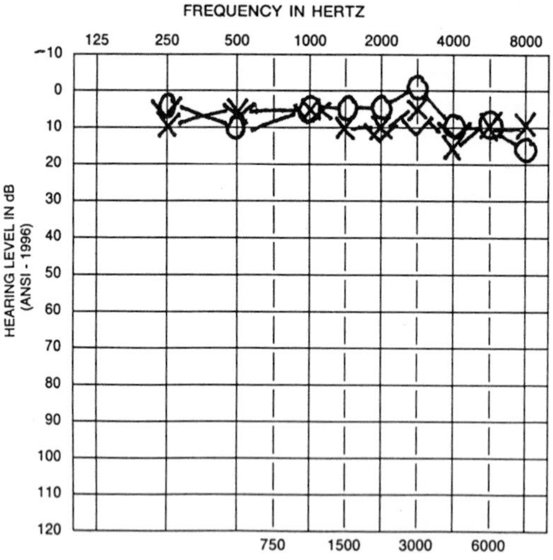

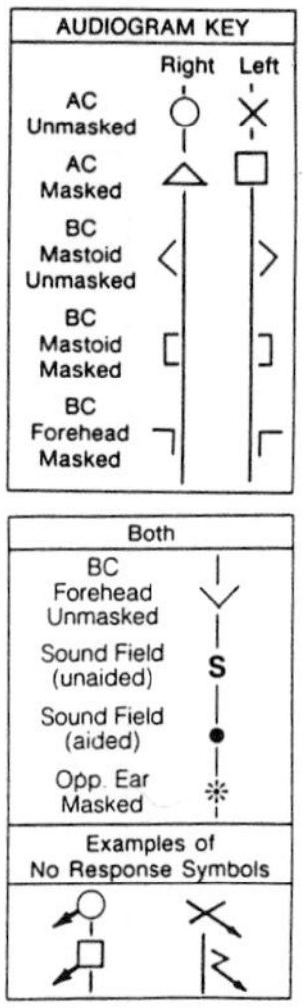

FIGURE 4.11 Audiogram illustrating normal hearing in both ears. Note that no hearing level by either air conduction or bone conduction exceeds 15 dB HL.

reference, has been compensated for in calibration of the audiometer, which uses a hearing level reference.

Bone-conduction Audiometry

The purpose of measuring hearing by bone conduction is to determine the patient's sensorineural sensitivity. The descriptions offered in Chapter 2 were very much oversimplified, as bone conduction is an extremely complex phenomenon. Actually, hearing by bone conduction arises from the interactions of at least three different phenomena.

When the skull is set into vibration, as by a bone-conduction vibrator or a tuning fork, the bones of the skull become distorted, resulting in distortion of the structures of hearing in the cochlea of the inner ear. This distortion activates certain cells and gives rise to electrochemical activity that is identical to the activity created by an air-conduction signal. This is called **distortional bone conduction.**

While the skull is moving, the chain of tiny bones in the middle ear, owing to its inertia, lags behind so that the third bone, the stapes, moves in and out of an oval-shaped window into the cochlea. Activity is generated within the cochlea as in air-conduction stimulation. This mode of inner-ear stimulation is appropriately called **inertial bone conduction.**

Simultaneously, oscillation of the skull causes vibration of the column of air in the outer-ear canal. Some of these sound waves pass out of the ear, whereas others go further down the canal, vibrating the eardrum membrane and following the same sound route as air conduction. This third mode is called **osseotympanic bone conduction.** Hearing by bone conduction results from an interaction of these three ways of stimulating the cochlea.

For many years the prominent bone behind the ear (the mastoid process) has been the place on the head from which bone-conduction measurements have been made. This was probably chosen for two reasons: (1) because bone-conducted tones are louder from the mastoid in normal-hearing persons and (2) because of each mastoid process' nearness to the ear being tested. Probably the bone-conducted tone is loudest from behind the ear because the chain of middle ear bones is driven on a direct axis, taking maximum advantage of its hinged action. The notion that placing a vibrator behind the right ear results in stimulation of only the right cochlea is false because vibration of the skull from any location results in approximately equal stimulation of both cochleas (Figure 4.12).

It has been demonstrated (Studebaker, 1962) that the forehead is in many ways superior to the mastoid process for measurement of clinical bone-conduction thresholds. Variations produced by vibrator-to-skull pressure, artifacts created by abnormalities of the sound-conducting mechanism of the middle ear, test-retest differences, and so on are all of smaller consequence when testing from the forehead than from the mastoid. It has recently been shown (Fagelson & Martin, 1994) that the greater amount of acoustic energy generated in the outer ear canal when the mastoid is the test site, as compared to the forehead, is further evidence of the advantage of forehead testing.

In addition to the theoretical advantages of forehead bone-conduction testing, there are numbers of practical conveniences. The headband used to hold the bone-conduction vibrator is much easier to affix to the head than the mastoid headband. Also, eyeglasses need not be removed when the vibrator is placed on the forehead, which is the case for mastoid placement.

The main disadvantage of testing from the forehead is that about 10 dB greater intensity is required to stimulate normal threshold, resulting in a decrease of the maximum level at which test-

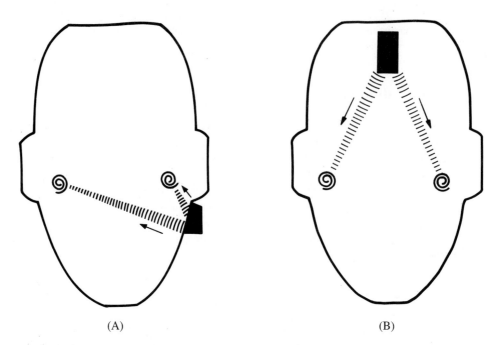

(A)   (B)

FIGURE 4.12   Vibrations of the skull result in bone-conducted stimulation of both inner ears, whether the vibrator is placed on (A) the mastoid or (B) the forehead.

ing can be carried out. Although bone-conduction testing should sometimes be done from both the forehead and the mastoid, the forehead is recommended here for routine audiometry. Despite negative reports on mastoid test accuracy and other problems that go back many years (e.g., Barany, 1938), a national survey (Martin, Champlin, & Chambers, 1998) shows that the mastoid process continues to be the preferred bone-conduction vibrator site among audiologists. It is hoped that this situation will change.

When the mastoid is the place of measurement, a steel headband crosses the top of the head (Figure 4.13A). If testing is to be done from the forehead, the bone-conduction vibrator should be affixed to the center line of the skull, just above the eyebrow line. A plastic strap encircles the head, holding the vibrator in place (Figure 4.13B). All interfering hair must be pushed out of the way, and the concave side of the vibrator should be placed against the skull.

Both ears must be uncovered during routine bone-conduction audiometry. When normal ears and those with sensorineural impairments are covered by earphones or occluded by other devices, there is an increase in the intensity of sound delivered by a bone-conduction vibrator to the cochlea, which occurs partly because of changes in osseotympanic bone conduction. This phenomenon, called the *occlusion effect (OE),* occurs at frequencies of 1000 Hz and below. The occlusion effect is rare in patients with conductive hearing losses (e.g., problems in the middle ear) because the increase in sound pressure created by the occlusion is attenuated by the hearing loss. The occlusion effect (Table 4.2) explains the results on the Bing tuning-fork test described in Chapter 2. Recent research findings confirm previous notions that the occlusion effect is the result of the increase in

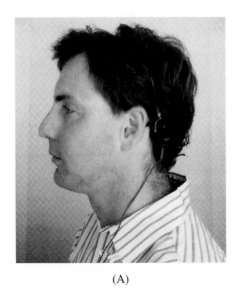
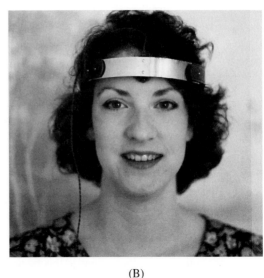

(A)   (B)

FIGURE 4.13   Bone-conduction vibrator placement on (A) the mastoid process and (B) the forehead.

sound pressure level in the external ear canal when the outer ear is covered (Fagelson & Martin, 1994; Martin & Fagelson, 1995).

Procedure for Bone-conduction Audiometry

The decision of which ear to test first in bone-conduction audiometry is unimportant. As a matter of fact, as is illustrated in Figure 4.12, clinicians really cannot be certain which cochlea they are testing. This is true regardless of whether the mastoid or the forehead is the vibrator placement site. The procedure for actual testing is identical to that for air conduction, although the range of frequencies to be tested and the maximum intensities are more limited for bone conduction than for air conduction.

Bone-conduction thresholds may be recorded in identical fashion to those for air conduction, using the appropriate spaces on the audiometric worksheet. Interpreting bone-conduction results from an audiogram is sometimes confusing, even though all audiograms should contain a key that

TABLE 4.2   Occlusion Effect for Bone Conduction Produced When a Supra-aural Earphone-cushion Arrangement (TDH-39 earphone in MX/41AR cushion) Is Placed over the Ear during Bone-conduction Tests*

Frequency (Hz)	250	500	1000	2000	4000
Occlusion effect (dB)	30	20	10	0	0

*The amounts shown indicate central tendencies and the range of occlusion effects may be considerable (Elpern & Naunton, 1963).

tells the reader the symbols used and what they represent. If the forehead is the test site, a red arrowhead pointing to the reader's left (<) is used for the right ear and a blue arrowhead pointing to the reader's right (>) for the left ear. If the printed page is viewed as the patient's face looking at the reader, the symbols for right and left are logical. When masking is used in the nontest ear, the symbols are changed to square brackets, [in red for the right ear and] in blue for the left ear. The symbol for forehead bone conduction is a black V when no masking is used. When the nontest ear is masked for forehead bone-conduction testing, a red ⌉ is used as a symbol for the right ear and a blue ⌈ for the left ear. Some audiologists prefer to connect the bone-conduction symbols on the audiogram with a dashed red line for the right ear and a dashed blue line for the left ear. Others prefer not to connect the symbols at all. The latter is the preference in this book. At times, a patient may give no response at the maximum bone-conduction limits of the audiometer. When this occurs, the appropriate symbol should be placed under the test frequency where that line intersects the maximum testable level. An arrow pointing down indicates no response at that level. Figure 4.11 shows the recording of results and plotting of an audiogram for a hypothetical normal-hearing individual. Note that the bone-conduction symbols, except for unmasked forehead, are placed to the side of the ordinate. All the audiometric illustrations in this book show that bone-conduction tests were performed with the vibrator on the forehead, which is, from most points of view, superior to the mastoid for testing.

Audiogram Interpretation

Whether the audiometric results have been recorded as numbers, or plotted on the graph, they are interpreted in the same way. Results must be looked at for each frequency in terms of (1) the amount of hearing loss by air conduction (the hearing level), (2) the amount of hearing loss by bone conduction, and (3) the relationship between air-conduction and bone-conduction thresholds. The audiometric test frequencies may be heard on the accompanying CD-ROM under *Audiograms*. The effects of different hearing loss configurations on the perceived clarity of speech may also be heard on the CD-ROM under *Simulated Hearing Loss*.

The audiometric results depicted in Figure 4.14 illustrate a conductive loss of hearing in both ears. There is approximately equal loss of sensitivity at each frequency by air conduction. Measurements obtained by bone conduction show normal hearing at all frequencies. Therefore, the air-conduction results show the loss of sensitivity (about 35 dB); the bone-conduction results show the amount of sensorineural impairment (none); and the difference between the air- and bone-conduction thresholds, which is called the **air-bone gap (ABG),** shows the amount of conductive involvement (35 dB).

Figure 4.15 shows an audiogram similar to that in Figure 4.14; however, Figure 4.15 illustrates a bilateral sensorineural hearing loss. Again, the air-conduction results show the total amount of loss (35 dB), the bone-conduction results show the amount of sensorineural impairment (35 dB), and the air-bone gap (0 dB) shows no conductive involvement at all.

The results shown in Figure 4.16 suggest a typical mixed loss of hearing in both ears. In this case the total loss of sensitivity is much greater than in the previous two illustrations, as shown by the air-conduction thresholds (60 dB). Bone-conduction results show that there is some sensorineural involvement (35 dB). The air-bone gap shows a 25 dB conductive component.

Sometimes high-frequency tones radiate from the bone-conduction vibrator when near-maximum hearing levels are presented by bone conduction. If the patient hears these signals by air conduction, the false impression of an air-bone gap may be made. Sensorineural hearing losses have

SPEECH AND HEARING CENTER
The University of Texas at Austin 78712
AUDIOMETRIC EXAMINATION

NAME: Last - First - Middle	SEX	AGE	DATE	EXAMINER	RELIABILITY	AUDIOMETER

AIR CONDUCTION

MASKING TYPE	RIGHT									LEFT								
	250	500	1000	1500	2000	3000	4000	6000	8000	250	500	1000	1500	2000	3000	4000	6000	8000
	35	30	40/40	40	35	35	40	45	45	35	30	40/40	35	35	45	40	45	50
EM Level in Opp. Ear																		

BONE CONDUCTION

MASKING TYPE	RIGHT						FOREHEAD						LEFT					
	250	500	1000	2000	3000	4000	250	500	1000	2000	3000	4000	250	500	1000	2000	3000	4000
NB	0*	-5*	5*	0*	5*	10*	0	-5	5	0	5	10	0*	-5*	5*	0*	5*	10*
EM Level in Opp. Ear	35	30	40	35	45	40							35	30	40	35	35	40

	2 Frequency	3 Frequency	WEBER							2 Frequency	3 Frequency
Pure Tone Average	33	35	M	M	M	M	M	M	Pure Tone Average	33	35

SPEECH AUDIOMETRY

MASKING TYPE	RIGHT					LEFT				
	SRT 1	SRT 2	Recognition 1	Recognition 2		SRT 1	SRT 2	Recognition 1	Recognition 2	
			List / SL	%	List / SL	%			List / SL	%	List / SL	%
EM Level in Opp. Ear										

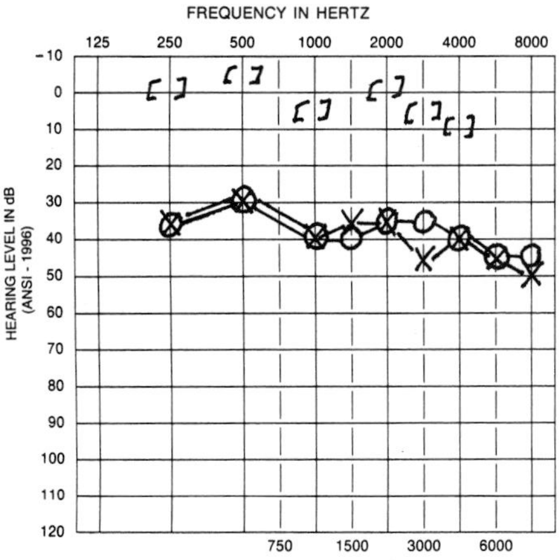

COMMENTS

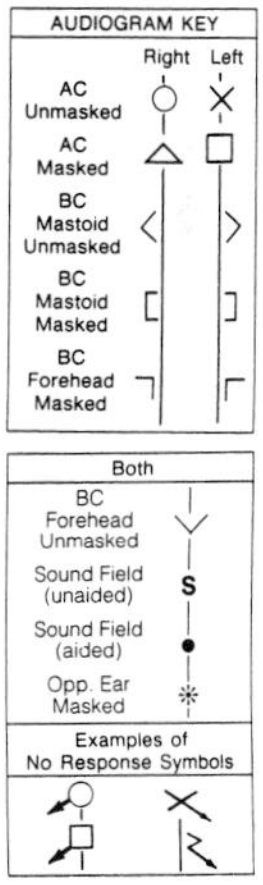

AUDIOGRAM KEY

	Right	Left
AC Unmasked	○	×
AC Masked	△	□
BC Mastoid Unmasked	<	>
BC Mastoid Masked	[	]
BC Forehead Masked	¬	⌐

	Both
BC Forehead Unmasked	∨
Sound Field (unaided)	S
Sound Field (aided)	●
Opp. Ear Masked	✳

Examples of No Response Symbols

FIGURE 4.14 Audiogram illustrating a conductive hearing loss in both ears. The three-frequency pure-tone averages are 35 dB HL in each ear. Bone-conduction thresholds were obtained from the forehead, first without masking and then with masking, and average 0 dB HL. Masking was required for all frequencies for bone conduction due to the air-bone gaps, and did not alter the original (unmasked) results. There are air-bone gaps of about 35 dB (conductive component) in both ears. An asterisk is used to denote that nontest-ear masking was used. Bone-conduction results obtained from the forehead with the left ear masked are assumed to come from the right cochlea, and bone-conduction results obtained from the forehead with the left ear masked are assumed to come from the right cochlea. No lateralization is seen on the Weber test at any frequency.

SPEECH AND HEARING CENTER
The University of Texas at Austin 78712
AUDIOMETRIC EXAMINATION

NAME: Last - First - Middle	SEX	AGE	DATE	EXAMINER	RELIABILITY	AUDIOMETER

AIR CONDUCTION

MASKING TYPE	RIGHT									LEFT								
	250	500	1000	1500	2000	3000	4000	6000	8000	250	500	1000	1500	2000	3000	4000	6000	8000
	25	30	35/35	40	40	50	55	65	65	20	25	30/30	40	50	60	65	65	70
EM Level in Opp. Ear																		

BONE CONDUCTION

MASKING TYPE	RIGHT						FOREHEAD						LEFT					
	250	500	1000	2000	3000	4000	250	500	1000	2000	3000	4000	250	500	1000	2000	3000	4000
							25	30	30	40	55	55						
EM Level in Opp. Ear																		

	2 Frequency	3 Frequency	WEBER						2 Frequency	3 Frequency
Pure Tone Average	33	35	M	M	M	M	M	M	Pure Tone Average 28	35

SPEECH AUDIOMETRY

MASKING TYPE	RIGHT					LEFT				
	SRT 1	SRT 2	Recognition 1 List/SL %	Recognition 2 List/SL %		SRT 1	SRT 2	Recognition 1 List/SL %	Recognition 2 List/SL %	
EM Level in Opp. Ear										

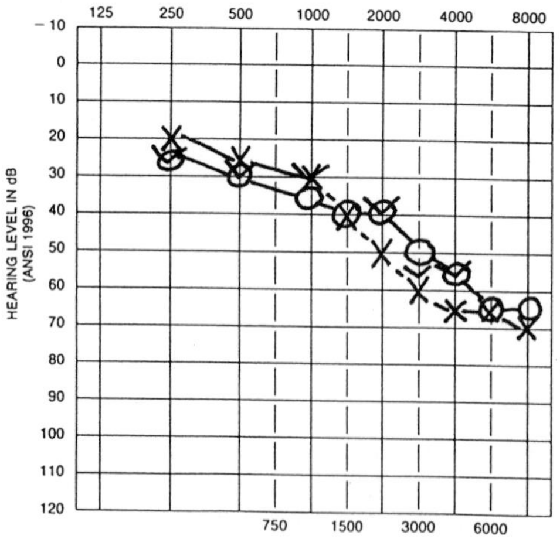

FREQUENCY IN HERTZ

COMMENTS

AUDIOGRAM KEY

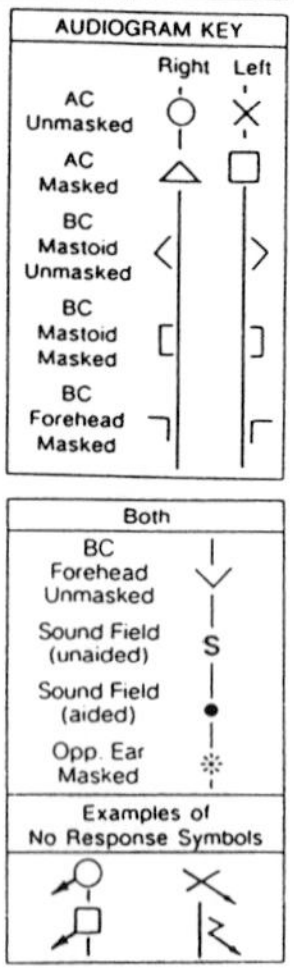

FIGURE 4.15 **Audiogram illustrating sensorineural hearing loss in both ears. The air-conduction thresholds average 35 dB HL and the bone-conduction thresholds (obtained from the forehead) about the same (33 dB HL). The lack of air-bone gaps indicates that masking is not needed for bone conduction. Tones are heard in the midline at all frequencies on the Weber test.**

SPEECH AND HEARING CENTER
The University of Texas at Austin 78712
AUDIOMETRIC EXAMINATION

NAME: Last - First - Middle	SEX	AGE	DATE	EXAMINER	RELIABILITY	AUDIOMETER

AIR CONDUCTION

MASKING TYPE	RIGHT									LEFT								
	250	500	1000	1500	2000	3000	4000	6000	8000	250	500	1000	1500	2000	3000	4000	6000	8000
	55	65	60/60	60	55	65	70	75	80	60	60	60/60	65	60	70	80	80	75
EM Level in Opp. Ear																		

BONE CONDUCTION

MASKING TYPE	RIGHT						FOREHEAD						LEFT					
	250	500	1000	2000	3000	4000	250	500	1000	2000	3000	4000	250	500	1000	2000	3000	4000
NB	25	35	35	35	40	45	25	35	35	35	40	45	25	35	35	35	40	45
EM Level in Opp. Ear	60	60	60	60	70	80							55	65	60	55	65	70

	2 Frequency	3 Frequency	WEBER							2 Frequency	3 Frequency
Pure Tone Average	58	60	M	M	M	M	M	M	Pure Tone Average	60	60

SPEECH AUDIOMETRY

MASKING TYPE	RIGHT				LEFT			
	SRT 1	SRT 2	Recognition 1	Recognition 2	SRT 1	SRT 2	Recognition 1	Recognition 2
			List / SL / %	List / SL / %			List / SL / %	List / SL / %
EM Level in Opp. Ear								

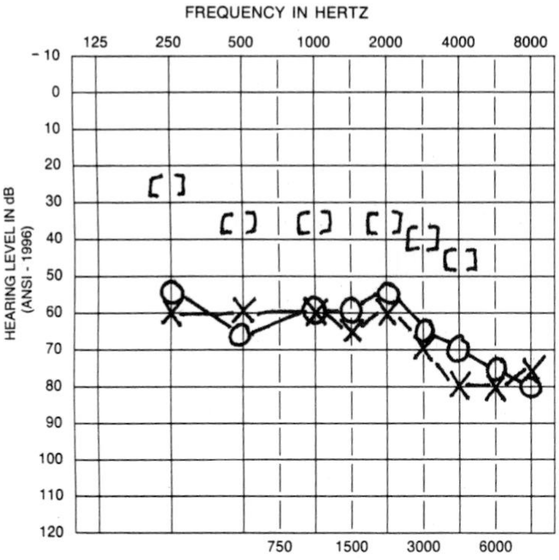

COMMENTS

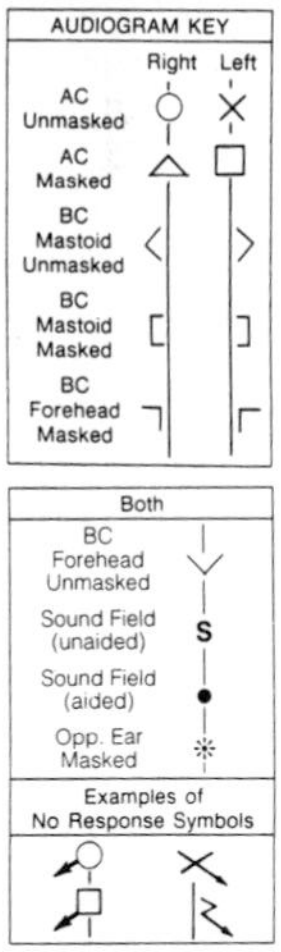

FIGURE 4.16 Audiogram illustrating a mixed hearing loss in both ears. The air-conduction thresholds average about 60 dB HL (total hearing loss), whereas the bone-conduction thresholds average 35 dB HL (sensorineural component). Masking was required for all frequencies for bone conduction due to the air-bone gaps. There is an air-bone gap of about 25 dB (conductive component). Tones on the Weber test do not lateralize.

been misdiagnosed as mixed losses in such cases. To avoid this problem, Frank and Crandell (1986) recommended that bone conduction be carried out a second time when an air-bone gap (greater than 10 dB) is observed at 3000 Hz and above. This second test is performed with an earplug in the external auditory canal to limit the effects of acoustic radiation. This is a safe thing to do in most cases since the occlusion effect is not present in the high frequencies.

Interpretation of the air-bone relationships can be stated as a formula that reads as follows: The air-conduction (AC) threshold is equal to the bone-conduction (BC) threshold plus the air-bone gap (ABG). With this formula, the four audiometric examples just cited would read

Formula: AC = BC + ABG
Figure 4.11:   5 = 5 + 0 (normal)
Figure 4.14:   35 = 0 + 35 (conductive loss)
Figure 4.15:   35 = 35 + 0 (sensorineural loss)
Figure 4.16:   60 = 35 + 25 (mixed loss)

Air-bone Relationships

Figure 2.2 suggests that (1) hearing by bone conduction is the same as by air conduction in those with normal hearing and in those with sensorineural impairment (no air-bone gap), (2) hearing by air conduction is poorer than by bone conduction in patients with conductive or mixed hearing losses (some air-bone gap), but (3) hearing by bone conduction poorer than by air conduction should not occur because both routes ultimately measure the integrity of the sensorineural structures. It has been shown that although assumptions 1 and 2 are correct, 3 may be false. There are several reasons why bone-conduction thresholds may be slightly poorer than air-conduction thresholds, even when properly calibrated audiometers are used. Some of these arise out of changes in the inertial and osseotympanic bone-conduction modes produced by abnormal conditions of the ears. In addition, Studebaker (1967b) has illustrated that slight variations are bound to occur based purely on normal statistical variability. Slight differences between air- and bone-conduction thresholds are to be anticipated (Barry, 1994) and are built into the most recent ANSI (1992) standard for bone conduction. Because no diagnostic significance is usually attached to air-conduction results being better than those obtained by bone conduction, the insecure clinician may be tempted to alter the bone-conduction results to conform to the usual expectations. Such temptations should be resisted because (in addition to any ethical reasons) they simply propagate the myth that air conduction can never be better than bone conduction.

Tactile Responses to Pure-tone Stimuli

At times, when severe losses of hearing occur, it is not possible to know for certain whether responses obtained at the upper limits of the audiometer are auditory or **tactile.** Nober (1970) has shown that some patients feel the vibrations of the bone-conduction vibrator and respond when intense tones are introduced, causing the examiner to believe the patient has heard them. In such cases a severe sensorineural hearing loss may appear on the audiogram to be a mixed hearing loss, possibly resulting in unjustified surgery in an attempt to alleviate the conductive component. Martin and Wittich (1966) found that some children with severe hearing impairments often could not differentiate tactile from auditory sensations. Nober found that it is possible for patients to respond to tactile stimuli to both air- and bone-conducted tones, primarily in the low frequencies, when the levels are near the maximum outputs of the audiometer. When audiograms show severe mixed hearing losses, the validity of the test should be questioned.

Since a severe mixed hearing loss may only *appear* to be the result of tactile stimulation, Dean and Martin (1997) describe a procedure for ascertaining whether this is the case. It is based on the fact that auditory thresholds are higher on the forehead, but tactile thresholds are lower on the forehead for the low frequencies. The procedure works as follows (assuming that original bone-conduction results were obtained from the forehead): Move the vibrator to the mastoid and retest at 500 Hz. If the threshold gets lower (better), the original response was auditory. If the threshold gets higher, the original response was tactile.

If the mastoid was the original test position and tactile response is suspected, move the vibrator to the forehead and retest at 500 Hz. If the threshold gets lower, the original response was tactile. If the threshold gets higher, the original response was auditory.

Cross-hearing in Air- and Bone-conduction Audiometry

It is logical to assume that if hearing sensitivity is considerably better in one ear than in the other (say 50 dB), it is possible that before the threshold of the poorer ear is reached, the intensity of the signal may be great enough for the sound to escape from beneath the air-conduction earphone into the room and be heard by the better ear. These audiograms have been called "shadow-grams." Sounds introduced by air conduction actually cross from one side of the head to the other, primarily by bone conduction (Chaiklin, 1967; Martin & Blosser, 1970). It is probable that whenever the intensity is raised to a high enough level, the air-conduction receiver vibrates sufficiently to cause deformations of the skull, giving rise to bone-conducted stimulation. If the level of a tone thus generated is above the bone-conduction threshold of the nontest ear during air-conduction audiometry, the patient will respond, signaling that the tone has been heard before the auditory threshold of the test ear has been reached.

As sounds travel from one side of the head to the other, a certain amount of energy is lost in transmission. This loss of intensity of a sound introduced to one ear and heard by the other is called **interaural attenuation (IA).** Interaural attenuation for air conduction varies with frequency and from one individual to another. Results of four studies of interaural attenuation using two different kinds of earphones are shown in Table 4.3.

TABLE 4.3   Interaural Attenuation for Pure Tones According to (A) Coles and Priede (1968), (B) Zwislocki (1950), (C) Sklare and Denenberg (1987)

Frequency in Hz	250	500	1000	2000	4000
Interaural attenuation in dB (A) (Supra-aural earphones)	61	63	63	63	68
Interaural attenuation in dB (B) (Supra-aural earphones)	45	50	55	60	65
Interaural attenuation in dB (C) (Insert earphones)	89+	94+	81	71	77

The danger of **cross-hearing** for air-conducted tones presents itself whenever the level of the tone in the test ear (TE) by air conduction, minus the interaural attenuation, is equal to or higher than the bone-conduction threshold of the nontest ear (NTE). Stated as a formula,

$$AC_{TE} - IA \geq BC_{NTE}$$

Since it is not possible to know in advance the interaural attenuation of a given patient, it is advisable to adopt a conservative approach and consider 40 dB as the minimum possible value when using supra-aural audiometer earphones.

Because there is rarely a way of knowing for certain which cochlea has been stimulated by a bone-conducted tone, regardless of where the vibrator is placed, cross-hearing during bone-conduction tests is always a possibility. Therefore, the minimum IA for bone conduction should, for clinical purposes, be considered to be 0 dB. There are many approaches to the problem of cross-hearing, only one of which is discussed in this book.

From a practical clinical viewpoint, it seems important to ask, "Does it matter which ear has responded during pure-tone audiometry?" In the case of air conduction, the answer is an emphatic "yes," for one must know for certain the hearing sensitivity of each ear. In the case of bone conduction, as illustrated in Figures 4.14 and 4.16, the answer is also yes because the bone-conducted thresholds of each ear tell the amount of conductive involvement (by comparing them to air conduction) and the amount of sensorineural involvement (by comparing them to 0 dB HL). If a bone-conduction response is obtained from the nontest ear, a completely incorrect diagnosis of the test ear may result. In the case of Figure 4.15, however, it really does not matter which ear has responded to the bone-conduction signal because both ears show an absent air-bone gap, resulting in a diagnosis of bilateral sensorineural hearing loss. Therefore, cross-hearing in bone-conduction testing is of concern only when there is an air-bone gap in the test ear. Because there is a certain amount of normal variability between air- and bone-conduction thresholds, even among patients without conductive hearing losses, bone conduction often appears to be slightly better (or poorer) than air conduction. It seems practical, therefore, to consider an air-bone gap of 5 or 10 dB to be insignificant. Thus, cross-hearing for bone conduction should be suspected whenever an air-bone gap greater than 10 dB is seen in the *test ear:*

$$ABG_{TE} > 10 \text{ dB}$$

Masking

Whenever cross-hearing is suspected, it is necessary to remove the nontest ear from the test procedure to determine (1) if the original responses were obtained through the nontest ear and (2) if they were, what the true threshold of the test ear really is. The only way to do this is to deliver a noise to the nontest ear to remove it from the test procedure by **masking.**

The alert audiologist will probably suspect the possibility of cross-hearing more often than it actually occurs. This is good, for it is better to mask unnecessarily than to fail to mask when a signal has been heard in the nontest ear. In clinical audiology the rule should be "When in doubt, mask."

The relative effectiveness of a masking noise on a pure tone is determined by several variables, including the spectrum of the noise, how the masking-level dial is calibrated (i.e., its decibel reference and the linearity of the attenuator), and the kind of earphone used to deliver the noise to the masked ear. When these variables are understood and controlled, the task of masking becomes considerably easier.

Noises Used in Pure-tone Masking

Several different kinds of masking noises are available on commercial pure-tone audiometers. Each noise has a characteristic spectrum and therefore provides a different degree of masking efficiency at different frequencies.

It is possible to generate a noise that has approximately equal energy per cycle and covers a relatively broad range of frequencies. Because of this analogy to white light, which contains all the frequencies in the light spectrum, this noise has been called **white noise.** White noise, which has also been called thermal and gaussian[1] noise, sounds very much like hissing. Since the earphones accompanying many audiometers are not of very high quality, they do not provide much response in the higher frequencies and therefore limit the intensity of white noise above about 6000 Hz. Hence, that which is labeled on the audiometer as white noise is more accurately termed *broadband* or *wideband* noise, as it emanates from the earphone.

Because it has been proven that the masking of a pure tone is most efficiently accomplished by frequencies immediately surrounding that tone, the additional frequencies used in a broadband noise are redundant. They supply additional sound pressure and loudness to the patient, with no increase in masking effectiveness. Through the use of band-pass analog filters it is possible to shape the spectrum of a broadband noise into **narrowband noise.** Modern digital technology now allows the generation of a digital noise that can be of any desired bandwidth and contain only the desired frequencies.

Surrounding every pure tone is a **critical band** of frequencies that provides **maximum masking** with minimum sound pressure. Narrowing the noise band to less than the critical bandwidth requires greater intensity for masking a given level of tone. Conversely, adding frequencies outside the critical band increases intensity (and therefore loudness) without increasing masking. Probably because of the expense of manufacture, the narrow noise bands found in most audiometers are usually considerably wider than the critical band.

The earphones usually employed to deliver a masking noise during clinical pure-tone testing are the ones provided with the audiometer, the TDH-39, TDH-49, or TDH-50P earphones, with MX-41/AR (supra-aural) cushions. There are many reasons to prefer the use of insert earphones, which decrease the occlusion effect evident in bone conduction when an ear is covered and have an advantage in masking during bone-conduction testing. In addition, because they are coupled to a smaller area of the skull, insert receivers provide 70 to 100 dB of interaural attenuation. When the foam rubber surrounding the tubing at the end of an insert receiver is inserted deeply into the external ear, an additional 15 to 20 dB of interaural attenuation can be achieved (Killion, Wilber, & Gugmundsen, 1985).

Calibration of Pure-tone Masking Noises

Calibration of the masking noise of an audiometer requires that the linearity of the masking-level dial be accurate and that the intensity reference be known. Linearity calibration is best accomplished through the use of a device called an **electronic voltmeter,** which measures differences in decibels.

---

[1]For Karl F. Gauss, 1777–1855, German mathematician and physicist.

By making measurements at the terminals of the earphones, the hearing-level dial can be moved in steps of 5 dB, and the accuracy of this 5 dB change can be checked throughout the entire range of the attenuator (–10 to 110 dB HL).

Some audiologists prefer that the decibel reference for masking be in sound-pressure level or hearing level. However, the concept of **effective masking (EM)** has become increasingly popular. Effective masking may be defined as the amount of threshold shift provided by a given level of noise. Thus, 20 dB EM at 1000 Hz is just enough noise to make a 20 dB HL 1000 Hz tone inaudible; 50 dB EM would just mask out a 50 dB tone, and so on. In the presence of 50 dB EM, a tone will not become audible until 55 dB HL, regardless of an individual's hearing loss (if it is less than 55 dB). This is true because any hearing loss attenuates both the tone and the masking noise equally.

The calibration of a noise in units of effective masking may be carried out electroacoustically on an artificial ear, if the concept of the critical band is thoroughly understood. In many clinics this calibration is carried out psychoacoustically. Using about a dozen normal-hearing subjects, calibration for effective masking may be accomplished as follows:

1. Present a tone to one ear by air conduction at 1000 Hz at 30 dB HL. Interrupt to prevent auditory fatigue.
2. Present a noise (preferably narrowband) to the same ear.
3. Raise the level of the noise in 5 dB steps until the 30 dB tone is no longer audible. The tone should be heard at 35 dB HL. Recheck several times for accuracy.
4. Take a median value of the masking-level dial setting at which the 30 dB HL tone was masked. This is 30 dB EM; 5 to 10 dB should be added as a safety factor.
5. Post a correction chart showing the number of decibels that must be added to 0 dB HL to reach 0 dB EM.
6. Repeat this procedure for all audiometric frequencies.

Once calibration has been completed, any level at any frequency can be masked out (in the same ear) up to the maximum masking limits of the audiometer simply by introducing a level of effective masking equal to the level of the tone to be masked. If, for example, a +25 dB correction is needed for 0 dB EM and a 40 dB tone is to be masked, the masking-level dial would be set to 40 dB EM, which is actually 65 dB HL (40 dB for the tone to be masked + 25 dB correction). Using this method builds the correction factor into the calibration and it should not be added again when determining the need for individual masking levels.

Central Masking

It has been shown (Wegel & Lane, 1924) that a small shift is seen in the threshold of a pure tone when a masking noise is introduced to the opposite ear. This threshold shift increases with increased noise but averages about 5 dB. It is believed that the elevation of threshold is produced by inhibition that is sent down from the auditory centers in the brain and has, therefore, been called **central masking.** Central masking must be differentiated from **overmasking (OM),** in which the noise is actually so intense in the masked ear that it crosses the skull and produces masking in the test ear.

Masking Methods for Air Conduction

Masking must be undertaken whenever the possibility of cross-hearing exists. A survey of clinical audiologists on contemporary clinical practices (Martin et al., 1998) showed more disagreement on masking methods, and apparently greater insecurity than on any other clinical procedure.

The "Shotgun" Approach

It is possible, in a large number of cases, for clinicians to mask by using some fixed or arbitrary level of noise in the masked ear, without really understanding what they are doing. In uncomplicated cases the procedure often appears to be satisfactory. Because of insufficient feedback about their errors, some individuals fail to profit by their mistakes and continue with such erroneous philosophies as "Just use 70 dB of noise," with no recognition of the properties of the noise or of its effectiveness. Clinicians may be unaware of when they have used too little or too much masking noise. This ignorance is abetted by those audiometer manufacturers whose masking-level dials are nonlinear and whose noise spectra are irregular, inadvertently relegating the masking procedure to a relatively unimportant one.

The Minimum-noise Method

Through calibration, it is possible to determine the minimum amount of noise necessary to mask a pure tone at a given intensity. There is no need to burden the patient with any more noise than is necessary to get the job done. The best way to do this is to regard the noise level in terms of decibels of effective masking.

Several methods have been developed using formulas for the determination of the minimum and maximum amounts of effective masking to be used (Liden, Nilsson, & Anderson, 1959; Studebaker, 1964). Although these formulas are accurate, they are time-consuming and not always practical for clinical use (Studebaker, 1967a). Martin (1974) has shown that the different formula approaches yield the same noise sound-pressure levels as does a simple, direct approach, requiring almost no calculation. This book describes one method that does not require much computation and that can be applied rapidly.

When test results suggest the possibility of cross-hearing, they should be examined closely. Consider the example in Figure 4.17. The criteria for masking are met for the left ear by air conduction since the threshold (60 dB HL) minus minimal IA (40 dB) is greater than the bone-conduction threshold of the right ear (10 dB HL). It is known, since the test was presumably performed carefully, that the 60 dB response was a threshold. However, the question that arises is "The threshold of which ear?" If the right (nontest) ear can be removed from the test by masking, and the threshold of the left (test) ear remains unchanged, this means that the original response was obtained through the test ear. If, however, eliminating the right ear from the test results in a failure of response at the left ear at the previous level (plus 5 dB for central masking), the right ear provided the hearing for the original response and further masking is required to determine the true threshold of the left ear.

The minimum amount of noise required for the screening described is an effective masking level equal to the AC threshold of the nontest ear, and may be referred to as **initial masking (IM).**

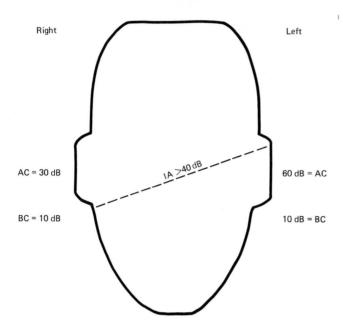

FIGURE 4.17   Illustration of the need to mask during air-conduction tests. Because the difference between the left-ear air conduction (60 dB HL) and the right ear bone conduction (10 db HL) exceeds the minimum possible interaural attenuation (40 dB), cross-hearing is a possibility. Note that the minimum interaural attenuation for this patient must be 50 dB (AC left minus BC right). Masking needed for the right ear is 30 dB EM.

This is just enough noise to shift the threshold of that ear 5 dB, by both air conduction and bone conduction. If the threshold of the tone presented to the test ear was originally heard by bone conduction in the nontest ear, raising the bone-conduction threshold of the nontest ear with masking will eliminate the possibility of this response.

Maximum Masking

Just as the test tone can lateralize from test ear to nontest ear, given sufficient intensity, so can the masking noise lateralize from masked ear to test ear, both by bone conduction. An individual's interaural attenuation cannot be less than the difference between the air-conduction level in the test ear and the bone-conduction level in the nontest ear at which threshold responses are obtained. For example, even though Figure 4.17 does not illustrate cross-hearing *per se,* but rather the danger of cross-hearing, the interaural attenuation for the individual illustrated cannot be less than 50 dB for the test frequency (air conduction of the test ear minus bone conduction of the nontest ear).

Whenever the level of effective masking presented to the masked ear, minus the patient's interaural attenuation, is above the bone-conduction threshold of the test ear, a sufficient amount of noise is delivered to the cochlea of the test ear to elevate its threshold. This is overmasking (Figure 4.18). The equation for overmasking for pure tones is

$$EM_{NTE} \geq BC_{TE} + IA$$

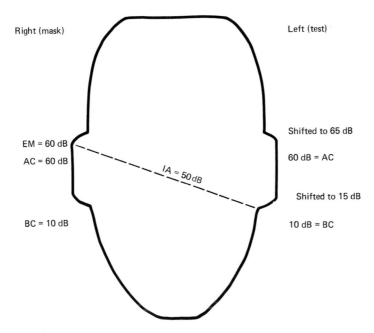

Right (mask)

Left (test)

Shifted to 65 dB

EM = 60 dB

AC = 60 dB

60 dB = AC

IA = 50 dB

Shifted to 15 dB

BC = 10 dB

10 dB = BC

FIGURE 4.18 **Example of overmasking. The effective masking level in the right ear (60 dB) is decreased by the interaural attenuation (50 dB) so that 10 dB EM is received by bone-conduction in the left ear. This shifts the bone-conduction threshold to 15 dB, plus any additional shift for central masking. Adding more noise to the right ear results in increased masking at the left ear, with further threshold shifts. In this case the minimum amount of noise required to mask out the right ear produces overmasking.**

Maximum masking is equal to the threshold of the test ear by bone conduction plus the interaural attenuation, minus 5 dB. When ears with large air-bone gaps are tested, minimum masking quickly becomes overmasking, sometimes making determination of masked pure-tone thresholds difficult. In such cases audiologists must recognize the problem and rely on other tests and observations to make their diagnoses.

The Plateau Method

Hood (1960) reported on a masking method that enjoys a great deal of popularity. When a tone seems to be heard through the nontest ear, a noise is delivered to that ear and the level of noise is increased in 5 dB steps until the tone is no longer audible. Then the threshold for the tone is measured again in the presence of the contralateral noise. The noise level is increased 5 dB, and the threshold is measured again. This often results in necessary increases in the tone level of 5 dB for every 5 dB increase in noise in order to keep the tone audible. The assumption is that the threshold of the tone in the test ear has not been reached and that both tone and noise are heard by the nontest ear (Figure 4.19A). When the threshold of the tone for the test ear has been reached (Figure 4.19B), the level of noise can be increased several times without affecting the level of tone that evokes a response. This is the **plateau.** If the noise level is raised beyond a certain point (the bone-conduction threshold of the test

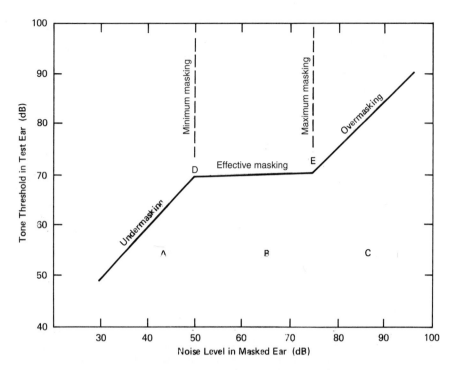

FIGURE 4.19   The plateau method for masking. (A) Undermasking: The tone (by cross-hearing) continues to be heard in the masked ear despite the noise since the tone level is below the threshold of the test ear. (B) The plateau: The tone has reached the threshold of the test ear. Therefore, raising the masking level in the masked ear does not shift the threshold of the tone. (C) Overmasking: The masking level is so intense that it crosses to the test ear, resulting in continuous shifts in the threshold of the tone with increases in the masking noise. Minimum (D) and maximum (E) masking are found at either side of the plateau.

ear plus the interaural attenuation), overmasking takes place and the tone and noise are mixed in the test ear. Further increases in noise will result in further shifts in the threshold of the tone (Figure 4.19C). Minimum and maximum masking are shown in Figure 4.19 D and E.

The plateau method is often used by introducing a masking noise at some low level, or some arbitrary beginning point. It is best combined with the minimum masking method, beginning with the initial masking level (the air-conduction threshold of the masked ear). Problems of overmasking plague all the masking methods, including the plateau system, whenever there are large air-bone gaps in both ears. The larger the air-bone gap, the narrower the plateau; the smaller the air-bone gap, the broader the plateau.

The width of the masking plateau is determined by three variables: (1) the air-conduction threshold of the nontest (masked) ear, (2) the bone-conduction threshold of the test ear, and (3) the patient's interaural attenuation. The higher the air-conduction threshold of the masked ear, the greater must be the initial masking level; the higher that level is, the greater are the chances that the noise will cross to the test ear. The lower the bone-conduction threshold of the test ear, the greater the likelihood that a noise reaching the cochlea of that ear from a masking receiver on the opposite ear will exceed its threshold, producing a threshold shift in the test ear. The smaller the interaural attenuation, the higher the level of the noise that reaches the test ear. By increasing interaural attenuation, insert receivers decrease the chances of overmasking and widen the masking plateau. These concepts are summarized in Table 4.4.

Masking Methods for Bone Conduction

Masking methods for bone conduction are very much the same as for air conduction, and their success depends on the training, interests, and motivation of the clinician. One problem in masking for bone conduction that does not arise for air conduction is the method of delivery of the masking noise. The matter is simple during air-conduction audiometry, as both ears have earphones already positioned, and one phone can deliver the tone while the other phone delivers the masking noise. Because both ears are uncovered during bone-conduction testing, an earphone must be placed over the nontest ear without covering the test ear. The test ear must not be covered because this may cause an occlusion effect and alter the zero reference for bone conduction. Figure 4.20 shows the proper positioning of supra-aural receivers and insert receivers for masking during bone conduction, with the vibrator on the mastoid and also on the forehead.

When an earphone is placed over the nontest ear, an occlusion effect may be created in that ear. This means that the intensity of the tone in the low frequencies is actually increased in the nontest ear, increasing the likelihood that the nontest ear will respond to the tone. Of course, if the masked ear has a conductive hearing loss, no additional occlusion effect is evidenced, but it is not always possible to know whether there is a conductive loss in the masked ear. After all, if we knew the conditions of the auditory pathway before testing, the tests themselves would be unnecessary.

Because the masking earphone may make the bone-conducted tone appear louder in the masked ear, the initial effective masking level must be increased by the amount of the occlusion effect. Failure to do this will result in **undermasking** in a significant number of cases. The initial effective level for bone-conduction masking is the air-conduction threshold of the tone in the masked ear, plus the occlusion effect (OE) for the tested frequency. Initial masking for bone conduction can be expressed as

$$EM = AC_{NTE} + OE$$

This increased amount of noise raises the chance of overmasking. In many cases it is advantageous to use insert receivers to deliver the masking noise because less noise needs to be delivered

TABLE 4.4 Factors That Influence the Width of the Masking Plateau

	Narrow Plateau	Wide Plateau
AC threshold of masked ear	High	Low
BC threshold of test ear	Low	High
Interaural attenuation	Smaller	Larger

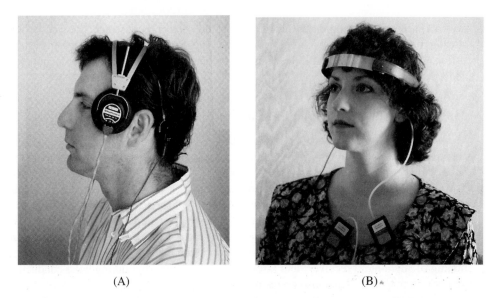

(A)   (B)

FIGURE 4.20   Masking noise delivered to the nontest ear during bone-conduction audiometry performed from (A) the mastoid, using a supra-aural earphone, and (B) the forehead, using an insert earphone.

to offset the smaller occlusion effect. The increased interaural attenuation provided by these small phones further decreases the probability of overmasking.

Martin, Butler, and Burns (1974) suggest a method by which the occlusion effect of the patient's masked ear may be determined and added to the initial masking level for air conduction. The procedure takes only moments and requires, after the need to mask for bone conduction has been determined, an audiometric version of the Bing test. After the patient's unoccluded bone-conduction thresholds have been measured, the masking receiver is placed over the ear to be masked (no noise is presented). With the nontest ear occluded, the thresholds at 250, 500, and 1000 Hz are redetermined. The occluded thresholds for each frequency are subtracted from the unoccluded thresholds. The difference is the patient's *own* occlusion effect. These differences should be added to the initial masking levels determined for air conduction. The bone-conduction vibrator may be placed either on the forehead or on the mastoid.

Use of the audiometric Bing test results in little or no additional masking for conductive losses, when higher noise levels present the danger of overmasking. When increased masking is required to offset the effect of having occluded the masked ear, the precise amount of noise may be added rather than some average figure that may be more or less masking than required for the individual patient.

The form shown in Figure 4.21 is useful for performing the audiometric Bing test. The results provide quantitative information about the amount of occlusion effect for each ear to be added to the initial effective masking level. In addition, the audiometric Bing test can be interpreted in the same way as the original tuning-fork test, to assist in the diagnosis of conductive versus sensorineural hearing loss.

Plotting Masked Results on the Audiogram

Before any threshold data are entered on the audiometric worksheet for either air conduction or bone conduction, 5 dB may be subtracted from the values obtained with the nontest ear masked to compensate for central masking. The appropriate symbols to indicate air conduction or bone conduction with and without masking are shown on the audiogram. The graph should contain only symbols that represent accurate thresholds; otherwise the audiogram will appear cluttered and misleading. The plotting of contralateral responses seems unnecessary, since they can readily be seen by examining the numerical insertions at the top of the audiometric worksheet.

Figure 4.22 illustrates a case of normal hearing in the right ear with a sensorineural hearing loss in the left ear. Note that the original test results suggested that the hearing loss in the left ear was conductive. The air-bone gap in the left ear was closed when proper masking was applied to the right ear.

The unmasked results shown in Figure 4.23 suggest a conductive loss in both ears, with poorer air conduction in the right ear. Using the criteria described earlier, masking was indicated for the right ear for air conduction and for both ears for bone conduction. Notice that the hearing loss in the left ear remains unchanged with masking, but the right ear actually has a severe mixed loss.

SPEECH AND HEARING CENTER
THE UNIVERSITY OF TEXAS AT AUSTIN 78712

Name: Last-First-Middle	Sex	Age	Examiner	Reliability	Date

	AUDIOMETRIC BING TEST				
	RIGHT			LEFT	
Frequency (Hertz)	250	500	1000	250	500	1000
1) Unoccluded						
2) Occluded						
3) Occlusion Effect (1-2)						

FIGURE 4.21   **Form for recording data obtained on the audiometric Bing test.**

SPEECH AND HEARING CENTER
The University of Texas at Austin 78712
AUDIOMETRIC EXAMINATION

NAME: Last - First - Middle	SEX	AGE	DATE	EXAMINER	RELIABILITY	AUDIOMETER

AIR CONDUCTION

MASKING TYPE	RIGHT									LEFT								
	250	500	1000	1500	2000	3000	4000	6000	8000	250	500	1000	1500	2000	3000	4000	6000	8000
NB	5	0	0/0	5	5	15	15	10	10	30	35	35/35	40	40	45	55	50	45
																55*		
EM Level in Opp. Ear																15		

BONE CONDUCTION

MASKING TYPE	RIGHT						FOREHEAD						LEFT					
	250	500	1000	2000	3000	4000	250	500	1000	2000	3000	4000	250	500	1000	2000	3000	4000
NB	5	0	5	5	15	10							5	5	5	10	15	10
													30*	35*	35*	40*	35*	55*
EM Level in Opp. Ear													60	50	35	35	40	55

	2 Frequency	3 Frequency	WEBER							2 Frequency	3 Frequency
Pure Tone Average	0	2	R	R	R	R	R	R	Pure Tone Average	35	37

SPEECH AUDIOMETRY

MASKING TYPE	RIGHT						LEFT					
	SRT 1	SRT 2	Recognition 1		Recognition 2		SRT 1	SRT 2	Recognition 1		Recognition 2	
			List / SL	%	List / SL	%			List / SL	%	List / SL	%
EM Level in Opp. Ear												

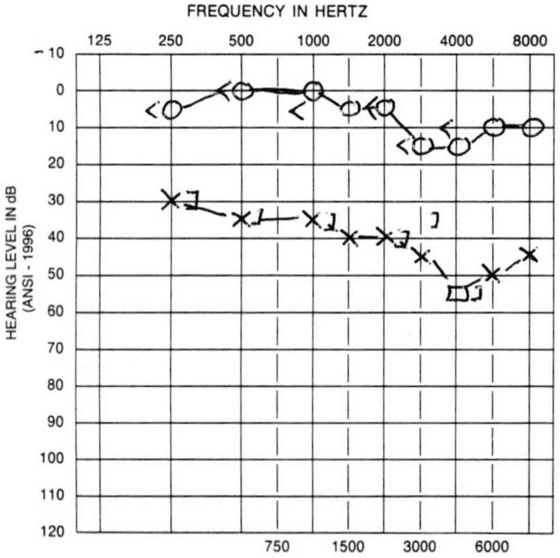

FREQUENCY IN HERTZ   COMMENTS   AUDIOGRAM KEY

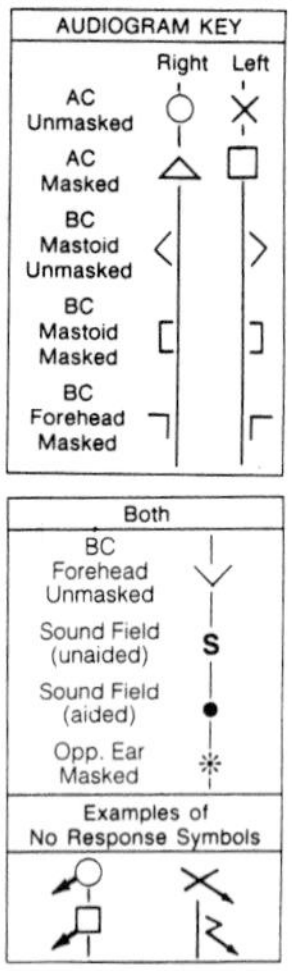

FIGURE 4.22   Audiogram showing normal hearing in the right ear and a sensorineural hearing loss in the left ear. The original (unmasked) results by air conduction and bone conduction suggested a conductive hearing loss in the left ear because of the air-bone gaps. When proper masking was administered to the right ear, the bone-conduction thresholds shifted, proving absence of any air-bone gaps in the left ear. Tones on the Weber test lateralize to the better-hearing right ear.

SPEECH AND HEARING CENTER
The University of Texas at Austin 78712
AUDIOMETRIC EXAMINATION

NAME: Last - First - Middle	SEX	AGE	DATE	EXAMINER	RELIABILITY	AUDIOMETER

AIR CONDUCTION

MASKING TYPE	RIGHT									LEFT								
	250	500	1000	1500	2000	3000	4000	6000	8000	250	500	1000	1500	2000	3000	4000	6000	8000
NB	50	55	45/50	50	55	65	70	70	75	45	40	45/45	45	45	50	60	60	70
	55	65	70	70	75	80	85	NR	NR									
EM Level in Opp. Ear	70	65	75	75	75	80	75	70	70									

BONE CONDUCTION

MASKING TYPE	RIGHT						FOREHEAD						LEFT					
	250	500	1000	2000	3000	4000	250	500	1000	2000	3000	4000	250	500	1000	2000	3000	4000
NB	25	35	40	45	45	50	5	0	10	15	10	20	5	0	10	15	10	20
EM Level in Opp. Ear	65	75	70	75	75	70							55	65	70	75	80	85

	2 Frequency	3 Frequency	WEBER							2 Frequency	3 Frequency
Pure Tone Average	68	70	<	<	<	<	<	<	Pure Tone Average	43	43

SPEECH AUDIOMETRY

MASKING TYPE	RIGHT								LEFT							
	SRT 1	SRT 2	Recognition 1		Recognition 2		SRT 1	SRT 2	Recognition 1		Recognition 2					
			List / SL	%	List / SL	%			List / SL	%	List / SL	%				
EM Level in Opp. Ear																

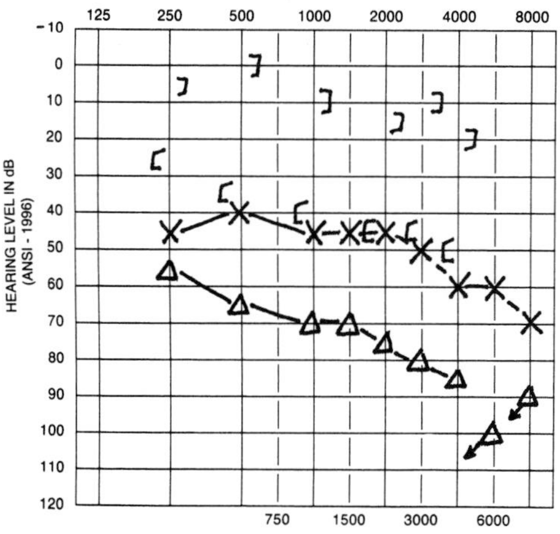

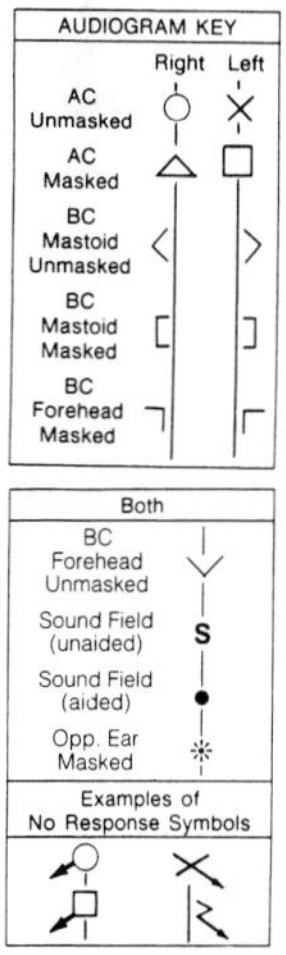

FIGURE 4.23 Audiogram showing a mixed hearing loss in the right ear and a conductive hearing loss in the left ear. Unmasked results showed conductive hearing losses in both ears. Masking was indicated for the right ear for air conduction, showing a slight threshold shift. Masking for bone conduction was indicated for both ears, resulting in a threshold shift for the right ear. The Weber test refers consistently to the left ear, which has the better sensorineural sensitivity. Note that no response is obtained in the right ear by air conduction at 6000 and 8000 Hz with masking in the left ear.

The Audiometric Weber Test

The Weber test, described in Chapter 2, can be performed by using the bone-conduction vibrator of an audiometer. The vibrator is placed on the midline of the skull, just as for forehead bone conduction, and the level of the tone is raised until it is above the patient's hearing threshold. Tones of different frequencies are then presented, and patients are asked to state whether they hear them in the left ear, in the right ear, or in the midline. Midline sensations are sometimes described as being heard in both ears or as unlateralized.

It is expected that when performing the Weber test, tones will be referred to the poorer hearing ear in a conductive loss, to the better ear in a sensorineural loss, and to the midline in symmetrical losses. It has been suggested that the **audiometric Weber test** be used to determine which ear to mask during bone-conduction testing. This notion is not encouraged here, as there are several reasons why the Weber may be misleading. Weber results help in the confirmation or denial of results obtained from standard pure-tone audiometry, and the probable results on this test are illustrated in all of the audiograms in this book.

Automatic Audiometry

Audiometers were devised that allowed patients to track their own auditory thresholds while they were automatically recorded in the form of a graph on a special form. Automatic audiometers that utilized an oscillator with a range from 100 to 10,000 Hz have been used. The tones were either automatically pulsed (200 msec on/200 msec off), or presented continuously. A special audiogram was placed on a movable stage on the audiometer, or on a fixed stage beneath a moving stylus. When the motor was engaged, the tone gradually increased in frequency while the intensity increased. The pen traced the precise frequency and hearing level emitted from an earphone as the stage or pen moved. When patients heard the tone they pressed a hand switch, which reversed the motor on the attenuator, causing the signal to get weaker. When the tone became inaudible, the hand switch was released and the tone was allowed to increase in intensity again. Frequency continued to increase whether the intensity was increasing or decreasing. This procedure was called **Békésy audiometry.**[2] Upon completion of the test, an audiogram had been drawn that represented the patients' thresholds over a continuous frequency range.

Although popular for a time, the use of automatic audiometry has faded from prominence, and it is now difficult to find a commercial version of one. Devices can be custom designed that allow for testing between the normal discrete audiometric frequencies, and this can be of value. Their use in industry, and as a test for auditory site of lesion, seems to have passed.

Computerized Audiometry

Computers may be programmed to control all aspects of administering pure-tone air- and bone-conduction stimuli, recognize the need for masking, determine the appropriate level of masking, reg-

---

[2]This test was suggested by Dr. Georg von Békésy, the Hungarian-born physicist (1899–1976), who won the Nobel Prize in 1961 for his contributions to the understanding of the human cochlea.

ulate the presentation of the masker to the nontest ear, analyze the subject's responses in terms of threshold-determination criteria, and present the obtained threshold values in an audiogram format at the conclusion of the test. **Computerized audiometry** may be performed on a device that is microprocessor-controlled, which allows it to be remotely operated by a computer. The audiometric data are "dumped" into a computer file for later retrieval. Stach (1988) states that computerized audiometry is used successfully to a greater extent for military, industrial, and educational applications than for individual diagnostic purposes. In the former cases the advantages lie, in part, in the rapid storage and retrieval of data that computers provide. In a pulse-count method the patient reports the number of tone pulses heard rather than the mere presence of the stimulus (Bragg & Collins, 1968). This method has been successful in minimizing the number of false positive responses that many patients give. This pulse-count method has been computerized (Meyer, Sutherland, & Grogan, 1975) and found to compare favorably with traditional manual audiometry (Sutherland, Danford, & Gasaway, 1976).

Despite its sophistication, the computer has not, nor is it likely to replace the clinical audiologist in the performance of pure-tone tests. The fact that computers can make step-by-step decisions in testing helps to prove that the majority of pure-tone tests can be carried out logically and scientifically.

Summary

For pure-tone hearing tests to be performed satisfactorily, control is needed over such factors as background noise levels, equipment calibration, patient understanding, and clinician expertise. The audiologist must be able to judge when responses are accurate, and to predict when a sound may have contralateralized to the ear not being tested. When cross-hearing occurs, proper masking procedures must be instituted to overcome this problem. Although at times the performance of pure-tone hearing tests is carried out as an art, it should, in most cases, be approached with a scientific attitude, using rigid controls.

STUDY QUESTIONS

1. Sketch an audiogram from memory. What is the proportional relationship between hearing level and the octave scale? Why?

2. Draw audiograms from memory illustrating normal hearing, conductive hearing loss, sensorineural hearing loss, and mixed hearing loss. What would the results for these hypothetical patients be on the tuning-fork tests described in Chapter 2?

3. Name the parts of a pure-tone audiometer.

4. How would you calibrate for air conduction and bone conduction, both with and without electro-acoustic equipment?

5. How would you calibrate for effective masking for pure tones?

6. Why does the occlusion effect change the initial masking levels you might use for bone conduction?

7. What are the advantages and disadvantages of insert receivers for air-conduction testing?

8. List the advantages and disadvantages of testing bone conduction from the forehead and the mastoid.

G L O S S A R Y

Air-bone gap (ABG) The amount by which the air-conduction threshold of a patient exceeds the bone-conduction threshold at any frequency in the same ear.

Audiogram A graphic representation of audiometric findings showing hearing levels as a function of frequency.

Audiometer (pure-tone) A device for determining the thresholds of hearing. Pure tones at various frequencies are generated, and their levels are increased and decreased until thresholds are found. Outputs may include earphones for air-conduction testing, a bone conduction vibrator for bone-conduction testing, and one or more loudspeakers for sound field testing.

Audiometric Weber test An extension of the tuning-fork Weber test. The bone-conduction vibrator of the audiometer is applied to the forehead of a patient, and tones are presented above threshold. The patient is directed to respond by stating whether the tone was heard in the right ear, the left ear, or the midline.

Békésy audiometry Automatic audiometry, wherein patients track their own auditory thresholds for pure tones by depressing a switch when the tone becomes audible and releasing it when the tone is inaudible. Results are traced on a special audiogram blank. This test is no longer popular.

Calibration The electroacoustic or psychoacoustic determination that an audiometer is performing properly in terms of its acoustic output, attenuator linearity, frequency accuracy, harmonic distortion, and so on.

Central masking The shift in the auditory threshold of a tone produced by a noise in the opposite ear when the level of the noise is not sufficient to cause peripheral masking by cross-conduction.

Computerized audiometry The process of testing human hearing sensitivity by having computers programmed to present the stimuli and interpret the threshold results.

Critical band A portion of a continuous band of noise surrounding a pure tone. When the sound-pressure level of this narrow band is the same as the sound-pressure level of the tone, the tone is barely perceptible.

Cross-hearing The reception of a sound signal during a hearing test (either by air conduction or bone conduction) at the ear opposite the ear under test.

Distortional bone conduction The response to a sound stimulus evoked when the skull is deformed by a bone-conduction vibrator, distorting the cochlea and giving rise to electrochemical activity within the cochlea.

Effective masking (EM) The minimum amount of noise required just to mask out a signal (under the same earphone) at a given hearing level. For example, 40 dB EM will just mask out a 40 dB HL signal.

Electronic voltmeter A device for measuring differences in decibels and voltages.

False negative response The failure of patients to respond during a hearing test when they have, in fact, heard the stimulus.

False positive response Response from a subject when no stimulus has been presented, or the stimulus is below threshold.

Inertial bone conduction Stimulation of the cochlea caused by lag of the chain of middle-ear bones, or inner-ear fluids, when the skull is deformed, resulting in movement of the stapes in and out of the oval window.

Initial masking (IM) The lowest level of effective masking presented to the nontest ear. For air-conduction tests, this level is equal to the threshold of the masked ear; for bone-conduction tests the IM is equal to the air-conduction threshold of the masked ear plus the occlusion effect at that frequency.

Interaural attenuation (IA) The loss of energy of a sound presented by either air conduction or bone conduction as it travels from the test ear to the non-test ear; the number of decibels lost in cross-hearing.

Masking The introduction of a noise into the nontest ear in an attempt to eliminate cross-hearing.

Maximum masking The highest level of noise that can be presented to one ear through an earphone before the noise crosses the skull and shifts the threshold of the opposite ear.

Narrowband noise A restricted band of frequencies surrounding a particular frequency to be masked; usually obtained by band-pass filtering a broadband noise.

Osseotympanic bone conduction The contribution to hearing by bone conduction created when the vibrating skull sets the air in the external ear canal into vibration, causing sound waves to pass down the canal, impinging on the eardrum membrane, and being conducted through the middle ear to the cochlea.

Overmasking (OM) Occurs when a masking noise presented to the nontest ear is of sufficient intensity to shift the threshold in the test ear beyond its true value. In overmasking, the masking noise crosses from the masked ear to the test ear by bone conduction.

Plateau The theoretical point in clinical masking at which the level of noise in the nontest ear may be raised or lowered about 15 dB without affecting the threshold of the signal in the test ear; the levels between undermasking and overmasking at which the true threshold of the test ear may be seen.

Pure-tone average (PTA) The average of the hearing levels at frequencies 500, 1000, and 2000 Hz for each ear, as obtained on a pure-tone hearing test. Sometimes the pure-tone average is computed by averaging the two lowest thresholds obtained at 500, 1000, and 2000 Hz.

Tactile responses The response obtained during bone-conduction (and occasionally air-conduction) audiometry to signals that have been felt, rather than heard by the patient.

Threshold In audiometry, the level at which a stimulus, such as a pure tone, is barely perceptible. Usual clinical criteria demand that the level be just high enough for the subject to be aware of the sound 50 percent of the times it is presented.

Undermasking Occurs when a masking noise presented to the nontest ear is of insufficient intensity to prevent the test signal from being heard in that ear.

White noise A broadband noise with approximately equal energy per cycle.

REFERENCES

American Academy of Ophthalmology and Otolaryngology Committee on Hearing and Equilibrium and the American Council of Otolaryngology Committee on the Medical Aspects of Noise (AAOO). (1979). Guide for the evaluation of hearing handicap. *Journal of the American Medical Association, 241,* 2055–2059.

American National Standards Institute (ANSI). (1992). *Standard reference zero for the calibration of pure-tone bone-conduction audiometers.* S3.43-1992. New York: Author.

———. (1996). *American National Standard specification for audiometers.* ANSI S3.6-1996. New York: Author.

American Speech-Language-Hearing Association (ASHA). (1978). Guidelines for manual pure-tone audiometry. *Asha, 20,* 297–301.

———. (1990). Guidelines for audiometric symbols. *Asha,* Supplement *32,* 25–30.

Barany, E. A. (1938). A contribution to the physiology of bone conduction. *Acta Otolaryngologica* (Stockholm), Supplement 26.

Barry, S. J. (1994). Can bone conduction thresholds really be poorer than air? *American Journal of Audiology, 3,* 21–22.

Békésy, G. v. (1947). A new audiometer. *Acta Otolaryngologica* (Stockholm), *35,* 411–422.

Bragg, V., & Collins, F. (1968, September). *Audiometer modification and pulse-tone technic for pure-tone threshold determination.* SAM-TR-68-91.

Carhart, R., & Jerger, J. F. (1959). Preferred method for clinical determination of pure-tone thresholds. *Journal of Speech and Hearing Disorders, 24,* 330–345.

Chaiklin, J. B. (1967). Interaural attenuation and cross-hearing in air-conduction audiometry. *Journal of Auditory Research, 7,* 413–424.

Clark, J. L., & Roeser, R. J. (1988). Three studies comparing performance of the ER-3A tube-phone with the TDH-50P earphone. *Ear and Hearing, 9,* 268–274.

Coles, R. R. A., & Priede, V. M. (1968). Clinical and subjective acoustics. *Institution of Sound and Vibration Research, 26,* Chapter 3A.

Dean, M. S., & Martin, F. N. (1997). Auditory and tactile bone-conduction thresholds. *Journal of the American Academy of Audiology, 8,* 227–232.

Elpern, B. S., & Naunton, R. F. (1963). The stability of the occlusion effect. *Archives of Otolaryngology, 77,* 376–382.

Fagelson, M., & Martin, F. N. (1994). Sound pressure in the external auditory canal during bone-conduction testing. *Journal of the American Academy of Audiology, 5,* 379–383.

Frank, T., & Crandell, C. C. (1986). Acoustic radiation produced by B-71, B-72, and KH-70 bone vibrators. *Ear and Hearing, 7,* 344–347.

Franks, J. R., Engel, D. P., & Themann, C. L. (1992). Real ear attenuation at threshold for three audiometric headphone devices: Implications for maximum permissible ambient noise level standards. *Ear and Hearing, 13,* 2–10.

Hood, J. D. (1960). The principles and practice of bone-conduction audiometry: A review of the present position. *Laryngoscope, 70,* 1211–1228.

Killion, M. C., Wilber, L. A., & Gugmundsen, G. I. (1985). Insert earphones for more interaural attenuation. *Hearing Instruments, 36,* 34–36.

Liden, G., Nilsson, G., & Anderson, H. (1959). Narrow band masking with white noise. *Acta Otolaryngologica* (Stockholm), *50,* 116–124.

Martin, F. N. (1974). Minimum effective masking levels in threshold audiometry. *Journal of Speech and Hearing Disorders, 39,* 280–285.

Martin, F. N., Champlin, C. A., & Chambers, J. A. (1998). Seventh survey of audiometric practices in the United States. *Journal of the American Academy of Audiology, 9,* 95–104.

Martin, F. N., & Blosser, D., (1970). Cross hearing—air conduction or bone conduction. *Psychonomic Science, 20,* 231.

Martin, F. N., Butler, E. C., & Burns, P. (1974). Audiometric Bing test for determination of minimum masking levels for bone-conduction tests. *Journal of Speech and Hearing Disorders, 39,* 148–152.

Martin, F. N., & Fagelson, M., (1995). Bone conduction reconsidered. *Tejas, 20,* 26–27.

Martin, F. N., & Wittich, W. W. (1966). A comparison of forehead and mastoid tactile bone conduction thresholds. *The Eye, Ear, Nose and Throat Monthly, 45,* 72–74.

Meyer, C. R., Sutherland, H. C., Jr., & Grogan, F. (1975, December). *The tone-count audiometric computer.* SAM-TR-75-50.

Nober, E. H. (1970). Cutile air and bone conduction thresholds of the deaf. *Exceptional Children, 36,* 571–579.

Reger, S. N. (1952). A clinical and research version of the Békésy audiometer. *Laryngoscope, 62,* 1333–1351.

Sataloff, J., Sataloff, R. T., & Vassallo, L. A. (1980). *Hearing loss* (2nd ed.). Philadelphia: Lippincott.

Sklare, D. A., & Denenberg, L. J. (1987). Interaural attenuation for Tubephone insert earphones. *Ear and Hearing, 8,* 298–300.

Stach, B. A. (1988). Computers and audiologic instrumentation. *Hearing Instruments, 39,* 13–16.

Stelmachowicz, P. G., Beauchaine, K. A., Kalberer, A., Kelly, W. J., & Jesteadt, W. (1989). High frequency audiometry: Test reliability & procedural considerations. *Journal of the Acoustical Society of America, 85,* 879–887.

Stewart, J. M., & Downs, M. P. (1984). Medical management of the hearing-handicapped child. In J. L. Northern (Ed.), *Hearing disorders* (2nd ed., pp. 267–278). Boston: Little, Brown.

Studebaker, G. A. (1962). Placement of vibrator in bone conduction testing. *Journal of Speech and Hearing Research, 5,* 321–331.

———. (1964). Clinical masking of air-and-bone conducted stimuli. *Journal of Speech and Hearing Disorders, 29,* 23–35.

———. (1967a). Clinical masking of the nontest ear. *Journal of Speech and Hearing Disorders, 32,* 360–371.

———. (1967b). Intertest variability and the air bone gap. *Journal of Speech and Hearing Disorders, 32,* 82–86.

Sutherland, H. C., Jr., Danford, R., Jr., & Gasaway, D. C. (1976, December). *Comparison of TCAS and manual audiometry.* SAM-TR-77-8.

Wegel, R. L., & Lane, G. I. (1924). The auditory masking of one pure tone by another and its probable relation to the dynamics of the inner ear. *Physiological Review, 23,* 266–285.

Zwislocki, J. (1953). Acoustic attenuation between ears. *Journal of the Acoustical Society of America, 25,* 752–759.

SUGGESTED READINGS

Dirks, D. D. (1994). Bone-conduction threshold testing. In J. Katz (Ed.), *Handbook of clinical audiology* (4th ed., pp. 132–146). Baltimore: Williams & Wilkins.

Yantis, P. A. (1994). Puretone air-conduction threshold testing. In J. Katz (Ed.), *Handbook of clinical audiology* (4th ed., pp. 97–108). Baltimore: Williams & Wilkins.

REVIEW TABLE 4.1 **Summary of Pure-tone Hearing Tests**

Test	Air Conduction (AC)	Bone Conduction (BC)
Purpose	Hearing sensitivity for pure tones	Sensorineural sensitivity for pure tones
When to mask	When difference between AC (test ear) and BC (nontest ear) exceeds minimal IA*	When there is an air-bone gap greater than 10 dB in the test ear
How to mask	Initial masking: IM = AC of nontest ear. If tone not heard, plateau	Same as AC plus occlusion effect
Overmasking occurs	When EM level in masked ear minus IA is equal to or greater than BC of test ear at same frequency	Same as AC
Interpretation	AC audiogram shows amount of hearing loss at each frequency	BC audiogram shows degree of sensorineural loss at each frequency
		Air-bone gap shows amount of conductive impairment at each frequency

*Minimal interaural attenuation is considered to be 40 dB for supra-aural earphones and 65 dB for insert earphones

5 Speech Audiometry

The hearing impairment inferred from a pure-tone audiogram cannot depict, beyond the grossest generalizations, the degree of disability in speech communication caused by a hearing loss. Because difficulties in hearing and understanding speech evoke the greatest complaints from patients with hearing impairments, it is logical that tests of hearing function should be performed with speech stimuli. Modern diagnostic audiometers include circuitry for measuring various aspects of receptive speech communication (Figures 3.19 and 3.20). Using speech audiometry, audiologists set out to answer questions regarding patients' degree of hearing loss for speech; the levels required for their most comfortable levels and uncomfortable loudness levels; the range of comfortable loudness; and, perhaps most important, their ability to recognize the sounds of speech.

Chapter Objectives

Chapter 4 introduced the concept of pure-tone audiometry and described its administration and interpretation. Chapter 5 acquaints the reader with speech audiometry and some of its ramifications. Upon completion of this chapter, the beginning student in audiology should have a fundamental knowledge of the measures obtained with speech audiometry, such as threshold for speech, most comfortable and uncomfortable loudness levels, and word-recognition ability. The reader should also be able to interpret speech audiometric results; relate them to pure-tone threshold tests; and after some supervised practice with an audiometer, actually perform the tests described in this chapter. The vocabulary supplied in the text, and reviewed in the glossary, is indispensable for understanding the concepts that follow in this book.

The Diagnostic Audiometer

In the early days of speech audiometry separate speech audiometers were used to perform the measurements to be described in this chapter. Modern devices have these circuits incorporated, along with circuitry for pure tones, into a single unit. Diagnostic audiometers are either accompanied by or have auxiliary inputs for testing with microphones, tape decks, or compact disks. A volume units (VU) meter is used to monitor the intensity of the input source visually.

All diagnostic audiometers contain a circuit for masking the nontest ear or for mixing a noise with a speech signal in the same ear. Tests can usually be carried out in either ear (**monaural**) or in both ears simultaneously (**binaural**). Hearing level controls that usually have a range of 120 dB (from −10 to 110 dB HL, according to ANSI-1996 values) are provided. Outputs to auxiliary amplifiers are available so that speech can be channeled to one or more loudspeakers for testing in the sound field. A talkback system is available for communication between separate rooms that hold the clinician and the patient.

Test Environment

Most speech audiometry is carried out with the patient isolated from the examiner in either one- or two-room sound-treated suites. This is mandatory when **monitored-live voice (MLV)** testing is used, because if examiners and patients are in the same room, there is no way to ensure that the patients are responding to sounds channeled to them through the audiometer, rather than directly through the air in the room. If prerecorded materials are used, same-room operation is possible, but this is probably an unusual procedure. Problems of ambient noise levels, as discussed in Chapter 4, are very much the same for speech audiometry as for pure-tone tests.

There are significant advantages to using recorded materials. Primarily, they provide a consistency of presentation that is independent of the expertise of the clinician. Most audiologists appear to prefer monitored live voice testing, as they feel it provides for more flexibility in delivering the stimuli and often takes less time. With the advent of the CD some of these objections have been overcome, and, for the most part, the CD should be used instead of live-voice testing.

The Patient's Role in Speech Audiometry

To use speech audiometry, patients must know and understand reasonably well the words with which they are to be tested. Depending on the type of test, a response must be obtainable in the form of an oral reply, a written reply, or the identification of a picture or object.

Although spoken responses are more necessary in some speech tests than in others, they have certain advantages and disadvantages. One advantage is in the speed with which answers can be scored. Also, a certain amount of rapport is maintained through the verbal interplay between the patient and the audiologist. One serious drawback is the possible misinterpretation of the patient's response. Many people seen for hearing evaluation have speech or language difficulties that make their responses difficult to understand. Also, discrepancies occur in the scoring of some speech tests when verbal responses are obtained, because audiologists tend to score some incorrect spoken responses as correct.

In addition, for reasons that have never become completely clear, the talkback systems on many audiometers are of poor quality, sounding very little better than inexpensive intercom systems. This creates an additional problem in interpreting responses.

Written responses lend themselves only to tests that can be scored upon completion. When responses require an instantaneous value judgment by the audiologist, written responses are undesirable. When used, however, written responses do eliminate errors caused by difficulties in discriminating the patient's speech; they also provide a permanent record of the kinds of errors made. Having patients write down or otherwise mark responses may slow down some test procedures and necessitate time at the end of the test for scoring. Difficulties with handwriting and spelling provide additional, though not insurmountable, problems.

The use of pictures or objects is generally reserved for small children, who otherwise cannot or will not participate in a test. Adults with special problems are sometimes tested by this method, in which the patient is instructed to point to a picture or object that matches a stimulus word.

False responses may occur in speech audiometry, as well as in pure-tone audiometry. False positive responses are theoretically impossible, because patients cannot correctly repeat words that have been presented to them below their thresholds, unless, through the carelessness of the examiner, they have been allowed some visual cues and have actually lipread the stimulus words. False negative responses, however, do occur. The audiologist must try to make certain that the patient completely understands the task and will respond in the appropriate manner whenever possible.

No matter how thorough the attempt to instruct patients, it is impossible to gain total control over the internal response criteria each individual brings to the test. It has been suspected, for example, that aging might affect the relative strictness of these criteria. Jerger, Johnson, and Jerger (1988), however, demonstrated that aging alone does not appear to affect the criteria that listeners use in giving responses to speech stimuli. All the alert clinician can do is to instruct patients carefully and be aware of overt signs of deviation from expected behaviors.

The Clinician's Role in Speech Audiometry

First and foremost in speech audiometry, through whatever means necessary, the audiologist must convey to patients what is expected of them during the session. A combination of written and verbal instructions is usually successful with adults and older children, whereas gestures and pantomime may be required for small children and certain adults. At times, the instructions are given to patients through their hearing aids or, if this is not feasible, through a portable amplifier or the microphone circuit of the audiometer.

It is just as important that the patient not observe the examiner's face during speech audiometry as it is during pure-tone audiometry, and even more so if monitored live-voice testing is used. The diagram in Figure 4.5 shows a desirable arrangement.

Speech-threshold Testing

The logic of pure-tone threshold testing carries over to speech audiometry. If a patient's thresholds for speech can be obtained, they can be compared to an average normal-hearing individual's thresholds to determine the patient's degree of hearing loss for speech. Speech thresholds may be of two kinds, the **speech-detection threshold (SDT)** and the **speech-recognition threshold (SRT).**

The terminology used in speech audiometry has been inconsistent. Konkle and Rintelmann (1983) feel that the word *speech* itself may be too general and that the specific speech stimuli in any test should always be specified. Likewise, they are concerned with the conventional term *speech-reception threshold,* since the listener is asked to *recognize,* rather than *receive,* the words used in the test. In the most recent "Guidelines for Determining Threshold Level for Speech," ASHA (1988) also recommends the term *speech-recognition threshold* as preferable to the traditional term *speech-reception threshold.*

Speech-detection Threshold

The speech-detection threshold (SDT) may be defined as the lowest level, in decibels, at which a subject can barely detect the presence of speech and identify it as speech. The SDT is sometimes called the speech-awareness threshold (SAT). This does not imply that the speech is in any way understood—rather, merely that its presence is detected. One way of measuring the SDT is to present to the patient, through the desired output transducer, some continuous-discourse stimulus. The level of the speech is raised and lowered in intensity until the patient indicates that he or she can barely detect the speech.

Sentences are preferable to isolated words or phrases for finding the SDT. The sentences should be read rapidly and monotonously so that there are few peaks above and below zero on the VU meter, or series of light-emitting diodes designed to control the input level of the speech signal. The materials should be relatively uninteresting.

Whether the right ear or the left ear is tested first is an arbitrary decision. Sometimes tests of SDT are run binaurally, or through the sound-field speakers, either with or without the use of hearing aids. Patients may respond verbally, with hand or finger signals, or with a push-button, indicating the lowest level, in dB HL, at which they can barely detect speech.

Speech-recognition Threshold

The speech-recognition threshold (SRT) may be defined as the lowest hearing level at which speech can barely be understood. Most audiologists agree that the speech should be so soft that about half of it can be recognized. For a number of reasons, the SRT has become more popular with audiologists than the SDT and is thus the preferred speech-threshold test. In this book very little attention is paid to the SDT, although it has some clinical usefulness. SRTs have been measured with a variety of speech materials using both continuous discourse, as in measurement of the SDT, and isolated words.

Cold running speech, a form of continuous discourse, may be used to determine the SRT by modifying instructions to the patient and altering response criteria. Today most SRTs are obtained with the use of **spondaic words,** often called **spondees.** A spondee is a word with two syllables, both pronounced with equal stress and effort. In setting up their list of spondees, Hirsh, Davis, Silverman, Reynolds, Eldert, and Benson (1952) reduced the list of 84 words originated by Hudgins, Hawkins, Karlin, and Stevens (1947) to 36 words to increase their homogeneity of audibility and their familiarity. Although spondees do not occur in spoken English, it is possible, by altering stress slightly, to force such common words as *baseball, hot dog,* and *toothbrush,* to conform to the spondaic configuration. Whether the spondees are spoken into the microphone, or introduced by tape or disk, both syllables of the word should peak at zero VU. Although it takes practice for the student to accomplish this equal peaking on the VU meter, most people can acquire the knack relatively quickly.

When a prerecorded list of spondaic words is to be used, it is common to find a calibration tone recorded on a special band. The calibration signal is played long enough so that the gain control for the VU meter can be adjusted with the needle at zero VU. On some prerecorded spondee lists, a **carrier phrase** precedes each word, for example, "Say the word," followed by the stimulus word. Although some clinicians prefer the use of a carrier phrase, many do not. No real advantage of using a carrier phrase with spondaic words has been proved. An alphabetized list of spondees may be found on the CD that accompanies this book.

SRT Testing with Cold Running Speech

When **connected speech** is used to measure the SRT, patients are instructed to indicate the level at which the speech is so soft that they can barely follow what is being said. Sometimes this involves using a verbal or hand signal. The level of the speech may be raised and lowered in steps of 2 or 5 dB, depending on the preferences of the audiologist. Several measurements should be taken to ensure accuracy.

SRT Testing with Spondaic Words

The SRT is usually defined as the lowest hearing level at which 50 percent of a list of spondaic words is correctly identified. This definition appears incomplete, however, for it does not specify how many words are presented at threshold before the 50 percent criterion is invoked. Also, many methods used for SRT measurement in the past were rather vague, suggesting that the level should be raised and lowered but not giving a precise methodology.

For some reason, most SRTs had been obtained in 1 or 2 dB steps until Chaiklin and Ventry (1964) proved that for clinical purposes, 5 dB steps are just as accurate. Using 5 dB steps speeds up the procedure and makes decisions regarding threshold easier without sacrificing the quality of test results.

Tillman and Jerger (1959) showed that familiarizing the patient with the list of spondaic test words lowers the measured SRT by 4 to 5 dB. Conn, Dancer, and Ventry (1975) found that only 15 of the original words from the 36 spondees in CID Auditory Test W-1 could be used without prior familiarization altering test results. Other studies (e.g., Frank & McPhillips, 1976) have shown that fewer than half of the original words are similar with respect to the intensity required for intelligibility.

Practice with the SRT procedure lowers the response interpreted as threshold by a very small amount, although guessing may lower that level more than 4 dB, at least for people with normal hearing. Burke and Nerbonne (1978) suggest that the guess factor should be controlled during SRT tests by asking the patient not to guess and thereby improving the agreement between the SRT and the PTA. Because no data have surfaced that reveal the effects of guessing on patients with actual hearing losses, the practice will probably continue to encourage guessing to increase attentiveness to the test stimuli. It is considered advisable, whenever possible, to give the patient a list of the words before the test begins, together with printed instructions for the entire test procedure (see the accompanying CD).

Although written instructions may serve as an adjunct, they should not routinely replace spoken directions for taking a test. Instructions are of great importance in test results. One usable set of instructions follows:

> *The purpose of this test is to determine the faintest level at which you can hear and repeat some words. Each word you hear will have two syllables, like hot dog or baseball, and will be selected from the list of words that you have been given. Each time you hear a word, just repeat it. Repeat the words even if they sound very soft. You may have to guess, but repeat each word if you have any idea what it is. Are there any questions?*

Until the work of Chaiklin and Ventry (1964), most descriptions of the measurement of the speech-recognition threshold were rather vague. Clinicians and students had been advised simply to use an up-down method in search of threshold. Chaiklin and Ventry, however, proposed a systematic approach. Tillman and Olsen (1973) refined the SRT test methodology into a series of steps that led to the use of a formula for deciding on SRT, thereby taking the arbitrary decision out of the clinician's hands. Martin and Stauffer (1975) modified the Tillman-Olsen method so that it could be used without prior knowledge of the pure-tone results, thereby increasing its objectivity as an independent measurement of hearing.

ASHA (1988) has recently revised its guidelines for determining the SRT. There has been evidence that audiologists were not using the guidelines advanced earlier (ASHA, 1979), probably because of the time-consuming nature of the recommended procedure (Martin, Champlin, & Chambers, 1998). The current ASHA guidelines are based on the findings of several studies (e.g., Beattie, Forrester, & Ruby, 1987). The ASHA (1988) method for determining SRT involves the following steps: (1) familiarizing the listener with the spondaic words in the word list to be used, (2) ensuring that the vocabulary is familiar, (3) establishing that each word can be recognized auditorily, and (4) ascertaining that the patient's responses can be understood by the clinician. These goals can be accomplished by allowing the patient to listen to the words as presented through the audiometer. Words that present any difficulty should be eliminated from the list.

The ASHA method involves a descending procedure that can be summarized as follows:

1. Set the *start level* at 30 to 40 dB above the estimated SRT. The pure-tone average can be used for this purpose, or if this is not known, the start level can be set at 50 dB HL (Martin & Stauffer, 1975). One spondee is presented.
2. If no response or an incorrect response is obtained, raise the level in 20 dB steps until a correct response is given or the intensity limit of the equipment is reached.
3. If the patient responds correctly, descend in 10 dB steps, presenting one spondee at each level until an incorrect response is obtained.
4. When an incorrect response is given, present a second spondee at the same level.
5. Continue to decrease the intensity in 10 dB decrements until a level is reached at which two spondees are incorrectly recognized at the same level.
6. Following step 5, increase the level by 10 dB. This is the *starting level*. Present two spondees at this level.
7. Each time both spondees are correctly identified, decrease the intensity in 2 dB steps.
8. The test is completed when the subject fails to respond correctly to five of the last six words presented.
9. "Threshold is calculated by subtracting the total number of correct responses from the starting level and adding a correction factor of 1. This calculation is based on a statistical precedent (Spearman, 1908) for estimating threshold at the 50% point of the psychometric function" (ASHA, 1988).

Stated as a formula,

SRT = starting level – # correct + correction factor

The ASHA method allows for substitution of five spondees and 5 dB steps in step 7, based on the recommendations of Martin and Stauffer (1975). Nevertheless, given the apparent reluctance with which previous ASHA methods have been adopted by the audiology profession (Martin et al., 1998), it is not surprising that this method also never enjoyed full acceptance.

Martin and Stauffer (1975) recommend beginning the SRT procedure at a given hearing level (50 dB), especially for cases in which pure-tone thresholds cannot be obtained. Additionally, if the SRT is to serve as an independent measurement of hearing, and a check of the reliability of pure-tone thresholds, it should be accomplished without knowledge of the pure-tone thresholds with which it is compared. For this reason, Martin and Dowdy (1986) recommend a different procedure.

They found that SRTs obtained with the ASHA (1979) method and one similar to the ASHA (1978) guidelines for pure-tone audiometry yielded very similar results. The latter method, however, could be completed in a fraction of the time, with many fewer word presentations and no loss of accuracy. An advantage of the Martin and Dowdy (1986) method is that the SRT can be determined before the pure-tone thresholds, or in the absence of pure-tone results, as when testing hearing aids. The Martin and Dowdy procedure is summarized as follows:

1. Set the start level at 30 dB HL. Present one spondee. If a correct response is obtained, this suggests that the word is above the patient's SRT.
2. If no correct response is obtained, raise the presentation level to 50 dB HL. Present one spondee. If there is no correct response, raise the intensity in 10 dB steps, presenting one spondee at each increment. Stop at the level at which either a correct response is obtained or the power limit of the equipment is reached.
3. After a correct response is obtained, lower the intensity 10 dB and present one spondee.
4. When an incorrect response is given, raise the level 5 dB and present one spondee. If a correct response is given, lower the intensity 10 dB. If an incorrect response is given, continue raising the intensity in 5 dB steps until a correct response is obtained.
5. From this point on the intensity is increased in 5 dB steps and decreased in 10 dB steps, with one spondee presented at each level until three correct responses have been obtained at a given level.
6. Threshold is defined as the lowest level at which *at least* 50 percent of the responses are correct, with a minimum of at least three correct responses at that intensity.

One reason for the selection of spondaic words for measuring SRT is that they are relatively easy to discriminate and can often be guessed with a high degree of accuracy. Once the threshold of spondees has been reached (50 percent response criterion), it does not take much increase in intensity before all the words can be identified correctly. This is illustrated by the curve in Figure 5.1, which shows the enhanced intelligibility of spondees as a function of increased intensity.

Recording SRT Results

After SRTs for each ear have been obtained, they should be recorded in the appropriate space on the audiometric worksheet (Figure 5.2K). Many audiologists prefer to make routine measurements of the SRT binaurally or in the sound field. The audiometric worksheet used in this book does not provide for such notation, but many forms are available that do.

Relationship of SRT to SDT and the Pure-tone Audiogram. The SRT is always higher (requires greater intensity) than the SDT. Egan (1948) showed that the magnitude of the difference between the SRT and SDT does not normally exceed 12 dB. However, this difference may change with the shape of the pure-tone audiogram.

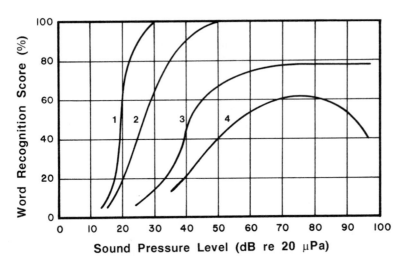

FIGURE 5.1   Theoretical performance-intensity (PI) functions for spondaic and PB words.
(1) Spondaic words. Note that at about 5 dB above the 50 percent correct point, almost all of the
words are intelligible. This shows an increase in recognition ability of approximately 10 percent per
decibel for scores between 20 percent and 80 percent. (2) PB word lists. Note the more gradual slope
for PB words than for spondees. The increase in intelligibility for the W-22 word lists averages
about 2.5 percent per decibel. The normal increase in word recognition scores with increased
intensity is to a maximum of approximately 100 percent (suggesting normal hearing or conductive
hearing loss). (3) PB word lists. Note the increase in word recognition scores with increased intensity
to a maximum of less than 90 percent (suggesting sensorineural hearing loss). (4) PB word lists. Note
the increase in word recognition scores with increased intensity to a given level, beyond which scores
decrease. This is the "rollover" effect, and it occurs in some ears when there are lesions in the higher
auditory centers (see Chapter 12).

For many years different methods have been used to predict the SRT from the pure-tone audiogram. Although some of these procedures have been quite elegant, most audiologists have agreed that the SRT can be predicted by finding the average of the lowest two thresholds at 500, 1000, and 2000 Hz (Fletcher, 1950). Carhart and Porter (1971) found that the SRT can be predicted from the pure-tone audiogram by averaging the thresholds at 500 and 1000 Hz and subtracting 2 dB. Although 500, 1000, and 2000 Hz have been called the "speech frequencies," Wilson and Margolis (1983) cautioned that such phrasing can be misleading if it is inferred that this narrow range of frequencies is all that is essential for the adequate discrimination of speech.

In some cases the SRT may be much lower (better) than the pure-tone average, such as when the audiogram falls precipitously in the high frequencies. In other cases the SRT may be higher (poorer) than even the three-frequency pure-tone average, for example, with some elderly patients or those with disorders of the central auditory nervous system. The special significance of pure-tone average-SRT disagreement regarding nonorganic hearing loss is discussed in Chapter 13.

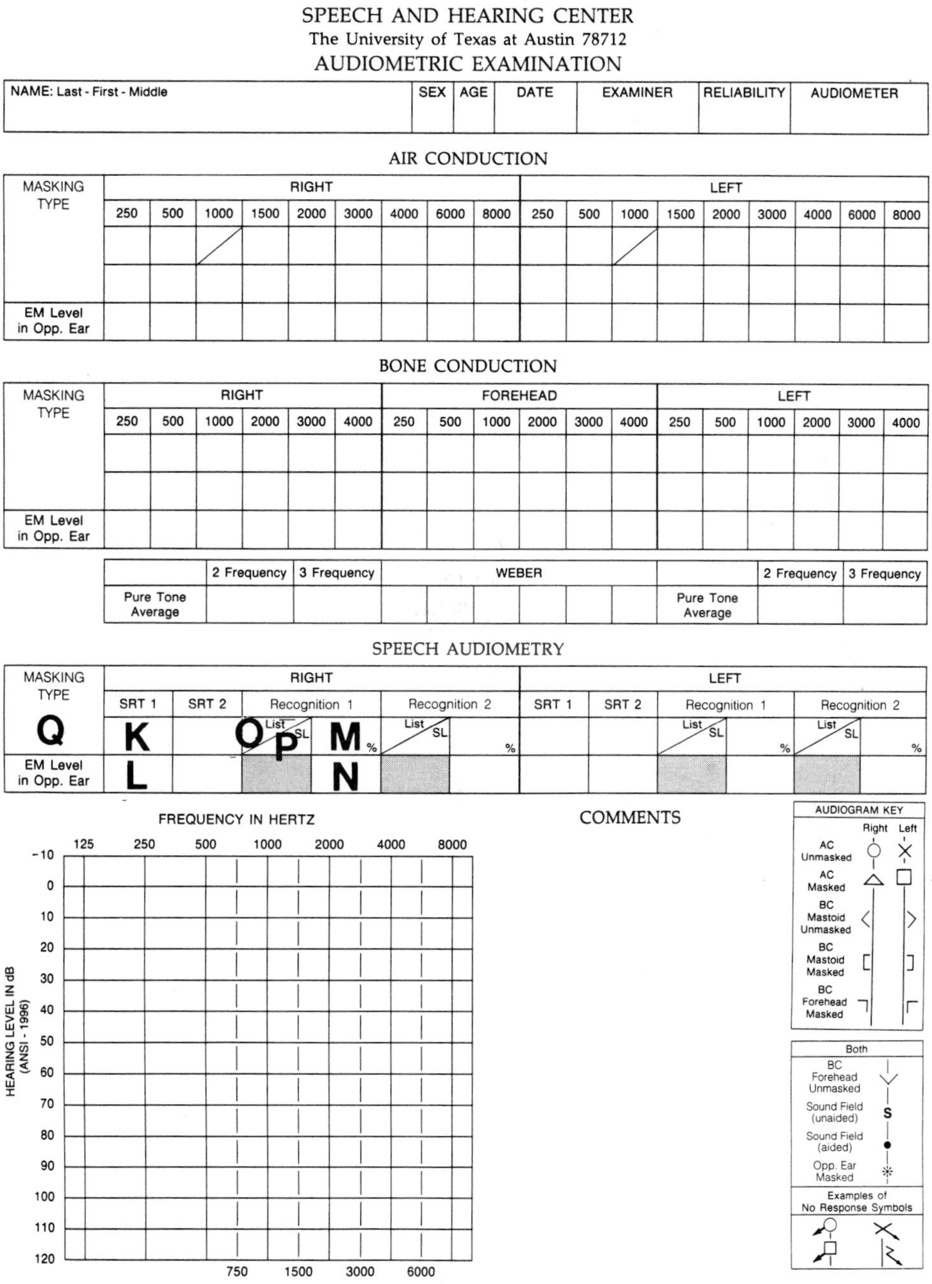

SPEECH AND HEARING CENTER
The University of Texas at Austin 78712
AUDIOMETRIC EXAMINATION

NAME: Last - First - Middle	SEX	AGE	DATE	EXAMINER	RELIABILITY	AUDIOMETER

AIR CONDUCTION

MASKING TYPE	RIGHT									LEFT								
	250	500	1000	1500	2000	3000	4000	6000	8000	250	500	1000	1500	2000	3000	4000	6000	8000
EM Level in Opp. Ear																		

BONE CONDUCTION

MASKING TYPE	RIGHT						FOREHEAD						LEFT					
	250	500	1000	2000	3000	4000	250	500	1000	2000	3000	4000	250	500	1000	2000	3000	4000
EM Level in Opp. Ear																		

	2 Frequency	3 Frequency		WEBER			2 Frequency	3 Frequency
Pure Tone Average						Pure Tone Average		

SPEECH AUDIOMETRY

MASKING TYPE	RIGHT				LEFT			
	SRT 1	SRT 2	Recognition 1	Recognition 2	SRT 1	SRT 2	Recognition 1	Recognition 2
Q	K		O List SL P	List SL M %			List SL	List SL
EM Level in Opp. Ear	L		N				%	%

FREQUENCY IN HERTZ

COMMENTS

AUDIOGRAM KEY

FIGURE 5.2   An example of an audiometric worksheet showing the following measurements that can be made during speech audiometry: (K) SRT; (L) effective masking level in the nontest ear used, when necessary, during SRT measurements; (M) word-recognition scores (WRS); (N) effective masking level in the nontest ear used for WRS; (O) test list number used for WRS; (P) level above the SRT for WRS test (SL); (Q) type of noise used for masking during speech audiometry.

Cross-hearing in SRT Tests

Problems involving cross-hearing exist for SRT measurements for the same reasons that they do for pure-tone air-conduction tests. In some cases the notion persists that there must be a significant difference between the SRTs of the two ears before suspicions of cross-hearing arise (Martin et al., 1998). This action ignores the current knowledge that sounds contralateralize by bone conduction rather than by air conduction. Cross-hearing is a danger whenever the SRT of the test ear, minus the interaural attenuation (conservatively set at 40 dB), is greater than or equal to the bone-conduction thresholds of the nontest ear. Because speech is a complex signal and bone-conduction thresholds are obtained with pure tones, it must be decided which frequency to use in computation. Martin and Blythe (1977) found that frequencies surrounding 250 Hz do not contribute to the recognition of spondees presented to the opposite ear until levels were reached that considerably exceeded normal interaural attenuation values. Their research supports the recommendations later made by ASHA (1988) that the SRT of the test ear should be compared to the lowest (best) bone-conduction threshold of the nontest ear at 500, 1000, 2000, or 4000 Hz.

$$SRT_{TE} - IA \geq best\ BC_{NTE}$$

Figure 5.3 illustrates the possibility of cross-hearing for SRT.

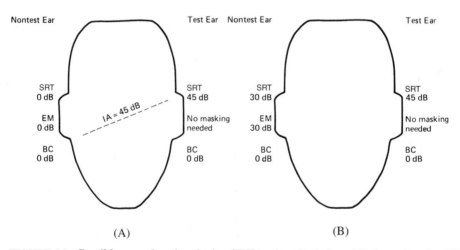

(A)   (B)

FIGURE 5.3   Possible cross-hearing during SRT testing. Both A and B show that the difference between the SRT of the test ear and the lowest bone-conduction threshold of the nontest ear exceed the minimum interaural attenuation found when speech sounds contralateralize (40 dB). Note that the SRT of the nontest ear in A is 0 dB HL and in B it is 30 dB HL. The SRTs of the nontest ears are unrelated to the danger of cross-hearing for speech. The SRT of the test ear must be compared to the lowest bone-conduction threshold of the nontest ear. The initial effective masking level for the SRT is equal to the SRT of the nontest ear (i.e., 0 dB EM for A; 30 dB EM for B).

Masking for SRT

Masking must be used in SRT testing to eliminate the influence of the nontest ear and to ascertain the true threshold of the test ear in precisely the same way as for pure-tone air-conduction audiometry. As in pure-tone testing, the audiologist should suspect the need to mask more often than cross-hearing actually occurs. Even in questionable cases of cross-hearing, masking is a prudent practice.

Most audiometers provide only the supra-aural earphone-cushion arrangements for testing and masking. The use of insert earphones can help to avoid some of the problems of overmasking by increasing interaural attenuation to at least 65 or 70 dB. The recent emphasis on their use holds promise for solving many masking dilemmas.

Noises Used in Masking for Speech

The types of masking noises used for speech audiometry are more limited than those used for pure tones. Because speech is a broad-spectrum signal, speech-masking noises must consist of a broad band of frequencies.

White noise is available on many diagnostic audiometers. Because it is a broad-spectrum noise, it masks speech satisfactorily, but is slightly less intense in the low frequencies.

Speech noise is obtained by filtering white noise above 1000 Hz at the rate of about 12 dB per octave. Speech noise provides more energy in the low-frequency spectrum than does white noise and is more like the overall spectrum of speech. Of the masking noises available on commercial audiometers, speech noise is usually preferred for masking speech.

Calibration of Speech-masking Noises

All of the needs for adequate control of the masking system for pure tones are identical to those for speech. The linearity of the masking-level dial must be proved. If the masking circuit is calibrated in decibels of effective masking, procedures for masking speech can be carried out in the same way as those used for pure tones. Field calibration for effective masking may be carried out in the following fashion on a group of normal-hearing subjects:

1. Present a series of spondees at 30 dB HL.
2. Present a noise (preferably speech noise) to the same ear.
3. Raise the level of the noise in 5 dB steps until subjects miss more than 50 percent of the words. Recheck this several times on each subject.
4. Obtain a median for the dial reading on the noise attenuator that masked speech at 30 dB HL. This is 30 dB EM for speech.
5. Subtract 30 dB from what was determined in step 4.
6. Add a safety factor of 5 or 10 dB to ensure masking effectiveness for most cases and this is 0 dB EM.
7. Post a correction chart showing the amount of noise that must be added to 0 dB HL to reach 0 dB EM for speech.

Once calibration is completed, speech at any level can be masked out when an effective masking level equal to the SRT is introduced into the same ear. Any correction factors must be added.

Central Masking for Speech

It has been demonstrated that threshold shifts for continuous discourse (Martin, Bailey, & Pappas, 1965) and for spondaic words (Martin, 1966) occur when a noise is presented to the nontest ear under earphones. Because the levels of noise need not be high enough to cause peripheral masking by cross-conduction, it is assumed that the same central masking phenomenon exists for speech as for pure tones. Martin and DiGiovanni (1979) found smaller threshold shifts due to central masking than had been previously reported, but it should be expected that a threshold shift of about 5 dB will be seen for speech in the presence of a contralateral noise, even if that noise is of relatively low intensity (Konkle & Berry, 1983).

Masking Methods for SRT

Figure 5.3 illustrates a case in which masking is needed for the nontest ear. The difference between the SRT of the test ear (45 dB) and the minimal interaural attenuation (40 dB) exceeds the bone-conduction threshold (0 dB) of the nontest ear. In this example, no specific frequency is referred to in terms of the bone-conduction threshold. In actual clinical practice, the SRT of the test ear is compared to the best (lowest) bone-conduction threshold of the nontest ear at 500, 1000, 2000, or 4000 Hz. If the nontest ear originally participated in the test, it should be removed by presenting an initial masking (IM) level equal to the SRT of the masked ear. If the SRT of the test ear does not shift by more than 5 dB (for central masking), the original threshold was correct as measured, and masking is completed. This is true because the nontest ear was rendered incapable of test participation. If the threshold shifted by more than 5 dB, the implication is that the nontest ear did, in fact, play a role in unmasked results by cross-hearing. When original speech stimuli have been cross-heard, further testing using the plateau method is required.

   Maximum masking for speech follows the same general rules noted previously for pure tones. If cross-hearing has taken place, the patient's interaural attenuation is no greater than the SRT of the test ear, minus the lowest bone-conduction threshold of the nontest ear. When a level of effective masking, minus the patient's interaural attenuation, is equal to or above the lowest bone-conduction threshold of the test ear, overmasking (OM) has occurred.

$$OM = EM_{NTE} - IA \geq Best\ BC_{TE}$$

The Plateau Method

The plateau method, described for pure tones in Chapter 4 and diagrammed in Figure 4.19, can be used when measuring the threshold for spondees. If the initial level of effective masking reveals that the SRT was obtained by cross-hearing, the SRT is determined with that level of noise in the nontest ear. Then, the intensity of the noise is raised 5 dB in the nontest ear, and spondaic words are presented to the test ear. If fewer than three out of six words can be repeated correctly, the level of the words is raised 5 dB, and so forth. The true SRT is reached when the intensity of the noise can be raised or lowered at least three times in 5 dB steps without affecting the threshold for the words. As in the case of pure tones, the plateau for speech is influenced by the patient's interaural attenuation, the bone-conduction thresholds of the test ear, and the SRT of the masked ear.

Recording Masked SRT Results

Before SRTs are recorded on the audiometric worksheet, a 5 dB correction for central masking may be subtracted from the SRT obtained with contralateral masking. The maximum level of effective masking required to obtain threshold should be recorded in the appropriate box below the SRT (Figure 5.2L).

Bone-conduction SRT

At times it is useful to determine the speech-recognition threshold by bone conduction. Because the bone-conduction circuits on diagnostic audiometers are not calibrated for speech, some degree of manipulation is required for bone-conduction speech audiometry (Barry & Gaddis, 1978). On most clinical audiometers the speech input may be used with the bone-conduction output.

Bone-conducted SRTs are especially useful in testing children who will "play a game" with words but not with tones. A comparison between children's hearing thresholds for speech by bone conduction and by air conduction may provide useful information regarding a possible conductive hearing loss. Hahlbrock (1962) found this method helpful in separating auditory from tactile responses by bone conduction. Goetzinger and Proud (1955) found a high correlation between the pure-tone average by bone conduction at 500, 1000, and 2000 Hz and the bone-conducted SRT. Other researchers have found the bone-conducted SRT to be of clinical value (Edgerton, Danhauer, & Beattie, 1977). Of course, with bone-conducted speech audiometry there is no way to be certain which ear is being tested unless proper masking is invoked, which is impossible with some patients. However, even the limited information derived from this procedure and the inferences it allows often justify the use of bone-conducted speech audiometry.

Most Comfortable Loudness Level

Some audiologists gain useful information from determining the hearing level at which speech is most comfortably loud for their patients. Most people with normal hearing find speech comfortable at 40 to 55 dB above threshold.

Measurement of **most comfortable loudness (MCL)** should be made with continuous discourse, so that the patient has an opportunity to listen to speech as it fluctuates over time. The use of cold running speech, as described for SRT or SDT measurements, is practical for this purpose.

The patient is instructed to indicate when the speech is perceived to be at a comfortable level. The test may start at a hearing level slightly above the SRT. From there the intensity is increased gradually. At each hearing level the patient should respond, indicating whether the speech is "too soft" "too loud," or "most comfortable." Several measurements should be made, approaching the MCL from both above and below the level first selected.

The MCL may be determined monaurally or binaurally under earphones or in the sound field. Martin and colleagues (1998) found that most audiologists do not use the MCL measurement, except in the evaluation of hearing aids.

Cross-hearing and Masking in MCL Tests

Because in the MCL test the level of speech is raised above threshold, the probability increases that the threshold of the ear not being tested will be reached or exceeded. This often happens without the patient's awareness. In most cases the inclusion of the opposite ear in an MCL measurement does not affect either the results or their interpretation. If it is decided that the nontest ear must be absolutely excluded from the test, this can be done, in most cases, with masking. It must be remembered that a noise presented to one ear may have an effect on the subjective impression of the loudness of speech in the other ear. The following formula shows when masking may be needed for measuring MCL under earphones.

$$MCL_{TE} - IA \geq best \ BC_{NTE}$$

As stated previously, masking is usually not used in determining the MCL. If it is desired, however, maximum masking should be used so the masking level can be set at the outset of the test and not varied thereafter. The maximum masking level for speech is equal to the lowest (best) bone-conduction threshold of the test ear plus 40 dB for interaural attenuation when supra-aural earphones are used. The equation for effective masking level for MCL is

$$EM = best \ BC_{TE} + 40 \ dB$$

Recording the MCL Test Results

After the MCL results are obtained, they should be recorded in the space provided for this purpose on the audiometric worksheet, with the proper masking levels indicated when necessary.

Uncomfortable Loudness Level

Under some conditions—for example, when a hearing aid is contemplated—it is important to find the level of speech that is uncomfortably loud for listeners. For normal-hearing subjects, this intensity often extends to the upper limit of the audiometer (100 to 110 dB HL). In some patients with hearing disorders the **uncomfortable loudness level (UCL)** is much lower, especially when expressed in decibels above the SRT. It is not known just how the abbreviation for uncomfortable loudness level became UCL, since "uncomfortable" is one word, but these kinds of derivations are often obscure. Some patients find a given level of speech uncomfortable because of its loudness, others because of discomfort produced by the physical pressure of the sound. When possible, it is helpful to determine which effect is active in a given case. The UCL is also called the **threshold of discomfort (TD)**, the **tolerance level,** and the **loudness discomfort level (LDL).**

Materials used for the UCL can be identical to those used for the MCL. Patients should be instructed to signal, either verbally or by some other method, when the speech is uncomfortably loud. They should be reminded that the UCL may be considerably above the level at which they find the loudness of speech most enjoyable, but that they should signal only when exceeding a given level would be intolerable. Acoustic feedback can be a real problem when UCLs are measured in the sound field.

Cross-hearing and Masking for UCL Tests

All the statements pertaining to cross-hearing and masking for MCL also pertain to UCL. Masking for UCL is not usually performed. However, if desired, the masking level may be determined in the same way as for MCL.

Recording UCL Test Results

The audiometric form used in this book has no space for the recording of the UCL. Appropriate space is provided on worksheets devised for sound-field speech audiometry that are sometimes used during hearing-aid evaluations. Audiologists who carry out UCL measurements under earphones design their own data sheets accordingly.

Range of Comfortable Loudness

The **range of comfortable loudness (RCL)** is the arithmetic difference between the SRT and the UCL. This difference is also called the **dynamic range (DR) for speech.** A normal-hearing person has an RCL of 100 dB or more. The RCL determination is sometimes used in selecting hearing aids and in other rehabilitative measures. When an SRT cannot be obtained, the difference between the SDT and the UCL provides a reasonable estimate of the RCL.

Word-recognition Testing

Many patients report that the difficulties they have in understanding speech are solved when speech is made louder. This can be accomplished by decreasing the distance from the listener to the speaker, by having talkers increase their vocal output, or by using a system of sound amplification. Most patients with conductive hearing losses show improved word recognition when loudness is increased.

A common complaint of many patients is difficulty in understanding what people are saying. Many patients with sensorineural problems, however, complain that even when sounds are made louder, they are not clearly recognizable. This difficulty in discriminating among the sounds of speech plagues patients much more than a reduction in loudness. These are the patients who claim, "I can hear, but I can't understand."

Through the years, a number of different expressions have been used to describe the measurement of speech discrimination. The expression **word-recognition score (WRS)** has appeared in the literature with increasing frequency in recent years and appears to be the current expression of choice. Konkle and Rintelmann (1983) contend that the word *discrimination* in this context implies distinguishing among different stimuli, whereas *recognition* suggests the report of a patient on what has been heard after the presentation of a single item. For the most part, throughout this book, the term word-recognition score will replace the older *speech-discrimination score* (SDS) to describe tests performed to determine an individual's understanding of speech stimuli.

The development of test materials to assess word-recognition ability has been arduous. For any test to be useful, it should be both reliable and valid. Reliability means that a test is able to reveal similar scores on subsequent administrations (test-retest reliability) and that different forms of the same test result in equivalent scores. The validity of any word-recognition test relates to the following:

1. How well it measures what it is supposed to measure (a person's difficulties in understanding speech).
2. How favorably a test compares with other similar measures.
3. How the test stands up to alterations of the signal (such as by distortion or presentation with noise) that are known to affect other speech tests in specific ways.

The quantitative determination of a patient's ability to discriminate speech helps the audiologist in several ways:

1. It determines the extent of the word-recognition difficulty.
2. It aids in diagnosis of the site of the disorder in the auditory system.
3. It assists in the determination of the need for and proper selection of amplification systems.
4. It helps the clinician to make a prognosis for the outcome of rehabilitative efforts.

Several methods have been advanced for measuring word recognition. These include testing with nonsense syllables, digits, monosyllabic words, and sentences, and prerecordings of many of these are commerically available. Procedures have included both open- and closed-response message sets. In the open-response format, the patient may select an answer from an infinite number of possible utterances. In a closed-response system, however, the patient must choose the correct response from a group of words, sentences, or pictures.

Egan (1948) showed a relationship between the number of sounds in a word and the ability to recognize that word. The more phonemes and the more acoustic redundancy contained in a word, the more easily it is recognized. Word recognition gets poorer as more and more high frequencies are eliminated from speech, which decreases intelligibility without affecting overall loudness very much. As frequencies below about 1900 Hz are removed from speech, the effect on discrimination is much less than when higher frequencies are removed (French & Steinberg, 1947).

Phonetically Balanced Word Lists

Original attempts at word-recognition testing (Egan, 1948) involved compiling lists of words that are **phonetically balanced (PB),** that is, lists that contain all the phonetic elements of connected English discourse in their normal proportion to one another. Egan's work at the Psychoacoustic Laboratories at Harvard University resulted in twenty lists of 50 words each. When these word lists are used today, a weight of 2 percent per word is allowed. The word-recognition score is determined by counting the number of correctly identified words out of 50 and multiplying this number by 2 percent.

Hirsh and others (1952) eliminated most of Egan's original 1000 words and were left with a total of 200 words, of which 180 were derived from Egan's list. These 200 words were divided into four lists of 50 words each, with each list scrambled into six sublists. The resultant PB word lists are known as CID Auditory Test W-22. Ross and Huntington (1962) found some slight differences among the W-22 word lists in terms of word-recognition scores, but the magnitude of the differences among lists is small enough that they may be used interchangeably in clinical practice. Four PB word lists from CID Auditory Test W-22 are included on the CD under *Forms* in the literature section.

Because many of the words in adult PB word lists are unfamiliar to children, Haskins (1949) developed four lists of fifty words, all within the vocabularies of small children. The test may be presented by tape, disc, or by monitored live voice, and it is scored in the same way as PB word lists when adults or older children are tested. Three PBK (for kindergarten) word lists are included on the CD; one of the original four (list 2) was found to be much easier than the other three and therefore is not included. The test difficulty increases sharply for children younger than $3\frac{1}{2}$ years of age (Sanderson-Leepa & Rintelmann, 1976).

Performance-intensity Curves for PB Word Lists

Many of the word lists currently used in speech-recognition testing were developed during World War II to test the efficiency with which electronic communications systems could transmit speech. Thus, the primary objective was to design military communication systems that would, while transmitting a minimum of acoustic content, enable the listener to understand the message. Hence, the term *articulation* was used to express the connection achieved between the listener and the speaker—that is, the joining together of the two by means of a communication system. Use of the word "articulation" in this context is sometimes confusing to students of speech-language pathology, who learn to use this word to mean the manner in which speech sounds are produced with such structures as the tongue, lips, palate, and teeth.

Research has been conducted to determine the articulation-gain functions of PB word lists—that is, the percentage of correct identifications of the words at a variety of sensation levels. As Figure 5.1 illustrates, for normal-hearing individuals, the maximum PB score (100 percent) is obtained about 35 to 40 dB above the SRT. For many people with sensorineural hearing losses, the maximum obtainable score is below 100 percent. The highest PB word score obtainable, regardless of intensity is called the **PB Max** (Eldert & Davis, 1951). The term **performance-intensity function for PB word lists (PI-PB)** has replaced the old articulation-gain function terminology. PI-PB functions are discussed again in later chapters of this book in terms of their diagnostic value.

Consonant-Nucleus-Consonant Word Lists

The phonetic construction of the English language is such that there is no way to truly balance a list of words phonetically, especially a relatively short list because of the almost infinite number of variations that can be made on each phoneme (allophones) as it is juxtaposed with other phonemes. Lehiste and Peterson (1959) prepared ten 50-word lists that were phonemically balanced, a concept they judged to be more realistic than phonetic balancing. Each monosyllabic word contained a consonant, followed by a vowel or diphthong, followed by another consonant. These were called **consonant-nucleus-consonant (CNC) words** and were scored the same way as the original PB word lists. Later, the CNC lists were revised (Lehiste & Peterson, 1962) by removing proper names, rare words, and the like.

Tillman, Carhart, and Wilber (1963) took 95 words from the CNC lists (Lehiste & Peterson, 1959) and added 5 of their own, thereby generating two lists of 100 words each. Tillman and Carhart (1966) later developed four lists of 50 words each (Northwestern University Test No. 6), which they found to have high intertest reliability. Each of the four lists is scrambled into four randomizations. The four main lists (alphabetized) are included on the CD. Auditory test NU-6 and CID- W-22 remain the most popular materials for word-recognition testing (Martin et al., 1998) and yield similar results on patients when testing in both quiet and with background noise, although scores are slightly higher on the NU-6 test. It is important to remember, however, that patients' responses to this test, as to other word recognition tests, may change on the basis of a number of variables, not the least of them being differences among the talkers who make the recordings. This problem is increased when the test is performed in the presence of background noise. An obvious solution to this would be for all audiologists to test with commercially available, prerecorded word lists.

High-frequency Emphasis Lists

Gardner (1971) developed two lists with 25 words on each (see the CD-ROM), each word carrying a value of 4 percent. The test used with these lists is designed to measure the word recognition scores of patients with high-frequency hearing losses who are known to have special difficulties in understanding speech. Each of the words contains the vowel /I/ (as in *kick*) and is preceded and followed by a voiceless consonant. Gardner suggested that the test is more useful if the words are spoken by a woman with a high-pitched voice. A similar approach to high-frequency word lists was taken by Pascoe (1975).

Nonsense-syllable Lists

Edgerton and Danhauer (1979) developed two lists, each with 25 nonsense syllables. Every item contains a two-syllable utterance, each syllable produced by a consonant, followed by a vowel (CVCV). Carhart (1965) earlier suggested that nonsense words are too abstract and difficult for many patients to discriminate, and this is sometimes true of the CVCV test. It does have the advantage that each phoneme can be scored individually, eliminating the obvious errors in the all-or-none scoring used in PB word tests.

Testing Word Recognition with Half Lists

Time can be saved in word-recognition testing by limiting the test lists to 25 words, using one-half of each list with a weight of 4 percent per word. Opposition to this procedure is based on the following arguments: (1) that one-half of a list may produce fewer audible sounds than the other half, (2) that there may be some real differences in difficulty of discrimination between the two halves of a list, but primarily (3) that splitting the lists causes them to lose their phonetic balance (which is not truly obtainable). Tobias (1964) pointed out that phonetic balancing is unnecessary in a "useful diagnostic test" and that half lists do measure the same thing as full lists. Thornton and Raffin (1978) showed half lists to be as reliable as the full 50-word lists. Martin and colleagues (1998) found that most audiologists prefer to test with 25-word lists.

It has been demonstrated that very good or very poor word-recognition scores may be found by using as few as 10 words (Hosford-Dunn, Runge, & Montgomery, 1983), if the word list is rank-ordered. Although this controversy is unresolved, it is probably advisable, when testing with monosyllables, to use all 50 words. When time is a factor, and a patient has achieved a high score on the first 25 words (i.e., has missed no more than 2 words), the second half of the list may be eliminated if this high score is consistent with other audiometric data, such as the type and amount of hearing loss present.

Short Isophonemic Word Lists

The Short Isophonemic Word Lists (Boothroyd, 1968) were designed to reduce word-recognition test time without sacrificing validity. Each of fifteen lists of 10 consonant-vowel-consonant words contains 30 phonemes. Rather than the traditional scoring of test words as correct or incorrect, each phoneme is scored individually, allowing for a potential of 30 speech recognition errors per list. The time saved in administration of the isophonemic lists can be considerable when multiple word lists are employed for attaining articulation-gain functions. No significant differences were found between measures of word recognition utilizing the Short Isophonemic Word Lists and the more commonly employed CID W-22 test (Tonry, 1988).

Testing of Monosyllables with a Closed-response Set

The closed-set paradigm for word-recognition testing followed the development of a rhyme test by Fairbanks (1958). House, Williams, Hecker, and Kryter (1965) developed the Modified Rhyme Test, in which the patients are supplied with six rhyming words from which they select the one they think they have heard. Fifty sets of items are presented to the patient, along with a noise in the test ear. Half of the word sets vary only on the initial phoneme, and the other half differ in the final phoneme.

A test designed to be sensitive to the discrimination problems of patients with high-frequency hearing losses is the **California Consonant Test** (Owens & Schubert, 1977). One hundred mono-syllabic words are arranged in two scramblings to produce two test lists. The subject, selecting from four possibilities, marks a score sheet next to the word that has been discriminated. Whereas normal-hearing individuals obtain high scores on this test, patients with high-frequency hearing losses show some difficulty.

The **Picture Identification Task (PIT)** was developed by Wilson and Antablin (1980) to test the word recognition of adults who could not produce verbal responses and had difficulty in select-ing items from a printed worksheet. The CNC words are represented by pictures that are arranged into sets of four rhyming words. The developers of the PIT found that it provides good estimates of word recognition for the nonverbal adult population.

Recognizing the need for testing the word-recognition abilities of small children who are either unable or unwilling to respond in the fashion of adults, Ross and Lerman (1970) developed the **Word Intelligibility by Picture Identification (WIPI) test.** The child is presented with a series of cards, each of which contains six pictures. Four of the six pictures are possibilities as the stimulus item on a given test, and the other two pictures on each card (which are never tested) act as foils to decrease the probability of a correct guess. Twenty-five such cards are assembled in a spiral binder. Children indicate which picture corresponds to the word they believe they have heard. This proce-dure is very useful in working with children whose discrimination for speech cannot otherwise be evaluated, provided that the stimulus words are within the children's vocabularies. Incorrect identi-fication of words simply because they are not known is common with children under three and one-half years of age. The test words are listed on the CD.

The Northwestern University Children's Perception of Speech (**NUCHIPS**) test (Elliott & Katz, 1980) is similar to the WIPI. Each child is presented with a series of four picture sets, includ-ing 65 items with 50 words scored on the test.

Testing Word Recognition with Sentences

Jerger, Speaks, and Trammell (1968) objected to the use of single words as a discrimination test on the basis that they do not provide enough information regarding the time domain of speech. Normal connected speech is constantly changing patterns over time, thus necessitating the use of longer samples than single words can provide for a realistic test. Jerger and colleagues also iterated the problems inherent in testing with an open-message set. Criticisms of sentence tests include the effects of memory and learning, familiarity with the items as a result of repetition, and the methods of scoring. Much of the opposition to sentence tests is that their structure enables a listener who is a good guesser to make more meaning of a sentence than does another patient with similar speech recognition abilities.

The test devised by Jerger and colleagues (1968) involves a set of 10 *synthetic* sentences. Each sentence contains 7 words, with a noun, predicate, object, and so on, but carries no meaning. All words were selected from Thorndike's list of the 1000 most familiar words. The sentences are recorded on CD or magnetic tape, and patients show their responses by indicating the number that corresponds to the sentence they have heard. Some sentences are more difficult than others. Because early experimentation showed that the test is not sufficiently difficult when presented in quiet, a competing message of connected speech is presented in the test ear, along with the synthetic sentences, and the intensity of the competing message is varied. Examples of 10 sentences used for **synthetic sentence identification (SSI)** are shown on the CD.

A number of different sentence tests have been devised to measure speech recognition. One that continues in use is the Central Institute for the Deaf (CID) Everyday Sentence Test (Davis & Silverman, 1978). Fifty key words are contained within ten sets of 10 sentences each. The percentage of correctly identified key words determines the score.

Kalikow, Stevens, and Elliott (1977) developed a test made up of eight lists of 50 sentences each; only the last word in each sentence is the test item, resulting in 200 test words. The test items are recorded on one channel of a two-channel tape, and a voice babble is recorded on the second channel. In this way the two hearing-level dials of an audiometer can control the ratio of the intensities of the two signals. This procedure, called the **Speech Perception in Noise (SPIN)** test, has undergone considerable modification (Bilger, Nuetzel, Rabinowitz, & Rzeczkowski, 1984). Schum and Matthews (1992) reported an interesting effect: A significant percentage of the elderly patients with hearing loss they tested did not use contextual cues as effectively on the SPIN as did their younger counterparts.

Another useful sentence test is the **Connected Speech Test (CST)** (Cox, Alexander, & Gilmore, 1987; Cox, Alexander, Gilmore, & Pusakulich, 1988). The most recent version of the test contains several practice passages and 48 test passages of continuous discourse, each approximately 30 seconds in length. On the second channel of a stereo recording is a babble of six simultaneous talkers, which is played to the same ear, thus serving as competition for the test sentences. Each passage contains 25 key words that are used for scoring—5 words at each of five levels of difficulty. Listeners are instructed to repeat each sentence within a given passage in its entirety. Intelligibility scores are based on the number of key words repeated correctly. The CST appears to meet many of the criteria for reliability and validity not found in other sentence tests, and thus holds promise as a diagnostic tool.

Cross-hearing and Masking in Word-recognition Tests

When word-recognition tests are delivered at suprathreshold levels, the danger of cross-hearing is even greater than during threshold tests. Because cross-hearing of an air-conducted signal occurs by bone conduction, the likelihood of opposite-ear participation in a word-recognition test increases as the level of the test signal increases. In addition, the better the bone-conduction threshold in the non-test ear, the greater the probability that it will be stimulated by the speech. In other words, whenever the hearing level of the words (PBHL) minus the interaural attenuation equals or exceeds the bone-conduction threshold of the nontest ear, cross-hearing is a strong probability. Expressed as a formula,

$$PBHL_{TE} - IA \geq best\ BC_{NTE}$$

As in the case of the SRT, the interaural attenuation is considered to be as little as 40 dB for supra-aural earphones, and the bone-conduction threshold inserted in the formula is the lowest (i.e., the best) one obtained in the nontest ear at 500, 1000, 2000, or 4000 Hz.

Whenever masking is needed during SRT testing, it will always be needed for word-recognition testing for the same ear. Often, however, masking becomes necessary only when the level of speech is raised above the SRT for the word-recognition test. Whatever masking noise is available for SRT should be used as well for finding the WRS. The noise should be calibrated as effective masking for speech. Although several masking methods have been suggested, the one described here has been found to be most useful (Martin, 1972). The effective masking level for the masked ear is equal to the hearing level at which the discrimination test is performed (PBHL), minus 40 dB for interaural attenuation, plus the largest air-bone gap in the masked ear:

$$EM = PBHL_{TE} - IA + ABG_{NTE}$$

The effective masking level thus derived is just sufficient to mask speech at the nontest ear if the interaural attenuation is as low as 40 dB, and it is more than enough noise if the IA is greater than 40 dB (a probability). If the interaural attenuation can be computed on the basis of masking needs for SRT, the larger number should be used in the formula, which lowers the effective masking level and decreases the chance of overmasking. The interaural attenuation can never be less than the SRT of the test ear, minus the lowest bone-conduction threshold of the nontest ear.

Insert receivers for word-recognition testing have several distinct advantages over supra-aural audiometer earphones, and the two types of receivers may be used interchangeably for measuring WRS (Martin, Severance, & Thibodeau, 1991). Presenting the words through the insert receiver increases the interaural attenuation from the test ear to the nontest ear. For example, substituting 70 dB for 40 dB as the minimum amount of interaural attenuation in the formula shown previously for determining the need to mask during word recognition testing will eliminate masking entirely for a large number of patients. When masking is required, if it is delivered through an insert receiver, the possibility of overmasking is reduced or eliminated because the interaural attenuation of the masking noise from nontest ear to test ear will likewise be increased. Seventy decibels can also replace 40 dB as interaural attenuation in the formulas used for determining the effective masking level needed for word-recognition testing. Finally, the attenuation of background noise that is provided by insert phones relative to supra-aural phones may result in improved word recognition when testing is done at low sensation levels or when background noise is a problem.

Whenever the nontest ear is masked for word recognition tests, just as for other audiometric measures, the level of effective masking should be indicated on the audiometric worksheet (Figure 5.2N). In this way, if someone other than the examiner should review the test results, the precise effective masking level that was used in testing can be seen.

Compensation for Central Masking

If the SRT was obtained with contralateral masking, the central masking correction of 5 dB may have been subtracted before the result was recorded. This correction must be borne in mind when setting the hearing level for the word-recognition test. If masking is required for finding the WRS, but not for determining the SRT, the clinician should assume that a 5 dB shift would have occurred if masking had been used when finding the SRT. In such cases the hearing level should be increased for word-recognition testing to compensate for the loss of loudness of the speech signal that results when noise is presented to the nontest ear.

Maximum Masking

Just as the need for masking increases as the hearing level is increased for the test stimuli, so does the necessary masking level increase. The possibility of overmasking increases as the level of noise is raised in the masked ear. Rules for maximum masking and overmasking for speech are given in the section on speech-recognition threshold and should be scrutinized carefully when masking for word recognition tests.

Administration of Word-recognition Tests

In administering word-recognition tests, audiologists must first help patients to understand what is expected of them, what the test will consist of, and how they are to respond. Audiologists must decide on

1. The method of delivery of the speech stimuli (prerecorded or monitored-live voice)
2. The type of materials to be used
3. The method of response
4. The intensity at which the test will be performed
5. Whether more than one level of testing is desired
6. Whether a noise is desired in the test ear (or loudspeaker) to increase the difficulty of the test and, if so, the intensity of the noise
7. Whether masking of the nontest ear is necessary and, if so, the amount and type of noise to use

Instructions to patients should be delivered orally, even if printed instructions have been read prior to the test. Gestures and pantomimes or the use of sign language may be necessary, although it is likely that any patient who is unable to comprehend oral instructions will be unable to participate in a word-recognition test. If responses are to be given orally, patients should be shown the microphone and the proper response should be demonstrated. If the responses are to be written, the proper forms and writing implements, as well as a firm writing surface, should be provided. Determining that the patient understands the task may save considerable time by avoiding test repetition.

Selection of Stimuli, Materials, and Response Method

Regardless of whether monitored-live voice or prerecordings are used, the level should be properly controlled and monitored on the VU meter of the audiometer. If a recording is used, it must contain a calibration signal of sufficient duration for the gain control of the VU meter to be adjusted so that the needle peaks at zero VU. If monitored-live voice is used, proper microphone technique is very important. The audiologist should be seated in front of the microphone and should speak directly into its diaphragm. If monosyllables are being tested, a carrier phrase should be used to prepare the patient for the stimulus word. The last word of the carrier phrase should be at the proper loudness so that the needle of the VU meter will peak at zero, corresponding to the calibration signal. The test word should be uttered with the same monotonous stress and should be allowed to peak where it will since words vary in acoustic power. Test words are not normally expected to peak at zero VU. Sufficient time (about five seconds) should be allowed between word presentations to permit the patient to respond.

Patients may respond by repeating the stimulus word, writing down their responses on a form (with 50 numbered spaces for PB word lists), circling or marking through the correct answer on a closed-message set, or pointing to a picture or object. It is difficult to gauge the criteria that patients use in determining their responses—that is, whether they are relatively strict or lax in expressing their recognition of specific items. Jerger and colleagues (1988) studied these criteria in elderly subjects and concluded that attempting to control for this variable is probably not essential. More research along these lines is obviously necessary.

Although no real satisfaction has been universally expressed for word recognition materials, audiologists have individual preferences. A survey on audiometric practices (Martin et al., 1998) showed the W-22 PB word lists to be most popular, with the NU-6 lists a close second. The theoretical word recognition scores illustrated throughout this book are the probable results on auditory test NU-6. One type of test material may be preferred for routine hearing tests under earphones and another type for special diagnostic tests.

Test Presentation Level

Some audiologists prefer to derive performance intensity functions for their word-recognition tests. Others prefer to test at MCL or some fixed level above the SRT. If testing is done at only one intensity or sensation level, there is no way to know that the WRS is the PB Max unless the score is 100 percent. Although there is no complete agreement on the ideal level for WRS testing, 30 dB sensation level seems to work well for the initial test. At times, other levels (higher or lower) are tested following the first test, in an attempt to obtain the maximum word-recognition score.

Testing Word Recognition with Competition.   Many audiologists feel that word-recognition tests carried out in quiet do not tax patients' word-recognition abilities sufficiently to diagnose the kinds of communication problems that are experienced in daily life. For this reason, a noise is often added to the test ear to make recognition more difficult. When this is done, the relative intensity of the signal (speech) and the noise is specified as the **signal-to-noise ratio (S/N).** The signal-to-noise ratio is not a ratio at all, but rather the difference in intensity between the signal (that which is wanted) and the noise (that which is not wanted) (see Table 5.1).

Signals used to help degrade the score include modulated white noise (Berry & Nerbonne, 1971), a mixture of noise in one or two speakers (Carhart, Tillman, & Greetis, 1969), one to three talkers (Carhart, Johnson, & Goodman, 1975), two- and four-talker combinations (Young, Parker, & Carhart, 1975), a single talker (Speaks & Jerger, 1965), and a multitalker babble (Cox et al., 1987).

TABLE 5.1   Examples of Three Signal-to-noise Ratios (S/N)

Signal	50 dB HL	50 dB HL	50 dB HL
Noise	40 dB HL	50 dB HL	60 dB HL
S/N	+10 dB	0 dB	−10 dB

Speech has been shown to be a better competing signal than electronically generated noise with a spectrum that resembles speech (Carhart et al., 1975).

Recording Word-recognition Test Results

After the word-recognition tests are completed, the results are recorded on the audiometric work-sheet in terms of the percentage of correctly identified words (Figure 5.2M), along with the test or list number (Figure 5.2O); the level at which the test was performed (Figure 5.2P); and, if opposite-ear masking was used, the effective masking level (Figure 5.2N) and the type of noise (Figure 5.2Q). If a second word-recognition test is carried out with a masking noise in the same ear, the S/N ratio is indicated, along with results and other identifying information.

Problems in Word-recognition Testing

Although the test-retest reliability of PB word tests is good for patients with normal hearing and conductive hearing losses, this reliability sometimes fails for patients with primarily sensorineural impairments (Engelberg, 1968). Estimates of expected test-retest agreement vary from 6 percent to 18 percent, but no justification has really been demonstrated for these estimates. Thornton and Raffin (1978) concluded that the significance of differences in word-recognition scores for a given individual depend on the number of items in the test and the true score for that test. From a statistical viewpoint, the greatest variability in scores should be found in the middle range of scores (near 50 percent) and the smallest variability at the extremes (near 0 percent and 100 percent). In general, the variability may be assumed to decrease as the number of test items increases. Therefore, it is sometimes risky for audiologists to assume that an increase or decrease in a given patient's word-recognition scores represents a real change in word-recognition ability.

Attempts have been made to relate the results obtained on word-recognition tests to the kinds of everyday difficulties experienced by patients. Statements such as "Our test shows you can understand 72 percent of what you hear," are oversimplified and naive, for they ignore such important variables as contextual cues, lipreading, ambient noise level, speaker intelligibility, and so on.

Bone-conduction Word-recognition Testing

At times, in cases of severe mixed hearing loss, a patient's best possible word-recognition score may not be attainable because of the severity of the air-conduction hearing loss. In many of these cases it is possible to test word recognition by bone conduction in the same way described earlier for testing SRTs. Goetzinger and Proud (1955) found PB word scores to be normal for bone-conducted

TABLE 5.2   General Guide for the Evaluation of Word-recognition Tests

Word-recognition Scores (in Percent)	General Word-recognition Ability
90 to 100	Normal limits
75 to 90	Slight difficulty, comparable to listening over a telephone
60 to 75	Moderate difficulty
50 to 60	Poor recognition; marked difficulty in following conversation
<50	Very poor recognition; probably unable to follow running speech

speech at 25 dB SL in normal-hearing subjects. Word-recognition testing by bone conduction has never become popular, but interest has been shown in this procedure from time to time.

Goetzinger (1978) generated a general guide for evaluating word-recognition scores, which is presented in Table 5.2. This table, though helpful, should not be interpreted rigidly. Many patients perform considerably better on recognition tests than they do in daily conversation, and others not nearly so well. Word-recognition tests are helpful in diagnosis, but are far from perfect for predicting real-world communication.

Computerized Speech Audiometry

Speech audiometry, like any behavioral measurement, must at times be practiced as more of an art than a science. In a majority of cases, however, it is possible to carry out these measurements in a methodical, scientific manner, using the process of logical decision making. To illustrate this, Wittich, Wood, and Mahaffey (1971) programmed a digital computer to administer SRT and WRS tests, including proper masking, to analyze the patient's responses and to present the results in an audiogram format at the conclusion of the test. Their results were compared to those of an experienced audiologist on a number of actual clinical patients, and very high correlations were observed.

Stach (1988) pointed out that the modern computer can improve the efficiency of speech audiometry in several ways. Speech materials may be presented by a digital tape player or compact disc, allowing for appropriate pacing of stimuli, and thus providing the flexibility of live-voice testing without its obvious limitations. Furthermore, the digital recordings do not deteriorate with time and use, and therefore the stimuli remain constant.

Summary

Speech audiometry includes measurement of a patient's thresholds for speech—speech-recognition threshold (SRT), speech-detection threshold (SDT), most comfortable loudness level (MCL), uncomfortable loudness level (UCL [or loudness discomfort level LDL]), range of comfortable loudness (RCL [or dynamic range DR]), and word-recognition score (WRS). Measurements may be made either monaurally or binaurally under earphones, through a bone-conduction vibrator or in the sound field through loudspeakers. Materials for speech audiometry may include connected speech, two-syllable (spondaic) words, monosyllabic words, or sentences. The materials may be presented by means of a microphone (using monitored-live voice), tape recorder, or CD player. At times the sensitivity of the nontest ear by bone conduction is such that it may inadvertently participate in a test under earphones. When cross-hearing is a danger, a masking noise must be presented to the nontest ear to eliminate its participation in the test.

Measurements using speech audiometry augment the findings of pure-tone tests and help to determine the extent of a patient's hearing loss, loudness tolerance, and word recognition. The knowledge gained from the use of speech audiometry is helpful in the diagnosis of the site of lesion in the auditory system, as well as in audiological rehabilitation.

The audiograms depicted in Chapter 4, illustrating normal hearing, conductive hearing loss, and sensorineural hearing loss, are repeated in Figures 5.4, 5.5, and 5.6. These figures show the probable results obtained during speech audiometry, including the use of masking, where indicated.

SPEECH AND HEARING CENTER
The University of Texas at Austin 78712
AUDIOMETRIC EXAMINATION

NAME: Last - First - Middle	SEX	AGE	DATE	EXAMINER	RELIABILITY	AUDIOMETER

AIR CONDUCTION

MASKING TYPE	RIGHT									LEFT								
	250	500	1000	1500	2000	3000	4000	6000	8000	250	500	1000	1500	2000	3000	4000	6000	8000
	5	0	5/5	5	0	5	10	5	5	0	5	5/5	5	5	0	0	0	5
EM Level in Opp. Ear																		

BONE CONDUCTION

MASKING TYPE	RIGHT						FOREHEAD						LEFT					
	250	500	1000	2000	3000	4000	250	500	1000	2000	3000	4000	250	500	1000	2000	3000	4000
							0	5	5	5	5	0						
EM Level in Opp. Ear																		

	2 Frequency	3 Frequency	WEBER							2 Frequency	3 Frequency
Pure Tone Average	0	2	M	M	M	M	M	M	Pure Tone Average	5	5

SPEECH AUDIOMETRY

MASKING TYPE	RIGHT				LEFT			
	SRT 1	SRT 2	Recognition 1	Recognition 2	SRT 1	SRT 2	Recognition 1	Recognition 2
	0		1A List 30 SL 100 %	List SL %	5		2A List 30 SL 98 %	List SL %
EM Level in Opp. Ear								

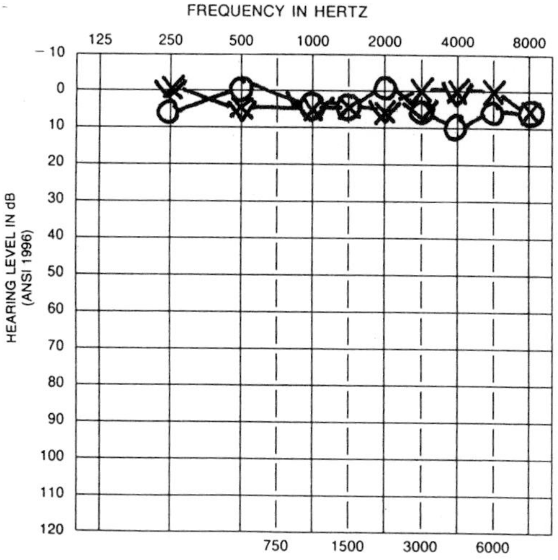

FREQUENCY IN HERTZ

COMMENTS

AUDIOGRAM KEY

	Right	Left
AC Unmasked	○	×
AC Masked	△	□
BC Mastoid Unmasked	<	>
BC Mastoid Masked	[	]
BC Forehead Masked	⌐	⌐

Both
BC Forehead Unmasked
Sound Field (unaided) S
Sound Field (aided) ●
Opp. Ear Masked
Examples of No Response Symbols

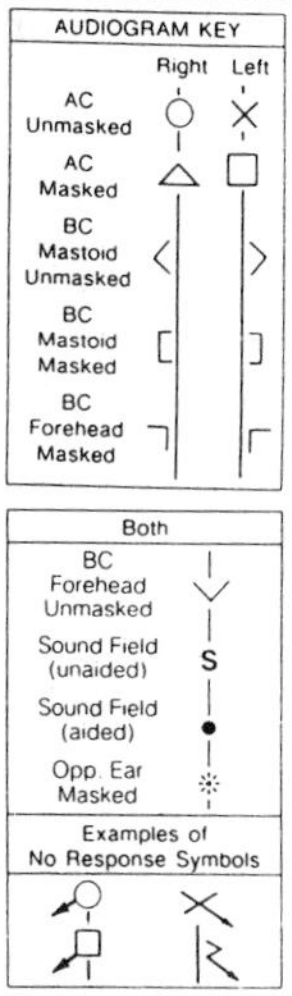

FIGURE 5.4 Audiogram illustrating normal hearing in both ears. Note that both the two- and three-frequency pure-tone averages compare favorably with the SRTs. The WRS in each ear is very high. No masking is indicated for any tests.

SPEECH AND HEARING CENTER
The University of Texas at Austin 78712
AUDIOMETRIC EXAMINATION

NAME: Last - First - Middle	SEX	AGE	DATE	EXAMINER	RELIABILITY	AUDIOMETER

AIR CONDUCTION

MASKING TYPE	RIGHT									LEFT								
	250	500	1000	1500	2000	3000	4000	6000	8000	250	500	1000	1500	2000	3000	4000	6000	8000
	35	40	45/45	40	40	50	45	50	55	40	40	45/45	45	50	55	55	60	60
EM Level in Opp. Ear																		

BONE CONDUCTION

MASKING TYPE	RIGHT						FOREHEAD						LEFT					
	250	500	1000	2000	3000	4000	250	500	1000	2000	3000	4000	250	500	1000	2000	3000	4000
NB	5*	5*	15*	20*	20*	15*	5	5	15	20	20	15	10*	5*	15*	20*	20*	20*
EM Level in Opp. Ear	40	40	45	50	55	55							50	40	45	40	50	60

	2 Frequency	3 Frequency	WEBER						2 Frequency	3 Frequency
Pure Tone Average	40	42	M	M	M	M	M	M	Pure Tone Average	43	45

SPEECH AUDIOMETRY

MASKING TYPE	RIGHT				LEFT			
	SRT 1	SRT 2	Recognition 1	Recognition 2	SRT 1	SRT 2	Recognition 1	Recognition 2
WB	45	45*	List 1A / SL 30 / 100%*	List / SL / %	45	45*	List 2A / SL 30 / 98%*	List / SL / %
EM Level in Opp. Ear		45	75			45	75	

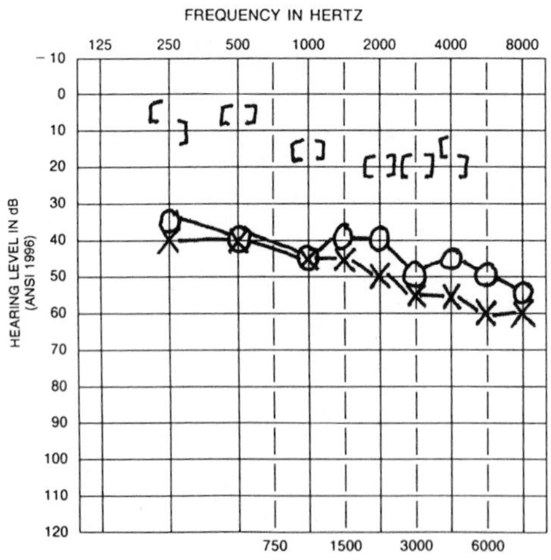

FREQUENCY IN HERTZ   COMMENTS

AUDIOGRAM KEY

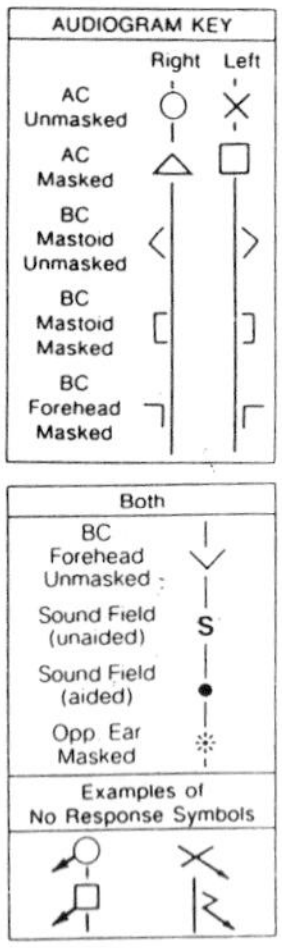

FIGURE 5.5   **Audiogram illustrating conductive hearing loss in both ears. The pure-tone averages are in close agreement with the SRTs. The WRSs are high in both ears. Because of the difference between the SRTs, and the opposite-ear bone-conduction thresholds, masking is required for testing SRTs and WRSs for both ears, although no evidence of cross-hearing was found. Speech noise was used for all speech masking.**

SPEECH AND HEARING CENTER
The University of Texas at Austin 78712
AUDIOMETRIC EXAMINATION

NAME: Last - First - Middle	SEX	AGE	DATE	EXAMINER	RELIABILITY	AUDIOMETER

AIR CONDUCTION

MASKING TYPE	RIGHT									LEFT								
	250	500	1000	1500	2000	3000	4000	6000	8000	250	500	1000	1500	2000	3000	4000	6000	8000
	35	35	40/40	45	50	60	70	70	75	40	35	45/45	50	55	60	65	65	60
EM Level in Opp. Ear																		

BONE CONDUCTION

MASKING TYPE	RIGHT						FOREHEAD						LEFT					
	250	500	1000	2000	3000	4000	250	500	1000	2000	3000	4000	250	500	1000	2000	3000	4000
							40	35	40	50	55	65						
EM Level in Opp. Ear																		

	2 Frequency	3 Frequency	WEBER						2 Frequency	3 Frequency
Pure Tone Average	38	42	M	M	M	M	M	M	Pure Tone Average 40	45

SPEECH AUDIOMETRY

MASKING TYPE	RIGHT				LEFT			
	SRT 1	SRT 2	Recognition 1	Recognition 2	SRT 1	SRT 2	Recognition 1	Recognition 2
	35		1C List / SL 30 78 %	List / SL %	40		2C List / SL 30 80 %	List / SL %
EM Level in Opp. Ear								

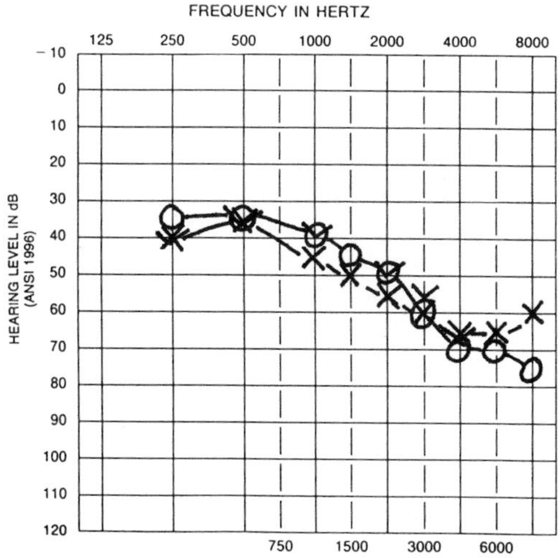

FREQUENCY IN HERTZ

COMMENTS

AUDIOGRAM KEY

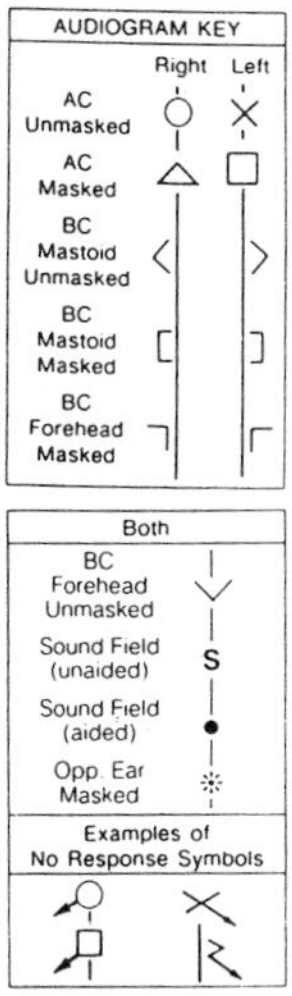

FIGURE 5.6 Audiogram illustrating sensorineural hearing loss in both ears. The pure-tone averages agree closely with the SRTs. WRSs show some word-recogniton difficulties in both ears. No masking is required for any speech tests.

STUDY QUESTIONS

1. Sketch, from memory, performance-intensity functions for spondaic words and PB word lists. Explain the differences in the curves on the basis of the words used.

2. Sketch audiograms illustrating normal hearing, as well as conductive, sensorineural, and mixed hearing losses. Predict the probable SRTs, WRSs, MCLs, UCLs, and RCLs.

3. What are the theoretical and practical values of the measures obtained in question 2?

4. Determine EM levels, if needed, for all speech tests in question 2.

5. List the different kinds of tests described in this chapter, and the different materials used for each test.

GLOSSARY

Binaural Listening with both ears to either the same or different stimuli.

California Consonant Test A closed-message word-recognition test, with the emphasis on unvoiced consonants to tax the abilities of patients with high-frequency hearing losses.

Carrier phrase A phrase, such as "Say the word _____," or "You will say _____," that precedes the stimulus word during speech audiometry. It is designed to prepare the patient for the test word and to assist the clinician (if a monitored live voice is used) in controlling the input loudness of the test word.

Cold running speech Rapidly delivered speech, either prerecorded or by monitored live voice, in which the output is monotonous and the peaks of the words strike zero on the VU meter.

Connected speech See *Cold running speech.*

Connected Speech Test (CST) A procedure by which the intelligibility of speech passages is measured on a sentence-by-sentence basis in the presence of a related background babble.

Consonant-nucleus-consonant (CNC) words Monosyllabic words used in testing word recognition. Each word has three phonemes; the initial and final phonemes are consonants, and the middle phoneme is a vowel or diphthong.

Dynamic range (DR) for speech See *Range of comfortable loudness.*

Loudness discomfort level See *Uncomfortable loudness level.*

Monaural Listening with one ear.

Monitored-live voice (MLV) Introduction of a speech signal (as in speech audiometry) through a microphone. The loudness of the voice is monitored visually by means of a VU meter (sometimes displayed as a series of light-emitting diodes).

Most comfortable loudness (MCL) The hearing level designated by a listener as the most comfortable listening level for speech.

Northwestern University Children's Perception of Speech (NUCHIPS) Test A picture-identification test for measuring the word-recognition abilities of small children.

PB Max The highest word-recognition score obtained with PB word lists on a performance-intensity function, regardless of level.

Performance-intensity function for PB word lists (PI-PB) A graph showing the percentage correct of word-recognition materials as a function of intensity. The graph usually shows the word-recognition score on the ordinate and the sensation level on the abscissa.

Phonetically balanced (PB) word lists Lists of monosyllabic words used for determining word-recognition scores. Theoretically, each list contains the same distribution of phonemes that occurs in connected English discourse.

Picture Identification Task (PIT) A word-recognition test using pictures of rhyming CNC words.

Range of comfortable loudness (RCL) The difference, in decibels, between the threshold for speech and the point at which speech becomes uncomfortably loud. It is determined by subtracting the SRT from the UCL. Also called the dynamic range (DR) for speech.

Signal-to-noise ratio (S/N) The difference, in decibels, between a signal (such as speech) and a noise presented to the same ear(s). When the speech has greater intensity than the noise, a positive sign is used; when the noise has greater intensity than the signal, a negative sign is used.

Speech-detection threshold (SDT) The hearing level at which a listener can just detect the presence of an ongoing speech signal and identify it as speech. Sometimes called the speech awareness threshold (SAT).

Speech Perception in Noise (SPIN) test A prerecorded sentence test with a voice babble recorded on the second channel of the same recording.

Speech-recognition threshold (SRT) The threshold of intelligibility of speech; the lowest intensity at which

at least 50 percent of a list of spondees can be identified correctly.

Spondaic word (spondee) A two-syllable word pronounced with equal stress on both syllables.

Synthetic sentence identification (SSI) A method for determining word recognition scores by means of seven-word sentences that are grammatically correct, but meaningless.

Threshold of discomfort (TD) See *Uncomfortable loudness level.*

Tolerance level See *Uncomfortable loudness level.*

Uncomfortable loudness level (UCL) That intensity at which speech becomes uncomfortably loud.

Word Intelligibility by Picture Identification (WIPI) test A test that uses pictures to determine word recognition ability in young children.

Word-recognition score (WRS) The percentage of correctly identified items on a word-recognition test.

REFERENCES

American National Standards Institute. (1996). *American National Standard specification for audiometers.* ANSI S3.6-1996. New York: Author.

American Speech-Language-Hearing Association (ASHA). (1978). Guidelines for manual pure-tone auditory. *Asha, 20,* 297–301.

———. (1979). Guidelines for determining the threshold level for speech. *Asha, 21,* 353–356.

———. (1988). Guidelines for determining threshold level for speech. *Asha, 30,* 85–89.

Barry, S. J., & Gaddis, S. (1978). Physical and physiological constraints on the use of bone conduction speech audiometry. *Journal of Speech and Hearing Disorders, 43,* 220–226.

Beattie, R. C., Forrester, P. W., & Ruby, B. K. (1987). Reliability of the Tillman-Olsen procedure for determination of spondaic word threshold using recorded and live voice presentation. *Journal of the American Audiology Society, 2,* 159–162.

Berry, R. C., & Nerbonne, C. P. (1971, October). *Comparison of the masking function of speech modulated and white noise.* Paper presented to the 82nd Meeting of the Acoustical Society of America, Denver.

Bilger, R. C., Nuetzel, J. M., Rabinowitz, W. M., & Rzeczkowski, C. (1984). Standardization of a test of speech perception in noise. *Journal of Speech and Hearing Research, 27,* 32–48.

Boothroyd, A. (1968). Developments in speech audiometry. *British Journal of Audiology, 2,* 3–10.

Burke, L. E., & Nerbonne, M. A. (1978). The influence of the guess factor on the speech reception threshold. *Journal of the American Auditory Society, 4,* 87–90.

Carhart, R. (1965). Problems in the measurement of speech discrimination. *Archives of Otolaryngology, 32,* 253–260.

Carhart, R., Johnson, C., & Goodman, J. (1975, November). *Perceptual masking of spondees by combination of talkers.* Paper presented to the 90th Meeting of the Acoustical Society of America, San Francisco.

Carhart, R., & Porter, L. S. (1971). Audiometric configuration and prediction of threshold for spondees. *Journal of Speech and Hearing Research, 14,* 486–495.

Carhart, R., Tillman, T. W., & Greetis, E. S. (1969). Perceptual masking in multiple sound backgrounds. *Journal of the Acoustical Society of America, 45,* 694–703.

Chaiklin, J. B., & Ventry, I. M. (1964). Spondee threshold measurement: A comparison of 2- and 5-dB methods. *Journal of Speech and Hearing Disorders, 29,* 47–59.

Conn, M., Dancer, J., & Ventry, I. M. (1975). A spondee list for determining speech reception threshold without prior familiarization. *Journal of Speech and Hearing Disorders, 40,* 376–388.

Cox, R. M., Alexander, G. C., & Gilmore, C. (1987). Development of the Connected Speech Test (CST). *Ear and Hearing, 8,* 1195–1265.

Cox, R. M., Alexander, G. C., Gilmore, C., & Pusakulich, K. M. (1988). Use of the Connected Speech Test with hearing-impaired listeners. *Ear and Hearing, 9,* 198–207.

Davis, H. & Silverman, S. R. (1978). *Hearing and deafness* (4th ed.). New York: Holt, Rinehart and Winston.

Edgerton, B. J., & Danhauer, J. L. (1979). *Clinical implications of speech discrimination testing using nonsense stimuli.* Baltimore: University Park Press.

Edgerton, B. J., Danhauer, J. L., & Beattie, R. C. (1977). Bone conduction speech audiometry in normal subjects. *Journal of the American Audiology Society, 3,* 84–87.

Egan, J. P. (1948). Articulation testing methods. *Laryngoscope, 58,* 955–991.

Eldert, M. A., & Davis, H. (1951). The articulation function of patients with conductive deafness. *Laryngoscope, 61,* 891–909.

Elliott, L. L., & Katz, D. (1980). *Development of a new children's test of speech discrimination.* St. Louis: Auditec.

Engelberg, M. (1968). Test-retest variability in speech discrimination testing. *Laryngoscope, 78,* 1582–1589.

Fairbanks, G. (1958). Test of phonemic differentiation: The rhyme test. *Journal of the Acoustical Society of America, 30,* 596–601.

Fletcher, H. (1950). Method of calculating hearing loss for speech from an audiogram. *Journal of the Acoustical Society of America, 22,* 1–5.

Frank, T., & McPhillips, M. A. (1976). *Relative intelligibility of the CID spondees for normal-hearing and hearing-impaired listeners.* Paper presented to the meeting of the American Speech and Hearing Association.

French, M. R., & Steinberg, J. C. (1947). Factors governing the intelligibility of speech sounds. *Journal of the Acoustical Society of America, 19,* 90–119.

Gardner, H. J. (1971). Application of a high frequency consonant discrimination word list in hearing-aid evaluation. *Journal of Speech and Hearing Disorders, 36,* 354–355.

Goetzinger, C. P. (1978). Word discrimination testing. In J. Katz (Ed.), *Handbook of clinical audiology* (2nd ed., pp. 149–158). Baltimore: Williams & Wilkins.

Goetzinger, C. P., & Proud, G. O. (1955). Speech audiometry by bone conduction. *Archives of Otolaryngology, 62,* 632–635.

Hahlbrock, K. H. (1962). Bone conduction speech audiometry. *International Audiology, 1,* 186–188.

Haskins, H. (1949). *A phonetically balanced test of speech discrimination for children.* Master's thesis, Northwestern University.

Hirsh, I., Davis, H., Silverman, S. R., Reynolds, E., Eldert, E., & Benson, R. W. (1952). Development of materials for speech audiometry. *Journal of Speech and Hearing Disorders, 17,* 321–337.

Hosford-Dunn, H., Runge, C. A., & Montgomery, P. (1983). A shortened rank-ordered word discrimination list. *The Hearing Journal, 36,* 15–19.

House, A. S., Williams, C. E., Hecker, M. H. L., & Kryter, K. D. (1965). Articulation testing methods: Consonantal differentiation with a closed-response set. *Journal of the Acoustical Society of America, 37,* 158–166.

Hudgins, C. V., Hawkins, J. E., Jr., Karlin, J. E., & Stevens, S. S. (1947). The development of recorded auditory tests for measuring hearing loss for speech. *Laryngoscope, 57,* 89.

Jerger, J., Johnson, K., & Jerger, S. (1988). Effect of response criterion on measures of speech understanding in the elderly. *Ear and Hearing, 9,* 49–56.

Jerger, J., Speaks, C., & Trammell, J. L. (1968). A new approach to speech audiometry. *Journal of Speech and Hearing Disorders, 33,* 318–328.

Kalikow, D. M., Stevens, K. N., & Elliott, L. L. (1977). Development of a test of speech intelligibility in noise using sentence materials with controlled predictability. *Journal of the Acoustical Society of America, 61,* 1337–1351.

Konkle, D. F., & Berry, G. A. (1983). Masking in speech audiometry. In D. F. Konkle & W. F. Rintelmann (Eds.), *Principles of speech audiometry* (pp. 285–319). Baltimore: University Park Press.

Konkle, D. F, & Rintelmann, W. F. (1983). Introduction to speech audiometry. In D. F. Konkle & W. F. Rintelmann (Eds.), *Principles of speech audiometry* (pp. 1–10). Baltimore: University Park Press.

Lehiste, I., & Peterson, G. E. (1959). Linguistic considerations in the study of speech intelligibility. *Journal of the Acoustical Society of America, 31,* 280–286.

———. (1962). Revised CNC lists for auditory tests. *Journal of Speech and Hearing Disorders, 27,* 62–70.

Martin, F. N. (1966). Speech audiometry and clinical masking. *Journal of Auditory Research, 6,* 199–203.

———. (1972). *Clinical audiometry and masking.* The Bobbs-Merrill Studies in Communicative Disorders. New York: Bobbs-Merrill.

Martin, F. N., Bailey, H. A. T., & Pappas, J. J. (1965). The effect of central masking on threshold for speech. *Journal of Auditory Research, 5,* 293–296.

Martin, F. N., & Blythe, M. (1977). On the cross-hearing of spondaic words. *Journal of Auditory Research, 17,* 221–224.

Martin, F. N., Champlin, C. A. & Chambers, J. (1998). Seventh survey of audiometric practices in the United States. *Journal of the American Academy of Audiology, 9,* 95–104.

Martin, F. N., & DiGiovanni, D. (1979). Central masking effects on spondee thresholds as a function of masker sensation level and masker sound pressure level. *Journal of the American Audiology Society, 4,* 141–146.

Martin, F. N., & Dowdy, L. K. (1986). A modified spondee threshold procedure. *Journal of Auditory Research, 26,* 115–119.

Martin, F. N., Severance, G. K., & Thibodeau, L. (1991). Insert earphones for speech recognition testing. *Journal of the American Academy of Audiology, 2,* 55–58.

Martin, F. N., & Stauffer, M. L. (1975). A modification of the Tillman-Olsen method for obtaining the speech reception threshold. *Journal of Speech and Hearing Disorders, 40,* 25–28.

Owens, E., & Schubert, E. D. (1977). Development of the California Consonant Test. *Journal of Speech and Hearing Research, 20,* 463–474.

Pascoe, D. R. (1975). Frequency responses of hearing aids and their effects on the speech perception of hearing impaired subjects. *Annals of Otology, Rhinology and Laryngology, 23* (Supplement), 1–40.

Ross, M., & Huntington, D. A. (1962). Concerning the reliability and equivalency of the CID W-22 auditory tests. *Journal of Auditory Research, 2,* 220–228.

Ross, M., & Lerman, J. (1970). A picture identification test for hearing impaired children. *Journal of Speech and Hearing Research, 13,* 44–53.

Sanderson-Leepa, M. E., & Rintelmann, W. F. (1976). Articulation function and test-retest performance of normal-hearing children on three speech discrimination tests: WIPI, PBK 50 and NU Auditory Test No. 6. *Journal of Speech and Hearing Disorders, 41,* 503–519.

Schum, D. J., & Matthews, L. J. (1992). SPIN test performance of elderly hearing-impaired listeners. *Journal of the American Academy of Audiology, 3,* 303–307.

Speaks, C., & Jerger, J. (1965). Method for measurement of speech identification. *Journal of Speech and Hearing Research, 8,* 185–194.

Spearman, C. (1908). The method of right and wrong cases ("Constant Stimuli") without Gauss's formulae. *British Journal of Audiology, 2,* 227–242.

Stach, B. A. (1988). Computers and audiologic instrumentation. *Hearing Instruments, 39,* 13–16.

Thornton, A. R., & Raffin, M. J. M. (1978). Speech discrimination scores modified as a binomial variable. *Journal of Speech and Hearing Research, 21,* 507–518.

Tillman, T. W., & Carhart, R. (1966). *An expanded test for speech discrimination utilizing CNC monosyllabic words.* Northwestern University Auditory Test No. 6, Technical Report, SAM-TR-66-55. Brooks Air Force Base, TX: USAF School of Aerospace Medicine, Aerospace Medical Division (AFSC).

Tillman, T. W., Carhart, R., & Wilber, L. (1963). *A test for speech discrimination composed of CNC monosyllabic words.* Northwestern University Auditory Test No. 4, Technical Report, SAM-TDR-62-135. Brooks Air Force Base, TX: USAF School of Aerospace Medicine, Aerospace Medical Division (AFSC).

Tillman, T. W., & Jerger, J. F. (1959). Some factors affecting the spondee threshold in normal-hearing subjects. *Journal of Speech and Hearing Research, 2,* 141–146.

Tillman, T. W. & Olsen, W. O. (1973). Speech audiometry. In J. Jerger (Ed.), *Modern developments in audiology* (2nd ed.; pp. 37–74). New York: Academic Press.

Tobias, J. V. (1964). On phonemic analysis of speech discrimination tests. *Journal of Speech and Hearing Research, 7,* 98–100.

Tonry, K. L. (1988). *A comparison of discrimination scores using the short isophonemic and CID W-22 word lists.* Unpublished masters thesis, University of Cincinnati.

Wilson, R. H., & Antablin, J. K. (1980). A picture identification task as an estimate of the word-recognition performance of nonverbal adults. *Journal of Speech and Hearing Disorders, 45,* 223–238.

Wilson, R. H., & Margolis, R. H. (1983). Measurements of auditory thresholds for speech stimuli. In D. F. Konkle & W. F. Rintelmann (Eds.), *Principles of speech audiometry* (pp. 79–126). Baltimore: University Park Press.

Wittich, W. W., Wood, T. J., & Mahaffey, R. B. (1971). Computerized speech audiometric procedures. *Journal of Auditory Research, 11,* 335–344.

Young, L. L., Parker, C., & Carhart, R. (1975, November). *Effectiveness of speech and noise maskers on numbers embedded in continuous discourse.* Paper presented to the 90th Meeting of the Acoustical Society of America, San Francisco.

SUGGESTED READING

Martin, M. (Ed.). (1997). *Speech audiometry* (2nd ed.). San Diego: Singular Publishing Group.

REVIEW TABLE 5.1   Summary of Tests Used in Speech Audiometry

Test	Purpose	Material	Unit	When to Mask	Initial Masking
SRT	HL for speech recognition Verify PTA	Spondees; Cold-running speech	dB	$SRT_{TE}-40 \geq BBC_{NTE}$	$EM = SRT_{TE}$ If over 5 dB, shift plateau
SDT	HL for speech awareness	Cold-running speech	dB	$SDT_{TE}-40 \geq BBC_{NTE}$	$EM = SDT_{TE}$
MCL	Comfort level for speech	Cold-running speech	dB	$SDT_{TE}-40 \geq BBC_{NTE}$	$EM = BBC_{TE} + 40$ dB
UCL	Level at which speech becomes un-comfortably loud	Cold-running speech	dB	$UCL_{TE}-40 \geq BBC_{NTE}$	$EM = BBC_{TE} + 40$ dB
RCL (DR)	Dynamic listening range for speech	Cold-running speech	dB		
WRS	Recognition of speech	PB words; CNC words; rhyming words; sentences	%	$HL_{TE}-40 \geq BBC_{NTE}$	$HL_{TE} - IA + ABG_{NTE}$

TE = test ear; NTE = nontest ear; PTA = pure-tone average; EM = effective masking; IA = interaural attenuation; BBC = best (lowest) bone-conduction threshold.

6

Electrophysiological Tests

Chapters 4 and 5 described measurements of hearing that can be made with pure tones and speech. These tests require the active cooperation of patients. The purpose of this chapter is to discuss some of the electrophysiological procedures that have been developed that serve both as indices of hearing sensitivity and as indications of the site of a lesion in the auditory system. For the most part, these tests do not require behavioral responses from patients.

All of the procedures to be described require the use of specially designed equipment. With this equipment audiologists can now accumulate valuable information for diagnostic purposes from a variety of procedures. These tests measure impedance and compliance in the plane of the eardrum membrane, changes in the pattern of electrical activity in the brain in response to acoustic stimuli, and tiny echoes whose presence can estimate the integrity of the inner ear.

Chapter Objectives

At this point the reader should have a good grasp of the tests described earlier, as well as a general knowledge of how the ear is constructed and how it responds to sound. An understanding of the procedures to follow is essential to the study of clinical audiology. It will allow readers to more fully comprehend the examples of different hearing disorders caused by damage to different parts of the auditory system that will be described in Chapters 9–12.

Acoustic Immittance

Measurements of acoustic **immittance** have become as routine in the audiometric battery as pure-tone and speech audiometry. Immittance measures guide the diagnostic audiologist in identifying abnormalities in the auditory system in numbers of ways. The introduction of acoustic immittance measures three decades ago was a milestone in audiology, and most audiologists would agree that this procedure is basic to the test battery.

For a number of years, interest has been directed toward the effects of various kinds of pathology on **acoustic impedance** in the plane of the eardrum membrane. Initially, most impedance measurements were made with mechanical devices too clumsy and too difficult to use routinely. A variety of commercial electroacoustic impedance meters (Figure 6.1), are commonly used by audiologists today. Most devices measure **compliance,** which is related to the dimensions of an enclosed volume

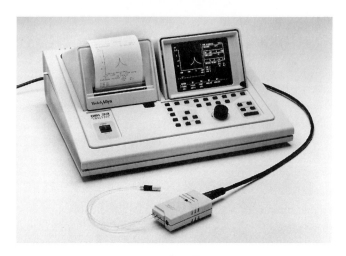

FIGURE 6.1 An electroacoustic immittance meter. (Courtesy of Grason-Stadler Co.)

of air as expressed on a scale of different units of measurement. Examples of the different units are cubic centimeters (cm^3) or milliliters (ml) of an equivalent volume of air in the middle ear.

Several terms have been used to describe the various measurements made in the plane of the eardrum membrane. The word immittance is used as an all-encompassing term to describe measurements made of eardrum membrane impedance, compliance, or admittance. The American National Standards Institute (ANSI, 1987) has adopted a set of standards that define both the characteristics of instruments used in the measurement of acoustic immittance and the associated terminology.

Immittance measures are often called "immittance audiometry," a term that is technically incorrect since audiometry is the measurement of hearing. Determinations of acoustic immittance are also frequently called "middle-ear measurements," which is also misleading since the measurements are not actually made of the middle ear. All determinations of middle-ear function are indirectly made by measurements made in the plane of the eardrum membrane.

Measurements Made on Acoustic Immittance Meters

Basically, three measurements are made in the plane of the eardrum membrane:

1. **Static acoustic compliance,** which is the mobility of the drum membrane in response to a given value of air pressure in the external ear canal.
2. **Tympanometry,** which is a measurement of middle-ear pressure, determined by the mobility of the membrane as a function of various amounts of positive and negative air pressure in the external ear canal (the more positive or negative the air pressure in the external ear canal the more the normal middle-ear system becomes immobilized, or "clamped").
3. Contraction of the middle-ear muscles, known as the **acoustic reflex,** in response to intense sounds, which has the effect of stiffening the middle ear system and decreasing its static acoustic compliance.

Factors Governing Acoustic Immittance

The reader will recall from Chapter 3 that the impedance (Z) of any object is determined by its frictional resistance (R), mass (M), and stiffness (S). The effects of mass and stiffness are critically dependent on the frequency (f) of the sound being measured. The formula for impedance is stated as

$$Z = \sqrt{R^2 + (2\pi f M - S/2\pi f)^2}$$

The combination of mass and stiffness (contained within the parentheses in the formula) is called complex resistance or **reactance.** Simple resistance is obviously independent of the rest of the formula, whereas mass reactance and stiffness reactance are inversely related to each other and are critically dependent on frequency. As frequency increases, the total value of the mass reactance factor also increases. Conversely, as frequency goes up, the effects of stiffness reactance diminish. Mass is therefore the important factor in the high frequencies, and stiffness is the important factor in the low frequencies. As the stiffness of a system increases, it is said to become less compliant; that is, it becomes more difficult to initiate motion. Compliance, therefore, is the inverse of the stiffness factor of the formula.

The anatomy of the ear was described in a cursory fashion in Chapter 2. Details are brought out in Chapters 9 through 12, and the effects of various disorders on immittance are discussed. For the present, however, the following general assignments of values can be made: Resistance is determined primarily by the ligaments that support the three bones in the middle-ear cavity. The mass factor is determined primarily by the weight of these three tiny bones, and the eardrum membrane. Stiffness is primarily determined by the load of fluid pressure from the inner ear on the base of the stapes, the most medial bone of the middle ear. The ear, therefore, is largely a stiffness-dominated system, at least in response to low-frequency sounds.

Equipment for Middle-ear Immittance Measurements

An electroacoustic immittance meter is diagrammed in Figure 6.2. Three small plastic or rubber tubes are attached to a metal probe, which is fitted into the external ear canal with an airtight seal. A

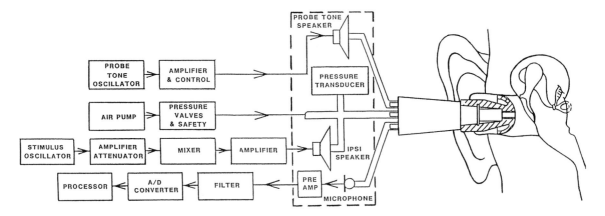

FIGURE 6.2 **Diagram of an electroacoustic immittance meter. (Courtesy of Grason-Stadler Co.)**

plastic or rubber cuff, placed around the probe, can be varied in size to accommodate most ears. The three tubes are connected to (1) a miniature loudspeaker, which emits a pure tone, usually at 220 or 226 Hz (the incident wave); (2) a tiny microphone, which picks up the sound in the ear canal (the sound comprising both the incident wave introduced to the ear from the speaker and the reflected wave as its returns from the eardrum membrane); and (3) an air pump, which can create either positive or negative air pressure within the canal. The air pump is calibrated in milliliters (ml), millimeters of water (mm H_2O), or dekapascals (daPa [tenths of a Pascal]). The units of measurement are very similar: 1 daPa = 1.02 mm H_2O, and 1 mm H_2O = 0.98 daPa, when measurements are made at standardized conditions of temperature and pressure. The devices must be calibrated so that 0 daPa (or 0 mm H_2O), is equal to atmospheric pressure at the site where measurements are to be made. The probe is attached to one side of a headset. An earphone connected to an acoustic reflex activator system, is attached to the opposite side (Figure 6.3), and functions as a built-in pure-tone audiometer.

Measurement of Static Acoustic Compliance

For static acoustic compliance to be measured, the ear canal should first be cleared of any occluding earwax or other debris. Even the smallest amount of material in the ear canal may clog one of the tiny probe tubes and make measurements impossible or very misleading. The ear tip is pressed into the ear canal, a tight seal is obtained, and positive pressure is increased with the air pump. Observation of the meter will indicate whether the necessary airtight seal has been obtained, or whether resealing, perhaps with a different-sized tip, is necessary. Once the seal is obtained, the pressure is increased to +200 daPa. On most instruments the intensity of the probe tone is automatically adjusted

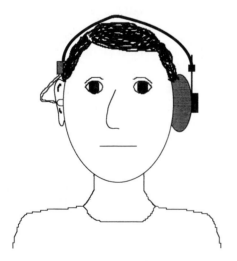

FIGURE 6.3   Configuration of the probe of an immittance meter in one ear and an audiometer earphone on the other ear.

until the desired sound-pressure level is obtained, usually 85 to 90 dB. The clinician can then determine the **equivalent volume** in cubic centimeters. This measurement, made with the eardrum membrane loaded with +200 daPa of pressure, is called c_1. This first measurement, c_1, therefore, is made with the eardrum membrane immobilized by positive air pressure, and it represents the compliance of the outer ear.

The second step in determining static acoustic compliance is attained when the pressure in the external ear canal is gradually decreased until the eardrum membrane achieves maximum compliance—that is, when pressures on both sides of the membrane are approximately equal. Another reading is taken, called c_2, which represents static acoustic compliance of the outer ear and middle ear combined. Many audiologists believe that c_2 should be measured with outer-ear pressure at 0 daPa (the ambient air pressure). The static acoustic compliance of the middle ear (c_x) can then be determined by working through the formula

$$c_x = c_2 - c_1$$

During conditions for measurement of c_1, the drum membrane's relative immobility causes a good deal of energy to be returned to the probe, raising the sound-pressure level in the external ear canal. The membrane's increased mobility during the c_2 measurement allows more energy to be admitted to the middle ear, lowering the sound pressure between the membrane and the probe. The static acoustic compliance of the middle ear (ME) mechanism is the difference between these two conditions, which cancels out the compliance of the external auditory canal (EAC). Stated as a formula,

$$c \text{ (ME)} = c \text{ (EAC + ME)} - c \text{ (EAC)}$$

Normal Values for Static Acoustic Compliance. Research over the years has not led to agreement on what values constitute normal static acoustic compliance. Studies have concluded that there are differences between adults and children, and among the various probe tone frequencies available. Most devices disregard the phase angle of the incident (original) and reflected waves in the ear canal. The fact that there is considerable variability for normal ears, often overlapping middle-ear conditions that cause high or low compliance, significantly reduces the value of this test. Values between 0.30 and 1.60 cm^3 may be considered the normal range (Hall & Chandler, 1994). Although this range is broad, a patient's middle-ear compliance values really cannot be considered abnormal unless one of the extremes is clearly exceeded. Even in individuals with normal middle ears the values of static compliance vary with both age and gender.

Recording and Interpreting Static Acoustic Compliance. Results of static acoustic compliance measures should be recorded on forms especially prepared for this purpose (Figure 6.4A). Some devices make these measurements automatically and provide a paper printout with the compliance values for each ear tested. However the numbers appear, they should become an integral part of the patient's record.

Compliance values below the normal range suggest some change in the stiffness, mass, or resistance of the middle ear, causing less than normal mobility of the eardrum membrane. This may result from fluid accumulation in the normally air-filled middle ear or immobility of the chain of middle-ear bones. High compliance suggests some interruption in the chain of bones, possibly caused by disease or fracture, or by abnormal elasticity of the eardrum membrane. Reduced elasticity of the eardrum membrane may be due to age or caused by partial healing of a previous perforation.

Although static acoustic compliance measures are an integral part of any audiological workup, like any diagnostic test they can be misleading. It is possible for different abnormalities of the ear to have opposing effects, resulting in what appear to be essentially normal immittance values (Popelka, 1983).

Tympanometry

The eardrum membrane vibrates most efficiently when the pressure on both sides is equal. This statement is basic to the understanding of tympanometry. As the membrane is displaced from its resting position by positive or negative pressure in the external ear canal, the vibratory efficiency of the membrane is decreased. Tympanometry is performed by loading the eardrum membrane with air pressure equal to +200 daPa, measuring its compliance, and then making successive measurements of compliance as the pressure in the canal is decreased. Pressure can be varied manually, in discrete steps of, for example, 50 daPa, or can be continuously varied by a motor-driven system. After the pressure has reached 0 daPa (atmospheric pressure), negative pressure is created by the pump and additional compliance measurements are made. The purpose of tympanometry is to determine the point and magnitude of greatest compliance of the eardrum membrane. Such measurements give invaluable information regarding the condition of the middle-ear structures. Performing tympanometry immediately after determining c_1 allows determination of both c_2 and the ear canal pressure required for measuring acoustic reflex thresholds.

Tympanometry is generally conducted with a low-frequency probe tone of 220 or 226 Hz. The use of higher-frequency probe tones, or a succession of different frequencies, can modify results in a variety of ways, making this test more valuable diagnostically (Shanks, Lilly, Margolis, Wiley, & Wilson, 1988). The difficulties encountered in the use of multifrequency tympanometry are mitigated by the newest generation of devices, which are microprocessor controlled.

Recording and Interpreting Tympanometric Results.   The compliance measurements may be recorded directly on a graph called a **tympanogram,** which shows compliance on the Y axis and pressure, in dekapascals, on the X axis (Figure 6.4F). Some clinicians find it useful to record their results numerically (Figure 6.4G) before drawing the graph. Popular today are units on which the tympanogram is recorded directly and automatically on a graph, showing pressure in dekapascals on the X axis and compliance on the Y axis. The advantage of this recording method is that it provides more accuracy than manually plotting discrete points on the tympanogram. The interpretation of the tympanograms is essentially the same.

Jerger (1970) has categorized typical tympanometric results into different types. To facilitate direct comparison, all five tympanogram types are illustrated on the same form (Figure 6.5).

Type A.   Type A curves are seen in patients who have normal middle-ear function. The point of greatest compliance is at 0 daPa (usually ± 50 daPa), and the curve is characterized by a rather large inverted V. Some clinics consider values of ± 100 daPa to represent a Type A.

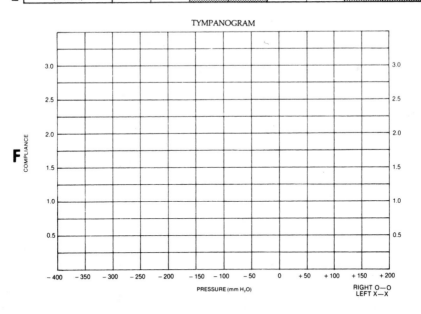

FIGURE 6.4   Form for recording results of immittance measures: (A) static compliance; (B) contralateral acoustic reflex thresholds; (C) behavioral thresholds obtained during standard pure-tone audiometry; (D) sensation levels of the reflexes (B minus C); (E) the number of seconds required for the reflex to decay to half of its original amplitude; (F) a graph (the tympanogram) showing the pressure-compliance function; (G) numerical data showing the amount of compliance observed with various amounts of positive and negative air pressure in the external auditory canal; (H) acoustic reflexes obtained with the probe tone and reflex eliciting stimulus presented to the same ear.

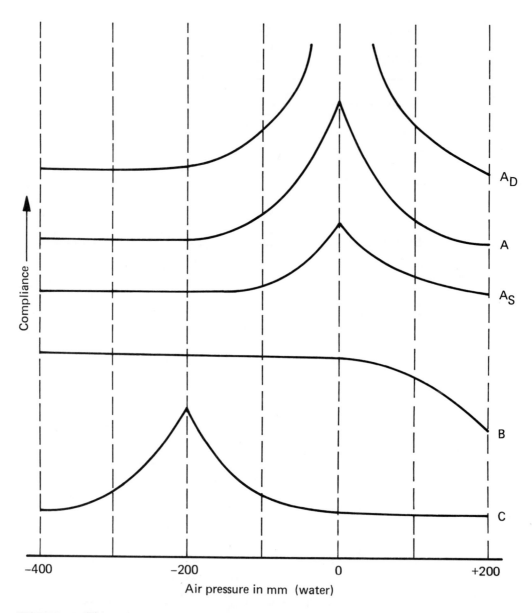

FIGURE 6.5 **Five typical tympanograms illustrating various conditions of the middle ear. Type A shows normal pressure-compliance functions and is typical of normal middle ears. Type AS curves are like the A curves but are much shallower and are associated with stiffness of the stapes, the smallest of the middle-ear bones. Type AD curves are much deeper than the normal Type A curves, and are symptomatic of interruptions in the chain of middle-ear bones or flaccidity of the eardrum membrane. Type B shows no pressure setting at which the eardrum membrane becomes most compliant, and suggests fluid in the middle-ear space. Type C shows the eardrum membrane to be most compliant when the pressure in the ear canal is negative, suggesting that the pressure within the middle-ear space is below atmospheric pressure.**

Type A$_S$.   Type A$_S$ curves show the same characteristic peak at or near 0 daPa, suggesting normal middle-ear pressure, however, the peak is much shallower than that of the usual Type A. Type A$_S$ curves are often seen in patients in whom the stapes has become partially immobilized. The "S" may stand for "stiffness" or for "shallow."

Type A$_D$.   In some cases the general Type A pattern is preserved; however, the amplitude of the curve is unusually high, or in some cases the positive and negative sides of the spike do not meet at all in Type A$_D$ curves. Such curves may be associated with flaccidity of the eardrum membrane or separation of the chain of middle-ear bones. The "D," therefore, may stand for "discontinuous" or for "deep."

Type B.   Type B curves are seen when the middle-ear space is filled with fluid. Because even wide variations of pressure in the ear canal can never match the pressure of fluid behind the tympanic membrane, the point of greatest compliance cannot be found. Type B curves may also be seen when a small amount of earwax or other debris occludes one of the tiny tubes within the probe, when a wax plug blocks the external ear canal, or when there is a hole in the eardrum membrane so that the meter measures the compliance of the rigid walls of the middle ear. Therefore, when Type B curves are evident, the clinician should make certain that these factors are not present.

Type C.   In certain conditions, discussed in Chapter 10, the pressure in the middle ear falls below normal. In such cases the tympanic membrane becomes most compliant when the pressure in the ear canal is negative, thus equaling the middle-ear pressure. When maximum membrane compliance occurs at a negative pressure of –100 daPa or greater, middle-ear pressure is considered to be abnormally negative.

At times it may erroneously appear that a tympanogram is flat, missing a peak pressure point. This can be due to negative middle-ear pressure that is so extreme that the peak pressure point does not appear. In cases of "flat" tympanograms it is often advisable to make immittance measures as low as –400 daPa. Such extremely negative middle-ear pressure may have significant medical effects on the patient, and they should be pointed out to the physician managing the case, or a medical referral should be made.

On occasion, a peak pressure point is observed in patients at positive pressures, greater than +50 daPa. This is sometimes seen in children who have been crying, patients who have blown their noses, and so on. It is likely that any such condition is short-lived and normal middle-ear pressure will become restored in a short time. If positive peak pressure is observed for longer than a brief period, it might be advisable to ask for a medical consultation.

A number of factors may influence the outcome of tympanometry. When pressure is varied from positive to negative, the peak of the wave is lower than when pressure is changed from negative to positive, although this rarely affects the interpretation of results. Performing tympanometry with different probe tone frequencies and even multifrequency testing can yield different results.

The shape of the tympanogram, or **gradient,** is a ratio between the height and width of the tympanogram (width over height). The steeper the ratio, the greater the amplitude of the tympanometric peak and the greater the inferred acoustic compliance. The American Speech-Language-Hearing Association (1990) has set up standards for measuring the tympanometric gradient, although it is not yet entirely agreed which types of measurement devices best accomplish this task.

Acoustic Reflexes

Definition of the Acoustic Reflex

Two small muscles, the **tensor tympani muscle** and the **stapedius muscle,** are involved in the operation of the middle-ear mechanism. The anatomy of these muscles is discussed in Chapter 10, but they are mentioned here because their action makes them an important part of the immittance battery. Although there is uncertainty about the role of the tensor tympani in response to sound in humans, it is generally accepted that the stapedius muscle in each middle ear normally contracts reflexively when an intense sound is introduced to either or both ears causing both tympanic membranes to stiffen. This has been called the acoustic reflex. Most normal-hearing individuals will effect a bilateral **intra-aural muscle reflex** when pure tones are introduced to either ear at 70 to 100 dB above threshold (median response level 85 dB SL) (Northern & Gabbard, 1994).

Measuring the Acoustic Reflex

The immittance meter enables the clinician to present a signal to one ear and detect a decrease in tympanic membrane compliance in either that ear (the ipsilateral acoustic reflex) or the opposite ear (the contralateral acoustic reflex). The signal used to produce the acoustic reflex is called the **reflex activating stimulus (RAS),** which can be any kind of sound from a pure tone to a noise band. Normally pure tones sampling the frequency range from 500 to 4000 Hz are used. A pure tone of the desired frequency should be introduced at 70 dB HL. If no compliance change is seen on the meter, the level should be raised to 80 dB, 90 dB, and so on, until a response is seen or the limit of the equipment is reached. Some commercial meters allow intensities up to 125 dB HL to be tested, but great care should be taken in introducing signals at such high levels. It is often inadvisable to exceed 115 dB HL.

If a response is observed, the level should be lowered 10 dB, then raised in 5 dB steps until the threshold can be determined. The tonal duration should be about one second, and measurements should be taken that sample the frequency range—for example, 500, 1000, 2000, and 4000 Hz, although, for no explainable reason, many normal-hearing individuals show no acoustic reflex at 4000 Hz. The lowest level at which an acoustic reflex can be obtained is called the **acoustic reflex threshold (ART).**

Criteria for the amount of compliance decrease required to constitute a response vary with different devices. At times a very small compliance change is observed, and the audiologist may be uncertain whether a response has truly been obtained. In such cases, when the level is raised 5 dB, an unequivocal response is usually observed. Extraneous compliance variations sometimes occur as the patient breathes, or occasionally the very sensitive probe microphone picks up a pulse from a blood vessel near the external ear canal. Of course, the patient must be completely silent during these measurements lest vocalizations be picked up by the microphone, masking changes in compliance. Proper recording of the intensity required to evoke an acoustic reflex assists in appropriate interpretation of results (Figure 6.4B).

Implications of the Acoustic Reflex

To understand the implications of acoustic reflex testing, it is important to have a basic knowledge of what is called the **acoustic reflex arc.** This pathway includes centers that are discussed in greater detail in Chapters 10 through 12 of this book, but they are mentioned here and diagrammed in Figure 6.6.

A sound presented to the outer ear is passed through the middle ear as mechanical energy, transduced to an electrochemical signal in the cochlea of the inner ear, and then conducted along the VIIIth

RIGHT   **LEFT**

CROSSOVER

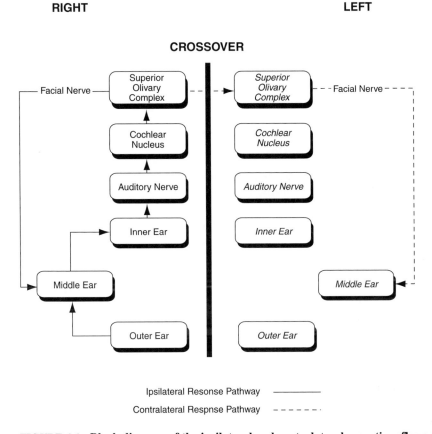

Ipsilateral Resonse Pathway ————
Contralateral Respnse Pathway – – – – – –

FIGURE 6.6   Block diagram of the ipsilateral and contralateral acoustic reflex pathways.

cranial (auditory) nerve to the brainstem. The impulse is received by the cochlear nucleus in the brainstem and is transmitted to the superior olivary complex. Here, some very interesting things occur: In addition to transmitting signals to higher centers in the brain (not shown in Figure 6.6), nerve impulses are sent from the superior olivary complex to the VIIth cranial (facial) nerve on the same side of the head, which in turn descends to innervate the stapedius muscle in the middle ear that originally received the sound, assuming that all systems are working properly. This is called the *ipsilateral response pathway*. In short, a sound presented to one ear can evoke an acoustic reflex in the same ear.

Almost simultaneously, neural impulses cross the brainstem to the opposite (contralateral) superior olivary complex, which in turn sends impulses by *that* facial nerve to the middle ear on the other side to evoke an acoustic reflex along the *contralateral response pathway*. Therefore, a stimulus presented to one ear evokes an acoustic reflex in the opposite middle ear as well as in the same ear. Although measurement of the acoustic reflex is made clinically in one ear at a time, in healthy ears, and in some pathological cases, responses occur in both ears in response to a stimulus presented to only one ear. Measurements are always made through the probe tip; however, the RAS may be presented through an earphone coupled to the ear opposite the probe assembly (the contralateral reflex), or through the probe tip itself (the ipsilateral reflex) (Figure 6.6). The measurement of ipsilateral and contralateral reflexes is extremely valuable in audiological diagnosis.

There are four possible outcomes on an acoustic reflex test:

1. The reflex may be present at a normal sensation level (about 85 dB SL).
2. The reflex may be absent at the limit of the reflex activating system (usually 110 to 125 dB HL).
3. The reflex may be present, in the case of a hearing loss, but at a low sensation level (less than 60 dB above the audiometric threshold).
4. The reflex may be present, but at a high sensation level (greater than 100 dB above the audiometric threshold).

Interpreting the Acoustic Reflex

Significance is placed on the presence or absence of the intra-aural muscle reflex and in terms of the level of the RAS above the audiometric threshold (Figures 6.4B and 6.4D) required to elicit the response. Abnormalities in the muscles themselves will, of course, affect the reflex in the ear to which the probe is affixed. In addition, the contraction of the muscles may not result in eardrum membrane stiffening if the chain of bones in the middle ear is immobile or interrupted, or if fluid is present in the middle-ear space.

Figure 6.7 illustrates theoretical findings on acoustic reflex tests with eleven possible conditions of the auditory and related systems. In each (lettered) example the condition is stated and the patients appear facing the reader as they would with the audiometer earphone over the right ear and the immittance meter probe in the left, and then with the earphone over the left ear and the probe in the right. During contralateral stimulation in each case the earphone delivers the RAS to one ear while the reflex is monitored via the probe in the opposite ear. During ipsilateral stimulation the RAS is delivered and monitored by the probe in the same ear. There are, of course, many other possibilities in addition to those shown and different constellations of responses may be attributed to a number of factors.

1. Middle-ear muscle reflexes will be present at about 85 dB SL in normal-hearing individuals (Figure 6.7A).
2. The middle-ear muscle reflex will be absent if the reflex activating tone presented to the ear is not sufficiently intense. The intensity of the tone will be attenuated if any of several types of hearing losses are present, especially those caused by conductive loss (Figure 6.7B, C).
3. Sometimes the reflex appears in an ear with a hearing loss when the stimulus is presented at a fairly low sensation level. Why would a person with a 50 dB hearing loss experience a reflex at 95 dB HL (45 dB SL)? A precise explanation for low-sensation-level acoustic reflexes, which are associated with cochlear lesions, is lacking at this time (Figure 6.7D, E).
4. When a severe cochlear hearing loss exists in the ear that receives the RAS there will often be no response at the limit of the equipment (Figure 6.7F). This is because the intensity of the signal reaching the brainstem is insufficient to produce the reflex.
5. When there is damage to the auditory (VIIIth cranial) nerve, acoustic reflexes are often absent or occur at higher than normal sensation levels, or the amplitude of the reflex is less than normal. This is probably due to alterations in the transmission of the RAS from the cochlea to the brainstem (Figure 6.7G).
6. The facial nerve supplies innervation to the stapedius muscle. If the facial nerve is in any way abnormal, the command supplied by the brain that mediates contractions may not be conveyed to the stapedius muscle. This occurs when the damage is in the ear to which the probe is affixed, regardless of whether the RAS is delivered ipsilaterally (Figure 6.7H) or contralaterally.

7. Even if the ipsilateral acoustic reflex pathway is normal, if damage occurs in the areas of the brainstem that house portions of the contralateral acoustic reflex pathway, ipsilateral reflexes may be present in both ears, but one or both of the contralateral reflexes may be absent, depending on the precise site and size of the lesion (Figure 6.7I, J).
8. Lesions in the higher centers of the auditory cortex usually produce no abnormalities in either contralateral or ipsilateral reflexes because these centers are above the acoustic reflex arc (Figure 6.7K).

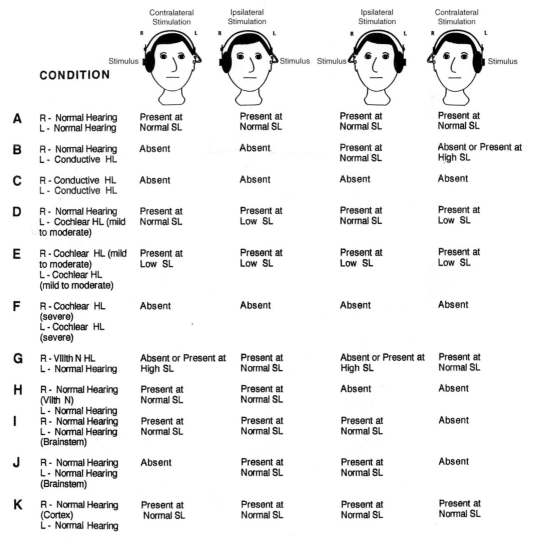

CONDITION		Contralateral Stimulation	Ipsilateral Stimulation	Ipsilateral Stimulation	Contralateral Stimulation
A	R - Normal Hearing L - Normal Hearing	Present at Normal SL	Present at Normal SL	Present at Normal SL	Present at Normal SL
B	R - Normal Hearing L - Conductive HL	Absent	Absent	Present at Normal SL	Absent or Present at High SL
C	R - Conductive HL L - Conductive HL	Absent	Absent	Absent	Absent
D	R - Normal Hearing L - Cochlear HL (mild to moderate)	Present at Normal SL	Present at Low SL	Present at Normal SL	Present at Low SL
E	R - Cochlear HL (mild to moderate) L - Cochlear HL (mild to moderate)	Present at Low SL	Present at Low SL	Present at Low SL	Present at Low SL
F	R - Cochlear HL (severe) L - Cochlear HL (severe)	Absent	Absent	Absent	Absent
G	R - VIIIth N HL L - Normal Hearing	Absent or Present at High SL	Present at Normal SL	Absent or Present at High SL	Present at Normal SL
H	R - Normal Hearing (VIIth N) L - Normal Hearing	Present at Normal SL	Present at Normal SL	Absent	Absent
I	R - Normal Hearing L - Normal Hearing (Brainstem)	Present at Normal SL	Present at Normal SL	Present at Normal SL	Absent
J	R - Normal Hearing L - Normal Hearing (Brainstem)	Absent	Present at Normal SL	Present at Normal SL	Absent
K	R - Normal Hearing (Cortex) L - Normal Hearing	Present at Normal SL	Present at Normal SL	Present at Normal SL	Present at Normal SL

FIGURE 6.7 Eleven theoretical examples of the results of ipsilateral and contralateral acoustic reflex testing. (Key: R = right ear; L = left ear; HL = hearing loss; SL = sensation level. In conditions H-K there is a lesion in the anatomical region in parentheses.)

Acoustic Reflex Decay Test

When the stapedius muscle is contracted by an intense sound in normal-hearing individuals, it will gradually relax as it is constantly stimulated. This is called **acoustic reflex decay,** and it is normal in the higher frequencies, but significant amounts of decay are usually seen only in lesions of the auditory nerve and some parts of the brainstem. Reflex decay is measured by sustaining a tone at 10 dB above the ART, and determining the number of seconds required for the amplitude of the reflex (the compliance change) to be reduced by 50 percent.

The test is completed when the reflex has decayed to half its original amplitude, or at the end of 10 seconds, whichever occurs first.

Recording and Interpreting Acoustic Reflex Decay Test Results.   This test is scored according to the number of seconds required for the amplitude of the reflex to decay to half magnitude. Test results may be printed automatically on a graph, so that changes in the amplitude of the response can be observed as a function of time, or they may be recorded on a form such as the one shown in Figure 6.4E.

In subjects with normal hearing there will be some decay of the reflex at 2000 and 4000 Hz, but not at 500 and 1000 Hz, and so this test is not performed in the higher frequencies. The slight decay sometimes evident in patients with cochlear hearing losses tends to occur more in the higher-frequency range. Lesions in the auditory nerve cause decay to half the original magnitude of the reflex, often within three to five seconds, even at 500 Hz (Anderson, Barr, & Wedenberg, 1970) because the nerve cannot maintain its continuous firing rate. Because the primary innervation of contraction of the middle-ear muscles is by way of the descending tract of the facial nerve, damage to that nerve may also cause an absent acoustic reflex or an initial response followed by rapid acoustic reflex decay.

Discussion of Acoustic Immittance Measurements

Both static compliance and tympanometry are measures of the mobility of the middle-ear mechanism. The acoustic reflex and reflex decay give information regarding probable disorders of different areas of the auditory system. These basic tests and their modifications are discussed in the appropriate portions of Chapters 10 to 12. Their inclusion in the test battery is a boon to the audiologist.

Under certain conditions bone-conduction audiometry may be unnecessary when acoustic immittance measures are combined with audiometric procedures. In the presence of normal hearing for pure tones, high word-recognition scores, Type A tympanograms, and normal acoustic reflex thresholds, normal hearing may be diagnosed without performance of bone conduction. When air-conduction thresholds are depressed, acoustic reflexes are present, and word-recognition scores are less than 90 percent, conductive hearing loss is eliminated as a possible finding, and bone-conduction audiometry will probably not produce an air-bone gap, resulting in a diagnosis of sensorineural hearing loss. If any signs of conductive loss do appear, such as absent acoustic reflexes or abnormal tympanograms, bone-conduction audiometry must be carried out. For these reasons, many audiologists prefer to do immittance measures among the first tests in the battery. The result, of course, is that bone-conduction testing may be eliminated when it is easiest to perform and least complicated (i.e., in patients with normal hearing and sensorineural loss). Bone conduction must be done to determine the amount of air-bone gap when it is most complicated by middle-ear artifacts and masking (in those with conductive and mixed hearing loss).

If contralateral acoustic reflexes and reflex decay are normal or provide information that confirms the audiometric findings, there is often no necessity to perform ipsilateral reflex testing. Of course, the way most immittance devices are designed (earphone on one ear, probe tip in the other), these results are not known until at least one ipsilateral reflex has been tested. The elimination of ipsilateral acoustic reflex testing saves very little time. However, many times contralateral testing is inconclusive or cannot be carried out at all. In such cases tests can be done ipsilaterally, although it should be noted that slightly different results may be found (Oviatt & Kileny, 1984) for acoustic reflex decay. When abnormal patterns are observed, a comparison of ipsilateral and contralateral tests can help to isolate lesions in the ascending tract versus the descending tract.

Acoustic immittance measurements have been called "impedance audiometry." Because audiometry *per se* is involved only with respect to the acoustic reflex, this term is not strictly accurate. There is no doubt that electroacoustic immittance measurements have reached a point of great importance in diagnostic audiology and the acoustic immittance meter has become as indispensable to the audiologist as the audiometer.

Auditory Evoked Potentials

From the time acoustic stimuli reach the inner ear, what is transmitted to the brain is not "sound" but rather a series of neuroelectric events. For many years there has been considerable interest in the measurement of the electrical responses generated within the cochlea. To this end, a procedure has evolved called **electrocochleography (ECoG).** Additionally, because hearing is a phenomenon involving the brain, it is only logical that whenever a sound is heard there must be some change in the ongoing electrical activity of the brain. These electrical responses have been referred to by several names, but when measured today they are commonly known as **auditory evoked potentials (AEPs).** AEPs can be subdivided on the basis of where and when they occur. They are better understood with the background provided in Chapter 12, which briefly reviews the auditory nervous system. Before attempting to measure AEPs, much more auditory anatomy and physiology, as well as other aspects of neuroscience, should be known than can be presented in an introductory text.

In Chapter 2, some mention was made of the connections between the brainstem and the higher centers for audition in the cerebral cortex. These connections occur via a series of way stations, called nuclei, within the central nervous system. When a signal is introduced to the ear, there are immediate electrical responses in the cochlea. As the signal is propagated along the auditory pathway, more time elapses before a response occurs, and thus the signal can be recorded at each subsequent nucleus in the pathway. The term **latency** is used to define the time period that elapses between the introduction of a stimulus and the occurrence of the response. Early AEPs, those that occur in the first 10 to 15 milliseconds after the introduction of a signal, are believed to originate in the VIIIth cranial nerve and the brainstem and are called the **auditory brainstem responses (ABRs).** AEPs occurring from 15 to 60 milliseconds in latency are called **auditory middle latency responses (AMLRs)** and probably originate in the midbrain. AEPs called **late evoked responses (LERs)** occur beyond 60 milliseconds and arise in the cortex. Responses recorded at 300 milliseconds or longer have been called **auditory event-related potentials (ERPs)** because they involve association areas in the brain.

AEPs are simply a small part of a multiplicity of electrical events measurable from the scalp. This electrical activity, which originates in the brain, is commonly referred to as electroencephalic and is measured on specially designed instruments called **electroencephalographs (EEGs),** which are used to pick up and amplify electrical activity from the brain by electrodes placed on the scalp. When changes in activity are observed on a computer monitor or printout, waveforms may be seen that aid in the diagnosis of central nervous system disease or abnormality.

In coupling the EEG to a patient to observe responses *evoked* by sounds, the ongoing neural activity is about 100 times greater than the auditory evoked potential and therefore obscures observation of the responses. The measurement of AEPs is further complicated by the presence of large electrical potentials from muscles (myogenic potentials). These obstacles were insurmountable until the advent of averaging computers, devices that allow measurement of electrical potentials, even when they are embedded in other electrical activity. A commercial device for measuring AEPs is shown in Figure 6.8.

Equipment for measurement of AEPs can range widely in price. More expensive units tend to provide greater flexibility in the number and variety of tests that can be performed; even relatively

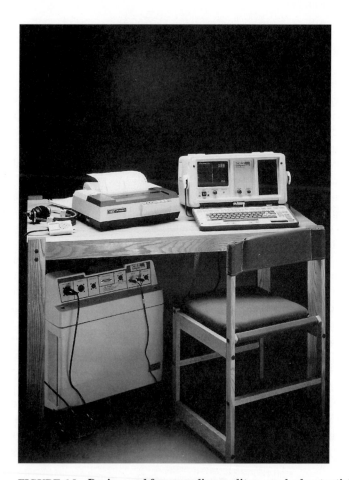

FIGURE 6.8   Device used for recording auditory evoked potentials. (Courtesy of Nicolet)

inexpensive units are generally acceptable to users. Calibration and maintenance of equipment is a major factor in the clinical measurement of AEPs. Normative data should be collected on every device before tests on patients can begin. Periodic recalibration is also necessary.

To measure AEPs, a series of auditory stimuli is presented to the subject at a constant rate by a transducer (earphone, bone-conduction vibrator, or loudspeaker). Insert earphones are gaining popularity for AEP testing because they are relatively comfortable to wear and help attenuate extraneous room noise. Also, their transducers are 250 millimeters from electrodes placed at the ear and therefore produce fewer electrical artifacts. The EEG equipment picks up the neural response, amplifies it, and stores the information in a series of computer memory time bins. Each bin sums neuroelectric activity that occurs at specific numbers of milliseconds after the onset of the stimulus. Of course, the computer is summing not only the response to the sound in any particular time bin, but also the random brain activity taking place at that precise moment. However, because the random activity consists of positive and negative voltages of varying amplitudes, summing reduces them to a value at or near zero. The polarity of the response is either positive or negative, and summing causes the magnitude of the response to increase in amplitude. It might be said that as the summing and averaging process continues, the signal-to-noise ratio improves. Even though the amplitudes of the responses are extremely small, often on the order of 1 to 5 microvolts (1 μV is equal to one-millionth of a volt), they can nevertheless be detected and interpreted.

Electrocochleography (ECoG)

The procedure for measuring electrical responses from the cochlea of the inner ear is called electrocochleography (ECoG, or sometimes ECochG). An active electrode may be placed in one of several positions: (1) on the promontory, the medial wall of the middle ear, which usually necessitates surgery to move the eardrum membrane aside; (2) on the promontory, using a needle electrode that is forced through the eardrum membrane; (3) in the skin of the outer-ear canal, using a needle electrode; (4) in saline-soaked cotton in the space of the outer-ear canal; (5) against the eardrum membrane, using a very thin electrode; (6) against the skin of the outer ear canal, using a silver ball electrode held in place by a plastic leaf; (7) in the outer ear canal using a disposable foam earplug covered by a very thin layer of gold foil, in which case the sound is delivered to the eardrum membrane through a plastic tube extending through the center of the foam. The further the active electrode is from the inner ear, the smaller the amplitude of the response and, consequently, the greater the number of stimuli that must be summed before the response can be identified with confidence.

The decision on whether to use more or less invasive electrodes during ECoG is largely determined by the types of workplaces in which audiologists find themselves, since all methods have their advantages and disadvantages (Ferraro, 1992). Transtympanic approaches, necessitating penetration of the eardrum membrane, are usually carried out in settings where physicians are on site since anesthesia is required. Extratympanic procedures, not requiring the risk or discomfort of minor surgery, can be performed in virtually any audiological setting. The primary focus for ECoG testing has moved from the determination of auditory sensitivity in difficult-to-test individuals (Cullen, Ellis, Berlin, & Lousteau, 1972), to neuro-otological applications, such as monitoring the function of the cochlea during some surgical procedures; enhancing the results of other electrophysiological tests; and probably most important, assisting in the diagnosis and monitoring of some conditions of the inner ear such as Méniére disease (see Chapter 11).

Auditory Brainstem Response (ABR) Audiometry

For measuring responses from the brain, the vertex (top of the skull) is the most common active electrode placement site. A reference electrode is usually placed on the mastoid process behind the outer
ear, and a ground electrode is placed on the opposite mastoid or on the forehead. Stimuli with rapid
rise times, such as clicks, must be used to generate these early responses. Tone pips, which provide
some frequency-specific information, can be used. Using the summing computer, seven small
wavelets generally appear in the first 10 milliseconds after signal presentation. Each wave represents
neuroelectrical activity at one or more generating sites along the auditory brainstem pathway.
Although disagreement persists on the site represented by each wave, Møller (1985) suggests the following simplified scheme of major ABR generators:

Wave Number	*Site*
I	VIIIth cranial nerve
II	VIIIth cranial nerve
III	Pons
IV	Pons
V	Midbrain
VI and VII	Undetermined

There are several ways in which routine ABR audiometry is performed, only one of which is
described here. The patient is first seated in a comfortable chair, often a recliner, which is placed in an
acoustically isolated, electrically shielded room. The skin areas to which electrodes will be attached are
carefully cleansed, and a conductive paste or gel is applied to the area. An **active electrode** is placed
on either the vertex or the forehead, and two other electrodes are attached to either the earlobes or the
mastoid processes behind the external ears. The ipsilateral electrode (nearest the ear to be stimulated)
is for **reference,** and the contralateral electrode (near the opposite ear) is for **ground.** After the electrodes are taped in place, electrical impedance is checked with an ohmmeter. The impedance between
the skin and the electrodes, and between any two electrodes, must be controlled for the test to be performed properly. An earphone is placed over or into the test ear, and the patient is asked to relax. The
lights are usually dimmed and the chair placed in a reclining position. The ABR is not affected by sleep
state, therefore the subject may sleep while the responses are being recorded. This characteristic of the
ABR is important as it allows anesthetized or comatose individuals to be evaluated.

One ear is tested at a time. A series of 1000 to 2000 clicks may be presented, at a rate of 33.1
clicks per second. The starting level is often 70 dB nHL (n is the reference to the normative group
threshold for click stimuli). Clear responses should be seen in the form of waves I, III, and V. If
responses are not present, the intensity is raised 20 dB; if responses are present, the level is lowered
in 10 or 20 dB steps until wave V becomes undetectable. With decreased intensity, wave amplitudes
become smaller and latencies increase. Since wave V normally has the largest amplitude of the first
seven waves and is the most impervious to change, the ABR threshold is considered to be the lowest intensity at which wave V can be observed. ABR threshold determinations can usually be ascertained to within 10 to 20 dB of behavioral thresholds.

After the test has been completed, a hard copy may be printed out and these data may be summarized on a special form (see Figure 6.9). A complete ABR test will provide the following information about each ear:

SPEECH AND HEARING CENTER
The University of Texas at Austin 78712

AUDITORY BRAINSTEM RESPONSE
(Adult Form)

NAME: Last · First · Middle	SEX	AGE	DATE	EXAMINER	RELIABILITY	INSTRUMENT

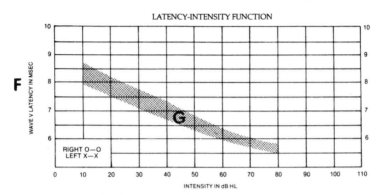

LATENCY-INTENSITY FUNCTION

SHADED AREA REPRESENTS Normal Wave V Range for patients older than 16 mos. for 30 clicks per second.

	STIMULUS			WAVE LATENCY IN MSEC						
EAR	RATE	dB HL	FILTER	I	II	III	IV	V	VI	VII
	A	B					C			

SUMMARY OF RESULTS   D

INTERWAVE INTERVALS . . . . R _____ L _____
AMPLITUDE RATIO (V SAME OR > I) . . . . R _____ L _____
LATENCY CHANGE WITH INCREASED CLICK RATE . . . . R _____ L _____
INTERAURAL DIFFERENCES . . . . _____

                                                                            E
ESTIMATED AIR CONDUCTION THRESHOLD IN dBHL (1-2 kHz) . . . . . . R _____ L _____
ESTIMATED BONE CONDUCTION THRESHOLD IN dB HL . . . . R _____ L _____

COMMENTS

_____
_____
_____
_____
_____

FIGURE 6.9   Form used for recording results of auditory brainstem response tests: (A) stimulus click rate; (B) intensity (in dB nHL) required to evoke the response; (C) latency (in milliseconds) to each of the seven peaks of the waves; (D) interpeak intervals (in milliseconds); (E) estimate of auditory thresholds for each ear; (F) graph showing the latency (in milliseconds) as a function of the intensity of the series of clicks presented to each ear; (G) shaded area showing a normal distribution of wave V latency values.

1. Absolute latencies of all identifiable waves I to V at different intensities
2. Interpeak latency intervals (i.e., I to V, I to III, III to V), or relative latencies
3. Wave amplitudes (absolute and relative)
4. Threshold of wave V

Interpreting the ABR.   The ABR may be used as a test of audiological or neurological function. If the ABR elicited by click stimuli is used as a test of hearing sensitivity, the auditory threshold in the frequency range from 2000 to 4000 Hz may be inferred from the lowest intensity at which wave V is identified. However, one must also look carefully at the wave V latency-intensity function and the absolute latencies of wave V. The closer the auditory stimulus is to a patient's threshold, the longer the latency of each wave. By plotting the latency of wave V at different intensities, general site-of-lesion information about a hearing loss may be inferred.

If a conductive hearing loss is present, the intensity required to produce the ABR is increased as the threshold is elevated, latencies of all waves are prolonged, but interpeak intervals are normal, and the slope of the latency-intensity function is similar to one showing normal hearing. If the lesion results in a high-frequency loss in the cochlea, wave V often shows a normal latency at high sensation levels if the intensity of the clicks is above threshold in the 2000 to 4000 Hz region, but it is prolonged near threshold, resulting in a steeply sloping latency-intensity function. With every 30 dB of hearing loss at 4000 Hz, there may be an increase of 0.2 milliseconds of wave V latency. When the lesion affects the auditory nerve, as in the case of a tumor, all waves subsequent to wave I are often delayed or absent at all intensities. Wave V and other waves may also be delayed or missing in cases of auditory brainstem tumors.

In addition to serving as a test for threshold and site of lesion, the ABR may be used as a neurological screening test, to assess the integrity of the central auditory pathway. The most significant finding in neurological lesions is an increase in interpeak intervals. If wave V can be observed at a slow click rate, for example, 11.1 clicks per second (often seen clearly at 70 dB nHL), a higher click rate may be presented, such as 89.1 clicks per second. Under this condition it is normal for the wave V latency to increase up to 0.8 milliseconds. In abnormal central nervous systems, however, such as those with demyelinating diseases like multiple sclerosis, the stress from rapid click rates often causes wave V to disappear entirely. An ABR is considered neurologically abnormal, indicating neuropathology affecting the auditory pathway of the brainstem, when any of the following occur:

1. Interpeak intervals are prolonged.
2. Wave V latency is significantly different between ears.
3. Amplitude ratios are abnormal (normally wave V is larger than wave I).
4. Wave V is abnormally prolonged or disappears with high click rate stimulation.

Normal ABR results are shown in Figures 6.10 and 6.11.

ABR measurements have been used with increasing frequency in the testing of infants and small children. Improvements in equipment and procedures have also brought ABR testing into the operating room, where it is used to monitor responses from the brain during delicate neurosurgical procedures (Kileny, Niparko, Shepard, & Kemink, 1988). Musiek, Gollegly, Kibbe, and Verkest (1988) find that ABR is often useful in the diagnosis of brainstem lesions when it is used in conjunction with some of the psychophysical procedures described in Chapter 12. The ABR has developed into the most important test in the diagnostic site-of-lesion battery and has proved to be

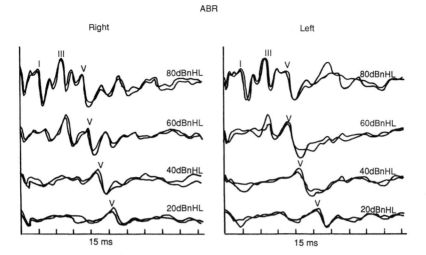

FIGURE 6.10   Auditory brainstem response testing on a normal-hearing individual. Absolute latencies are shown in Figure 6.11.

sensitive, specific, and efficient in detecting lesions affecting the auditory pathways through the brainstem.

Auditory Middle Latency Response (AMLR) Audiometry

For some time it was uncertain whether the middle latency responses, which occur between 15 and 60 milliseconds after signal presentation, are *myogenic* (produced by changes in electrical potential generated in muscles on the scalp and behind the ear) or *neurogenic* (produced by electrical potentials in nerve units within the auditory pathways). This controversy is not completely resolved, but it is now generally accepted that the AMLR has a neurogenic component. The generator sites within the brain have not yet been absolutely determined, but they may include several areas of the auditory cortex, as well as other areas between the auditory brainstem and the cortex.

Patient setup for measurement of the AMLR is essentially the same as for ABR. A major difference lies in the importance of keeping the patient inactive to minimize myogenic artifacts. Patients must remain calm but alert. Clicks, filtered clicks, or tone bursts are delivered through an earphone. It may be necessary to deliver 1000 to 2000 stimuli to discern a clear AMLR.

Interpreting the AMLR.   Because the ABR gives information about hearing primarily in the 2000 to 4000 Hz range, the AMLR is a nice complement in that it can provide information about hearing for the lower frequencies when performed with tone bursts (Fifer & Sierra-Irizarry, 1988). The AMLR is useful in the assessment of neurological function of the higher central auditory nervous system. This information can be very helpful, but AMLR is often of least utility in the patients where it is needed most, such as in the diagnosis of infants and other uncooperative individuals. It is affected by state—that is, whether the patient is awake or asleep. Further refinement of AMLR

SPEECH AND HEARING CENTER
The University of Texas at Austin 78712

AUDITORY BRAINSTEM RESPONSE
(Adult Form)

NAME: Last - First - Middle	SEX	AGE	DATE	EXAMINER	RELIABILITY	INSTRUMENT

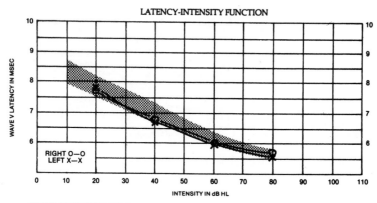

LATENCY-INTENSITY FUNCTION

RIGHT O—O
LEFT X—X

SHADED AREA REPRESENTS Normal Wave V Range for patients older than 16 mos. for 30 clicks per second.

	STIMULUS			WAVE LATENCY IN MSEC						
EAR	RATE	dB HL	FILTER	I	II	III	IV	V	VI	VII
R	33.1	80	150-1500	1.8		3.75		5.7		
L	33.1	80	150-1500	1.6		3.62		5.6		

SUMMARY OF RESULTS

INTERWAVE INTERVALS.. R _3.9_ L _4.0_
AMPLITUDE RATIO (V SAME OR > I)............................. R _NORMAL_ L _NORMAL_
LATENCY CHANGE WITH INCREASED CLICK RATE................. R _____ L _____
INTERAURAL DIFFERENCES.................................... _____

ESTIMATED AIR CONDUCTION THRESHOLD IN dBHL (1-2 kHz)....... R _≤20_ L _≤20_
ESTIMATED BONE CONDUCTION THRESHOLD IN dB HL............ R _____ L _____

COMMENTS

_____
_____
_____
_____
_____

FIGURE 6.11   Latency-intensity functions for wave V derived from the auditory brainstem response tracings shown in on a normal-hearing individual (Figure 6.10). All the latencies are normal.

measurement techniques will probably increase its use as a neurodiagnostic procedure. An AMLR response is shown in Figure 6.12.

Late Evoked Responses (LERs)

The earliest work done on AEPs was on the cortical evoked response, which was involved with those responses that appear at least 60 milliseconds after signal presentation (Figure 6.13). Problems in interpreting LER test results, along with improvements in microcomputers and averaging systems, led to a much greater interest in the earlier components of the evoked response (ABR and AMLR), but in subsequent years renewed interest has been found in the later components. A major advantage of measuring the later responses is that it is possible to use frequency-specific stimuli, such as pure tones, as well as short segments of speech. The responses are considerably larger than the earlier waves and therefore can be tracked closer to the individual's behavioral threshold; however, the responses are affected by a patient's attention, and therefore the procedure has limitations when used with children. These potentials are dependent on state of consciousness; that is, significant degradation occurs with sleep, whether natural or induced.

The first late response (P1) often occurs at approximately 60 milliseconds latency. P1 is followed by a series of negative (N) and positive (P) waves (N1, P2, N2) occurring between 100 and

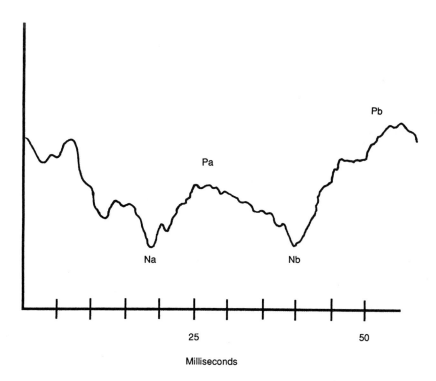

FIGURE 6.12   **Auditory evoked potentials showing the middle latency response.**

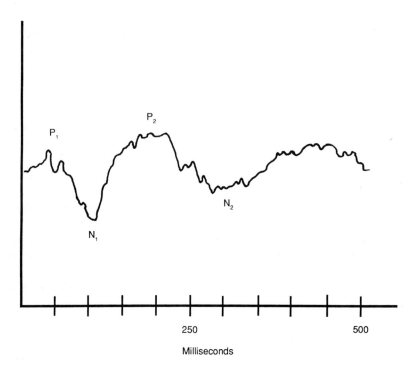

FIGURE 6.13   Auditory evoked potentials showing the late evoked response.

250 milliseconds. At approximately 300 milliseconds a larger (10 to 20 μv) positive wave, which has become known as P300, is seen in response to rare or novel stimuli that are embedded in more frequent stimuli. This has been called an "oddball paradigm." For example, rare 2000 Hz tones may be presented 15 percent of the time along with standard 1000 Hz tones, which are presented 85 percent of the time (Kibbe-Michal, Verkest, Gollegly, & Musiek, 1986). The subject is instructed to attend only to the (rare) higher-pitched tones by, for example, counting them or signaling each time one is heard. Also called the auditory event-related potential, the P300 is the earliest AEP that requires active participation by the subject to generate the response.

Another late-evoked response, the **mismatch negativity (MMN)** has produced significant interest. This is a small negative response using an oddball paradigm. However, unlike the P300, the subjects are instructed to ignore both the rare and standard stimuli, which may both be present in the same ear or presented individually to different ears. The effect is that different responses are evoked by the rare and standard signals, resulting in the acquisition of two different waveforms that are combined to obtain the waveform containing the MMN. It is believed that the different responses to the rare and standard stimuli are due to the brain noticing a difference between the two stimuli, hence the term "mismatch" (Picton, 1995). The MMN, whose multiple generator sites include the temporal cortex, holds great promise for the understanding of how the brain conducts its cognitive functions (Naatanen, 1995).

Interpreting the Late Evoked Responses. Late evoked responses may aid in the estimation of threshold for pure tones over a wide frequency range and in the assessment of neurological function. Of course, if patients are awake and cooperative enough to allow LERs, they can often be tested voluntarily. The P300 potential is called *event-related* because it depends on discrimination of target stimuli by the listener (Figure 6.14). For this reason the P300 is thought to be related to the perception or processing of stimuli rather than to the mere activation of the auditory nervous system by a stimulus. Late evoked, P300, and MMN responses offer great promise for practical applications in diagnosis of neurological disease and injury.

Intraoperative Monitoring

Many of the electrical responses described above have been used during neurosurgical procedures for **intraoperative monitoring** of the physiological state of the patient. During these delicate operations surgeons often require reports on the condition of the patient, so that they may be alerted to possible damage to the auditory system before it occurs, thus averting both hearing loss and damage to other structures in the brain. Some operations that can benefit from this kind of monitoring include surgery on the auditory and facial nerves, as well as on the inner ear.

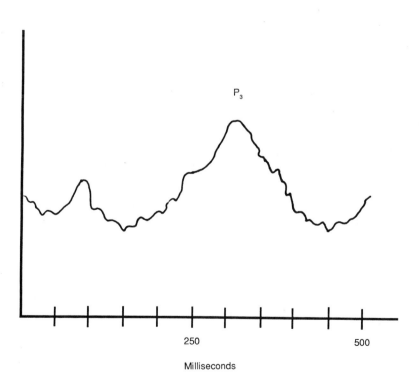

250   500

Milliseconds

FIGURE 6.14   Auditory evoked potentials showing the P300 (event-related) response.

The modern operating room is filled with many people in addition to the surgeon and patient (anesthesiologists, technicians, and nurses) as well as a lot of electrical equipment that can put out signals that can interfere with monitoring of neuroelectrical responses. The operating room is not an easy work environment, and the persons performing these duties, who are increasingly audiologists, require very special training and skills. Intraoperative monitoring usually involves ECoG and ABR and is becoming part of the professional role of many audiologists.

Discussion of Auditory Evoked Potentials

Using computer averaging techniques and a series of acoustic stimuli, it is possible to evoke responses on the basis of neuroelectric activity within the auditory system. By looking at the kinds of responses obtained during electrocochleography and auditory brainstem response audiometry, along with the later components of electroencephalic audiometry, it is often possible to predict the site of lesion and estimate auditory threshold. Many of these tests are finding their way into the operating room for monitoring during neurosurgery. Although the ABR should be considered to be more of a test of synchronous neural firings than of hearing per se, its value to diagnostic audiology and to neurological screening is growing rapidly.

Otoacoustic Emissions (OAEs)

The fact that many normal cochleas are capable of producing sounds in the absence of external stimulation came as a surprise to researchers and clinicians in audiology when it was first described by Kemp in 1979. These **spontaneous otoacoustic emissions (SOAEs)** occur in over half the population of persons with normal hearing as a continuous tonal signal that can be recorded in the external auditory canal. The typical frequency range of SOAEs is 1000 to 3000 Hz, although some have been reported well above and below this range. While there is considerable variation in the amplitude of an SOAE, it is often found to be between ± 10 dB SPL and is generally inaudible to the person in whom it is measured. It is possible to have more than one SOAE in a given ear, and to have OAEs in both ears.

A second class of OAE occurs either during or immediately following acoustic stimulation. These responses are called **evoked otoacoustic emissions (EOAEs)** and there are several types. EOAEs have come into clinical prominence, the two major types being **transient** and **distortion-product EOAEs.**

Transient-evoked Otoacoustic Emissions (TEOAEs)

TEOAEs are produced by brief acoustic stimuli, such as clicks or tone pips. Signal-averaging equipment, similar to that described in the section on auditory-evoked potentials, must be used to separate the emission from ongoing noise in the ear. Anywhere from 260 to 500 stimuli are presented, and the waveforms of the responses are averaged, along with the ongoing noise in the ear, in order to improve the signal-to-noise ratio. Responses should be observable from virtually all individuals with normal outer, middle, and inner ears. As hearing loss due to cochlear damage increases, the amplitude of the response decreases until a hearing loss of about 40 dB, where the response usually disappears altogether.

When a click stimulus is used, the entire cochlea is stimulated and a wide range of frequencies is normally present in the TEOAE. If a broadband TEOAE can be observed, it may be inferred that the pathway up to the cochlea, the auditory periphery, is unimpaired. It cannot be known whether there is a disorder in the auditory nerve or other structures beyond the cochlea. Therefore, a normal TEOAE does not guarantee normal hearing. When a TEOAE is not seen, the suggestion is that a hearing loss is present, but does not reveal whether the problem is in the conductive pathway or the cochlea. A commercial version of an OAE measurement device can be seen in Figure 6.15, and a typical response is shown in Figure 6.16.

Distortion-product Otoacoustic Emissions (DPOAEs)

When two "primary tones" that vary in frequency by several hundred hertz (F1 and F2, where F2>F1) are presented to the ear, the normal cochlea responds by producing energy at additional frequencies. These are called "distortion products." By varying the primary-tone frequencies, responses are generated from different areas of the cochlea. Typically, the levels and the frequency ratio of the primary tones are not varied. These responses often compare favorably with voluntary audiometric results, provided that the hearing loss does not exceed 40 to 50 dB. As with TEOAEs, the conductive pathway must be normal to obtain DPOAEs.

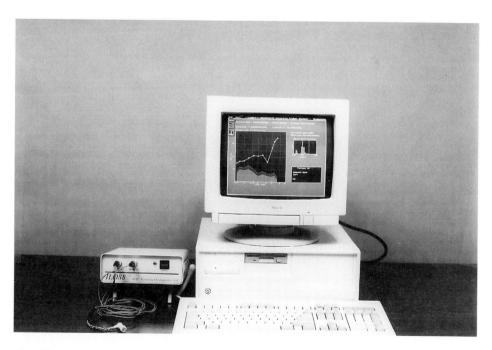

FIGURE 6.15   Commercial device for measurement of otoacoustic emissions. (Photo courtesy of Eye Dynamics, Inc. and JEDMED Instrument Company)

TEOAE Waveform

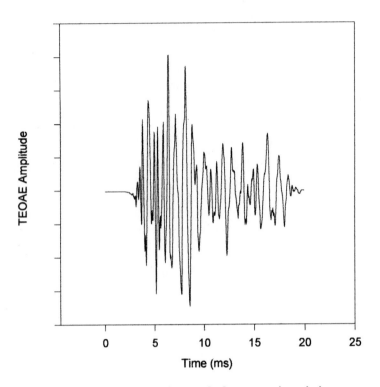

FIGURE 6.16   A typical transient-evoked otoacoustic emission.

Measuring OAEs

Advances in microcircuitry have allowed for accurate measurement of OAEs. A probe containing a miniature loudspeaker to present the evoking stimulus and also a tiny microphone to pick up the emission and convert it from a sound into an electrical signal is placed in the external auditory canal. The device that delivers the stimuli for DPOAE testing differs from the one for measuring TEOAEs, in that the probe that is fitted to the ear must have two openings that can deliver the two primary tones. Because DPOAEs are separate in frequency from the evoking stimuli, averaging background noise is less of a problem for measurement of DPOAE than for TEOAE, and fewer stimulus presentations are required, which may reduce test time slightly. Acoustic control of the test environment for OAE testing is less critical than might be imagined, since the noise that must be averaged out is the noise contained in the ear of the subject. If subject noise levels are too high, for example, in crying babies, they may mask the emission, since the sensitive microphone used cannot differentiate one acoustic signal from another.

Interpreting OAEs

Otoacoustic emissions (OAEs) are thought to reflect the activity of an intact cochlea and a brief physiological explanation of this phenomenon can be found in Chapter 11 on the inner ear. For any type of OAE to be observed, the conductive pathway must be normal because the strength of a signal traveling from the inner ear to the outer ear canal may be attenuated by an abnormality of the middle ear in the same way as an externally generated signal traveling from the outer ear to the inner ear.

The presence of an EOAE suggests that there is very little or no conductive hearing loss caused by middle-ear abnormality. It further suggests that responding frequency regions of the cochlea are normal, or exhibit no more than a mild hearing loss. It reveals essentially nothing about the auditory structures that lie beyond the inner ear, except for possible insights into the efferent neural pathways.

Discussion of Otoacoustic Emissions

The introduction of otoacoustic emissions to the test battery is a giant leap in the direction of testing patients who cannot or will not cooperate during voluntary hearing tests. Perhaps more than this, the procedure will probably provide important insights in the differential diagnosis of cochlear versus retrocochlear disorders.

The advantages to using OAEs with children are obvious. This procedure is both noninvasive and requires no patient cooperation, except to remain relatively motionless. Data collection time has been estimated to be from one to five minutes per ear, which is very advantageous considering that children tend to be active. OAEs may be used in combination with evoked potential measures to help to differentiate sensory from neural lesions and may also be utilized as a cross-check of middle-ear status, as determined by acoustic immittance measures.

Summary

Acoustic immittance measurements and tympanometry give remarkably reliable information regarding the function of the middle ear, and acoustic reflex measurements have become essential in diagnostic audiometry. Auditory brainstem response (ABR) audiometry has become an important part of the site-of-lesion test battery, and some of the other evoked potential techniques are becoming more valuable as they are improved. Otoacoustic emissions have added significantly to the battery of tests for site of lesion and it is expected that refinement of the present techniques and new experimental findings will add greatly to the practical use of this procedure.

STUDY QUESTIONS

1. Describe the equipment needed for each of the tests described in this chapter.

2. Why is the term "impedance audiometry" inaccurate?

3. What are the relationships between OAE and ABR thresholds to voluntary thresholds?

4. What are the theoretical and practical values of the measures described in this chapter?

5. Describe the limitations of the tests described in this chapter.

GLOSSARY

Acoustic impedance The total opposition to the flow of acoustic energy (as in the plane of the eardrum membrane). It consists of mass, stiffness, and frictional resistance and is influenced by frequency.

Acoustic reflex Contraction of one or both of the middle-ear muscles in response to an intense sound.

Acoustic reflex arc The path of an acoustic stimulus that ascends from the outer ear to the brainstem and then descends via the facial nerves on both sides of the head to innervate the stapedial muscles in both middle ears.

Acoustic reflex decay A decrease in the magnitude of the middle-ear reflex that occurs with constant acoustic stimulation.

Acoustic reflex threshold (ART) The lowest intensity at which a stimulus can produce the acoustic reflex.

Active electrode The electrode used in testing auditory evoked potentials in conjunction with a reference electrode. It is placed on an area of the scalp, such as the vertex, where electrical activity is high. The potential difference between these electrodes is amplified, thus canceling out unwanted signals.

Auditory brainstem response (ABR) The seven wavelets that appear within 10 milliseconds after signal presentation.

Auditory event-related potentials (ERPs) AEPs that occur after latencies of about 60 milliseconds, with the largest positive wave at about 300 milliseconds. Patients must cooperate by counting "oddball" stimuli.

Auditory evoked potentials (AEPs) The use of summing or averaging computers to observe the very small electrical responses to sound from the cochlea, brainstem, and cortex.

Auditory middle latency response (AMLR) Responses that occur 10 to 50 milliseconds after signal onset and are thought to arise from the upper brainstem.

Compliance The inverse of stiffness.

Distortion product otoacoustic emission (DPOAE) The emission of a sound from the cochlea, measured in the external auditory canal, which is the result of inner-ear distortion generated when two tones of different frequencies are introduced to the ear.

Electrocochleography (ECoG) Response to sound in the form of electrical potentials that occur within the first few milliseconds after signal presentation. The responses that arise from the cochlea are small in amplitude and must be summed on a computer after a number of presentations of clicks or tone pips.

Electroencephalograph (EEG) A tracing showing changes in the electrical potentials in the brain.

Equivalent volume A method of approximating the compliance component of impedance; the volume (in cm^3) with a physical property equivalent to a similar property of the middle ear.

Evoked otoacoustic emission (EOAE) A measurable echo produced by the cochlea in response to signals presented to the ear.

Gradient The width of a tympanogram, defined as a horizontal line extending 50 daPa either side of a line drawn vertically down from the peak pressure point, divided by the height of the peak pressure point.

Ground electrode The third electrode used in testing auditory evoked potentials to ground subjects so that their bodies cannot serve as an antenna.

Immittance A term used to describe measurements made in the plane of the tympanic membrane.

Intra-aural muscle reflex The contraction of the stapedius muscles produced by introduction of an intense sound to one ear. The reflex is a bilateral phenomenon.

Intraoperative monitoring The use of auditory evoked potentials, such as ECoG and ABR for monitoring some of the electrophysiological states of the patient during neurosurgery.

Late evoked responses (LERs) Those auditory evoked potentials evident after about 60 milliseconds. They are usually of larger amplitude than the earlier responses. Pure tones may be used as stimuli, and frequency-specific information may be available.

Latency The time delay between the presentation of a stimulus and the measured physiological response to that stimulus.

Mismatch negativity (MMN) A small negative response evoked when subjects are instructed to attend to a set of stimuli in one ear, while different signals are presented to the other ear.

Reactance The contribution to total acoustic impedance provided by mass, stiffness, and frequency.

Reference electrode An electrode placed on an area of the scalp that is relatively unaffected by electrical activity in the brain.

Reflex activating stimulus (RAS) A pure tone or other acoustic signal of high intensity designed to cause the stapedial muscle to contract. The RAS can be presented through the probe assembly of an immittance meter to observe an acoustic reflex in the ear that houses the probe tip (the ipsilateral reflex), or it can be presented via an earphone in the ear opposite the probe (the contralateral acoustic reflex).

Spontaneous otoacoustic emission (SOAE) A weak sound, emanating from the cochlea with no external stimulation, that travels through the middle ear and can be measured by a sensitive microphone placed in the external auditory canal.

Stapedius muscle A small muscle in the middle ear. Both stapedius muscles normally contract, causing a change in the resting position of the eardrum membrane, when either ear is stimulated by an intense sound.

Static acoustic compliance A measurement of the mobility of the eardrum membrane.

Tensor tympani muscle One of two small muscles in the middle ear that contract in response to intense acoustic stimulation.

Transient-evoked otoacoustic emission (TEOAE) An otoacoustic emission evoked in the cochlea by very brief acoustic stimuli like clicks or tone pips.

Tympanogram A graphic representation of a pressure-compliance function.

Tympanometry Measurement of the pressure compliance function of the eardrum membrane.

REFERENCES

American National Standards Institute (ANSI). (1987). *American National Standard specifications for instruments to measure aural acoustic impedance and admittance (aural acoustic immittance).* ANSI S3.39-1987. New York: Author.

American Speech-Language-Hearing Association (ASHA). (1990). Guidelines for screening for hearing impairment and middle ear disorders. *Asha, 32* (Supplement 2), 17–24.

Anderson, H., Barr, B., & Wedenberg, E. (1970). Early diagnosis of VIIIth nerve tumors by acoustic reflex tests. *Acta Otolaryngologica, 263* (Supplement).

Cullen, J. K., Ellis, M. S., Berlin, C. I., & Lousteau, R. J. (1972). Human acoustic nerve action potential recordings from the tympanic membrane without anesthesia. *Acta Otolaryngologica, 74,* 15–22.

Ferraro, J. A. (1992). Electrocochleography: What and why. *Audiology Today, 4,* 25–27.

Fifer, R. C., & Sierra-Irizarry, M. A. (1988). Clinical applications of the auditory middle latency response. *The American Journal of Otology, 9,* 47–56.

Hall, J. W. III, & Chandler, D. (1994). Tympanometry in clinical audiology. In J. Katz (Ed.), *Handbook of clinical audiology* (4th ed., pp. 283–299). Baltimore: Williams & Wilkins.

Jerger, J. (1970). Clinical experience with impedance audiometry. *Archives of Otolaryngology, 92,* 311–324.

Kemp, D. T., (1979). Evidence of mechanical nonlinearity and frequency selective wave amplification in the cochlea. *Archives of Oto-Rhino-Laryngology, 221,* 37–45.

Kibbe-Michal, K., Verkest, S. B., Gollegly, K. M., & Musiek, F. E. (1986). Late auditory potentials and the P300. *Hearing Instruments, 37,* 22–24.

Kileny, P. R., Niparko, J. K., Shepard, N. T., & Kemink, J. L. (1988). Neurophysiologic intraoperative monitoring: I. Auditory function. *The American Journal of Otology, 9,* 17–24.

Møller, A. R. (1985). Physiology of the ascending auditory pathways with special reference to the auditory brain stem response (ABR). In M. L. Pinheiro & F. E. Musiek (Eds.), *Assessment of central auditory dysfunction: Foundations and clinical correlates* (pp. 23–41). Baltimore: Williams & Wilkins.

Musiek, F. E., Gollegly, K. M., Kibbe, K. S., & Verkest, S. B. (1988). Current concepts on the use of ABR and auditory psychophysical tests in the evaluation of brain stem lesions. *The American Journal of Otology, 9,* 25–35.

Naatanen, R. (1995). The mismatch negativity: A powerful tool for cognitive neuroscience. *Ear and Hearing, 16,* 6–18.

Northern, J. L., & Gabbard, S. A. (1994). The acoustic reflex. In J. Katz (Ed.), *Handbook of clinical audiology* (4th ed., pp. 300–316). Baltimore: Williams & Wilkins.

Oviatt, D. L., & Kileny, P. (1984). Normative characteristics of ipsilateral acoustic reflex adaptations. *Ear and Hearing, 5,* 145–152.

Picton, T. W. (1995). The neurophysiological evaluation of auditory discrimination. *Ear and Hearing, 16,* 1–5.

Popelka, G. R. (1983). Basic acoustic immittance measures. *Audiology: A Journal for Continuing Education, 8,* 1–16.

Shanks, J. E., Lilly, D. J., Margolis, R. H., Wiley, T. L., & Wilson, R. H. (1988). Tympanometry. *Journal of Speech and Hearing Disorders, 53,* 354–377.

SUGGESTED READINGS

Jacobson, J. T. (1994). *Principles and applications in auditory evoked potentials.* Boston: Allyn & Bacon.

Northern, J. L. (1996). Acoustic immittance measurements. In J. L. Northern (Ed.), *Hearing disorders* (3rd ed., pp. 57–72). Boston: Allyn & Bacon.

Robinette, M. S., & Glattke, T. J. (1997). *Otoacoustic emission: Clinical applications.* New York: Thieme.

REVIEW TABLE 6.1   Summary of Electrophysiological Tests

Test	Purpose	Unit
Tympanometry	Pressure-compliance function of TM	cm^3
Static compliance	Compliance of TM	cm^3
ART	Sensation level of acoustic reflex	dB
ABR	Latency-intensity function of early AEP	msec
OAE	Check cochlear function	dB

REVIEW TABLE 6.2   Typical Interpretation of Electrophysiological Tests

	Normal Hearing	Conductive Loss	Sensory Loss	Neural Loss
Tympanogram Type	A	A$_D$, A$_S$, B, or C	A	A
Static Compliance (cm^3)	.3 to 1.6	<.3 or >1.6	.3 to 1.6	.3 to 1.6
ART	Present at 85 to 100 dB SL	Absent or >100 dB SL	Present at <65 dB SL	Absent or >100 dB SL
ABR	Normal wave V & interpeak latencies	All wave latencies prolonged.	Slightly increased wave V & interpeak latencies	Very increased wave V & interpeak latencies
OAE	Present	Absent	Absent	Present

7 Behavioral Tests for Site of Lesion

The **site of a lesion** producing a hearing loss is of more than casual interest to audiologists. Separating conductive from sensorineural hearing losses is not difficult on the basis of the pure-tone and speech tests described in Chapters 4 and 5, but the distinction between *sensory* and *neural* is more difficult to determine. Lesions of the auditory portions of the inner ear (*cochlear*) are said to be sensory, and lesions beyond the inner ear (*retrocochlear*) are often called neural. The purpose of this chapter is to present some of the original tests used to help differentiate cochlear from retrocochlear pathology.

At one time, the tests to be described in this chapter were extremely popular among audiologists. There is evidence that many of them are used today with much less frequency than in the past (Martin, Champlin, & Chambers, 1998); however, they are important, not only from an historical perspective, but also because they illustrate principles that are important to the understanding of normal and impaired auditory systems. In many cases, performance of these diagnostic hearing tests requires the use of specially designed equipment. With this equipment, audiologists could accumulate valuable information for diagnostic purposes prior to the advent of the elecrophysiological measures described in Chapter 6. These procedures allow measurement of the growth of loudness in pathological ears as compared to normal ears, the rates at which tones fade from audibility, different kinds of tracking behavior using automatic audiometers, and the detection of brief changes in intensity.

Behavioral site-of-lesion tests of the past, like their contemporary electrophysiological counterparts, were helpful in determining the kinds of medical referrals that needed to be made, and their urgency. As is discussed in subsequent chapters, these tests can even uncover disorders that are potentially fatal to the patient.

Although there are now many tests to determine the site of an auditory lesion, each must be subjected to scrutiny to determine its specific usefulness in a particular situation. Questions arise about two factors—reliability and validity. *Reliability* has to do with how well a test score is repeatable. Poor reliability can make a test useless, but good reliability does not necessarily make it valuable unless it is also valid. Questions of *validity* ask whether a test measures what it is supposed to measure—in this case, the power with which a test reveals the locus of a disorder in the auditory system.

Because no diagnostic procedure is infallible, any single test will turn out in one of four ways:

1. *True positive:* The test indicates a lesion site correctly.
2. *True negative:* The test correctly eliminates an anatomical area as a potential locus of the problem.
3. *False positive:* The test indicates a lesion site incorrectly.
4. *False negative:* The test incorrectly eliminates an anatomical area as causing the hearing problem.

Jerger and Jerger (1983) and Turner and Nielsen (1984) have suggested that audiological tests for site of lesion can be subjected to a set of mathematical models by **clinical decision analysis (CDA).** The CDA asks questions about each test's **sensitivity** (how well it correctly identifies a lesion site—true positive), its **specificity** (the inverse of sensitivity—how well it rejects an incorrect diagnosis, or true negative), its **efficiency** (the percentage of false positive and false negative results), and its **predictive value** (the percentage of true positive and true negative results). These issues will be discussed with respect to the behavioral site-of-lesion tests covered in this chapter.

Chapter Objectives

At this point the reader should have a good grasp of the tests described in earlier chapters, as well as a general knowledge of how the ear is constructed and how it responds to sound. This chapter reviews a number of early behavioral site-of-lesion tests for diagnostic purposes.

Loudness Recruitment

Loudness increases with intensity in a logical and lawful manner. As the intensity of a sound is increased, so is the experience of loudness. It is possible to compare this *growth of loudness* in the two ears of an individual with normal hearing by pulsing a tone alternately from one ear to the other. The subject's task consists of matching the loudness of the tone in one ear (the test ear) to that of the other (reference) ear. This loudness-balancing procedure is usually performed at several suprathreshold levels. For purposes of illustration let us create a hypothetical individual with normal hearing sensitivity in both ears. The **laddergram** in Figure 7.1A shows that as the intensity of a tone is increased in one ear, a similar increase in loudness in the opposite ear requires the same increase in intensity. This is the normal increase in loudness with increased intensity.

If a hearing loss is imposed on the right ear of our hypothetical subject, greater intensity is required to reach threshold in that ear; but after the threshold has been reached, increases in intensity (in decibels) above the threshold for the impaired ear result in increases in loudness identical to those in the unimpaired ear (Figure 7.1B). Nothing is very surprising about these statements, for logic tells us that a tone of 40 dB SL in a normal ear should sound as loud as the same tone at 40 dB SL in a pathological ear, even though the hearing thresholds are different. There are, however, a number of exceptions to the normal growth of loudness just described.

Recruitment

Figure 7.1C shows a patient with the same degree of hearing loss as that in Figure 7.1B; but note that as intensity increases in the normal ear, the same amount of intensity results in an unusually rapid growth of loudness in the impaired ear. It seems as though a great deal of loudness is compressed into a relatively small amount of intensity increase for this individual. Such findings are observed for some patients with unilateral hearing losses by using a binaural loudness-balancing procedure. The disproportionate increase in loudness as a function of intensity is called **recruitment.** Recruitment has been shown to be symptomatic of the majority of hearing losses that are caused by damage to the delicate sensory cells of the inner ear. Although loudness recruitment is a very helpful symptom in

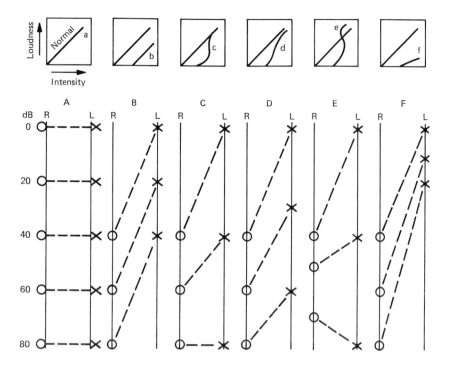

FIGURE 7.1 Growth of loudness in the left ear relative to the growth of loudness in the right ear in the following hypothetical cases where the left ear has normal hearing and the right ear has (A) normal hearing; (B) a 40 dB hearing loss without recruitment; (C) a 40 dB hearing loss with recruitment; (D) a 40 dB hearing loss with partial recruitment; (E) a 40 dB hearing loss with hyperrecruitment; (F) a 40 dB hearing loss with decruitment.

the diagnosis of the site of lesion in the auditory system, it presents a number of difficulties in audiological rehabilitation.

Partial Recruitment

Frequently, performance of the loudness-balancing procedure shows that loudness grows more rapidly than normal in the impaired ear but without complete recruitment (Figure 7.1D). Such individuals are said to exhibit **partial recruitment.** Some audiologists believe that partial recruitment has the same diagnostic significance as complete recruitment—that is, damage to the inner ear.

Hyperrecruitment

In some pathological cases, loudness grows so rapidly with small increases in intensity that a tone may appear to be louder in the impaired ear than it is in a normal ear at the same (high) intensity. People showing this phenomenon are said to exhibit **hyperrecruitment,** or **overrecruitment.** Hyperrecruitment, illustrated in Figure 7.1E, may be a dramatic diagnostic finding, or it may be a variation on recruitment caused by differences in performance on the test.

Decruitment

In some hearing losses, nerve units in the auditory system are missing or damaged, and loudness grows more *slowly* in the impaired ear than it does in a normal ear as intensity is increased. To individuals with this problem, even very intense sounds may not produce much loudness. Such difficulties, illustrated in Figure 7.1F, are called **decruitment.** Decruitment is frequently associated with lesions of the auditory nerve.

Implications of Loudness Recruitment

Some examples of the growth of loudness are illustrated in Figure 7.1. Hearing loss in only one ear is shown so that the normal ear can serve as a reference to which the growth of loudness might be compared at a number of sensation levels. Not all patients manifesting different loudness growths have hearing losses in only one ear. In fact, most hearing losses are bilateral. Many different procedures have been developed to test for loudness recruitment since it was first described by Fowler (1936).

Measures of Loudness Growth

The procedure that is preferred by most audiologists as a direct test for recruitment in patients with unilateral hearing losses is the **alternate binaural loudness balance (ABLB) test.** A candidate for the ABLB procedure must have normal hearing in one ear for the frequencies to be tested. The ABLB is administered by pulsing a tone of a single frequency from one ear to the other, and, by controlling the intensity of the tones delivered to the ears through a two-channel audiometer, the patient is guided toward a perceived loudness balance. While clinical practice survey results for the past twenty-five years (most recently, Martin et al., 1998) have shown a steady decline in the clinical use of the ABLB, circuitry for the administration of this test is still included on most two-channel audiometers. Some clinics record results of the ABLB test directly on an audiogram, placing the symbols for the right and left ears on either side of the ordinate, indicating the test frequency. Other clinics develop special forms for this purpose, such as the one shown in Figure 7.2A. Details on ABLB testing procedures may be found in clinical audiometer instruction manuals and will not be presented here.

Two other loudness balance procedures that enjoyed brief popularity are the *alternate monaural loudness balance (AMLB) test* and the *simultaneous binaural loudness balance (SBLB) test.* The AMLB (Reger, 1936) was developed to measure the growth of loudness of one frequency (that demonstrates a hearing loss) to the growth of loudness of another frequency (at which the patient has normal hearing) in the same ear.

Unlike the alternate delivery of tones between the ears in the ABLB, in the SBLB, the tone, fed through separate attenuaters to each earphone, is presented simultaneously to both ears. Jerger and Harford (1960) showed that the ABLB and the SBLB do not measure the same functions. Although the SBLB test may have value in determining lesions that are higher in the auditory system, it should not be used as a test for recruitment.

Measures of loudness growth for site-of-lesion assessment have been largely supplanted by electrophysiological measures of the auditory system that can lead more easily to the same diagnosis with a significant decrease in invested clinical time. Loudness growth measures have, however, found more recent clinical utility in fitting hearing aids to patients with recruitment.

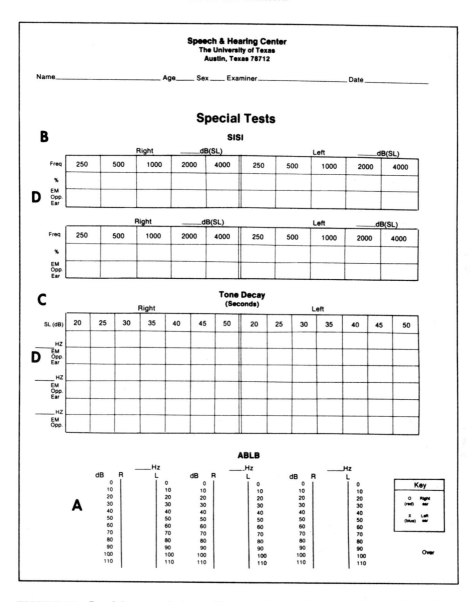

FIGURE 7.2   Special test worksheet with space allocated for recording results on the following tests: (A) alternate binaural loudness balance (ABLB); (B) short increment sensitivity index (SISI); (C) tone decay. Spaces next to the letter D allow for the recording of effective masking levels in the nontest ear.

Discussion of Loudness Recruitment

As a rule, recruitment is more likely to be demonstrated in the higher than in the lower frequencies. Often, only one or two frequencies lend themselves to ABLB testing, and decisions regarding the presence of recruitment must be based on these. Disagreement persists regarding the diagnostic value of recruitment tests. This chapter, as throughout this book, emphasizes that no single procedure or set of procedures in audiology may be relied on completely to determine the site of a hearing disorder.

As was mentioned in Chapter 6, acoustic reflexes are often observed at low sensation levels in patients who have lesions of the cochlea. This has been interpreted by some audiologists as a manifestation of loudness recruitment, which occurs because a tone presented at, say, 45 dB SL sounds as though it is very loud (as loud as a 95 dBHL tone to a normal listener). There is no evidence that recruitment, *per se*, produces an acoustic reflex at low sensation levels, although both phenomena are often found in the same patients.

The Short Increment Sensitivity Index

For some time it has been known that as intensity is increased in a normal ear, the ability to detect small changes in intensity in that ear also increases. That is, at low sensation levels a tone might change in intensity several decibels before the listener becomes aware of any change in loudness. When that same tone is very loud, a change in intensity equal to a fraction of a decibel can often be detected. The smallest change in intensity that can be recognized as a change in loudness is the **difference limen for intensity (DLI).** Because increased loudness of a tone improves the normal listener's ability to tell when the tone has changed in intensity, it was once a popular belief that the DLI is an indirect measurement of loudness recruitment. That is, if a patient with a hearing loss has a small DLI at a low sensation level, that sound must be perceived as loud. The conventional wisdom is that although both loudness recruitment and small DLIs near threshold suggest a cochlear lesion, a cause-and-effect relationship does not necessarily exist between the two.

In the 1950s a number of variations on the DLI theme developed. Many audiometers came equipped with special controls for performing DLI measurements. Audiologists eventually began to despair over the lack of reliability of these tests. A procedure as delicate as the DLI requires, for one thing, a great deal more practice and familiarization on the part of the patient than is practical in most clinical situations.

Clinical experience with the DLI suggested that patients with disorders of the cochlea can detect small intensity changes in an otherwise steady-state signal. Patients with normal hearing and those with disorders other than in the cochlea do not have this ability. Jerger, Shedd, and Harford (1959) developed a test based on this principle, the **short increment sensitivity index (SISI).** Rather than measuring the size of the DLI, the SISI procedure is designed to test the ability of a patient to detect the presence of a 1 dB increment superimposed on a tone presented at 20 dB SL (Figure 7.3).

Any patient can be tested with the SISI procedure as long as a hearing loss at the frequency tested does not exceed the maximum limit of the audiometer. Because the sensation level for the standard SISI test is 20 dB, the patient's hearing threshold should be at least 20 dB below the audiometer's limit for the frequency tested.

Because the SISI is a suprathreshold procedure, the problem of cross-hearing presents itself often. When the hearing level of the SISI carrier tone is above the bone-conduction threshold of the

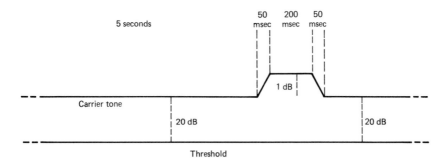

FIGURE 7.3 **Diagram of the stimulus of the SISI. The carrier tone is presented at 20 dB above the patient's threshold for the test frequency. Every 5 seconds a 1 dB increment is superimposed that rises to maximum in 50 milliseconds, remains at that level for 200 milliseconds, and then returns to the 20 dB SL in 50 milliseconds.**

opposite ear by an amount equal to or greater than the patient's interaural attenuation, the nontest ear is involved in the test. Masking for the SISI is similar to masking for word recognition testing.

Just as recruitment is more likely to be found in the higher frequencies on the ABLB test, SISI scores tend to be higher for the high frequencies. The higher the SISI score, the greater the likelihood that a hearing disorder is in the cochlea. At frequencies of 1000 Hz and above, 100 percent SISI scores are common in patients with cochlear hearing losses. Below 500 Hz, scores above 20 percent are rare, even in cochlear disorders. As a general rule, hearing losses of 30 dB or less do not show high SISI scores. Although patients with recruitment on the ABLB tend to have high SISI scores, and those without recruitment tend to have low SISI scores, it is probably best, from a clinical viewpoint, to look at the two tests in terms of the diagnostic information they provide, rather than to regard the SISI as an indirect recruitment test.

Several modifications of the SISI have been suggested. One procedure uses a high-level SISI at 75 dB HL (Sanders, Josey, & Glasscock, 1974). It has also been suggested that the SISI be performed with increment sizes larger than 1 dB when scores at 20 dB SL are low. In some cases of pathology in the higher centers of the auditory system, even increasing the increment size does not allow the patient to identify the increment.

As with the ABLB, the SISI is rarely used clinically today (Martin et al., 1998), although circuitry for the administration of the SISI is still included on most clinical audiometers. Details on SISI testing procedures may be found in clinical audiometer instruction manuals and will not be presented here.

Tone Decay

In most cases, even among people with normal auditory systems, listening to sustained signals will bring about a certain amount of shift in an individual's thresholds for those signals. For many years it has been noted that patients with some forms of hearing disorder find it impossible to hear sustained tones for more than a brief time. To many of these patients, a tone heard clearly at a level 5 dB above threshold fades rapidly to inaudibility. If the level of the tone is increased, the tone may be heard again, only to disappear quickly to silence. Although a number of different names have been ascribed to this phenomenon, perhaps the most popular one among audiologists is **tone decay.**

Since it has been recognized that extreme threshold tone decay may be a powerful symptom of some serious medical conditions, audiologists have become interested in developing tests to quantify its presence. Of all the special tests described in this chapter, none requires less esoteric equipment than the tone decay tests; only a standard audiometer and a stopwatch are necessary. Compared to the other behavioral site-of-lesion measures discussed here, tone decay testing has retained some clinical utility given its relatively high sensitivity and the limited clinical time required to administer.

The Tone Decay Tests

A number of tone decay tests have been proposed since the earliest procedure developed by Carhart (1957). Of these, one of the more popular is a modification of the original Carhart method proposed by Olsen and Noffsinger (1974). Because some tone decay is usually evident in patients with damage to the cochlea, these investigators recommended the test be started at 20 dB above threshold rather than at threshold as recommended by Carhart. Olsen and Noffsinger's study found that the same information was obtained with this procedure as with the Carhart method in terms of diagnosis, but with some time savings.

The *Olsen-Noffsinger tone decay test* is begun by presenting a tone to the patient through an earphone at 20 dB SL. Patients are asked to signal as soon as they hear a tone and again when they no longer hear it. As soon as the patient signals that the tone is heard, the stopwatch is started; it is stopped when the patient signals that the tone is no longer heard. The number of seconds that the tone is heard at 20 dB HL is recorded. The stopwatch is reset, and the level of the tone is raised by 5 dB *without interrupting the tone*. This procedure is continued until (1) the patient can hear the tone for a full 60 seconds; (2) 30 dB above the starting level has been reached, and the patient fails to hear the tone at that level for at least 60 seconds; or (3) the maximum limit of the audiometer has been reached. As in the Carhart procedure, the amount of tone decay is expressed as the number of decibels above threshold that the tone can be heard for a full minute.

Rosenberg (1969) described an earlier modification to the tone decay test that he felt provided all the information derived from the Carhart method, but in only one minute for each frequency tested. In the *Rosenberg tone decay test* the tone is introduced at 5 dB SL and timing is begun with a stopwatch. When the patient signals that the tone is no longer heard, the level is immediately raised by 5 dB, but the stopwatch is allowed to continue to run. If the patient signals silence again, the level is raised another 5 dB, and so forth, until the entire 60 seconds has elapsed. The test is scored as the number of decibels of decay in the 60-second period. This procedure can even further conserve clinical time with no loss of test accuracy when used with a 20 dB SL starting level as advocated by Olsen and Noffsinger.

Clinical observation of some patients with disorders of the higher auditory centers (beyond the cochlea) caused Green (1963) to approach tone decay from another viewpoint. Green noticed that although some patients could continue to hear the tone presented to them, there was a change in its *quality*. Some patients have remarked that pure tones may be devoid of their tonality shortly after introduction. Following Green's recommendation, clinicians often, in addition to having the patients signal when they no longer hear a tone, instruct patients to notify the examiner if the tone loses its tonal quality. Apparently, some patients do experience loss of tonality much before and even in the absence of threshold shift. However, many patients have difficulty in determining their criteria for loss of tonality.

Another modification of early tone decay measures arose from the observation that many patients with lesions in areas central to the inner ear, such as tumors of the auditory nerve, show greater amounts of tone decay when the presentation of the stimulus is at a high intensity. This is the premise of the **suprathreshold adaptation test (STAT)** (Jerger & Jerger, 1975). Instructions for this test are the same as for all tone decay tests—that the patient continue to signal as long as the tone is audible.

The STAT is done with the tone presented at 110 dB SPL, rounded off to 100 dB HL at 500 and 2000 Hz and to 105 dB HL at 1000 Hz. Timing begins as soon as the patient signals that the tone is heard, and the test is concluded when 60 seconds have elapsed, or when the patient signals that the tone is inaudible. The STAT is interpreted as positive for a neural lesion if complete adaptation occurs within one minute.

Cross-hearing and Masking in Tone Decay Tests

It is only logical that as the level of a signal is raised in the test ear, that level, minus the patient's interaural attenuation, may reach the bone-conduction threshold of the nontest ear. As soon as the nontest ear has been stimulated, assuming it has no tone decay, the patient's tone decay in the test ear will *appear* to have reached a plateau. Cross-hearing for tone decay tests (TDT) is stated as

$$TDT\ HL_{TE} - IA = BC_{NTE}$$

Because the signal may be initially at a high intensity, or constantly increased in level during a tone decay test, minimum masking is not advocated here. The use of maximum masking seems to be a practical approach for these tests and may be stated as the bone-conduction threshold of the test ear plus the patient's interaural attenuation, minus a 5 dB safety factor:

$$EM = BC_{TE} + IA - 5$$

When masking during any tone decay test, the tone should be turned off before the noise to make certain that the patient is signaling the audibility of the tone and not that of the noise. Masking may often be unnecessary for tone decay tests when insert receivers are used.

Interpreting Tone Decay Tests

Although all the tone decay tests are useful, the Olsen-Noffsinger method is used to illustrate typical test results for the different kinds of hearing disorders described in Chapters 9 through 12. Interpretation of the Olsen-Noffsinger and similar tone decay methods that are begun near threshold is shown in Table 7.1. Three types of tone decay appear (Owens, 1971):

Type I. No tone decay in 60 seconds at any frequency. This is seen in patients with normal auditory systems, in those with conductive hearing losses, and in some with lesions of the cochlea.

Type II. Progressively slower tone decay as the level is raised in 5 dB steps. Type II tone decay is strongly suggestive of cochlear pathology.

Type III. Type III tone decay is the most dramatic. Even with increased intensity, the patient is unable to sustain hearing of the tone for increasing periods of time. Type III tone decay patterns are strongly suggestive of lesions of the auditory nerve.

TABLE 7.1 Typical Tone Decay Patterns (responses in seconds)

Sensation Level dB	Type I	Type II	Type III
5	60	14	3
10		26	12
15		39	8
20		48	15
25		60	10
30			8

In addition to rates of decay, tone decay patterns appear with respect to stimulus frequency. In Type I patterns no significant decay is seen at any frequency. In Type II patterns more decay is generally observed for higher than for lower frequencies, suggesting the advisability of testing several different frequencies. Type III patterns show rapid tone decay, even in the low frequencies.

Rosenberg (1958) described some useful criteria in interpreting tone decay tests:

1. Normal—0 to 5 dB in 60 seconds
2. Mild—10 to 15 dB in 60 seconds
3. Moderate—20 to 25 dB in 60 seconds
4. Marked—30 dB or more in 60 seconds

Békésy Audiometry

The use of a modern version of Békésy's automatic audiometer was once a popular audiological procedure that allows patients to track their own auditory thresholds. During **Békésy audiometry** the patient presses a button when a tone becomes audible in an earphone, keeps the button depressed as long as the tone is heard, and then releases it when the tone becomes inaudible. The tone is allowed to increase in intensity until the button is pressed, which causes the tone to be attenuated. A pen, controlled by the attenuator of the audiometer, traces the level of the tone on an audiogram as a function of both time and either fixed or constantly changing frequency.

Békésy Tracing Types

The initial report of Jerger (1960) led to the use of Békésy audiometry as a clinical tool in the differential diagnosis of site of lesion. Observations were made of responses to continuous and to pulsed tones. The result of these observations was a series of four different types of Békésy audiograms; a fifth was subsequently noted by Jerger and Herer (1961) (Figure 7.4).

Although observed in some patients with cochlear lesions, the Type I Békésy tracing is most often seen in patients with normal hearing and those with conductive hearing losses. These patients produce audiograms in which the pulsed and continuous tracings overlap; that is, the thresholds are the same whether the tone is continuously on or pulsing on and off.

Sweep Frequency Tracings

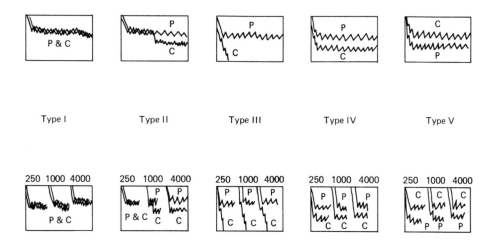

Type I   Type II   Type III   Type IV   Type V

Fixed Frequency Tracings

FIGURE 7.4   Five Békésy types: *Type I* sweep- and fixed-frequency Békésy audiogram showing
continuous and pulsed tracings to interweave, with swing width about 10 dB. *Type II* sweep- and
fixed-frequency Békésy audiograms showing continuous and pulsed tracings to interweave in the
low frequencies. At about 1000 Hz the continuous-tone tracing drops below the pulsed tracing,
suggesting that it is harder to hear a continuous tone. The swing width becomes narrower in the
higher frequencies, indicating that the patient can make sharp distinctions between audibility and
inaudibility, with very small changes in intensity. *Type III* sweep- and fixed-frequency audiograms
showing the continuous tone to be difficult to hear even in the low frequencies. The pulsed-tone
trace follows the pattern of the conventional audiogram. *Type IV* sweep- and fixed-frequency
audiograms showing the continuous tone to drop below (become harder to hear than) the pulsed
tone throughout the frequency range. Unlike the *Type III* tracing, the *Type IV* continuous tracing
never completely fades to inaudibility. *Type V* sweep- and fixed-frequency Békésy tracings showing
the pulsed tone to be more difficult to hear than the continuous tone. This tracing is not explainable
on the basis of typical organic pathology.

The pulsed tracings of patients with cochlear disorders generally follows the audiometric configuration obtained using conventional pure-tone audiometry, as do both the pulsed and continuous
Type I tracings. However, the Type II tracings typical of cochlear pathology differ sharply in the
continuous-tone trace, when at about 1000 Hz the tracing for the continuous tone drops below the
interrupted one. The continuous tracing often becomes significantly narrower and tends to run not
more than 20 dB below the pulsed tone.

The most dramatic, but least common of all the Békésy types, is the Type III. In this pattern,
as in the others, the interrupted trace follows the pattern of manual audiometry; however, the continuous tone reveals marked adaptation to the signal. This pronounced separation of the continuous
from the pulsed tracing occurs at all frequencies. Type III tracings are associated with lesions medial
to the cochlea, although not all such lesions manifest Type III tracings.

Type IV tracings appear similar to Type IIs, with the differentiation that Type IV tracings often exhibit the continuous tone breakaway below 500 Hz, with a separation of at least 20 dB. Type IV tracings were originally ascribed to lesions medial to the inner ear, although observations of patients with cochlear disorders exhibiting Type IV tracings have been noted.

Jerger and Herer (1961) observed unusual Békésy tracings on a series of patients who were believed to be exaggerating their hearing thresholds for financial or other gain. In these tracings, called Type V, the hearing for continuous tones appears to be better than for pulsed tones, a phenomenon that defies explanation on the basis of organic pathology. Although Type V tracings might alert the audiologist to a nonorganic disorder, they are by no means evidence of this. Type V tracings are mentioned again in Chapter 13 in the discussion on nonorganic hearing loss.

Variations on Békésy Audiometry

Several modifications of the standard Békésy procedure described earlier have been suggested. Some of these procedures include: change in frequency direction (sweeping from the high frequencies to the low frequencies), changing the intensity direction (beginning at a high level instead of below the patient's threshold), change in stimulus duration (presenting brief tones of 20 msec, instead of the normal pulse duration of 200 msec), and having the patient track most comfortable listening levels (rather than threshold). All of these variations have been said to increase the separation between the pulsed and continuous tracings.

Discussion of Békésy Audiometry

Though Békésy audiometry was never used routinely with small children, it can be carried out successfully with the majority of patients for whom diagnosis is needed. Experience and research suggest that the slower the attenuation rate, the more information may emerge from this test. Because of the significant clinical time investment to complete Békésy testing, coupled with the procedure's low test sensitivity, this test has been largely supplanted by electrophysiologic audiometric procedures. Today, Békésy is rarely used and it is difficult to purchase a Békésy audiometer.

Summary

The presence of loudness recruitment is a strong indicator of lesions of the cochlea and may best be measured by the alternate binaural loudness balance (ABLB) test. Decruitment is considered to be a strong symptom of neural lesions. The absence of recruitment suggests a lesion elsewhere than the cochlea or normal hearing.

High scores on the SISI test at 20 dB SL and acoustic reflexes at low sensation levels are other strong indicators of cochlear disorders. The modified SISI test, performed at high intensities, reveals low scores when retrocochlear lesions are present. Tone decay tests and the rarely used Békésy audiometry produce patterns suggestive of hearing loss in the conductive, sensory, or neural pathways of hearing.

None of the tests described in this chapter is infallible. Roeser (1986), on the basis of the findings of Jerger and Jerger (1983), has pointed out that some tests, like Békésy audiometry and the suprathreshold adaptation test (STAT), have high specificity but low sensitivity (i.e., they rule out

TABLE 7.2 Sensitivity, Specificity, and Efficiency of Seven Popular Site-of-lesion Auditory Tests

Procedure	Sensitivity (%)	Specificity (%)	Efficiency (%)
ABR	97	88	90
AR/Decay	86	86	86
PI-PB	93	98	97
Tone Decay	75	91	88
SISI	68	90	85
ABLB	51	88	64
Békésy	42	95	52

(From Worthington, 1988)

the wrong lesion but do not correctly identify the right lesion), whereas others, like performance intensity functions for PB word lists (PI-PB) have high specificity and moderate sensitivity. Still other tests, like ABR, are both highly specific and highly sensitive, and are both efficient and possessive of high predictive value. On the basis of his own clinical observations, and the findings of other clinicians, Worthington (1988) prepared a summary of various site-of-lesion tests, comparing their sensitivity, specificity, and efficiency (Table 7.2).

The trends pointed out by Martin and colleagues (1998) suggest that the older psychophysical tests have all but given way to the newer electrophysiological procedures discussed in Chapter 6. The results of any special diagnostic testing must always be compared to pure-tone and speech results and, above all, to the patient's history.

STUDY QUESTIONS

1. For each site-of-lesion test described in this chapter, indicate whether it may be performed with (a) unilateral losses, (b) bilateral losses, or (c) both. Explain why.

2. For the tests described in question 1, list the equipment required and consider the performance and interpretation of each test.

3. Draw audiograms for unilateral conductive and sensorineural hearing losses. What are the probable results of the site-of-lesion tests described in this chapter, based on the type of hearing loss and the probable site of lesion?

4. What are the theoretical and practical values of the measures obtained in question 3?

5. Determine the effective masking levels, if needed, for all the tests described in question 3.

GLOSSARY

Alternate binaural loudness balance (ABLB) test A procedure that tests for recruitment in unilateral hearing losses. The growth of loudness of pure tones in the impaired ear is compared with that of the opposite (normal) ear as a function of increasing intensity.

Békésy audiometry A procedure utilizing the Békésy automatic audiometer during which tracings are obtained for both pulsed and continuous tones.

Clinical decision analysis (CDA) Procedures by which tests can be assessed in terms of their sensitivity, specificity, efficiency, and predictive value.

Decruitment The less than normal growth in loudness of a signal as the intensity is increased. Also called *subtractive hearing loss,* it is suggestive of a loss of nerve units.

Difference limen for intensity (DLI) A test designed to determine a subject's ability to detect small changes in the intensity of a pure tone. In the 1950s a small DLI was considered a symptom of recruitment.

Efficiency The percentage of time that a test correctly identifies a site of lesion and correctly eliminates an anatomical area as the site of lesion.

Hyperrecruitment A condition of some pathological hearing disorders in which a tone of a given intensity produces a sensation of greater loudness than that same intensity would produce for a normal ear.

Laddergram The plotting of results on the ABLB test. The relative loudness at each ear is shown at several intensities at the test frequency.

Overrecruitment See *Hyperrecruitment.*

Partial recruitment The condition in which a given amount of intensity in a pathological ear produces almost as much loudness as the same amount of intensity produces in a normal ear.

Predictive value The percentage of all positive test results that are truly positive and the percentage of all negative test results that are truly negative.

Recruitment A large increase in the perceived loudness of a signal produced by relatively small increases in intensity above threshold; symptomatic of some hearing losses produced by damage to the inner ear.

Sensitivity The percentage of time a test correctly identifies a site of lesion.

Short increment sensitivity index (SISI) A test designed to determine a patient's ability to detect small changes (1 dB) in intensity of a pure tone presented at 20 dB SL.

Site of lesion The precise area in the auditory system producing symptoms of abnormal auditory function.

Specificity The percentage of time a test correctly rejects an incorrect diagnosis.

Suprathreshold adaptation test (STAT) A tone decay test that begins at intensities near the limit of the audiometer. If the patient hears the tone for a full 60 seconds, the test result is considered to be negative for a lesion of the auditory nerve.

Tone decay The loss of audibility of a sound produced when the ear is constantly stimulated by a pure tone.

REFERENCES

Carhart, R. (1957). Clinical determination of abnormal auditory adaptation. *Archives of Otolaryngology, 65,* 32–39.

Fowler, E. P. (1936). A method for early detection of otosclerosis. *Archives of Otolaryngology, 24,* 731–741.

Green, D. S. (1963). The modified tone decay test (MTDT) as a screening procedure for eighth nerve lesions. *Journal of Speech and Hearing Disorders, 28,* 31–36.

Jerger, J. F. (1960). Békésy audiometry in analysis of auditory disorders. *Journal of Speech and Hearing Research, 3,* 275–287.

Jerger, J. F., & Harford, E. R. (1960). The alternate and simultaneous balancing of pure tones. *Journal of Speech and Hearing Research, 3,* 17–30.

Jerger, J. F., & Herer, G. (1961). Unexpected dividend in Békésy audiometry. *Journal of Speech and Hearing Disorders, 26,* 390–391.

Jerger, J., & Jerger, S. (1975). A simplified tone decay test. *Archives of Otolaryngology, 101,* 403–407.

Jerger, J., & Jerger, S. (1983). The evaluation of diagnostic audiometric tests. *Audiology, 22,* 144–161.

Jerger, J. F., Shedd, J., & Harford, E. R. (1959). On the detection of extremely small changes in sound intensity. *Archives of Otolaryngology, 69,* 200–211.

Martin, F. N., Champlin, C. A., & Chambers, J. A. (1998). Seventh survey of audiometric practices in the United States. *Journal of the American Academy of Audiology, 9,* 95–104.

Olsen, W. O., & Noffsinger, D. (1974). Comparison of one new and three old tests of auditory adaptation. *Archives of Otolaryngology, 99,* 94–99.

Owens, E. (1971). Audiologic evaluation in cochlear versus retrocochlear lesion. *Acta Otolaryngologica, 283* (Supplement).

Reger, S. N. (1936). Differences in loudness response of normal and hard-of-hearing ears at intensity levels slightly above threshold. *Annals of Otology, Rhinology, and Laryngology, 45,* 1029–1039.

Roeser, R. (1986). *Diagnostic audiology.* Austin, TX: Pro-Ed.

Rosenberg, P. E. (1958, November). *Rapid clinical measurement of tone decay.* Paper presented at the American Speech and Hearing Association convention, New York.

———. (1969). *Tone decay.* Maico Audiological Library Series, Report 6.

Sanders, J. W., Josey, A. F., & Glasscock, M. E. (1974). Audiologic evaluation in cochlear and eighth nerve disorders. *Archives of Otolaryngology, 100,* 283–289.

Turner, R. G., & Nielsen, D. W. (1984). Application of clinical decision analysis to audiological tests. *Ear and Hearing, 5,* 125–133.

Worthington, D. W. (1988). *Site of lesion: Special auditory tests.* Presentation at the Scott Haug Audiology Retreat, Kerrville, Texas.

SUGGESTED READINGS

Brunt, M. A. (1994). Tests of cochlear function. In J. Katz (Ed.), *Handbook of clinical audiology* (4th ed., pp. 165–175). Baltimore: Williams & Wilkins.

Green, D. S., & Huerta, L. (1994). Tests of retrochoclear function. In J. Katz (Ed.), *Handbook of clinical audiology* (4th ed., pp. 176–180). Baltimore: Williams & Wilkins.

REVIEW TABLE 7.1   Summary of Site-of-lesion Tests

Test	Purpose	Unit	When to Mask	How to Mask
ABLB	Recruitment	dB	N/A	
SISI	Detect 1 dB Increment	dB	SISI HL_{TE}-IA $\geq BC_{NTE}$	EM = SISI HL – IA + ABG_{NTE}
TDT	Perstimulatory adaptation	Seconds	Routinely	EM = BC_{TE} + IA – 5
Békésy Audiometry	Tracking pulsed & continuous tones	Seconds or dB	Same as TDT	Same as TDT

REVIEW TABLE 7.2   Typical Interpretation of Site-of-lesion Tests

	Normal Hearing	Conductive Loss	Sensory Loss	Neural Loss
ABLB or AMLB	No recruitment	No recruitment	Partial, full, or hyperrecruitment	No recruitment or decruitment
SISI (%)	0–30	0–30	70–100	0–30
Tone Decay Type	I	I	II	III
Békésy Type	I	I	II	III or IV

CHAPTER

8

Hearing Tests for Children

Most of the audiometric procedures described earlier in this text can be applied with great reliability to children beyond ages four or five years. In such cases, the examination is often no more difficult than it is with cooperative adults. However, in many instances, because of the level at which a particular child functions, special diagnostic procedures must be adopted. Since the prevalence of hearing loss in children has been estimated to range from between 1 and 2.5 per 1000 (Davidson, Hyde, & Alberti, 1989; Mauk & Behrens, 1993) up to 6 per 1000 (Hayes & Northern, 1996), the need for pediatric audiology is self evident.

Chapter Objectives

This chapter presents a variety of techniques that have proved helpful in obtaining information about the auditory function of children who cannot be tested using usual audiometric procedures. Methods are described to determine the presence, type, and extent of hearing loss in children. Some insights should be gained about cases presenting special diagnostic difficulty, such as central disorders and nonorganic hearing loss.

Auditory Responses

It has been stated in this book that what is measured with hearing tests is not "hearing" itself, but rather a patient's ability and/or willingness to respond to a set of acoustic signals. Therefore, whatever determination is made about the hearing of any individual is made by inference from some set of responses. The hearing function itself is not observed directly.

The manner of a patient's response to some of the tests described earlier has not been considered to be of great concern. For example, it is not important whether the patient signals the awareness of a tone by a hand signal, by a vocal response, or by pressing a button. With small children, however, the manner and type of response to a signal may be crucial to diagnosis. It is also important to remember that most small children do not respond to acoustic signals at threshold; rather, sounds must be more clearly audible to them than to their older counterparts. It is safe, therefore, to assume that during audiometry, small children's responses must be considered to be at their **minimum response levels (MRLs),** which in some cases may be well above their thresholds.

Responses from small children may vary from voluntary acknowledgment of a signal to involuntary movement of the body, or from an overt cry of surprise to a slight change in vocalization.

Response to sound may be totally unobservable, except for some change in the electrophysiological system of the child being tested. If a clear response to a sound is observed by a trained clinician, it may be inferred that the sound has been heard, although the sensation level of the signal may be very much in question. Conversely, if no response is observed, it cannot be assumed that the sound has not been heard.

Obviously, a number of factors contribute to the responses offered by a child. Of primary concern is the physiological and psychological state prior to stimulation. Shepherd (1978) describes prestimulus activity levels as a range consisting of alert attentiveness, relaxed wakefulness, drowsiness, light sleep, and deep sleep. Students of audiology should spend time observing normal children to understand motor development, language and speech acquisition, and auditory behaviors.

Even though audiologists may have preferences for certain kinds of responses from a child, they must be willing to settle for whatever the child provides. Audiologists must also be willing to alter, in midstream, the kind of procedure used if it seems that a different system might be more effective. Modification of a procedure may be the only way to evoke responses from a child, and flexibility and alertness are essential. Response to a sound may appear only once, and it may easily be lost to the inexperienced or unobservant clinician.

Identifying Hearing Loss in Infants under Three Months of Age

Speech and language are imitative processes, acquired primarily through the auditory sense. A hearing defect, either congenital or acquired early in life, can interfere with the development of concepts that culminate in normal communication. For a variety of reasons, many children with abnormal hearing proceed into the third year of life or beyond before a hearing problem is suspected. A hearing disorder in a child is often not detected because parents believe that if their own child had a hearing loss, they would somehow know it because he or she would be obviously different from other children.

There has also been a mistaken notion that babies with hearing loss do not babble. It is probable that the act of babbling is a kind of vegetative activity that is reinforced by a child's tactile and proprioceptive gratification from the use of the mouth and tongue. Around the age of six months, children with normal hearing begin to notice that those interesting cooing sounds have been coming from their own mouths, and they begin to amuse themselves by varying rate, pitch, and loudness. Often, children with impaired hearing, who do not receive adequate auditory feedback, will gradually decrease their vocalizations. In contrast, children with normal hearing will begin to repeat, in parrotlike fashion, the sounds they hear. Eventually, meaning becomes attached to sounds, and the projective use of words is initiated. Usually the normal-hearing child is speaking well before the age of two years; the child with an auditory deficit is not.

The average age at which children with hearing losses were identified in the United States in the early 1990s was nearly three years of age (National Institutes of Health, 1993), whereas in Israel it has been between seven and nine months (Gustafson, 1989). This significant difference can be attributed primarily to the differences in the health-care delivery systems in the two countries and the auditory screening procedures used. With the knowledge that profound hearing loss in children is declining, whereas mild losses are on the increase, and that these mild losses produce more difficulties for children than had been supposed (Tharpe & Bess, 1991), it is generally agreed that early identification of hearing loss is of paramount importance. The earlier in the life of a child that specific educational and training procedures can be initiated, the greater the chance that they will be successful. There is, of course, no earlier time that testing can begin than immediately after birth. It is for these reasons that a universal infant hearing screening bill was finally introduced in the United States Congress in 1997.

A number of criteria must be met before newborn screening of any disorder can be justified. These include (1) a sufficient prevalence of the disorder to justify the screening, (2) evidence that the disorder will be detected earlier than would be the case without screening, (3) the availability of follow-up diagnostics immediately after the failure of a screening, (4) treatment accessibility immediately following diagnosis, and (5) a documented advantage to early identification. All of these criteria are easily met in the argument for newborn hearing screening.

Infant Hearing Screening

Hearing screening procedures can be justified on several bases, including cost efficiency. When compared with other disorders routinely screened for, such as phenylketonuria (PKU) or neonatal hypothyroidism, the yield is considerably higher for hearing loss. As a matter of fact, hearing loss of varying degrees has been ranked sixth in prevalence of chronic conditions in the United States (U.S. Department of Health and Human Resources, 1993). Simmons, McFarland, and Jones (1980) found hearing loss in 1 out of 50 infants who graduated from an intensive care nursery. Within the general population, reported prevalence data vary because of differences among studies in screening procedures and definition of hearing impairment, but prevalence may be as high six babies with significant hearing loss in every 1000 births (Hayes & Northern, 1996). From a purely objective and financial viewpoint, the fact that hundreds of millions of dollars might be saved each year if early identification and habilitation of hearing impairments were in place, seems to justify neonatal hearing screening, even if the obvious humanitarian aspects are ignored.

Inexperienced audiologists enter their professional careers with little time spent in observing the behaviors of normal infants. Their initial professional experiences are often with children who have problems, which they must diagnose without a satisfactory standard for comparison. Learning the sometimes subtle differences in the appearance and behaviors between children with and without normal hearing is one of the vast benefits of clinical experience since diagnostic decisions are often based on subjective impressions.

Apgar[1] (1953) developed a system for evaluating newborns that is used in many hospitals today. The procedure now utilizes an acronym based on her name: A (appearance), P (pulse), G (grimace), A (activity), R (respiration). Basically the **Apgar Test** score evaluates the normalcy of respiratory effort, muscle tone, heart rate, color, and reflex irritability. The evaluation of the newborn is usually carried out by trained nurses who assign values of 0 to 10 at 1, 5, and 10 minutes after birth. These evaluations help to determine whether the child requires additional oxygen, and whether there is a likelihood of central nervous system damage. Children with low Apgar scores should also be suspected of having sensorineural hearing loss.

---

[1]Dr. Virginia Apgar, American anesthesiologist, 1909–1974.

The History of Screening Children

Wedenberg (1956) screened 150 infants between the ages of one and seven days by hitting a cow-bell with a hammer close to the child's head. Of the infants, 149 responded with an **auropalpebral reflex (APR),** which is a contraction of the muscles surrounding the eyes. Wedenberg subsequently used an audiometer, which powered a small loudspeaker positioned near a sleeping child's head. Testing with a variety of frequencies, he observed responses (in the intensity range from 104 to 112 dB SPL) from normal-hearing infants in light sleep. He noted that premature children do not respond well to external stimuli, and that arousal responses depend, to a large extent, on the sleep level of the child.

Downs and Sterritt (1967), using a specially designed device to produce a 3000 Hz **warble tone,** found that they could observe responses of most infants at about 90 dB SPL. Responses consisted primarily of APRs, movement of the hands or head, or overall startle responses. These researchers tested about 10,000 infants using this procedure, with only 150 failing, 4 of whom were subsequently identified as having hearing losses.

For a time, these kinds of results suggested that screening the hearing of neonates before they leave the hospital might be the method by which early identification and follow-up could be achieved. There were, however, several problems. The training of the individual performing the test is of great importance. Attendance by a separate observer is often useful, but disagreements on acceptance of responses occur. Because a number of children with normal hearing may fail the screening, informing their parents of possible hearing loss may produce undue alarm and concern. Additionally, startle responses to high-intensity sounds may be observed from children with moderate hearing losses who show loudness recruitment. In large measure because of the lack of sophisticated means of testing the hearing of neonates, it looked for a time that the goal of large-scale screening, noble though it was, was just too impractical to implement.

A joint committee of the American Speech-Language-Hearing Association (ASHA), the American Academy of Otolaryngology-Head and Neck Surgery, the American Academy of Pediatrics (AAP), the American Academy of Audiology (AAA), and directors of speech and hearing programs in state health and welfare agencies, revised their previous positions and endorsed the goal of universal hearing screening. They felt that the **high-risk registry,** which contains a list of indicators of hearing loss previously described (Joint Committee, 1991) should be maintained, but that due to certain drawbacks it lacked the specificity required to find the majority of children at risk for hearing loss. Mehl and Thomson (1998) state that selective hearing screening based on high-risk criteria fails to detect at least half of all infants with congenital hearing loss.

The registry, as revised in 1994 (Joint Committee, 1994), separated the risk factors for neonates (birth through 28 days) from those of infants (29 days through 2 years and 29 days through 3 years). These risk criteria are listed in Tables 8.1, 8.2, and 8.3.

Since some hearing losses are **hereditodegenerative,** a child falling on the high-risk registry because of family history might pass an early screening, lulling the family into a false sense of security about the potential for later development of a hearing loss. An obvious additional difficulty in using the high-risk registry lies in the fact that many hereditary hearing losses are of a recessive nature, and the genetic potential for hearing loss may exist without an obvious family history of this disorder.

With the realization of the many drawbacks of the high-risk registry and the advent of new testing technology, opinions began to swing back to the desirability of universal hearing screening

TABLE 8.1   Risk Factors Suggesting Inclusion on a High-risk Registry for Neonates (birth through 28 days) Requiring Hearing Screening

1. Family history of congenital or delayed-onset childhood sensorineural hearing loss.
2. In utero infection known or suspected to be associated with sensorineural hearing impairment (e.g., cytomegalovirus, rubella, herpes, toxoplasmosis, syphilis).
3. Craniofacial anomalies, including abnormalities of the pinna and ear canal.
4. Birth weight less than 1500 grams (~ 3.3 pounds).
5. Hyperbilirubinemia (excess amounts of certain bile pigments in the blood) at levels exceeding indications for exchange transfusion.
6. Ototoxic medications including, but not limited to, the aminoglycosides (e.g., gentamycin, kanamycin, streptomycin), and certain diuretics used in combination with these drugs.
7. Bacterial meningitis.
8. Severe depression at birth, which may include infants with Apgar scores of 4 or lower at 1 minute, or 6 or lower at 5 minutes.
9. Prolonged mechanical ventilation for a duration equal to or greater than 5 days.
10. Stigmata or other findings associated with a syndrome known to include sensorineural and/or conductive hearing loss.

TABLE 8.2   Risk Factors Suggesting Inclusion on a High-risk Registry for Infants (age 29 days through 2 years) Requiring Hearing Screening

1. Parent or caregiver concern regarding hearing, speech, language, and/or developmental delay.
2. Bacterial meningitis and other infections associated with sensorineural hearing loss.
3. Head trauma associated with loss of consciousness or skull fracture.
4. Stigmata or other findings associated with a syndrome known to include sensorineural and/or conductive hearing loss.
5. Ototoxic medications and certain diuretics.
6. Recurrent or persistent otitis media with effusion for at least three months.

TABLE 8.3   Risk Factors Suggesting Inclusion on a High-risk Registry for Infants (age 29 days through 3 years) Requiring Periodic Monitoring of Hearing

1. Indicators associated with delayed onset of sensorineural hearing loss:
   a. Family history of hereditary childhood hearing loss.
   b. In utero infection, such as cytomegalovirus, rubella, syphilis, herpes, or toxoplasmosis.
   c. Neurofibromatosis and certain neurodegenerative disorders.

2. Indicators associated with conductive hearing loss:
   a. Recurrent or persistent otitis media with effusion.
   b. Anatomic deformities and other disorders that affect eustachian tube function.
   c. Neurodegenerative disorders.

for all neonates (National Institutes of Health, 1993). Impetus for this thinking was, at least in part, due to the enthusiasm generated by the Rhode Island project using otoacoustic emissions for screening hearing (Vohr, White, Maxon, & Johnson, 1993; White, Vohr, Maxon, & Behrens, 1993; White, Vohr, Maxon, Behrens, McPherson, & Mauk, 1994). Although the cost per child for newborn hearing screening is significantly higher than screening tests performed on blood, the higher incidence of congenital hearing loss results in a comparable cost per case diagnosed. In fact, the incidence of bilateral congenital hearing loss is many times greater than the combined incidence of all newborn screening tests currently conducted on blood samples (Mehl & Thomson, 1998)

Automated Detection Devices

From a historical perspective, two devices for testing neonates, while they remain in the hospital, are of interest. The crib-o-gram (Simmons, 1976; Simmons & Russ, 1974) and the neonatal auditory response cradle (Bennett, 1979) both used motion-sensitive transducers capable of sensing an infant's movements in response to calibrated signals. Time required for testing and equipment difficulties, along with the development of more successful means for neonatal screenings, led to the virtual discontinuation of these early screening devices.

Screening with ABR

Auditory brainstem response (ABR) audiometry has become increasingly popular as a neonatal testing system (Figure 8.1). Some of the disadvantages of this procedure have been discussed previously in this book, for example, the lack of frequency specificity evident when click stimuli are used. When testing infants on the high-risk registry, it is important to compare responses to norms that correspond to children's gestational ages, rather than to their chronological ages, because immaturity of the central nervous system in a premature child can have a profound effect on results and must be taken into account.

Although the Committee on Hearing, Bioacoustics, and Biomechanics (National Research Council, 1987) concluded that "ABR is the most objective measure currently available with which to assess the functional integrity of the peripheral auditory system in neonates," they also cautioned that the ABR is "only a moderately effective predictor of the behavioral audiogram." Research emphasizes the need for data over a period of years to determine the percentage of false positive and false negative findings of neonatal hearing loss based on ABR testing. Follow-up testing is essential when ABR results are either positive or negative for infants on the high-risk registry. However, combining ABR with acoustic reflex testing appears to produce a sensitive and specific approach to the testing of high-risk infants (Hirsch, Margolis, & Rykken, 1992).

Equipment used for measuring ABRs in infants was initially rather costly and more sophisticated than what was required in the neonatal nursery. This equipment has been replaced by less expensive, dedicated units that have a higher degree of portability without sacrifice in quality. In recent years automated systems have been developed that are easy to use, require little in the way of interpretation of results, and can be used by trained technicians, including volunteers. Electrodes and earphones are disposable and easy to apply and remove. Results with this kind of equipment have been very encouraging and can have a pronounced effect on lowering the cost of neonatal screening.

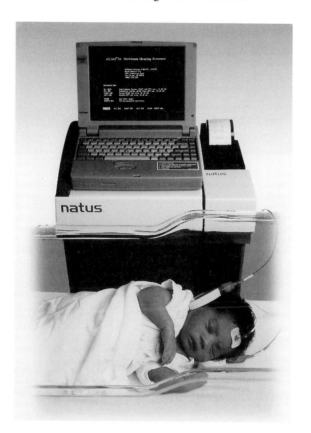

FIGURE 8.1   Auditory brainstem response measurement is one method for screening neonatal hearing. (Courtesy of Natus Medical, Inc.)

Screening with Otoacoustic Emissions

The use of otoacoustic emissions (OAE) as a neonatal screening method has emerged rapidly in recent years (see Bonfils, Dumont, Marie, Francois, & Narcy, 1990; Bonfils, Vziel, & Pujol, 1988; Kemp & Ryan, 1993; Norton, 1994). Over 6000 infants were investigated in the Rhode Island Hearing Assessment Project (RIHAP) (Maxon, White, Vohr, & Behrens, 1992). The OAEs have been shown to be specific, sensitive, and cost-effective measures in infants.

If all the requirements can be met, including a tightly fitting ear piece, quiet test environment, and so on, it can be assumed that children whose ears produce evoked emissions have normal hearing, or no worse than a 30 dB hearing loss. Those who fail the screenings should be followed up with ABR or other testing as deemed by the attending clinician. The first few days of life are ideal for measuring OAEs, since bodily movement makes it difficult to perform and evaluate, and neonates spend many hours each day in sound sleep. However, the presence of even a slight conductive hearing loss eliminates the measurable emission.

It must be remembered that the probable origin of the otoacoustic emission is the outer hair cells of the cochlea. Therefore, if the cochlea is normal and a lesion exists in a retrocochlear area, there is a good chance for normal-appearing emissions to be evoked. This fact produces a cogent argument in favor of a combination of OAE and ABR testing.

Acoustic Reflexes

Obviously, the more hearing screening tests performed on a neonate the less fallible the approach becomes. Hirsch, Margolis, and Rykken (1992) suggest testing acoustic reflexes along with ABR to increase reliability. Margolis (1993) recommends acoustic reflex threshold (ART) testing of infants, increasing the reliability of this test by using probe tone frequencies above the usual 226 Hz, and comparing ARTs for pure tones to ARTs for broadband noise. This procedure does not reveal actual hearing thresholds, but helps to categorize the child as either having normal hearing or greater than a 30 dB sensorineural hearing loss.

For normal-hearing individuals, the ART for a broadband noise is approximately 15 dB lower than the average ARTs at 500, 1000, and 2000 Hz (Jerger, Burney, Mauldin, & Crump, 1974). This difference does not exist in patients with cochlear hearing losses, and so comparisons of the two allow for sensitivity prediction from the acoustic reflex (SPAR). Margolis (1993) has found the SPAR excellent for use with adults, and promising for use with children. A combination of ABR, OAE, and ART should further increase the probability of correct identification of neonatal hearing loss, although the practicality of the screening decreases with the increased screening time and expense associated with such combinations.

Testing Children from Birth to Approximately One Year of Age

Experienced audiologists do not launch quickly into hearing tests with small children. First, they spend some time casually observing each child. They should notice such factors as the children's relationships with the adults who have taken them to the clinic; their gaits, standing positions, and other indications of general motor performance; and their methods of communication. Compiling complete and detailed case histories is of paramount importance.

It has been frequently observed that in general the broader the frequency spectrum of a sound, the better it is at catching the attention of a small child. For this reason, many clinicians use speech or other broadband signals in testing. One of the great dangers of accepting an obvious response to a sound with a broad acoustic spectrum lies in the fact that many children with hearing loss have reasonably good sensitivity in some frequency ranges and impaired sensitivity in other ranges. Many children, for example, have sharply falling high-frequency hearing losses and respond quite overtly to sounds containing low-frequency energy like the clapping of hands or the calling of their names. In addition, there is a smaller but significant number of children who have congenital low-frequency sensorineural hearing losses (Ross & Matkin, 1967).

Ewing and Ewing (1944) were pioneers in the testing of young children. They used a wide variety of noisemakers, such as bells, rattles, rustling paper, and xylophones. They advocated stirring a spoon in a cup, which produces a soft sound from a child's daily life that may evoke a response when a loud sound does not. Stress on using meaningful sounds is most closely associated with the work of the Ewings.

Hardy, Hardy, Brinker, Frazier, and Doughtery (1962) tested a large group of babies ranging in age from four to eight months. The procedure they used requires two clinicians. One clinician sits before the child, who is usually seated on the parent's lap, to occupy the child's attention with a toy or puppet. The second clinician, who is behind and to the side of the mother, utters phonemes such as S, S, S, S. Toys and other noisemakers may also be used; crinkling cellophane or onionskin paper makes the sort of soft, annoying sound that is extremely useful in techniques such as these, but provides little or no information about the configuration of the hearing loss.

Many pediatric audiologic procedures involve the child's response to a sound through auditory localization. For a sound to be localized, hearing thresholds must be similar in both ears, although not necessarily normal. As a child's ability to localize sound matures, it progresses from eye and head movement seen horizontally, then vertically, then on an arc and finally in a direct line to the sound source (Figure 8.2).

If a child does not turn to locate a sound by the age of eight months, it can be suspected that something is wrong, although not necessarily hearing loss. Mental retardation and some childhood symbolic disorders may manifest themselves in a similar lack of response. The general approach described here constitutes what has been called **behavioral observation audiometry (BOA).**

Sound-Field Audiometry

Several approaches for the testing of infants use multiple loudspeakers in a sound-field situation. Recordings of animal noises and baby cries have been effective in eliciting responses, even when

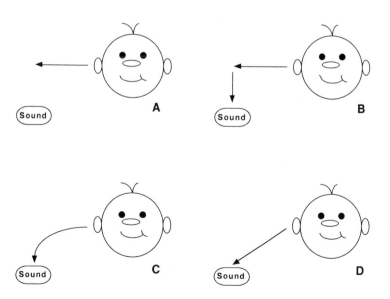

FIGURE 8.2   Development of auditory localization in infants. (A) At three months the head moves somewhat jerkily along a horizontal plane. (B) At five months localization is in straight lines, first horizontally and then vertically. (C) At six months the head and eyes move in an arc toward the sound source. (D) At eight months the eyes and head move directly to the sound source.

filtered into narrow bands. Although a sound such as a whistle, bell, drum, or some vocal utterance may appear subjectively to represent a specific frequency range, this often turns out not to be true. What may seem to be a high-pitched sound may have equal intensity in the low- and high-frequency ranges, as verified by spectral analysis. One exception to this is the Manchester high-pitch baby rattle (Kettlety, 1987), which has been used extensively in Great Britain as a specially designed infant screening device whose intensity is primarily above 5000 Hz.

Several kinds of responses may be observed when sounds are presented to a child from different directions in the sound field. The child may look for the sound source, cease ongoing activity, awaken from a light sleep, change facial expression, or offer a cry or other vocalized response. Once again, a response to sound has considerable significance, whereas a lack of response is not necessarily meaningful. A useful setup for sound-field localization has been diagrammed by Hodgson (1987) and is shown in Figure 8.3.

Frequently, children will respond to the off-effect of a sound but not to the on-effect. Evaluation of responses to the cessation of sound often goes well with the use of noisemakers, but it can be adapted to sound-field audiometry. A high-intensity pure tone or narrow noise band can be introduced for a minute or so and then abruptly interrupted. This interruption may produce a response whereas the initial presentation of the sound will not.

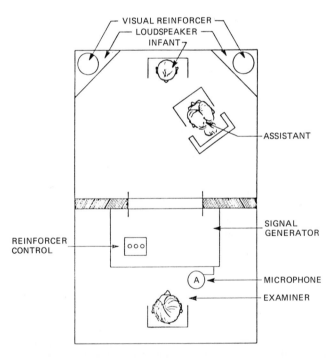

FIGURE 8.3   Diagram of a room useful for sound-field localization tests with small children. (Adapted from W. R. Hodgson, *Hearing Disorders in Children*, F. N. Martin (Ed.), 1987, p. 201. Reprinted by permission of Prentice-Hall, Englewood Cliffs, NJ.)

It is generally the case that at age two months a soft voice begins to become a better stimulus than a loud voice. At one to three months, percussion instruments are best at eliciting APRs, startle responses such as the **Moro reflex,**[2] and overall increases in activity or crying. At four months, percussion instruments are less successful than they were earlier, but the human voice gains in effectiveness. By six months of age much reflex activity begins to disappear.

Relying on the localization ability of normal-hearing babies more than four months old, Suzuki and Ogiba (1961) developed a sound-field procedure called **conditioned orientation reflex (COR).** Children are seated between and in front of a pair of loudspeakers, each of which holds an illuminated doll within the children's peripheral vision. Pure-tone and light introductions are paired; after several of these paired presentations, children will begin to glance in the direction of the light source in anticipation of the light whenever a tone is presented. The introduction of the light may then be delayed until after children have glanced at the speaker; this can serve as a reinforcement for their orientation to the signal. This procedure works well with some small children and has been modified in several ways, including the "puppet in the window illuminated" (PIWI) procedure (Haug, Baccaro, & Guilford, 1967).

Rewarding children's auditory responses with visual stimuli has led to the use of **visual reinforcement audiometry (VRA)** (Liden & Kankkonen, 1961). The reinforcer may be anything from a light to a picture, as long as it evokes the children's interests. Matkin (1973) reports that VRA works with earphones, if the children will tolerate them, as well as in the sound field, with or without hearing aids. Speech as well as tones may serve as signals. It can be expected that responses to VRA may be obtained from children whose corrected age (chronological age minus the estimated number of weeks of prematurity, if any) reaches six months (Moore, Thompson, & Folsom, 1992).

Audiologists do not completely agree on the best acoustic stimuli for testing small children. Many, but not all, authorities believe that pure tones are probably not the ideal stimuli because they are not meaningful to children. Pure tones have the obvious advantage of supplying information about children's hearing sensitivity at specific frequencies. If, however, a child shows no interest in pure tones, other carefully controlled acoustic stimuli may be used.

The justification for narrowband filtering of a signal for a small child is obvious, and many clinicians use the narrowband noise generators on their clinical audiometers. The belief is that this provides specific frequency information if the child responds. Such an approach may be very misleading. The narrow bands on many audiometers are not very narrow at all, and they may reject frequencies on either side of the center frequency at rates as little as 12 dB per octave. This allows sufficient energy in the side bands to produce a response when a child has not heard the frequency in the center of the band. It is obvious that audiologists must understand the nature of the equipment they use, and if they elect to test with narrow bands, they should ascertain for themselves just what the bandwidths are.

A potential problem, present whenever screening responses involving high-intensity stimuli are used, is the effect of loudness recruitment on startle responses. If recruitment is present, a child could conceivably respond to a sound as if it were loud, when in fact it might be only slightly above auditory threshold. If this occurs, a child with a cochlear hearing loss with loudness recruitment may pass early screening tests because of the very nature of the disorder. The criteria for minimum response level may be very different for children with hearing impairment.

---

[2]Named for Ernst Moro, German pediatrician, 1874–1951.

Testing Children Approximately One to Five Years of Age

At one year of age the hard-of-hearing child may begin to lose the potential for normal spoken-language development. Lack of speech often brings the problem to the attention of the parents or other caretakers. At eighteen months, the normal child usually obeys simple commands. Speech tests are useful to evaluate children at this age, as a child may give good responses to soft speech while apparently ignoring loud sounds, such as percussion instruments. It is interesting that quiet voiced speech will sometimes elicit a response when whispered speech will not. At two to three years of age, tests with voice, whispers, pitch pipes, and other special stimuli may be unnecessary with children who have no problems other than hearing loss, because they can often be taught to respond to pure tones, especially warble tones.

Early reports in the literature on testing children indicated that it was not possible to get pure-tone threshold responses from children under five years of age. It is now quite common to test children age three years or under. It is naturally necessary to work rapidly and smoothly to keep such a young child's attention and cooperation. A child with a "pure" hearing loss (i.e., no other significant problems) should be testable well before three years of age.

If a child cannot be tested by using formal methods, an imitation of vocalization can be tried. The clinician can babble nonsense syllables, without the child watching, to see if the child will imitate. If imitation does take place, it indicates that hearing is good enough to perceive voice. If no response is noted, and the clinician babbles again in the child's line of vision, the child with a severe hearing impairment may attempt to imitate, but may do so without voice. This is a most important diagnostic sign. In addition to being a strong indication of hearing loss, silent imitation indicates that the child's perceptual function is probably intact. If the child vocalizes, the voice quality can be evaluated. Although the vocal quality of individuals with hearing loss is sometimes different from that of those with normal hearing, it must be remembered that the voice of the very young child who has a hearing impairment frequently cannot be differentiated from that of the child with normal hearing.

It is possible to observe a child's reaction to the examiner's imitation of the child's sounds. In this case a response is made by the examiner to the child's babbling or other vocalizations. A child with normal hearing may cease vocalization and may sometimes repeat it. There are instances in which this procedure works when nothing else does, as the child may stop and listen, the interpretation being that the examiner's voice was heard. The child may also be tested by asking such questions as "Where is Mommy?" "Where are your hands?" The question "Do you want to go home now?" often evokes a clear response, but it should be reserved as a last resort, for if children do hear that question, it may become impossible to keep them longer. Often a whisper may cause 2- or 3-year-old youngsters to whisper back. If they can hear their own whisper, this may indicate good hearing for high-pitched sounds.

Speech Audiometry

Some children will not respond to pure tones, and by their almost stoic expressions, it appears that they cannot hear. A large number of these children can be conditioned to respond to speech signals. If they possess the appropriate language skills, many children will point to parts of their bodies or to articles of clothing. If this kind of response can be obtained, the clinician can recite a list of items to which the child points. The level of the signal can be raised and lowered until speech threshold is approximated.

Pictures or objects that can be named with spondaic stress can be used to test children. A child will often point to a "cowboy" or "hot dog." The clinician may first demonstrate the procedure and then reward the child's appropriate behavior with a smile, a nod, or a wink. SRTs can frequently be obtained with pictures by age two years. Word-recognition tests, such as the WIPI (Ross & Lerman, 1970) described in Chapter 5, may be accomplished in the same way.

Speech audiometry is often possible with children, even when they have very severe hearing losses. Use of the Ling Six Sound Test (Ling, 1989; Ling & Berlin, 1997) can provide frequency specific hearing loss information even when reliable tonal responses cannot be attained. The six sounds /a/, /u/, /i/, /ʃ/, /s/, and /m/ are representative of the speech energy contained within all the speech sounds of English. In particular, audibility of /a/, /u/, and /i/ indicates usable hearing through 1000 Hz; audibility of /ʃ/ suggests hearing through 2000 Hz; and audibility of /s/ indicates hearing through 4000 Hz. How well children can recognize those phonemes, and the formant frequencies they represent, can illustrate how well a hearing aid may meet their acoustic needs. At times the Six Sound Test is the only speech measurement that a child can or will perform. It is most useful when carried out in conjunction with other speech and pure-tone audiometric procedures.

Speech audiometry has revealed hearing abnormalities, or their absence, in children who were unable or unwilling to take pure-tone tests. This has resulted, in many cases, in a substantial savings of time in initiating remedial procedures. Of course, failure of children to respond during speech audiometry may occur because they do not know what the item (picture or object) is, rather than because they have not heard the word. The clinician should ask the adults accompanying their children to the examination whether specific words are in the children's vocabularies. It is essential to assure that it is word recognition ability and not receptive vocabulary that is being tested.

Pure-tone Audiometry

Many times, in testing small children, the problem is to get them to respond. The ingenuity of the clinician can frequently solve this problem. For a child to want to participate, usually the procedure must offer some enjoyment. Some children, however, are so anxious to please that they deluge the clinician with many false positive responses on pure-tone tests, so that it is difficult to gauge when a response is valid. In such cases, slight modifications of adult-like tests may prove workable with some older children. A child may be asked to point to the earphone in which a tone is heard. The ears may be stimulated randomly, and in this way the appropriateness of the response can be determined. The same result may be achieved by using pulsed-tone procedures, asking the child to tell how many tones have been presented.

Operant Conditioning Audiometry

Many times it appears that no approach to a given child will produce reliable results. This is particularly true of children with mental retardation. However, Spradlin and Lloyd (1965) suggested that given sufficient time and effort, no child is "untestable," and they recommend that this term be replaced by the phrase *difficult to test*.

In **operant conditioning audiometry (OCA),** food is often used as a reward for proper performance. A child may be seated in the test room before a table that contains a hand switch. Sounds are presented either through the sound-field speaker or through earphones. The child is encouraged to press the switch when the sound, which can be either a pure tone or a noise band, is presented. If the child's response is appropriate, a small amount of food, such as a candy pellet, some fruit juice, or a token, is released from a special feeder box. Once children see that pressing the switch will result in a reward, they will usually continue to press it in pursuit of more. It is essential that the switch that operates the feeder be wired in series with the tone-introducer switch so that no reward is forthcoming without presentation of the sound. In this way the child gets no reinforcement for pushing the switch unless a tone is actually introduced and, presumably, heard. Signals that are thought to be above the child's threshold must be introduced first, after which the level may be lowered until threshold is reached. If severe hearing loss is suspected, a good starting point is 500 Hz at 90 dB HL because there is a strong likelihood of hearing at this frequency and level.

Operant conditioning audiometry requires much time and patience if it is to work. Often, many trials are required before the child begins to understand the task. As in other audiometric procedures, it is essential that the signals be introduced aperiodically, for the child may learn to predict a signal and to respond to a sound that has not been heard. Often operant conditioning audiometry can be successful when other procedures have failed. The term **tangible reinforcement operant conditioning audiometry (TROCA)** was coined by Lloyd, Spradlin, and Reid (1968) to describe specifics of operant conditioning to audiometry.

For a number of years clinicians have been using *instrumental conditioning* in testing younger children—that is, teaching the children to perform in a certain way when a sound is heard. This requires a degree of voluntary cooperation from the children, but the clinician can select a method that will evoke appropriate responses.

A number of devices for operant audiometry have been described in the literature dating back to the earliest years of audiology. The peep show (Dix & Hallpike, 1947) gives children the reward of seeing a lighted picture when they respond correctly to a tone presented through a small loudspeaker below the screen. The pediacoumeter (Guilford & Haug, 1952) works on a similar principle, except that the child may wear earphones to increase the accuracy of the test. If the child hears a tone and responds correctly by pushing a button, one of seven puppets pops up to startle and amuse. Similar approaches have been used with animated toys, pictures, slides, motion pictures, and computers.

Martin and Coombes (1976) applied the principles of operant audiometry to the determination of speech thresholds. A brightly colored clown was devised whose body parts (e.g., hand, mouth, nose, leg) were wired to microswitches that triggered a candy-feeder mechanism (Figure 8.4). Children were shown how to touch a part of the clown. Reinforcement of the correct response was the immediate delivery of a candy pellet to a cup, which was momentarily lighted in the clown's hand. Preprogramming of the proper switch on a special device in the control room ensured that false responses would not be rewarded. Speech thresholds were obtained on very young children in a matter of several minutes. Weaver, Wardell, and Martin (1979) found this procedure for obtaining speech thresholds useful with children with mental retardation.

Play Audiometry

Often, using elaborate devices and procedures is unnecessary to test the hearing of young children (Figure 8.5). Many can simply be taught by demonstration to place a ring on a peg, a block in a box, or a bead in a bucket when a sound is introduced. The more enthusiasm the clinician shows about the procedure, the more likely the child is to join in. Children seem to enjoy the action of the game. Tones can be presented through earphones if children will tolerate them, or through the sound-field

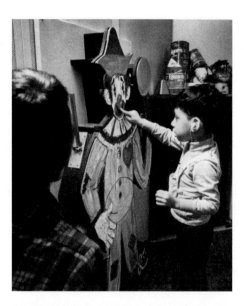

FIGURE 8.4 Photograph of a young child with a hearing impairment whose speech thresholds are being tested in the sound field. The clown serves as a device for delivering a tangible reward (candy pellets) when the part of the clown named by the clinician is pressed by the child.

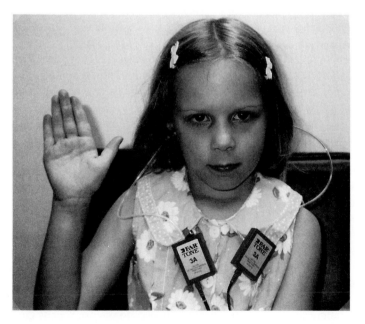

FIGURE 8.5 A small child taking a voluntary pure-tone hearing test. Use of insert earphones increases interaural attenuation thereby decreasing the need for masking. (Courtesy of HearCare)

speaker if they will not. Some children will readily accept insert receivers because they are light and do not encumber movement.

The probable reason that some clinicians do not embrace play audiometric techniques is that they feel these techniques can easily become boring to children, and that conditioning will therefore extinguish rapidly. This is probably a case of projection of adult values, since many alert children can play the "sound game" for long periods of time without boredom. When asking children to move beads or other objects from one container to another, it is a good idea to have a large supply on hand because many children will refuse to play further once the first bucket has become empty, even if they have appeared to enjoy the game up to this point.

One problem in using play audiometry is to find suitable rewards for prompting the children to maintain interest and motivation in the test. DiCarlo, Kendall, and Goldstein (1962) felt that conditioning in audiometry depends on the following: (1) motivation, (2) contiguity (getting the stimulus and response close together in time and space), (3) generalization (across frequency and intensity), (4) discrimination (between the stimulus and any background activity), and (5) reinforcement (conveying to children that they are doing what is wanted).

It often becomes apparent to a clinician that a limited amount of time is available to test a small child and that, even though some reliable threshold results are forthcoming, the test should best be abbreviated before the child ceases to cooperate. In such cases, it may be advisable to test one frequency in each ear both by air conduction and by bone conduction. This will provide information about the relative sensitivity of each ear, and about the nature of the disorder (conductive or sensorineural). If an SRT is obtained that suggests normal hearing, the frequency to be tested may be a higher one, say 3000 or 4000 Hz, to make certain that the normal SRT does not mislead in cases of high-frequency hearing loss. If only three to six thresholds are to be obtained, it is often more meaningful to get readings at one or two frequencies in each ear by both air and bone conduction than to obtain six air-conduction thresholds in one ear. Accurate threshold readings at only 500 and 2000 Hz will give some evidence of degree, configuration, and type of hearing loss.

Sometimes it is impossible, for a variety of reasons, to teach a child to take a hearing test in one session. In such cases the child should be rescheduled for further testing and observation. It is often worthwhile to employ the talents and interests of the child's parents or other adults. They can be instructed in methods of presenting sounds and evoking responses. Children may also be more amenable to training in the comfort and security of their homes than in the strange and often frightening environment of sound-treated rooms. One parent may use a noisemaker, such as a bell, in full view of the child, while the other parent responds by dropping a block in a bucket, or by some other enjoyable activity. Children can be encouraged to join in the game and, after beginning to participate by following the parents' lead, can be encouraged to go first. Once they participate fully, the sound source can be gradually moved out of the line of vision so that it can be determined that responses are to auditory, and not visual, stimulation. A few minutes a day of such activities may allow the audiologist at the next clinic appointment to use the same procedure, preferably with the same materials, which are already familiar to the child. After professional observation of the child's responses, the audiologist can substitute other sound stimuli in an attempt to quantify the hearing loss, if any. It has also been found useful to have the parents borrow an old headband and set of earphones to accustom the child to wearing them without fear.

Small children's failure to produce observable responses to intense sounds during informal testing may or may not be due to profound hearing loss. The lack of response during formal testing, such as pure-tone audiometry, may mean either that the children have not heard the sounds or that they have not responded correctly when they have heard them. Deciding between these two possibilities is often difficult. It is sometimes advisable to teach children to respond to some other stimulus, such as to a light, or to the vibrations of a hand-held bone-conduction vibrator, which delivers a strong low-frequency tone. If a child can be taught to give appropriate responses to one sensory input, the inference is that the child can be conditioned to respond, and that lack of response to a sound probably means that it was not heard.

Immittance Measures

The use of acoustic immittance measurements with children has great clinical utility. Tympanometry can determine a number of middle-ear disorders, including abnormal middle-ear pressure, eustachian tube function, effusion, mobility and integrity of the middle ear ossicles, thin or perforated tympanic membrane, and patency of pressure equalization tubes. Additionally, the sensation level or absence of the acoustic reflex can give general kinds of information about a possible sensorineural hearing loss.

A major problem with immittance tests with very small children results when they move about or cry. For a test to be accurate, the patient must be relatively motionless. Furthermore, any vocalizations—for example, crying—will be picked up by the probe microphone. An experienced team of clinicians can often work so efficiently that children are distracted and tested before they have time to object. Immittance measurements should almost always be attempted on small children.

Electrophysiological Hearing Tests

It has been obvious for some time that objective tests for measuring hearing in young children are highly desirable. Such tests must embody methods that require no active participation from the child, and they must result in clear-cut responses of an objective nature. An obvious approach would seem to be to monitor one or more of the child's electrophysiological mechanisms for any changes that might be induced by the introduction of a sound. Changes in pulse rate, breathing pattern, heart rhythm, skin resistance, and electrical brain activity have all been investigated.

For a number of years electrodermal audiometry (EDA) was very popular for testing young children (Hardy & Pauls, 1952). Although some clinicians reported high correlation between electrodermal response and behavioral thresholds, others reported confusing results and poor reliability. The trauma to the child caused by the electric shocks that are used in this test as a conditioning stimulus are not justified by the presumed value of the procedure, which is rarely if ever used today (Martin & Gravel, 1989).

Differences of opinion also exist about the reliability of respiration audiometry in testing young children, as well as another procedure, cardiotachometry (Eisenberg, 1975), which has been suggested. Heart rate seems to decelerate when speech stimuli are presented to a listener; no such effects are evident with nonspeech signals. Respiration audiometry and cardiotachometry have not gained the status for testing children that had been predicted.

Electrophysiological tests today primarily involve auditory evoked potentials, and a great deal of satisfaction has been achieved using auditory brainstem response (ABR) audiometry (Chapter 6). A primary advantage is that the procedure is effective during sleep, and the child may be anesthetized with no effects on test accuracy.

There is little doubt that continuing research brings us closer to the goal of an efficient and reliable index of auditory function in uncooperative children. Until that goal is reached, audiologists will still have to confirm their findings with behavioral tests. It should be assumed that the diagnosis is never complete until a voluntary hearing test is obtained from the child.

Language Disorders

Small children are frequently seen in audiology centers because they show some deficiencies in the normal development of speech and language. Because language and speech depend on interactions between the peripheral and central nervous systems, a detailed history must be taken. Special attention should be paid to such things as onset of different kinds of motor development, the age at which meaningful speech or an alternative communication system was acquired, social development, communication of needs, and pre- and postnatal developmental factors. Pertinent data should also include prenatal diseases, the length of the pregnancy, difficulties at birth, and early distress—for example, that seen in cyanotic ("blue") babies, in babies with jaundice, and so on. Notations should be made of childhood illnesses, especially those involving high or prolonged fevers, and medications taken. Attention should be paid to any illnesses or accidents and any regressions in development associated with them. Some objective data may be obtained from tests of hearing, symbolic behavior, intelligence, and receptive and expressive language.

A young child's unwillingness to cooperate may be common to all sensory modalities, and could indicate a disorder or combination of disorders other than hearing loss (e.g., mental retardation, or emotional maladjustment). If a child does not respond to visual stimuli, such as lights or shadows, or to touching or vibration, one might wonder whether the problem is in fact behavioral. However, if a positive response is obtained in one modality and a negative one in another, a certain patterning appears, which is more significant than a generalized response (or lack of response).

Although long lists of possible causes for significant language delay have been postulated, such delay is usually produced by hearing loss, some congenital or early acquired symbolic disorders, attention deficit hyperactivity disorder, mental retardation, emotional disturbance, or **autism.** A common error committed by clinicians is to consider causes as an either-or condition, and to attempt differential diagnosis to rule out all but one cause. The experienced clinician will have observed that the presence of one significant disorder increases, rather than decreases, the probability of another.

When a small child has a language disorder, and hearing loss cannot be eliminated as a possible causal factor, the resources and experience of the clinician are called on for an appropriate diagnosis. The behavioral characteristics of the clinical entities mentioned here can frequently be ruled out on the basis of observation of behavior and developmental history. The problem then remains to differentiate between the hard-of-hearing and the otherwise language-disordered child. Even though the child with brain injury is said to manifest such symptoms as impatience, hyperactivity, poor judgment, **perseveration,** and **dysinhibition,** often there is a symbolic disorder without the presence of bizarre behavior.

Audiologists frequently see children who are either believed to have hearing losses or whose auditory behavior is so inconsistent as to cast doubt on the presence of normal hearing. A parent or teacher may complain that a child's responses to sound are inconsistent, that performance is better when background noises or competing messages are at a minimum, and that it is possible that the child "just doesn't pay attention." Sometimes auditory test results appear normal on such a child, and the parents are mistakenly assured that all is fine. The audiologist must constantly be alert for auditory-processing disorders that can coexist with other learning and language disabilities. A child with such disorders should be referred to the proper specialists, such as speech-language pathologists.

So as not to over-refer cases to language pathologists, Martin and Clark (1977) developed a screening procedure using a dichotic listening task with the WIPI test as discrimination stimuli. Children with intact central auditory nervous systems seemed to do as well diotically (high- and low-frequency filtered bands to both ears) as they did dichotically (high band to one ear and low band to the other). Children with confirmed language-learning disorders showed significant diotic enhancement, indicating that they have difficulty in fusing the signals from the two ears. More screening tests are needed so that children with central auditory disorders, however mild, will not be overlooked, but will be properly referred for complete diagnosis and therapy. Many of the tests for central auditory disorders, described in Chapter 12, can be performed accurately on children as young as six years old.

In the final analysis, the diagnosis of the "difficult case" must often be made subjectively by a highly qualified, experienced examiner. Despite the initial diagnosis, it must be remembered that until a pure-tone audiogram is accomplished on the language-impaired child, hearing loss cannot be ruled out as a possible contributory element.

Central Auditory Processing Disorders

Recent years have brought a focus on an auditory disorder in children with otherwise normal hearing sensitivity. The term **central auditory processing disorder (CAPD)** has been applied to children whose recognition or use of language is not age-appropriate, and/or is inconsistent with their level of intelligence. Many of these children also have learning disabilities, which prevent them from progressing normally in their education. The assumption that all CAPD children have normal peripheral hearing is bound to be incorrect, at least in some cases, which leads to additional problems in diagnosis and treatment.

Since CAPD has become recognized, it may be a favored diagnostic category, and there may be reason to be concerned that overdiagnosis of this condition can lead to inappropriate educational methods. These children, despite normal intelligence, often have poor listening skills, short attention spans, seemingly poor memories and reading comprehension, difficulty in linguistic sequencing, and problems in learning to read and spell. One of the most frequently reported dysfunctions is difficulty in recognizing speech in the presence of background noise. All of these deficits, in addition to a number of others not listed, contribute to delays in speech and language, and poor performance in school. As a result, these children may suffer from lowered self-esteem, which further complicates the disorder. Many children with central auditory disorders make inappropriate social contacts since their failures with children in their age group lead them to seek playmates who are younger than they are. Often parents and other adults report these children prefer to play alone.

Several screening measures have been designed for CAPD (see Chapter 12), although these often cannot lead to an appropriate diagnosis because they are not sufficiently comprehensive. Perhaps the diagnosis of the site of lesion should be considered less important than descriptions of how children function in the classroom, at home, in different listening situations, and with other aspects of the world around them. For communicating with other professionals, such as teachers, technical diagnostic statements are less useful than those that describe the kinds of difficulties a child may have in learning and suggestions for specific remedies. Diagnostic entities such as CAPD, ADHD (attention deficit/hyperactivity disorder), dyslexia, emotional disturbance, and so on, may be more threatening than useful to professionals who must assist these children. Management suggestions for a more structured learning environment can be a useful addendum to reports to the classroom teacher (Clark, 1980; Hall & Mueller, 1997).

Psychological Disorders

Hearing loss that is congenital, or acquired early in life, can have an effect on social, intellectual, and emotional development, including "egocentricity, difficulty in empathizing with others, rigidity, impulsivity, coercive dependency and a tendency to express feelings by actions rather than by symbolic communication" (Rose, 1983). As a child continues to develop without normal hearing, the normal parent-child relationship is invariably affected, lending further justification for intervention at the earliest possible time.

Developmental Disabilities

Children with developmental disabilities may include those with mental retardation, cerebral palsy, epilepsy, or autism. While a high percentage of children with developmental disability have cognitive impairments as well, many have normal or greater than normal intelligence. Hearing loss among these children may go undetected, as behaviors of auditory inattention may be attributed to the child's more overt handicap.

Evaluation of children with developmental disabilities presents a true challenge to the audiologist. Responses from children who are profoundly multidisabled may be more reflexive than representative of true attention behaviors (Flexer & Gans, 1985). Such responses may be best evaluated in the context of the child's developmental age than chronological age. Hearing may be considered normal if the development of auditory responses is generally consistent with the age level of the child's other developmental behaviors. This judgment becomes more difficult if the child's cognitive and developmental ages have not yet been determined.

The physiologic measures described in Chapter 6 provide a dimension to the evaluation of the difficult-to-test patient that was not available in the past. However, the sometimes ambiguous results of physiologic measures of hearing increase with central nervous system involvement, thereby increasing the value of any behavioral results that may be obtained (Martin & Clark, 1996).

Identifying Hearing Loss in the Schools

The exact number of school-age children who have hearing impairments is not known. Surveys that attempt to come up with figures are also confounded by such factors as geographic location and season of the year; there are more failures during cold weather (Gardner, 1988). It is probable that more than 5 percent of the public school population will have a hearing impairment at any given time. This does not count the students enrolled in residential and day schools for children with profound hearing impairments. Clearly, there is a need for testing methods that identify school children with hearing loss.

Equipment accuracy and the use of acceptable workspaces are mandatory in hearing loss identification programs. Audiometers should be calibrated annually by a factory-trained technician, with outputs checked on an artificial ear every three months (Patrick, 1987). Of course, if an audiometer or its earphones are jarred or dropped, calibration should be checked before any further hearing tests are done. Listening checks should be performed at the start of every test day, with special attention to breaks in the receiver cords.

Hearing Screening Measures

Early school hearing screenings were conducted in groups, thereby decreasing the demands on personnel, space, and equipment. Problems arising from difficulties in maintaining equipment calibration, and from the many false positive responses from children striving to pass due to fear of nonacceptance, eventually led to discontinuation of group screening measures. School screenings are carried out today on an individual basis. They are usually done by fixing the intensity of the audiometer and changing frequencies. Obviously, screenings may be performed more rapidly if a restricted number of frequencies is sampled and screening is done at a level high enough to be attended to easily by young children. Some authorities have recommended screening only at 4000 Hz because this frequency is often affected by hearing loss. Other people believe that screening with immittance meters will uncover the major source of hearing disorders in the schools—otitis media. It is possible that this approach could catch middle-ear disorders in the early stages, perhaps averting any conductive hearing loss at all. The combination of tympanometry and ipsilateral acoustic reflex screenings is most useful for this purpose. Utilizing a pulsed tone to elicit the reflex has been demonstrated to significantly increase the utility of the ipsilateral acoustic reflex within a screening protocol (Sells, Hurley, Morehouse, & Douglas, 1997). Of course, middle-ear problems are not the *only* cause of hearing loss in school children. Cooper, Gates, Owen, and Dickson (1975) suggested a combination of pure-tone screening at 4000 Hz (to find children with high-frequency sensorineural losses) and immittance screenings (to find children with middle-ear problems).

A study of a large number of students in Pittsburgh over a four-year period (Eagles, Wishik, Doerfler, Melnick, & Levine, 1963) revealed poor correlations between positive physical findings on otological examination and hearing losses. The obvious conclusion is that the best way to know if a hearing loss is present is through audiometry, and the best way to know if an otological abnormality is present is by otoscopic examination. Given the impracticality of including diagnostic otoscopy within a screening program, the use of acoustic immittance measures, not available at the time of the Pittsburgh study, can overcome the poor correlation between the outcome of audiometric screening and the presence of otitis media.

In 1975 ASHA published guidelines for identification audiometry in the schools. Proposed revisions of these guidelines that have since appeared (ASHA, 1993) state that the goals of such programs are to incorporate acoustic immittance measures with pure-tone audiometry to identify students who are in need of audiological and/or medical services. Patrick (1987) states that 80 to 90 percent accuracy is obtained when acoustic immittance is combined with pure-tone screenings, as compared to 60 to 70 percent accuracy when pure tones are used alone. New, automated, portable, easily used immittance screening devices (Figure 8.6) produce a tympanogram, and screen for acoustic reflexes in a matter of seconds on each ear tested (Figure 8.7). The most recent ASHA guidelines (ASHA, 1997) are summarized in Table 8.4.

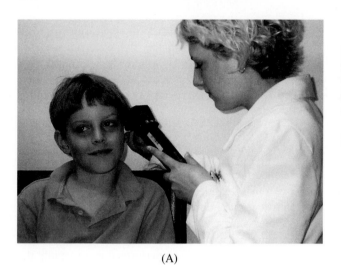

(A)

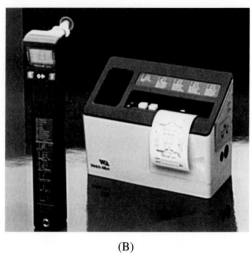

(B)

FIGURE 8.6   Portable acoustic immitance device in use (A) and with its holder (B) stores, recharges the unit, and prints the tympanogram and acoustic reflex results (see Figure 8.7). (Courtesy of HearCare and Welch-Allyn, Inc.)

Patient name:_____

    Date: 22-Aug-89   Time: 10:06

Left ear: Compliance:

1.0

                              0.4 ml pk

                              25 daPa

                              0.7 ml Vol

                              I Reflex C

                              ... .5k ...

                              90 1k ...

                              ... 2k ...

0   ... 4k ...

-400   -200   0   200

American Electromedics Corp.

AE-106 Tympanometer Serial #360147

Calibration date: 30-May-89

Tester: _____

Comments:

FIGURE 8.7   Printout of a tympanogram and acoustic reflex screening done on a school child with normal hearing.

TABLE 8.4 Summary of ASHA (1997) Guidelines for Audiologic Screening of the Pediatric Population

1. **Screening for outer and middle ear disorders, birth through 18 years**
   A. Combination of visual identification of structural defects of the ear or ear canal abnormalities and tympanometric screening.
   B. Failure if visual abnormality noted or tympanogram reveals reduced peak admittance (compliance) (<0.2 mmho for infants / <0.3 mmho for one year to school age / <0.4 mmho for children > 6 years of age) or tympanometric width >235 daPa for infants or >200 daPa above one year.
   C. Immediate medical referral for otalgia or otorrhea or tympanometric findings consistent with TM perforation. Otherwise rescreen within 6 to 8 weeks for failed tympanogram.

2. **Hearing-impairment screening for birth to 6 months of age**
   A. Recommend screening in quiet or sleeping state with ABR or OAE.
   B. Refer in absence of reliable response in either ear with confirmation of auditory status within 1–3 months.

3. **Hearing-impairment screening for 7 months to two years of age**
   A. When can condition to VRA screen with earphones (supra-aural or insert) using 1000, 2000, and 4000 Hz at 30 dB HL.
   B. When can condition to play audiometry screen with earphones using 1000, 2000, and 4000 Hz at 20 dB HL.
   C. Sound field can be substituted for earphone screening, recognizing limitations.
   D. OAE suggested as an alternative procedure when behavioral methods are ineffective.
   E. Screenings failed at any frequency in either ear should be referred for audiologic confirmation of hearing status within 1–3 months.

4. **Hearing-impairment screening for 3 to 5 years of age**
   A. If can reliably participate in conditioned play audiometry or conventional audiometry, screen with earphones using 1000, 2000, and 4000 Hz at 20 dB HL.
   B. Screenings failed at any frequency in either ear should be referred for audiologic confirmation of hearing status within 1–3 months.

5. **Hearing-impairment screening for school-age children, 5 through 18 years of age**
   A. Screen on initial entry to school, entrance to special education, or grade repetition, and annually in kindergarten through 3rd grade and in 7th and 11th grades.
   B. Screen via conventional audiometry or conditioned play audiometry with supra-aural or insert earphones using 1000, 2000, and 4000 Hz at 20 dB.
   C. Reinstruct and rescreen within the same screening session in which a child fails.
   D. Refer all who fail the rescreen or fail to condition to the screening task.
   E. Screenings failed at any frequency in either ear should be referred for audiologic confirmation of hearing status within 1–3 months.

Note: All referrals for hearing-impairment screening should ensure prompt completion of the diagnostic process and timely initiation of habilitative procedures. Screenings should be completed within appropriate settings as defined within the comprehensive guidelines with calibrated equipment. Screenings may be carried out by support personnel under the supervision of an audiologist.

Testing the Reliability of Screening Measures

For a hearing screening to be useful, it must be both sensitive and specific. The sensitivity of a test may be determined by dividing the number of children with hearing loss who fail the screening by the number who actually have a hearing loss. This yields the percentage of those who have been correctly identified as positive. The specificity of a screening procedure is calculated by dividing the number of children who pass the screening and do not have a hearing loss by the total number who do not have a hearing loss. This is the percentage of true negative results. A comparison of the sensitivity and specificity of a screening test to the overall population with hearing loss determines the predictive value of a screening procedure, which will account for the inevitable overreferrals and underreferrals for follow-up.

Any screening carries the danger of misclassification. No matter how cleverly a screening measure is designed, it is not possible to determine its shortcomings without submitting it to some empirical verification. A procedure described by Newby (1948) involves the use of a **tetrachoric table** and appears to serve this purpose well (Figure 8.8). One hundred children who have taken the screening are selected at random and given threshold tests under the best possible test conditions. The threshold test serves as the criterion for the accuracy of the screening measure. Cells A and D in Figure 8.8 represent agreement between threshold assessments and screenings, showing correct identification of those children with and without hearing losses. Cells B and C represent disagreement between the two measures; the larger the number in those two cells, the poorer the screening is at doing its job. Cell C seems to be the biggest offender, passing children on the screening who fail the individual test thereby missing their hearing losses. This suggests that the criteria, such as the

		THRESHOLD ASSESSMENT	
		Failed	Passed
SCREENING MEASURE	Failed	A	B
	Passed	C	D

FIGURE 8.8 Tetrachoric table used to validate the efficiency of a hearing screening measure. The children correctly identified as having hearing losses by the screening and verified by the threshold assessment are shown in cell A (true positive). Those properly identified as having no hearing loss are shown in cell D (true negative). Those children with normal hearing incorrectly identified by the screening as having hearing losses are shown in cell B (false positive). Cell C shows the children with hearing losses who were missed by the screening (false negative).

screening level, are too lax. A large number in cell B shows that time and energy are being wasted by identifying children with normal hearing as having hearing losses. In such cases, screening criteria may be too stringent, failing children who should have passed.

No matter how carefully a screening is conceived, the numbers in cells B and C will probably never reach the ideal zero. If the criteria are so stringent that no child passes who should fail, the penalty is to retest a lot of children with normal hearing, or to make many overreferrals. On the other hand, decreasing the number in cell B at the expense of missing children with hearing losses seems unthinkable.

In the real world, the person in charge of any screening program must balance factors of money, personnel, and the number of children to be tested against the efficiency of the screening measure. There appears to be an inverse relationship between efficiency and accuracy in any screening if one defines "efficiency" in terms of the number of screenings performed with the least expenditure of time and money.

Public school environments for hearing screenings are often less than satisfactory. Often the testing is done in large rooms with poor acoustics and with considerable background noise. Many children may be tested before an audiometer calibration defect is detected. Unless all the criteria for adequate testing are met, the purpose of the procedure is defeated.

Nonorganic Hearing Loss in Children

There are numerous reports in the literature of nonorganic (false or exaggerated) hearing losses among children. The causes may range from misunderstanding of the test, to malingering, to psychogenic disorders. While nonorganic hearing loss may be easily missed in a screening measure, as a general rule, it is not difficult for alert clinicians to detect nonorganicity in children and, with some clever manipulation, to determine the true organic hearing thresholds. The earlier nonorganic problems can be detected, the sooner they can be managed. It is important to quickly eliminate the reliance on a false hearing loss, before it becomes a crutch to solve or avoid emotional, social, or academic problems.

Dixon and Newby (1959) observed a series of forty children with nonorganic hearing loss. These children had normal hearing, yet they behaved on hearing tests as though they had hearing losses. The children did not appear to have hearing difficulty in normal conversation situations and often showed normal speech thresholds, despite apparent hearing losses for pure tones. Dixon and Newby felt that motivation for nonorganic hearing loss in children may be very different from that in adults, and that psychological or psychiatric consultation may be indicated in some cases.

Although many schoolchildren try diligently to pass their hearing tests, others manifest nonorganic symptoms. Ross (1964) has pointed out the dangers of reinforcing children's notions that they have a hearing loss. They may consciously or unconsciously see the advantages of hearing loss and may decide that the risk is worth the secondary gains to be realized in the forms of favors and excuses. Ross advised that children should not be referred for follow-up examinations by physicians unless the person in charge of the school tests is reasonably certain that a hearing problem exists. Most experienced audiologists can probably recall specific incidents in which a child has become committed to continued fabrication of a hearing loss, no matter how the problem got started.

Summary

While pediatric audiology can be stimulating and rewarding, it can also be time-consuming and frustrating. Often clinicians do not have the feeling, as they have with most adults, of complete closure on a case at the end of a diagnostic session. Nevertheless, the proper identification and management of hearing loss in children is one of the most solemn responsibilities of the audiologist. Truly, work with children is often carried out more as an art than a science, testing the cleverness and perseverance of clinicians, and calling on all their training and experience.

Pediatric audiology includes the use of those tests and diagnostic procedures designed especially for children who cannot be tested by conventional audiometry. Approaches vary with both the chronological and mental ages of children. Some tests, designed merely to elicit some sort of startle reaction, may be carried out on children as young as several hours of age. Other tests employ play techniques, or use special rewards to encourage proper performance. Still other procedures involve measuring changes in electrophysiological states in response to sound, or the detection of sounds emitted from the ear. With some children it is possible to test by making slight alterations in conventional audiometric techniques used with adults. Hearing testing is designed to determine the nature and extent of a child's communicative problem and is virtually useless unless some (re)habilitative path is pursued, as discussed in Chapter 15.

STUDY QUESTIONS

1. What are the first five questions you would ask the parents of a small child being seen for a hearing evaluation?

2. A child under one year of age is to be seen for an evaluation. How would you prepare before the child's arrival in the clinic? List the procedures you would use, in the order you would use them.

3. List the pros and cons of neonatal screening.

4. What are the major steps you would take as an audiologist organizing a school hearing test program? Once begun, how would you test its efficiency?

5. Consider the major causes for the lack of speech development. List some of the typical symptoms for each cause.

GLOSSARY

Apgar Test A method for evaluating the status of infants immediately and shortly after birth. Observations are made of the child's respiration, heart rate, muscle tone, color, and reflex irritability.

Auropalpebral reflex (APR) Contraction of the ring muscles of the eyes in response to a sudden, unexpected sound.

Autism A condition of withdrawal and introspection manifested by asocial behavior.

Behavioral observation audiometry (BOA) Observation of changes in the activity state of an infant in response to sound.

Central auditory processing disorders (CAPD) Difficulty in the development of language and other communication skills associated with disorders of the auditory centers in the brain.

Conditioned orientation reflex (COR) A technique for testing young children in the sound field by having them look in the direction of a sound source in search of a flashing light.

Dysinhibition Bizarre behavior patterns often associated with brain-damaged individuals.

Hereditodegenerative hearing loss A hearing loss of genetic origin, with onset after birth.

High-risk registry A set of criteria designed to help identify neonates whose probability of hearing loss is greater than normal.

Minimum response level (MRL) The lowest level of response offered by a child to an acoustic stimulus. Depending on a variety of circumstances, the signal responded to may be either barely audible or well above threshold.

Moro reflex A sudden embracing movement of the arms and drawing up of the legs of infants and small children in response to sudden loud sounds.

Operant conditioning audiometry (OCA) The use of tangible reinforcement, such as edible items, to condition difficult-to-test patients for pure-tone audiometry.

Perseveration Persistent repetition of an activity.

Tangible reinforcement operant conditioning audiometry (TROCA) A form of operant audiometry using tangible reinforcers, such as food or tokens.

Tetrachoric table A table containing four cells designed to test the efficiency and accuracy of group hearing tests.

Visual reinforcement audiometry (VRA) The use of a light or picture to reinforce a child's response to a sound.

Warble tone A pure tone that is frequency modulated. The modulation is usually expressed as a percentage (e.g., a 1000 Hz tone warbled at 5 percent would vary from 950 to 1050 Hz).

REFERENCES

American Speech-Language-Hearing Association (ASHA). (1984). Proposed guidelines for identification audiometry. *Asha, 26,* 47–50.

———. (1993). Guidelines for audiology services in the schools. *Asha, 35* (Supplement 10), 24–32.

———. (1997). *Guidelines for audiologic screening.* American Speech-Language-Hearing Association publication. Rockville, MD: Author.

Apgar, V. (1953). A proposal for a new method of evaluation of the newborn infant. *Anesthesia Analgesia, 32,* 260–266.

Bennett, M. J. (1979). Trials with the auditory response cradle I: Neonatal responses to auditory stimuli. *British Journal of Audiology, 13,* 125–134.

Bonfils, P., Dumont, A., Marie, P., Francois, M., & Narcy, P. (1990). Evoked otoacoustic emission in newborn hearing screening. *Laryngoscope, 100,* 186–189.

Bonfils, P., Vziel, A., & Pujol, R. (1988). Screening for auditory dysfunction in infants by oto-acoustic emissions. *Archives of Otolaryngology-Head and Neck Surgery, 114,* 887–890.

Clark, J. G., (1980). Central auditory dysfunction in school children: A compilation of management suggestions. *Speech, Language, and Hearing Services in Schools, 11*(4), 208–213.

Cooper, J. C., Gates, G. A., Owen, J. H., & Dickson, H. D. (1975). An abbreviated impedance bridge technique for school screening. *Journal of Speech and Hearing Disorders, 40,* 260–269.

Davidson, J., Hyde, M. L., & Alberti, P. W. (1989). Epidemiologic patterns in childhood hearing loss: A review. *International Journal of Pediatric Otorhinolaryngology, 17,* 239–266.

DiCarlo, L. M., Kendall, D. C., & Goldstein, R. (1962). Diagnostic procedures for auditory disorders in children. *Folia Phoniatrica, 14,* 206–264.

Dix, M. R., & Hallpike, C. S. (1947). The peep show: A new technique for pure tone audiometry in young children. *British Medical Journal, 2,* 719–723.

Dixon, R. F., & Newby, H. A. (1959). Children with nonorganic hearing problems. *Archives of Otolaryngology, 70,* 619–623.

Downs, M. P., & Sterritt, G. M. (1967). A guide to newborn and infant screening programs. *Archives of Otolaryngology, 85,* 15–22.

Eagles, E., Wishik, S., Doerfler, L., Melnick, W., & Levine, H. (1963). Hearing sensitivity and related factors in children. *Laryngoscope,* Monograph Supplement.

Eisenberg, R. B. (1975). Cardiotachometry. In L. J. Bradford (Ed.), *Physiological measures of the audio-vestibular system* (pp. 319–348). New York: Academic Press.

Ewing, I., & Ewing, A. (1944). The ascertainment of deafness in infancy and early childhood. *Journal of Laryngology, 59,* 309–333.

Flexer, C., & Gans, D. (1985). Comparative evaluation of the auditory responsiveness of normal infants and profoundly multihandicapped children. *Journal of Speech and Hearing Research, 28,* 163–168.

Gardner, H. J. (1988). Moderate vs. cold weather effects on hearing screening results among preschool children. *The Hearing Journal, 41,* 29–32.

Guilford, F. R., & Haug, C. O. (1952). Diagnosis of deafness in the very young child. *Archives of Otolaryngology, 55,* 101–106.

Gustafson, G. (1989, October/November). Early identification of hearing-impaired infants: A review of Israeli and American progress. *Volta Review,* 291–294.

Hall, J. W., & Mueller, H. G. (1997). *Audiologists' Desk Reference, Vol. I.* San Diego: Singular Publishing Group.

Hardy, W. G., Hardy, J. B., Brinker, C. H., Frazier, T. M., & Doughtery, A. (1962). Auditory screening of infants. *Annals of Otology, Rhinology and Laryngology, 71,* 759–766.

Hardy, W. G., & Pauls, M. D. (1952). The test situation of PGSR audiometry. *Journal of Speech and Hearing Disorders, 17,* 13–24.

Haug, O., Baccaro, P., & Guilford, F. (1967). A pure-tone audiogram on the infant: The PIWI technique. *Archives of Otolaryngology, 86,* 435–440.

Hayes, D., & Northern, J. L. (1996). *Infants and hearing.* San Diego: Singular Publishing Group.

Hirsch, J. E., Margolis, R. H., & Rykken, J. R. (1992). A comparison of acoustic reflex and auditory brain stem response screening of high-risk infants. *Ear and Hearing, 13,* 181–186.

Hodgson, W. R. (1987). Tests of hearing—The infant. In F. N. Martin (Ed.), *Hearing disorders in children* (pp. 185–216). Austin, TX: Pro-Ed.

Jerger, J., Burney, P., Mauldin, L., & Crump, B. (1974). Predicting hearing loss from the acoustic reflex. *Journal of Speech and Hearing Disorders, 39,* 11–22.

Joint Committee. (1991). Joint Committee on Infant Hearing 1990 position statement. *Asha, 33* (Supplement 5), 3–6.

———. (1994). Joint Committee on Infant Hearing 1994 position statement. *Asha, 38,* 38–41.

Kettlety, A. (1987). The Manchester high pitch rattle. *British Journal of Audiology, 21,* 73–74.

Kemp, D. T., & Ryan, S. M. (1993). The use of transient evoked otoacoustic emissions in neonatal hearing screening programs. *Seminars in Hearing, 14,* 30–45.

Liden, G., & Kankkonen, A. (1961). Visual reinforcement audiometry. *Acta Otolaryngologica* (Stockholm), *67,* 281–292.

Ling, D. (1989). *Foundations of spoken language for hearing impaired children.* Washington, DC: Alexander Graham Bell Association for the Deaf.

Ling, D., & Berlin, C. (1997). The six sound test. In D. Ling (Ed.), *Acoustics, audition and speech reception.* Alexandria, VA: Auditory-Verbal International.

Lloyd, L. L., Spradlin, J. E., & Reid, M. J. (1968). An operant audiometric procedure for difficult-to-test patients. *Journal of Speech and Hearing Disorders, 33,* 236–245.

Margolis, R. H. (1993). Detection of hearing impairment with the acoustic stapedius reflex. *Ear and Hearing, 14,* 3–10.

Martin, F. N., & Clark, J. G. (1977). Audiologic detection of auditory processing disorders in children. *Journal of the American Audiology Society, 3,* 140–146.

Martin, F. N., & Clark, J. G. (1996). Behavioral hearing tests with children. In F. N. Martin & J. G. Clark (Eds.), *Hearing care for children,* (pp. 115–134). Boston: Allyn & Bacon.

Martin, F. N., & Coombes, S. (1976). A tangibly reinforced speech reception threshold procedure for use with small children. *Journal of Speech and Hearing Disorders, 41,* 333–338.

Martin, F. N., & Gravel, K. L. (1989). Pediatric audiological practices in the United States. *The Hearing Journal, 42,* 33–48.

Matkin, N. D. (1973, June). *Some essential features of a pediatric audiological evaluation.* Talk presented to the Eighth Danavox Symposium, Copenhagen.

Mauk, G. W., & Behrens, T. R. (1993). Historical, political, and technical context associated with early identification of hearing loss. *Seminars in Hearing, 14,* 1–17.

Maxon, A. B., White, K. R., Vohr, B. R., & Behrens, T. R. (1992). *Evoked otoacoustic emissions in neonatal screening: From data to implementation.* Short course presented at the Annual Convention of the American Speech-Language-Hearing Association, San Antonio, TX.

Mehl, A. L., & Thomson, V. (1998). Newborn hearing screening: The great omission. *Pediatrics, 101,* 4e (www.pediatrics.org).

Moore, J. M., Thompson, G., & Folsom, R. C. (1992). Auditory responsiveness of premature infants utilizing visual reinforcement audiometry. *Ear and Hearing, 13,* 187–194.

National Institutes of Health. (1993). Early identification of hearing impairment in infants and young children. *NIH Consensus Statement, 11* (1).

National Research Council. (1987). Committee on Hearing, Bioacoustics, and Biomechanics, Commission on Behavioral and Social Sciences and Education. Brainstem audiometry of infants. *Asha, 29,* 47–55.

Newby, H. A. (1948). Evaluating the efficiency of group screening tests of hearing. *Journal of Speech and Hearing Disorders, 13,* 236–240.

Norton, S. J. (1994). Emerging role of evoked otoacoustic emissions in neonatal hearing screening. *American Journal of Otology, 15* (Supplement 1), 4–12.

Patrick, P. E. (1987). Identification audiometry. In F. N. Martin (Ed.), *Hearing disorders in children* (pp. 399–425). Austin, TX: Pro-Ed.

Rose, D. S. (1983). The fundamental role of hearing in psychological development. *Hearing Instruments, 34,* 22–26.

Ross, M. (1964). The variable intensity pulse count method (VIPCM) for the detection and measurement of the pure-tone thresholds of children with functional hearing losses. *Journal of Speech and Hearing Disorders, 29,* 477–482.

Ross, M., & Lerman, J. (1970). A picture identification test for hearing impaired children. *Journal of Speech and Hearing Research, 13,* 44–53.

Ross, M., & Matkin, N. (1967). The rising audiometric configuration. *Journal of Speech and Hearing Disorders, 32,* 377–382.

Sells, J. P., Hurley, R. M., Morehouse, C. R., & Douglas, J. E. (1997). Validity of the ipsilateral acoustic reflex as a screening parameter. *Journal of the American Academy of Audiology, 8,* 132–136.

Shepherd, D. C. (1978). Pediatric audiology. In D. E. Rose (Ed.), *Audiological assessment* (2nd ed., pp. 261–300). Englewood Cliffs, NJ: Prentice-Hall.

Simmons, F. (1976). Automated hearing screening test for newborns: The crib-o-gram. In G. Mencher (Ed.), *Proceedings of the Nova Scotia Conference on Early Identification of Hearing Loss* (pp. 171–180). Basel: S. Karger.

Simmons, F., & Russ, F. (1974). Automated newborn hearing screening: Crib-o-gram. *Archives of Otolaryngology, 100,* 1–7.

Simmons, F. B., McFarland, W. H., & Jones, F. R. (1980). Patterns of deafness in newborns. *Laryngoscope, 90,* 448–453.

Spradlin, J. E., & Lloyd, L. L. (1965). Operant conditioning audiometry with low level retardates: A preliminary report. In L. L. Lloyd & D. R. Frisina (Eds.), *The audiological assessment of the mentally retarded: Proceedings of a national conference* (pp. 45–58). Parsons, KS: Parsons State Hospital and Training Center.

Suzuki, T., & Ogiba, Y. (1961). Conditioned orientation reflex audiometry. *Archives of Otolaryngology, 74,* 84–90.

Tharpe, A. M., & Bess, F. H. (1991). Identification and management of children with minimal hearing loss. *International Journal of Otorhinolaryngology, 21,* 41–50.

U. S. Department of Health and Human Resources. (1993). Prevalence of selected chronic conditions: United States, 1986–88. Centers for Disease Control and Prevention, National Center for Health Statistics.

Vohr, K. R., White, K. R., Maxon, A. B., & Johnson, M. J. (1993). Factors affecting the interpretation of transient evoked otoacoustic emission results in neonatal hearing screening. *Seminars in Hearing, 14,* 57–72.

Weaver, N. J., Wardell, F. N., & Martin, F. N. (1979). Comparison of tangibly reinforced speech-reception and pure-tone thresholds of mentally retarded children. *American Journal of Mental Deficiency, 33,* 512–517.

Wedenberg, E. (1956). Auditory test in newborn infants. *Acta Otolaryngologica, 46,* 446–461.

White, K. R., Vohr, B. R., Maxon, A. B., & Behrens, T. R. (1993). Universal newborn hearing screening using transient evoked otoacoustic emissions: Results of the Rhode Island Hearing Assessment Project. *Seminars in Hearing, 14,* 18–29.

White, K. R., Vohr, B. R., Behrens, T. R., McPherson, M. G., & Mauk, G. W. (1994). Screening of all newborns for hearing loss using transient evoked otoacoustic emissions. *International Journal of Pediatric Otorhinolaryngology, 29,* 203–217.

SUGGESTED READINGS

Hayes, D., & Northern, J. L. (1996). *Infants and hearing.* San Diego: Singular Publishing Group.

Martin, F. N., & Clark, J. G. (Eds.). (1996). *Hearing care for children.* Boston: Allyn & Bacon.

Northern, J. L., & Downs, M. P. (1991). *Hearing in children* (4th ed.). Baltimore: Williams & Wilkins.

REVIEW TABLE 8.1   Procedures Used in Pediatric Audiometry

Procedure	Age Group Most Suitable	Probability of Success
Warblet	Infants	Fair
Speech sounds	4 to 8 months	Good
COR, VRA	6 months to 2 years	Good
Imitation of vocalization	Under 1 year	Fair
Play audiometry	$2\frac{1}{2}$ to 6 years	Good
Operant conditioning	2 to 5 years	Good
Noisemakers	Under 3 years	Fair
Immittance measures	All ages	Very good
AEP	All ages	Very good
OAE	All ages	Very good
Pure-tone audiometry	Over 3 years	Good

PART III

Hearing Disorders

In Chapters 9 through 12 the description of the auditory system is divided into four separate parts for study of the outer ear, the middle ear, the inner ear, and the auditory nerve and central auditory pathways. The anatomy and physiology are described, as well as different disease processes that produce auditory disorders, their causes, and appropriate treatments. Chapter 13 discusses patients who are either pretending to have a hearing loss or exaggerating the loss they do have for some special gain. Examples are given of actual and theoretical findings on a variety of auditory tests described in Chapters 4 through 8, so that each disorder is exemplified from a diagnostic point of view. Additional tests are described where appropriate.

9

The Outer Ear

When laypersons think of the "ear," it is the outer ear that comes to mind. The outer ear is responsible for gathering sounds from the acoustical environment, and funneling them into the auditory mechanism. Some of the outer-ear structures found in humans are absent in such animals as birds and frogs, whose hearing sensitivity is nevertheless similar to that of humans. It is, of course, the outer ear of humans with which this chapter is concerned.

Chapter Objectives

This chapter requires no previous knowledge of human anatomy, but it does assume an understanding of the physics of sound and the various tests of hearing described earlier. All the minuscule details of the anatomy of the outer ear are not provided here. These may be obtained readily from books on anatomy.

Upon completion of Chapter 9, the reader should have a basic grasp of outer-ear anatomy and purpose. Knowledge should be acquired about some aspects of genetics, common disorders that affect the outer ear, how they are caused and treated, and how they manifest on a variety of audiometric tests.

Anatomy and Physiology of the Outer Ear

The Auricle

The most noticeable portion of the outer-ear mechanism is the **auricle** or **pinna** (Figure 9.1). The auricle varies from person to person in size and shape and its funnel-like action plays a substantial role in gathering sound waves from the environment. The auricle is made entirely of cartilage, with a number of individually characteristic twists, turns, and indentations. The entire cartilage is covered with skin, which is continuous with the face. The bottom-most portion of the auricle is the *lobule,* or ear lobe. Extending up from the lobule, the outer rim of the auricle folds over outwardly, forming the *helix.* Above the lobule is the *antitragus.* Another elevation running closer to the center of the auricle is the *antihelix.* A small triangular protrusion, which points slightly backward and forms the anterior portion of the auricle, is called the *tragus,* Latin for "goat's beard." The tragus is so named because in older men, a number of bristly hairs appear in this region. Depression of the tragus into the opening of the external ear canal is an efficient means of blocking sounds. This occlusion

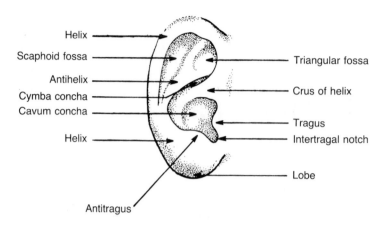

FIGURE 9.1   The human pinna (auricle).

provides more efficiency than plugging the ear with a finger, clasping the hands over the auricle, or even using some ear plugs specifically designed for sound attenuation. Although humans cannot voluntarily close off the tragus, as can some animals, vestiges of muscles designed for this purpose remain in the human ear.

The middle-most portion of the ear, just before the opening into the head, is called the *concha* because of its bowl-like shape. The concha is divided into two parts, the lower *cavum concha,* and the upper *cymba concha.* This portion of the external ear aids in the human ability to localize the sources of sounds that come from front, behind, below, and above the head. The concha helps to funnel sounds directed to it from the surrounding air into the opening of the **external auditory canal (EAC),** or *external auditory* **meatus.** The anatomy of the auricle is such that it is more efficient at delivering high-frequency sounds than low-frequency sounds, and it helps in the localization of sounds delivered to the head.

The External Auditory Canal

In discussing this portion of the ear, it is important not to omit the word *external* to avoid confusion with the internal auditory canal, discussed in Chapter 12. The external auditory canal is a tube, formed in the side of the head, beginning at the concha and extending inward at a slight upward angle for approximately 1 inch (2.5 cm) in adults. Although it appears round, the EAC is actually elliptical and averages about 9 mm in height and 6.5 mm in width. It is lined entirely with skin (Figure 9.2).

The outer portion of the EAC passes through cartilage. The skin in this area supports several sets of glands, including the sebaceous glands, which secrete sebum, an oily, fatty substance. The major product of these secretions is earwax, or **cerumen,** which is usually soft, moist, and brown, but can be light in color, flaky, and dry. Cerumen exits the ear naturally when the walls of the EAC are distorted by movement of the jawbone during chewing or speaking. The outer third of the EAC contains a number of hair follicles. The combination of hairs and cerumen helps to keep foreign objects, such as insects, from passing into the inner two-thirds of the canal.

The inner area of the EAC passes through the tympanic portion of the temporal bone. There are no glands and no hair in this area. The two portions of the EAC meet at the **osseocartilaginous**

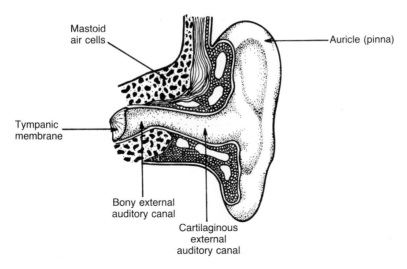

FIGURE 9.2   Cross section of the external ear.

junction. The **condyle,** a protrusion of the mandible (jawbone), comes to rest just below the osseo-cartilaginous junction when the jaw is closed. If the mandible overrides its normal position, as in the case of missing or worn molar teeth or a misaligned jaw, the condyle will press into the junction, causing pain. The term **temporomandibular joint (TMJ) syndrome** has been coined for this neuralgia. The TMJ syndrome produces a referred pain, perceived in the ear, which constitutes a significant amount of **otalgia** (ear pain) in adults.

The term *myofacial pain dysfunction (MPD)* syndrome is sometimes used to describe pain in the temporomandibular joint, along with headaches; grating sounds (crepitus); dizziness; and back, neck, and shoulder pain. At times, emotional stress and tension have been associated with MPD syndrome, and treatment has ranged from emotional therapy to biofeedback training, the use of prosthetic devices, and major maxillofacial surgery.

In infants and small children, the angle of the EAC is quite different from that in adults. The canal angles downward, rather than upward, and is at a more acute angle. For this reason, it is advisable to examine children's ears from above the head, rather than from below. When one looks into an ear, the adult pinna is pulled up and back, whereas the child's is pulled down and back.

The EAC serves several important functions. The **tympanic membrane** is situated at the end of the canal, where it is protected from trauma and where it can be kept at a constant temperature and humidity. The canal also serves as a filter to reduce low frequencies and a tube resonator for frequencies between 2000 and 7000 Hz, thereby creating an efficient transfer of energy to the tympanic membrane.

The Tympanic Membrane

The external auditory canal terminates in a concave, disk-like structure called the tympanic membrane (Figure 9.3). The term *eardrum* is commonly used to describe this structure, although properly speaking a drum would include the space below a vibrating membrane (in this case the middle ear),

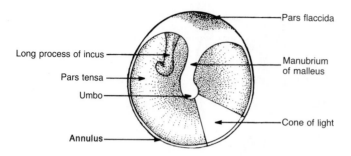

FIGURE 9.3   A right tympanic membrane.

and so the term *eardrum membrane* is more accurate. The tympanic membrane is discussed in this book under the heading of the outer ear because it can be viewed along with the outer-ear structures. Because the tympanic membrane marks the border between the outer ear and the middle ear, how-ever, it is really a common boundary between both areas. Whether the tympanic membrane is thought of as part of the outer ear or the middle ear is not important as long as its structure and func-tion are understood.

The total area of the tympanic membrane is about 63.3 mm^2 (Harris, 1986) and is constructed of three layers. The outer layer, as viewed from the external auditory canal, is made up of the same skin that is stretched over the osseous meatus. Below the skin is a layer of tough, fibrous, connec-tive tissue, which contributes most to the membrane's ability to vibrate with impinging sound waves. Behind the tympanic membrane is the middle-ear space, which is completely lined with **mucous membrane,** including the third layer of the tympanic membrane.

The tympanic membrane is extremely thin, averaging about 0.07 mm. Harris (1986) describes it as "a little conical loudspeaker." It is an extremely efficient vibrating surface. Movement of one-billionth of a centimeter is sufficient to produce a threshold response in normal-hearing individuals in the 800 to 6000 Hz range (Harris, 1986). The entire area of the tympanic membrane is very rich in blood supply, which is why it appears so red when infection is present and blood is brought to the area.

Embedded in the fibrous portion of the tympanic membrane is the *malleus,* the largest bone of the middle ear (described in Chapter 10). The tip of the malleus ends in the approximate center of the tympanic membrane and angles downward and backward (see Figure 9.3). If an imaginary line is drawn through the tympanic membrane at a 180-degree angle to the handle of the malleus and that line is bisected through the center of the tympanic membrane at right angles, the two intersecting imaginary lines thus drawn conveniently divide the tympanic membrane into four quadrants: *anterior-superior, posterior-superior, anterior-inferior,* and *posterior-inferior.*

The tip of the handle of the malleus is so poised as to cause the center of the tympanic mem-brane to be pulled inward, resulting in its concave configuration. The point of greatest retraction is called the **umbo.** To observe the tympanic membrane it is necessary to direct a light, as from an **oto-scope** (Figure 9.4) into the external auditory canal. Because the tympanic membrane is semitrans-parent, such a light allows some of the structures of the middle ear to become visible. However, some of the light rays directed against the membrane are reflected and refracted away. The concavity of the tympanic membrane usually causes the light reflex to appear in a cone shape directed inferiorly and anteriorly.

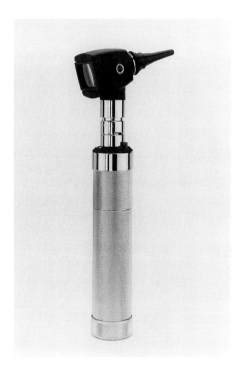

FIGURE 9.4 A hand-held otoscope. (Courtesy of Welch-Allyn, Inc.)

One of the many modern breakthroughs in medical instrumentation is the video otoscope (Figure 9.5). It combines an otoscope with a separate light source, fiberoptic cable, video camera, and color monitor. Viewing of the tympanic membrane takes place not through the otoscope in conventional ways, but by watching the video monitor, where the structures can be seen not only by the examiner, but also by the patient and other interested parties. Attachments for the device allow for still photography or videotaping for later viewing.

The tympanic membrane is held in position at the end of the EAC by a ring of tissue called the tympanic **annulus.** The slight stretching of the tympanic membrane into the middle ear results in its tension and conical appearance. The greatest surface area of the tympanic membrane is taut and is appropriately called the **pars tensa.** At the top of the tympanic membrane, above the malleus, the tissues are looser because they contain only the epidermal and mucous membrane layers, resulting in the name **pars flaccida.** The pars flaccida is also called **Shrapnell's membrane.**[1]

The auricle and external auditory canal provide a resonant tube through which sound waves may pass, and the tympanic membrane is the first mobile link in the chain of auditory events. Pressure waves, which impinge on the tympanic membrane, cause it to vibrate, reproducing the same spectrum of sounds that enters the external auditory canal. Movement of the tympanic membrane

---

[1]For Henry Jones Shrapnell, 19th century British anatomist.

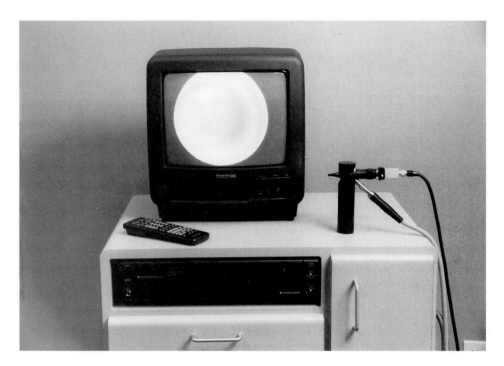

FIGURE 9.5   A Star Med video-otoscope. (Courtesy of Starkey laboratories.)

causes identical vibration of the malleus, to which it is attached. The further transmission of these sound waves is discussed in ensuing chapters.

Development of the Outer Ear

About 28 days after conception of the human embryo, bulges begin to appear on either side of the tissue that will develop into the head and neck. These are the **pharyngeal arches.** Although there may be as many as six arches, separated by grooves or clefts, significant information is available only about the first three: the *mandibular arch,* the *hyoid arch,* and the *glossopharyngeal arch.* These arches are known to have three layers, the **ectoderm,** or outer layer; the **entoderm,** or inner surface; and the **mesoderm,** or inner core. Each arch contains four components: an artery, muscle and cartilage that come from the mesoderm, and a nerve that forms from the ectoderm.

The auricle develops from the first two pharyngeal arches. The tragus forms from the first arch, and the helix and antitragus from the second arch. Development of the auricle begins before the second fetal month.

The external auditory canal forms from the first pharyngeal groove and is very shallow until after birth. A primitive meatus forms in about the fourth gestational week, and a solid core forms near the tympanic membrane in the eighth week. The solid core canalizes (forms a tube or canal) by the twenty-eighth gestational week, although the entire osseous meatus is not complete until about the time of puberty. **Pneumatization** of the temporal bone surrounding the external auditory canal begins in the thirty-fifth fetal week, accelerates at the time of birth, and is not complete until puberty.

The tympanic membrane annulus forms in the third fetal month. The outer layer of the membrane itself forms from ectoderm; the inner layer, from entoderm; and the middle layer, from **mesenchyme,** which is a network of embryonic tissue that later forms the connective tissues of the body, as well as the blood vessels and the lymphatic vessels. The tympanic membrane has begun formation by the beginning of the second embryonic month.

Hearing Loss and the Outer Ear

When conditions occur that interfere with or block the normal sound vibrations transmitted through the outer ear, conductive hearing loss results. Except in rare cases, the loss of hearing is rarely severe and never exceeds a 60 dB air-bone gap, because beyond that intensity supra-aural earphones vibrate the skull and generate bone-conduction signals. Because some of the disorders alter the normal resonance frequency of the outer ear, or otherwise interfere with the osseotympanic mode of bone conduction, the bone-conduction audiogram may be slightly altered; however, this does not, in itself, suggest abnormality of the sensorineural system.

Disorders of the Outer Ear and Their Treatments

Some abnormalities of the external ear do not result in hearing loss. They are mentioned, nonetheless, because of the audiologist's usual curiosity about disorders of the ear in general, and because abnormalities in one part of the body, specifically congenital ones, are frequently related to other abnormalities.

Disorders of the Auricle

Since hearing tests performed with earphones ignore the auricle, they do not reveal any effects it may have on hearing sensitivity, word recognition, and localization. For example, people who have had a portion or an entire auricle removed by accident or surgery, as in the case of cancer, appear to have no apparent hearing loss. At times, one or both ears may be of very small size (**microtia**), or the pinna may be very prominent and stand away from the head, or be entirely absent (**anotia**). Congenital malformations of the auricle have also been associated with other disorders, such as **Down syndrome.**[2]

When the auricle protrudes markedly from the head, or when it is pressed tightly against the skull, a simple surgical procedure called **otoplasty** or **pinnaplasty** may be performed. These operations may improve the patient's appearance, which often has a beneficial psychological effect. In cases of missing auricles in children, plastic surgery is often inadvisable because the scar tissue formed from the grafts does not grow as does normal tissue. Plastic auricles can be made that are

---

[2]Named for John Langdon Haydon Down, British physician, 1828–1896.

affixed to the head with adhesive and are amazingly realistic. Hairstyles can sometimes be arranged to conceal malformed auricles entirely.

Atresia of the External Auditory Canal

In some patients, either the cartilaginous portion, the bony portion, or the entirety of the external auditory canal has never formed at all. Such congenital abnormalities may occur in one or both ears. This lack of canalization is called **atresia** and can occur in the EAC either in isolation or in combination with other anomalies. One condition, Treacher Collins syndrome, which is inherited and sex-linked, involves the facial bones, especially the cheek and lower jaw; the auricle; and congenital atresia of the EAC. At times, patients with Treacher Collins syndrome present with preauricular tags, which represent incomplete embryological development, and appear just in front of the auricle and do not, in themselves, cause hearing difficulties. Sometimes these tags contain a core of cartilage and are large enough to be called accessory auricles. A number of abnormalities of the middle ear and temporal bone are seen with Treacher Collins syndrome, making surgical correction quite difficult.

Not all closures of the external auditory canal are congenital; some may occur as the result of trauma or burns. Trauma to the outer ear may result in an unsightly blood blister, called a hematoma. Since the pinna protrudes from the side of the head, it can be damaged by sunlight or extreme cold. Frostbite can appear rather like a severe burn. Either condition can lead to loss of the pinna.

Sometimes, when an ear is malformed in a small child, it is difficult to determine whether the condition is one of congenital atresia or a marked **stenosis** (narrowing) of the canal. Surgical procedures for correction of atresia of the EAC have improved in recent years, and surgeons have been assisted greatly by the advent of modern imaging techniques. Chances for success are better when only the cartilaginous canal is involved, and when the middle ear and tympanic membrane are normal. Drillouts of the bony canal have led to some serious aftercare problems. Although, in some cases, it may appear that it is better to treat a child with a congenital external ear canal atresia with a hearing aid, rather than with surgery, the ultimate decision on such matters is always left to the family in consultation with a physician.

Stenotic EACs do not produce hearing loss, as does atresia, although the very narrow lumen can easily be clogged by earwax or other debris and thus cause a conductive problem. In cases of atresia of the canal, the hearing loss is directly related to the area and the amount of occlusion. The loss may be mild if only the cartilaginous area is involved, and certainly will be more severe if the bony canal is occluded. As stated earlier, a congenital anomaly in one part of the body increases the likelihood of another anomaly elsewhere. For this reason, when an atresia is seen, it must be suspected that the tympanic membrane and middle ear may likewise be involved. Figure 9.6 shows the test results for a theoretical patient with atresia of both external ear canals. Notice that the conductive loss reaches near maximum (about 60 dB). In cases of atresia, the valuable information from measurements of acoustic immittance is unobtainable, because the probe cannot be inserted into the EAC.

Foreign Bodies in the External Ear Canal

For unexplained reasons, children, and sometimes adults, place foreign objects, such as paper, pins, and crayons, into their mouths, noses, and ears. If the object is pushed past the osseocartilaginous junction of the external ear canal, swelling at the isthmus formed by this junction may result.

SPEECH AND HEARING CENTER
The University of Texas at Austin 78712
AUDIOMETRIC EXAMINATION

NAME: Last - First - Middle	SEX	AGE	DATE	EXAMINER	RELIABILITY	AUDIOMETER

AIR CONDUCTION

MASKING TYPE	RIGHT									LEFT								
	250	500	1000	1500	2000	3000	4000	6000	8000	250	500	1000	1500	2000	3000	4000	6000	8000
NB	55	60	60/60	60	55	60	65	65	70	60	55	55/55	60	60	60	65	65	60
	55	60	60	60	60	60	65	65	70	60	55	55	60	60	60	65	65	60
EM Level in Opp. Ear	60	55	55	60	60	60	60	65	60	55	60	60	60	55	60	65	65	70

BONE CONDUCTION

MASKING TYPE	RIGHT						FOREHEAD						LEFT					
	250	500	1000	2000	3000	4000	250	500	1000	2000	3000	4000	250	500	1000	2000	3000	4000
NB	10	10	15	20	20	20	10	10	15	20	20	20	10	10	15	20	20	25
EM Level in Opp. Ear	60	55	55	60	60	65							70	60	60	55	60	80

	2 Frequency	3 Frequency	WEBER								2 Frequency	3 Frequency
Pure Tone Average	60	60	M	M	M	M	M	M		Pure Tone Average	55	57

SPEECH AUDIOMETRY

MASKING TYPE	RIGHT					LEFT			
	SRT 1	SRT 2	Recognition 1	Recognition 2		SRT 1	SRT 2	Recognition 1	Recognition 2
WB	60	60	1A List 30 SL 100%	List SL %		60	60 24 List 30 SL	96% List SL %
EM Level in Opp. Ear		60	95				60	95	

FREQUENCY IN HERTZ / COMMENTS

AUDIOGRAM KEY

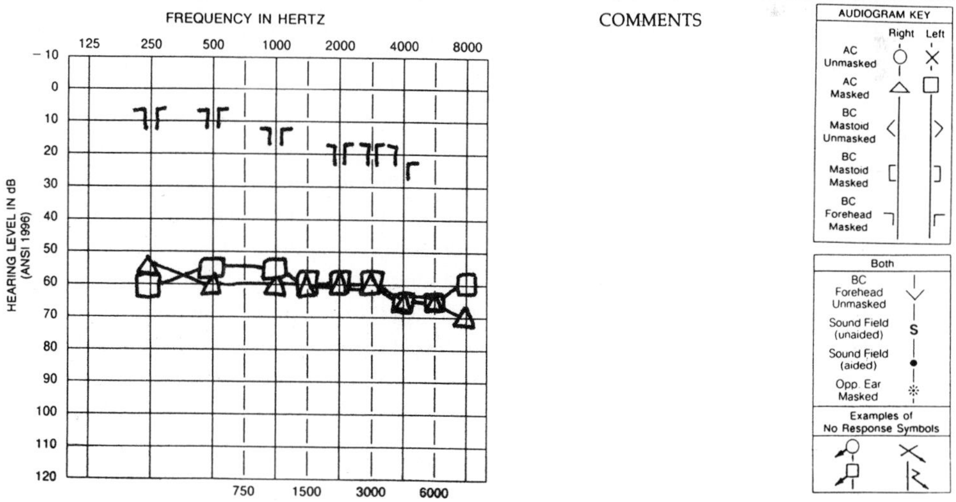

FIGURE 9.6 **Audiogram showing a moderately severe conductive hearing loss consistent with Treacher Collins syndrome. Note the large air-bone gaps with essentially normal bone conduction. The SRTs and pure-tone averages are in close agreement, and the word-recognition scores are normal.**

Although hearing loss may result from such an incident, it is of secondary importance to prompt and careful removal of the object, which may be a formidable task and may require surgery in some cases.

External Otitis

An infection that occurs in the skin of the external auditory canal is called **external otitis.** The condition is often called "swimmer's ear," because it frequently develops in people who have had water trapped in their ears. External ear infections are often called "fungus," although bacterial infections are more common. **Otomycosis,** or fungal external ear infections, are rare and may be caused by the overuse of ear drops. External otitis is quite common in tropical areas.

External otitis may originate from allergic reactions, as to ear plugs, hearing-aid earmolds, soap or other allergens. **Furunculosis,** infection of hair follicles, may begin with infection of a single hair in the lateral third of the external auditory canal and spread to involve the entire area.

Systemic antibiotics or eardrops are frequently unsuccessful in the treatment of external otitis, because the pocket of infection may be inaccessible, either topically, or through the bloodstream. Itching is a common complaint in early or mild infections. Patients with more advanced infections are sometimes in extreme pain, especially upon touch to the infected area, which may become red and swollen and may produce a discharge. Often body temperature elevates. The condition may be successfully treated by irrigating the canal with warm saltwater, drying it carefully, and applying topical antibiotics. Sometimes a cotton wick is inserted into the canal, which is saturated with antibiotic drops. The skin may be treated topically with steroids to curtail the inflammation.

Hearing tests often cannot be performed on patients with external otitis because the ear is too painful to allow the pressure of the earphones. It is suspected that if the lumen of the canal is closed, either by the accumulation of infectious debris or by the swelling of the canal walls, a mild conductive loss is likely, as shown in Figures 9.7 and 9.8. Some concern has been expressed by audiologists regarding the contamination by bacteria of earphones and their rubber cushions. Large colonies of certain organisms may be found on earphone cushions (Kemp, Roeser, Pearson, & Ballachanda, 1995), which can often be controlled using ultraviolet light.

Sometimes the tympanic membrane itself becomes inflamed, often in response to systemic viral infection. The patient may develop blood blisters on the surface of the tympanic membrane, which in turn produce fever and pain. Often these blebs must be carefully lanced to relieve the pain. Inflammations of the tympanic membrane are called **myringitis.**

Several forms of external otitis are considered particularly dangerous to the patient and require rather aggressive therapy. For example, *necrotizing,* or *malignant, external otitis* is often initially a routine infection of the skin of the external auditory canal. The condition is particularly threatening to diabetic and elderly patients, and may result in massive bone destruction in the external, middle, and inner ears. It can also result in **osteitis** and in **osteomyelitis** of the temporal bone. Patients suffering from this condition, which is often fatal, may be hospitalized and treated with systemic antibiotics. Surgery is sometimes required to stop the spread of infection through the bone.

Growths in the External Auditory Canal

Tumors, both benign and malignant, have been found in the EAC. Bony tumors, called *osteomas,* do not present hearing problems unless their size is such that the lumen of the canal is occluded and conductive hearing loss results; however, they may result in serious infection of the EAC.

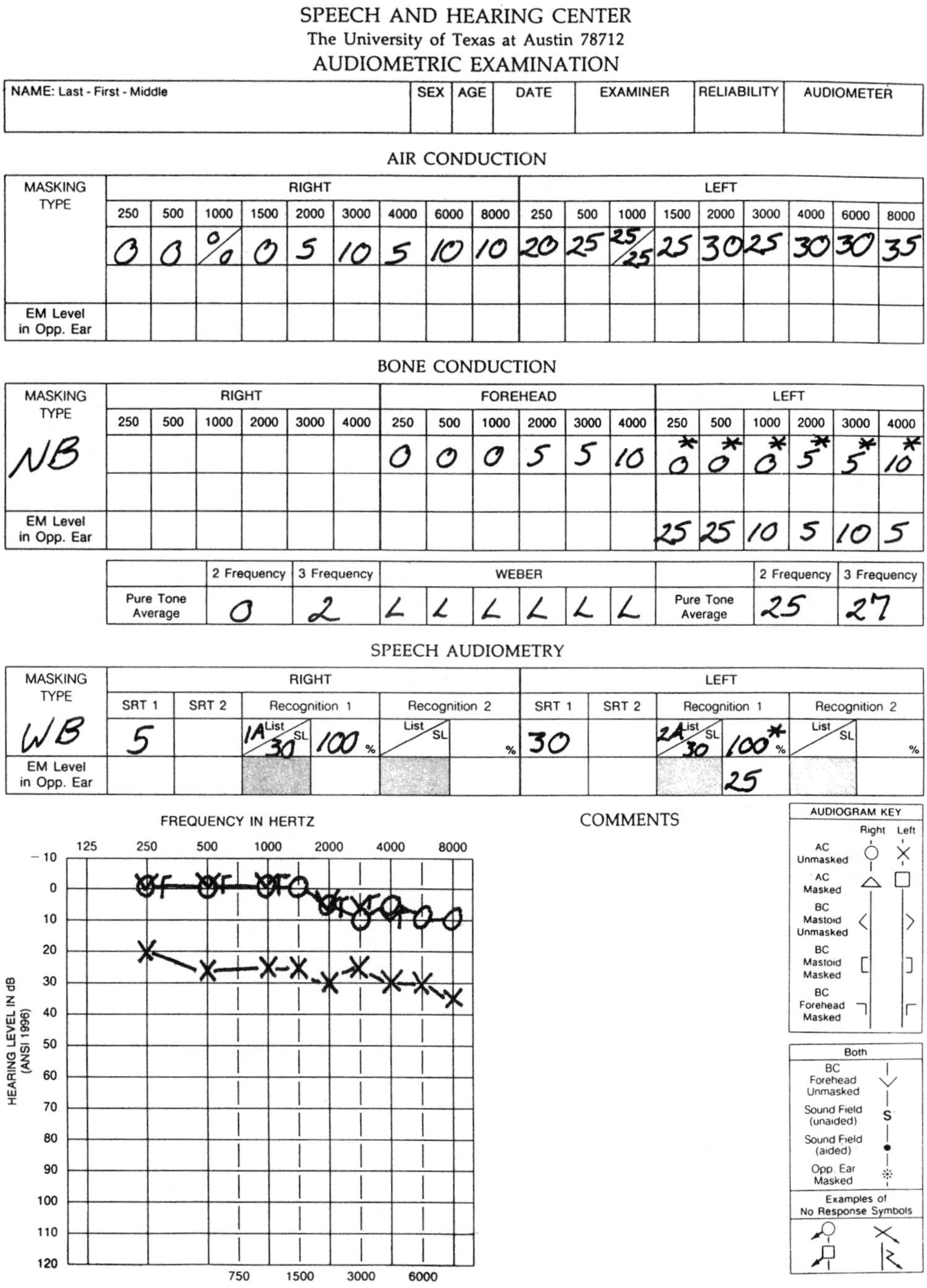

SPEECH AND HEARING CENTER
The University of Texas at Austin 78712
AUDIOMETRIC EXAMINATION

NAME: Last - First - Middle	SEX	AGE	DATE	EXAMINER	RELIABILITY	AUDIOMETER

AIR CONDUCTION

MASKING TYPE	RIGHT									LEFT								
	250	500	1000	1500	2000	3000	4000	6000	8000	250	500	1000	1500	2000	3000	4000	6000	8000
	0	0	0/0	0	5	10	5	10	10	20	25	25/25	25	30	25	30	30	35
EM Level in Opp. Ear																		

BONE CONDUCTION

MASKING TYPE	RIGHT						FOREHEAD						LEFT					
	250	500	1000	2000	3000	4000	250	500	1000	2000	3000	4000	250	500	1000	2000	3000	4000
NB							0	0	0	5	5	10	0*	0*	0*	5*	5*	10*
EM Level in Opp. Ear													25	25	10	5	10	5

	2 Frequency	3 Frequency	WEBER							2 Frequency	3 Frequency
Pure Tone Average	0	2	∠	∠	∠	∠	∠	∠	Pure Tone Average	25	27

SPEECH AUDIOMETRY

MASKING TYPE	RIGHT				LEFT			
	SRT 1	SRT 2	Recognition 1	Recognition 2	SRT 1	SRT 2	Recognition 1	Recognition 2
WB	5		1A List 30 SL / 100 %	List SL / %	30		2A List 30 SL / 100* %	List SL / %
EM Level in Opp. Ear							25	

FREQUENCY IN HERTZ

COMMENTS

AUDIOGRAM KEY

FIGURE 9.7 A mild unilateral (left) conductive hearing loss, due to external otitis. SRT and pure-tone findings are in close agreement, and word-recognition scores are normal. Masking is needed for the left ear for bone conduction and WRS. The Weber results show lateralization to the left ear.

SPEECH AND HEARING CENTER
THE UNIVERSITY OF TEXAS AT AUSTIN 78712

Name: Last-First-Middle	Sex	Age	Examiner	Reliability	Date

	AUDIOMETRIC BING TEST					
	RIGHT			LEFT		
Frequency (Hertz)	250	500	1000	250	500	1000
1) Unoccluded	0	0	0	0	0	0
2) Occluded	-25	-15	-10	0	0	0
3) Occlusion Effect (1-2)	25	15	10	0	0	0

FIGURE 9.8   Results on the Bing test for a patient with unilateral conductive hearing loss caused by external otitis (see Figure 9.7). Note the absence of the occlusion effect in the left ear on the Bing test.

Exostoses, the outward projections for the surfaces of bone, are sometimes seen in the ears of people who have done a great deal of swimming in cold water. To the untrained eye such protrusions in the bony wall of the EAC may be confused with osteomas. As with osteomas, exostoses only require treatment when their size produces a conductive hearing loss, or when they block the normal cleansing action of the EAC, resulting in infection.

Earwax in the External Auditory Canal

In some cases the glands in the EACs are extremely active, producing copious amounts of cerumen. When the canal is small, it may become blocked and produce a hearing loss. Even when a large amount of wax is found in the ear, hearing may remain normal as long as there is a tiny opening between the tympanic membrane and the outside environment. Overzealous cleaning of the external ears, however, may result in cerumen being pushed from the cartilaginous canal into the bony canal, where natural cleansing cannot take place. Cotton swabs and wadded tissues are often used for such purposes, frequently by well-meaning parents, on the ears of their children.

Once the wax is deposited in the bony canal, it must remain there until it is properly removed. Wax deposited in the bony canal becomes dry, causing itching, which encourages the individual to push still more wax down from the cartilaginous canal by instruments such as cotton swabs. Sometimes water pressure during diving forces wax deep into the canal.

Because more and more audiological procedures—such as testing with insert receivers, immittance measures, electrocochleography, and the fitting of hearing aids, require patients' external ear canals to be clear, the role of the audiologist has changed concerning cerumen removal. ASHA (1992) suggests that audiologists become proficient at careful removal of earwax.

A complete history must be taken to rule out possible tympanic membrane perforation, ear disease, or the presence of pressure-equalizing tubes (see Chapter 10). If anything in the history seems to contraindicate the audiologist's removal of the cerumen (e.g., diabetes, AIDS, previous ear surgery), the patient should be referred to a physician to have the wax removed.

Careful otoscopic examination must be performed, in part, to determine that it is cerumen and not some other substance or object occluding the canal. If the tympanic membrane can be seen, its integrity should be ascertained.

An approved **cerumenolytic,** a chemical substance known to safely soften earwax, may be used. This substance should be placed into the ear at least an hour before removal is attempted, although it is preferable for patients to use the substance several times a day for several days. The harder and dryer the cerumen is found to be at examination, the longer the wax will take to soften.

Although many audiologists use water irrigation to flush the cerumen from the external auditory canal, many others prefer the use of suction and curettes for mechanical removal. Of course, proper illumination is essential, as from a headlamp, or, preferably, a surgical microscope or video otoscope.

As in the case of external otitis, the amount of hearing loss produced by impacted cerumen is directly related to the amount of ear canal occlusion. Hearing losses may range from very mild to moderate. Audiologists must be careful whenever they insert any object or perform any procedure on a patient's external ear, and all procedures should be duly noted in the patient's chart.

Perforations of the Tympanic Membrane

The tympanic membrane may become perforated in several ways. Excessive pressure buildup during a middle-ear disorder may cause rupturing of the membrane. Sometimes, in response to infection, usually in the middle ear, the membrane may become necrosed (dead) and perforate.

A frequent cause of perforation is direct trauma from a pointed object such as a cotton swab or hairpin. This may happen if patients are attempting to cleanse their own ears, and either misjudge the length of the EAC, or are jarred or startled while probing in it. Such accidents are extremely painful, as well as embarrassing. The tympanic membrane may also be perforated from sudden pressure in the external ear canal, as created by a hand clapped over the ear or an explosion.

Because traumatic perforations alter what is essentially normal tissue, they tend to show spontaneous closure better than do perforations resulting from disease. Perforations in the inferior portion of the tympanic membrane heal more rapidly than those in the superior portion, because the normal epithelium migration is more active inferiorly. The migration of tissue has been encouraged by placing a thin piece of cigarette paper over the perforation. Often, when a perforation is thus healed, the mucosal and skin layers close off the opening, but a thin area remains in the fibrous layer, which does not migrate as well. Such thin areas in the tympanic membrane lend themselves to easy reperforation, as from water irrigation of the external canal, or even a strong sneeze.

Surgical repair of a perforated tympanic membrane is called **myringoplasty.** In early versions of myringoplasty, skin grafts, usually taken from the inner aspect of the arm, were placed over the perforation. Even though the grafts often "took" initially, they tended to desquamate (flake off), with consequent reperforation. Skin grafts were later replaced by vein grafts, taken from the patient's hand or arm. Vein works well for this purpose because its elasticity is similar to that of the fibrous layer of the tympanic membrane, although narrow veins are inadequate for large perforations. Most middle-ear surgeons today prefer to use fascia, the tough fibrous protective covering over muscle. Results with myringoplasty have been very gratifying.

The amount of hearing loss produced by a perforated tympanic membrane depends on several variables. The exact size and place of the perforation can cause variations, not only in the amount of hearing loss, but in the audiometric configuration as well. Measurements on acoustic immittance meters are sometimes impossible because an airtight seal cannot be formed as a consequence of leakage of pressure from the air pump of the meter through the perforation into the middle ear. At times perforations, not readily visible with the naked eye because of their small size, can be detected by the immittance meter. If a seal can be obtained when there is a tympanic membrane perforation, the C1 value will be very large because the outer-ear cavity is continuous with the middle-ear cavity.

Thickening of the Tympanic Membrane

Often, in response to infection, usually of the middle ear, the tympanic membrane becomes thickened and scarred. At times calcium plaques appear, adding to the mass of the tympanic membrane and interfering with its vibration, but sometimes causing no appreciable hearing loss. Such conditions are called **tympanosclerosis** and they do not respond well to medical or surgical treatment.

Often the tympanic membrane can become quite thickened. The thickening can be coincidental with disorders of the middle ear, thus making it impossible to determine the amount of hearing loss each disorder contributes.

Collapsing External Auditory Canals

At times a conductive hearing loss appears because the pressure of the earphone causes the auricle to move forward, blocking the opening of the canal, and attenuating sound entering it. Often the patient does not experience the loss subjectively. Inspection of the ear prior to testing can often avoid the finding of a false conductive hearing loss. Collapsing external ear canals are common in the elderly because of a lack of sturdy supporting cartilage. When this is suspected, a plastic tube can be inserted into the canal with a strong string attached for easy retrieval, or a wedge of foam rubber can be put behind the pinna before the headset is placed in position. Often insert earphones can be used for this purpose as well.

Summary

The outer ear, including the auricle, external auditory canal, and tympanic membrane, is the channel by which sounds from the environment are first introduced to the hearing mechanism. The auricle helps gather the sound, the external auditory canal directs it, and the tympanic membrane vibrates in sympathy with the airborne vibrations that strike it. When portions of the outer ear are abnormal or diseased, hearing may or may not become impaired, depending on which structures are involved, and the nature of their involvement.

Abnormalities of the external ear do not affect the sensorineural mechanism. However, alterations in the canal may cause a change in the osseotympanic mode of bone conduction, which may alter the bone-conduction curve slightly. Audiometric findings on word recognition and site-of-lesion tests are the same as expected for persons with normal hearing. Measurements on the acoustic immittance meter are frequently impossible in external-ear anomalies, by virtue of the disorder itself.

Whenever an audiologist sees a patient with an external-ear disorder, an otological consultation should be recommended. If hearing is impaired and no medical therapy is available, other habilitative or rehabilitative avenues should be investigated, depending on the extent of hearing loss, and the needs of the patient.

STUDY QUESTIONS

1. Make sketches of the outer ear and tympanic membrane. Label from memory as many parts as you can. Compare your drawings with the ones in Figures 9.1, 9.2, and 9.3.

2. List as many disorders of the outer ear as you can remember. Divide them into two columns, those that produce hearing loss and those that do not.

3. For each of the disorders you listed that produce hearing loss, draw a pure-tone audiogram. Predict the probable SRT, word-recognition scores, and results on the site-of-lesion tests discussed earlier.

GLOSSARY

Anotia Absence of the pinna.

Annulus The ring of tissue around the periphery of the tympanic membrane that holds it in position at the end of the external auditory canal.

Atresia Congenital closure of a normally open body orifice, such as the external auditory canal.

Auricle The cartilaginous appendage of the external ear.

Cerumen Earwax.

Cerumenolytic A chemical substance (such as carbamide peroxide and glycerin) that is used to soften cerumen prior to removal.

Condyle The rounded projection, or process, of a bone. The condyle of the mandible comes to rest in a fossa (a hollowed or depressed area) just below the osseocartilaginous junction of the external auditory canal.

Down syndrome Sometimes called "trisomy 21 syndrome," Down disorder is characterized by mental retardation; a small, slightly flattened skull; low-set ears; abnormal digits; and other unusual facial and body characteristics.

Ectoderm The outermost of the three primary embryonic germ layers.

Entoderm The innermost of the three primary embryonic germ layers.

Exostoses Projections for the surfaces of bone, as the external auditory canal, which are usually covered with cartilage.

External auditory canal (EAC) The channel in the external ear from the concha of the auricle to the tympanic membrane.

External otitis Infection of the outer ear. Also called *otitis externa*.

Furunculosis Infection of hair follicles, as in the external auditory canal.

Meatus A passage, such as the external auditory canal.

Mesenchyme   A network of embryonic connective tissue in the mesoderm, which forms the connective tissue, blood vessels, and lymph vessels of the body.

Mesoderm   The middle-most of the three primary embryonic germ layers, lying between the ectoderm and the entoderm.

Microtia   A congenitally abnormally small external ear.

Mucous membrane   The moist lining of cavities of the body, such as the middle ear.

Myringitis   Any inflammation of the tympanic membrane.

Myringoplasty   Surgery for restoration or repair of the tympanic membrane.

Osseocartilaginous junction   The union between the bony and cartilaginous portions of the external auditory canal.

Osteitis   Inflammation of bone marked by tenderness, enlargement, and pain.

Osteomyelitis   Inflammation of bone caused by a purulent infection.

Otalgia   Pain in the ear.

Otomycosis   Fungal infection of the external ear.

Otoplasty   Any plastic surgery of the outer ear.

Otoscope   A special flashlight device with a funnel-like speculum on the end, designed to observe the tympanic membrane.

Pars flaccida   The loose folds of epithelium of the tympanic membrane above the malleus.

Pars tensa   All of the remaining (taut) portion of the tympanic membrane besides the pars flaccida.

Pharyngeal arches   Paired embryonic arches that modify, in humans, into structures of the ear and neck. In fish they modify into gills.

Pinna   The auricle of the external ear.

Pinnaplasty   A cosmetic operation designed to improve the appearance of the pinna.

Pneumatization   The formation of air cavities in tissues, as in the temporal bones of the skull.

Shrapnell's membrane   The pars flaccida of the tympanic membrane.

Stenosis   An abnormal narrowing, as of the external auditory canal.

Temporomandibular joint (TMJ) syndrome   Pain felt in the ear, but referred from a neuralgia of the temporomandibular joint.

Tympanic membrane   The separation between the outer and middle ears, located at the end of the external auditory canal. It comprises an outer layer of skin, a middle layer of connective tissue, and an inner layer of mucous membrane.

Tympanosclerosis   Formation of whitish plaques in the tympanic membrane and masses of hard connective tissue around the bones of the middle ear. This occurs secondary to otitis media and may result in fixation of the ossicular chain.

Umbo   The point at the approximate center of the tympanic membrane at which it is most retracted.

REFERENCES

American Speech-Language-Hearing Association (ASHA). (1992). External auditory canal examination and cerumen management. *Asha, 34* (Supplement), 22–24.

Harris, J. D. (1986). Anatomy and physiology of the peripheral auditory mechanism. In *The Pro-Ed Studies in Communication Disorders*. Austin, TX: Pro-Ed.

Kemp, R. J., Roeser, R. J., Pearson, D., & Ballachanda, B. B. (1995). *Infection control for the professions of audiology and speech-language pathology*. San Diego: Singular Publishing Group.

SUGGESTED READINGS

Hirsch, B. E. (1996). Diseases of the external ear. In C. D. Blue-stone, S. E. Stool, & M. A. Kenna (Eds.), *Pediatric otolaryngology* (pp. 378–387). Philadelphia: W. B. Saunders Co.

Kenna, M. A. (1996). Embryology and developmental anatomy of the ear. In C. D. Bluestone, S. E. Stool, & M. A. Kenna (Eds.), *Pediatric otolaryngology* (pp. 113–126). Philadelphia: W. B. Saunders Co.

REVIEW TABLE 9.1   The Outer Ear

Anatomical Area	Disorder	Causes Hearing Loss	Treatment
Auricle	Missing, small, or malformed	No	Plastic Surgery
External auditory canal	Wax	Sometimes	Removal
	Infection	Sometimes	Medical treatment
	Atresia	Yes	Surgery
	Stenosis	Sometimes	Observation/surgery
	Foreign bodies	Sometimes	Removal
Tympanic membrane	Perforation	Yes	Yes
	Thickening	Sometimes	Sometimes

10 The Middle Ear

The development of the middle ear was no doubt one of evolution's most splendid engineering feats. The middle ear carries vibrations from the outer ear to the inner ear by transferring the sound energy from the air in the outer ear to the fluids of the inner ear. The middle ear overcomes the loss of energy that results when sound passes from one medium (in this case, air) to another medium (fluid).

Chapter Objectives

This chapter assumes a basic understanding of hearing loss as introduced in Chapter 2, the physics of sound in Chapter 3, and the details of hearing tests and their interpretation in Chapters 4 to 8. Oversimplifications of the anatomy of the middle ear and its function, provided as an introduction earlier in this book, should be clarified.

At the completion of this chapter, readers should understand the anatomy and physiology of the middle ear, and they should be familiar with the etiologies and treatments of common disorders that produce hearing loss. In addition, they should be able to predict what the typical audiometric results for each of the pathologies might be, and they should be able to make a reasonable attempt at diagnosing the etiology of the hearing loss based on audiometric and other findings.

Anatomy and Physiology of the Middle Ear

An average adult middle ear is an almost oval, air-filled space of roughly 2 cm^3 (about one-half inch high, one-half inch wide, and one-quarter inch deep). The roof of the middle ear is a thin layer of bone, separating the middle-ear cavity from the brain. Below the floor of the middle ear is the **jugular bulb,** and behind the anterior wall is the **carotid artery.** The labyrinth of the inner ear lies behind the medial wall, and the mastoid process is beyond the posterior wall. The lateral portion of the middle ear is sometimes called the *membranous wall,* as it contains the tympanic membrane. The space in the middle ear above the tympanic membrane is called the **epitympanic recess.**

As is shown in Figure 10.1, the middle ear is separated from the external auditory canal by the tympanic membrane. The middle ear is connected to the **nasopharynx,** that area where the back of the throat and the nose communicate, via the **eustachian tube.** The eustachian tube and middle ear form the **middle-ear cleft.** The entire middle-ear cleft, including the surface of the tympanic membrane that is within the middle ear, is lined with **mucous membrane,** the same lining found in the nose and paranasal sinuses. Much of this mucous membrane is ciliated; that is, the topmost cells con-

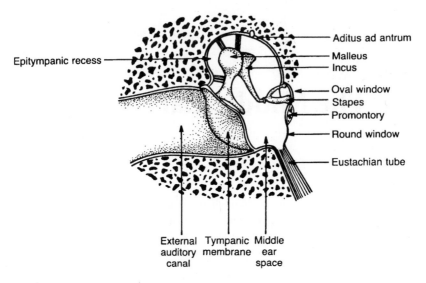

FIGURE 10.1   The human middle ear in cross section.

tain **cilia,** small hair-like projections that provide a motion similar to that of a wheat field in the wind. The motion of the cilia creates a wiping action that helps to cleanse the middle ear by moving particles down and out of the eustachian tube.

The Eustachian Tube

The eustachian tube[1] enters the middle ear anteriorly at a 30-degree angle and passes down into the nasopharynx. In adults the tube is normally kept closed by the spring mechanism of cartilage. It is opened by the action of three sets of muscles at the orifice of the tube in the nasopharynx. This opening occurs during yawning, sneezing, or swallowing, or when excessive air pressure is applied from the nose. While we are awake, our eustachian tubes open about once per minute; during sleep, on an average of once every five minutes. In infants the eustachian tube is shorter and wider in relation to its length and in a more horizontal plane than it is in adults. The orifice of the eustachian tube in the nasopharynx tends to remain open in infants up until the age of about six months.

The air pressure of the middle ear must match that of the external auditory canal to keep the pressure equal on both sides of the tympanic membrane to maximize its mobility. The absorption of air by middle-ear tissues is the major reason for the need for a pressure-equalization system. The only way for this pressure equalization to be maintained is through the eustachian tube. At one time or another most people have had the experience of fullness in the ear—for example, when flying or driving to a higher or lower elevation. During ascension this fullness results when the air in the external ear canal becomes rarefied (thin), while the middle ear remains at ground-level pressure. The full sensation occurs when the tympanic membrane is pushed outward by the greater pressure

---

[1]For Bartolommeo Eustachio, 16th century Italian anatomist.

from within the middle ear. Upon descent, the pressure in the middle ear may be less than in the external ear canal, so that the tympanic membrane is pushed in. The sensations are the same whether the tympanic membrane is pushed in or out. The simple solution is to swallow, yawn, or otherwise open the eustachian tube so that the pressure may be equalized. Because the normal function of the tube is to replenish air pressure, moving from lesser to greater air pressure is more traumatic. At extreme pressures the eustachian tube will lock shut, making pressure-equalization impossible, and great pain and tympanic membrane rupture likely. A new type of earplug has been developed for people who experience eustachian-tube difficulties during flying. The plugs are flanged and gradually release pressure during ascent and descent, providing decreased discomfort for many flyers.

The Mastoid

Figure 10.1 shows that some of the bones of the skull that surround the ear are not solid but rather are honeycombed with hundreds of air cells. Each of these cells is lined with mucous membrane, which, though nonciliated, is similar to that of the middle-ear cleft. These cells form the pneumatic mastoid of the temporal bone. The middle ear opens up, back, and outward in an area called the **aditus ad antrum** to communicate with the mastoid. The bony protuberance behind the auricle is called the **mastoid process.**

Windows of the Middle Ear

A section of the bony portion of the inner ear extends into the middle-ear space. This is caused by the basal turn of the cochlea, which is described in Chapter 11. This protrusion is the **promontory** and separates two connections between the middle and inner ear. Above the promontory is the **oval window** and below it the **round window,** both of whose names are derived from their shapes. The round window is covered by a very thin, but tough and elastic, membrane. The oval window is filled by a membrane that supports the base of the stapes, the tiniest bone of the human body.

Bones in the Middle Ear

To accomplish its intended function of carrying sound waves from the air-filled external auditory canal to the fluid-filled inner ear, the middle ear contains a set of three very small bones called **ossicles.** Each of these bones bears a Latin name descriptive of its shape: **malleus, incus,** and **stapes.**

The **manubrium** (handle) of the malleus is embedded in the middle (fibrous) layer of the tympanic membrane; it extends from the upper portion of the tympanic membrane to its approximate center (the **umbo**). The head of the malleus is connected to the incus, and this area of connection extends upward into the aditus ad antrum (or epitympanic recess). Details of the anatomy of the malleus are shown in Figure 10.2. The incus (Figure 10.3) has a long process, or **crus,** which turns abruptly to a very short crus, the lenticular process. The end of the lenticular process sits squarely on the head of the stapes. As is shown in Figure 10.4, the stapes comprises a head, neck, and two **crura** (plural of crus). The posterior crus is longer and thinner than the anterior crus to aid in its rocking motion. The base, or **footplate,** of the stapes occupies the space in the oval window. Additional schematic illustrations of the middle ear ossicles and their ligaments may be found on the CD-ROM under *Anatomy.*

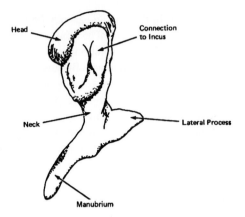

FIGURE 10.2   Anatomy of the human malleus.

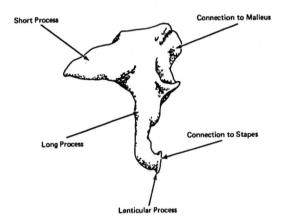

FIGURE 10.3   Anatomy of the human incus.

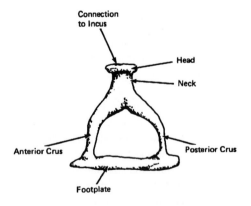

FIGURE 10.4   Anatomy of the human stapes.

Because the malleus and incus are connected rather rigidly, inward and outward movement of the umbo of the tympanic membrane causes these two bones to rotate, which transfers this force to the stapes, which in turn results in the inward and outward motion of the oval window. Each of the ossicles is so delicately poised by its ligamental connections within the middle ear that their collective function is unaltered by gravity when the head changes in position. The photograph in Figure 10.5 illustrates the very small size of the ossicles.

Vibrations of the tympanic membrane are conducted along the ossicular chain to the oval window. The chain (2 to 6 mm in length) acts much like a single unit when transmitting sounds above about 800 Hz. It is the action of these ossicles that provides the energy transformation for which the middle ear is designed.

The Middle-ear Impedance Matcher

Fish have an organ called the *lateral line* that is similar in some ways to an unrolled version of the cochlea of the inner ear of humans. This fluid-containing structure runs along the sides of the fish's body. The water in which the fish swims conducts waves that distort the membranes covering the lateral lines, setting the fluids within them into motion. Distortion of the membranes causes wave motion within the fluids of the lateral line. This leads to perception in the fish's brain, the nature of which is not understood. Fish have no need for an impedance matcher.

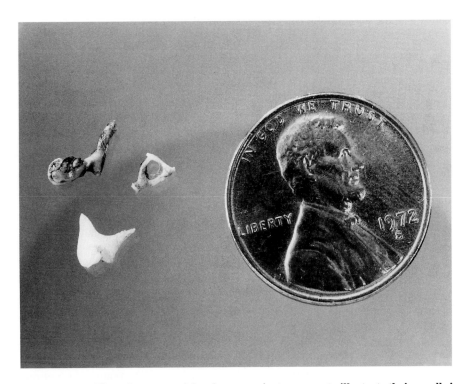

FIGURE 10.5 Three human ossicles shown against a penny to illustrate their small size.

The average adult tympanic membrane is 85 to 90 mm², but the effective vibrating area is only about 55 mm². This vibrating area is seventeen times that of the oval window. Therefore, the sound pressure collected over the entire area of the tympanic membrane is concentrated on the oval window. This concentration increases the sound pressure in the same way that a hose increases water pressure when a thumb or a finger is placed over the opening. What results is not a greater volume of water but greater pressure. The drawing in Figure 10.6 illustrates this action. Despite the exquisite engineering of the middle ear, all sound pressure delivered to the tympanic membrane is not made available to the inner ear; the middle-ear mechanism is not 100 percent efficient as an impedance-matching device .

The mass of the ossicular chain (malleus = 25 mg, incus = 25 mg, stapes = 2.5 mg) is poised to take advantage of the physical laws of leverage. Figure 10.7 illustrates this simple principle. Through leverage, the force received at the footplate of the stapes is greater than that applied at the malleus. In this way the ratio of tympanic membrane displacement to oval window displacement is increased by about 1.3:1. The ossicular chain actually rocks back and forth on an imaginary axis, and the action of the stapes in the oval window is not that of a piston but, rather, like a pivot.

The combined effects of increased pressure and the lever action of the malleus result in a pressure increase at the oval window twenty-three times what it would be if airborne sound impinged on it directly. This value is equivalent to approximately 30 dB, remarkably close to the 28 dB loss that would be caused by the air-to-fluid impedance mismatch without the ossicular chain. The fact that the tympanic membrane is conical, rather than flat, assists slightly in the process of impedance matching by increasing the force and decreasing the velocity, because the handle of the malleus does not move with the same amplitude as the tympanic membrane.

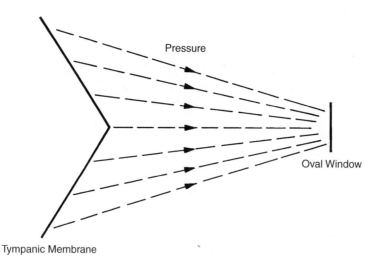

FIGURE 10.6 Sound pressure collected over the surface area of the tympanic membrane is concentrated on the (smaller) surface area of the oval window, thus increasing the pressure.

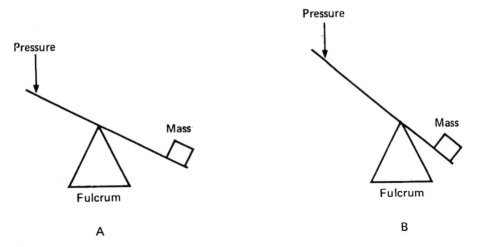

FIGURE 10.7 Demonstration of the advantage of lever action. Note that the advantage is increased in (B) when the fulcrum is moved closer to the mass to be lifted.

Nonauditory Structures in the Middle Ear

The middle ear contains several structures that are unrelated to hearing. The **fallopian canal,** containing the **facial (VIIth cranial) nerve,** passes through the middle ear as a protrusion on its medial wall. The fallopian canal is a bony channel covered with mucous membrane. The facial nerve runs beside the auditory (VIIIth cranial) nerve as the two travel to the brainstem, about which more is said in Chapter 12.

The **chorda tympani nerve** is a branch of the facial nerve that passes through the middle-ear space. This nerve carries information about the sensation of taste from the anterior two-thirds of one side of the tongue. Unfortunately, the chorda tympani frequently acts as an obstruction during middle-ear surgery. Sometimes the nerve is accidentally or intentionally sacrificed to increase visibility of the operative field. Taste changes caused by surgical severance of the chorda tympani nerve frequently disappear after several months.

The Middle-ear Muscles

Two muscles, the primary functions of which continue to be debated, are active in each middle ear. It has been thought that contractions of these muscles may serve a protective function for the inner ear by stiffening the ossicular chain and attenuating loud, and therefore potentially damaging sounds, that enter it. It is known, however, that the latency of the reflex is too long to protect the inner ear from impulsive sounds such as gunshots. Contraction of these muscles may additionally serve to decrease the loudness of sounds generated within the head, for example, by chewing or speaking.

The **stapedius muscle** (length 7 mm, cross section 5 mm^2) originates in the posterior (mastoid) wall of the middle ear. The stapedius tendon emerges through a tiny hole in a pyramidal eminence, but the muscle itself is in a canal beside the facial canal. The tendon attaches to the posterior portion of the neck of the stapes. When the stapedius muscle is contracted, the stapes moves to the side and tenses the membrane in the oval window, reducing the amplitude of vibration. It is possible that contraction of the stapedius muscle may help to improve word recognition in noise by attenuating the low-frequency components of the noise. The stapedius muscle is innervated by a branch of the facial (VIIth cranial) nerve. In addition to its function of attaching the stapedius muscle to the stapes, the stapedius tendon also supplies blood to the lenticular process of the incus.

The **tensor tympani muscle** (length 25 mm, cross section 5 mm^2) is also encased in a small bony cavity. The tendon from this muscle inserts into the manubrium of the malleus and, upon contraction, moves the malleus in such a way that the tympanic membrane becomes tense. The innervation of the tensor tympani is from the **trigeminal** (Vth cranial) **nerve.**

Both the stapedius and tensor tympani muscles respond reflexively and bilaterally, but in humans only the stapedius is thought to respond to sound. For example, introduction of a loud sound into the right ear will cause both stapedius muscles to contract. The tensor tympani can be caused to contract by a jet of air in the external auditory canal or the eye and by changes in temperature or touch in the external auditory canal.

Development of the Middle Ear

During embryonic or fetal development, specific anatomical areas form or differentiate. Like the outer ear, the middle ear and eustachian tube form from the pharyngeal arch system, limited to the first two arches. As in the outer ear and all areas of the body, developmental milestones are somewhat variant and times should be viewed as approximate.

Both the middle-ear space and the eustachian tube form the first pharyngeal pouch, which is lined with entoderm. During gestation, the middle-ear space is filled with mesenchyme as the ossicles are developing. The ciliated epithelium that lines these spaces also arises from the entoderm. The oval window is formed by about the forty-seventh gestational day.

The ossicles first form as cartilage of the first and second pharyngeal arches. The superior portions of the incus and malleus, which form the incudomalleal joint, come from the first arch. The lower parts of the incus and malleus, and the superstructure of the stapes, come from the second arch. The base of the stapes forms from the otic capsule.

At about 29 to 32 days tissue forms that will become the malleus and incus. By the twelfth fetal week the ossicles differentiate and are fully formed by the sixteenth week as cartilaginous structures that have begun to ossify. Almost total ossification of the malleus and incus has taken place by the twenty-first week. The twenty-fourth week shows rapid ossification of the incus and stapes. The middle-ear muscles derive from mesenchyme, the tensor tympani from the first arch, and the stapedius from the second arch.

Hearing Loss and the Middle Ear

Abnormalities of the middle ear produce conductive hearing losses. The air-conduction level drops in direct relationship with the amount of attenuation produced by the disorder. Theoretically, bone conduction should be unchanged from normal unless the inner ear becomes involved; however, our knowledge of middle-ear anatomy and physiology should make our understanding of the effects of inertial bone conduction even clearer. Conductive hearing losses produced by middle-ear disorders may show alteration in the bone-conduction thresholds even without sensorineural involvement. The amount of sensorineural impairment in mixed hearing losses may be exaggerated by artifacts of bone conduction. These facts were demonstrated in a report by Orchik, Schumaier, Shea, and Xianxi (1995), where, in one case, the bone-conduction thresholds were significantly altered by a displacement of a prosthetic device used in middle-ear surgery.

Disorders of the Middle Ear and Their Treatments

Suppurative Otitis Media

One of the most common disorders of the middle ear causing conductive hearing loss is infection of the middle-ear space, or **otitis media.** Otitis media is any infection of the mucous-membrane lining of the middle-ear cleft. It is seen in nearly 70 percent of children born in the United States before they are two years old, with more than half of these children experiencing further episodes. The common cold is the only illness seen more frequently in children (Brooks, 1994).

Factors that predispose an individual to otitis media include poorly functioning eustachian tubes, **barotrauma** (sudden changes in air pressure, as when flying or diving), abnormalities in the action of the cilia of the mucous membranes, anatomical deformities of the middle ear and eustachian tube, age, race, socioeconomic factors, and the integrity of the individual's immune system. This last fact suggests that the growing epidemic of acquired immune deficiency syndrome (AIDS) will probably increase the incidence of otitis media. External factors associated with otitis media include exposure to cigarette smoke or other fumes. A link has been found between otitis media and Haemophilus influenza in the nasal passages of children.

Although otitis media is primarily a disease of childhood, it can occur at any age. There are clear seasonal effects (otitis media is most common in the winter months), but it is less clear why the disease is more common in males than in females. Also difficult to explain is the difference in incidence among racial groups; otitis media is most common in Eskimos and Native Americans, less common in whites, and least common in blacks (Giebink, 1984). The interrelationships between socioeconomic and anatomical (genetic) differences are unclear.

As a rule, organisms gain access to the middle ear through the eustachian tube from the nasopharynx. They travel as a subepithelial extension of a sinusitis or pharyngitis, spreading the infection up through the tube. Often the infection is literally blown through the lumen of the tube by a stifled sneeze or by blowing the nose too hard. In general, it is probably a good idea not to teach small children to blow their noses at all. They should also be encouraged to minimize pressure through the eustachian tube when sneezing by keeping their mouths open. Infection may also enter the middle ear through the external auditory canal if there is a perforation in the tympanic membrane. Bloodborne infection from another site in the body may occur, but this source of middle-ear infection is unusual.

As stated earlier, infection usually begins at the orifice of the eustachian tube and spreads throughout the middle-ear cavity. When the tube is infected it becomes swollen, interfering with its middle-ear pressure-equalization function. Also, when the tubal lining becomes swollen, the cleansing action of the cilia is compromised, and the infection is spread to adjacent tissues. A major contributing cause of otitis media, especially in children, is exposure to tobacco smoke. One study shows that in households in which more than three packages of cigarettes are smoked in a day, the risk to children of otitis media and other respiratory infections is four times more than it would be without such exposure (Kraemer, Richardson, Weiss, Furukawa, Shapiro, Pierson, & Bierman, 1983).

Patients often report that as little as several hours may elapse between the appearance of initial symptoms and a full-blown infection in their children. In such rapidly progressing cases, it is probable that fluids that functioned as a culture medium for pus-producing (**purulent**) organisms had previously been deposited in the middle ear, perhaps from an earlier bacterial or viral infection. The rate of spread is also related to the virulence of the organisms.

In cases of otitis media, medical treatment is imperative. Proper diagnosis of the several usual stages can result in appropriate therapy. In the initial stage of eustachian tube swelling, causing occlusion of the tube, negative middle-ear pressure may be set up. The tympanic membrane may appear to be retracted (sucked in). Often audiometric examination reveals normal hearing on all tests. The tympanometric function may appear as a Type C, suggesting that the pressure within the middle ear is lower than that of the external auditory canal.

Before the actual accumulation of pus in the middle ear, the tympanic membrane and middle-ear mucosa may become very vascular. This inflammation produces the so-called "red ear" described by many physicians. If the condition is allowed to continue beyond this stage, suppuration (production of pus) may result. Enzymes are usually produced by bacterial infections, some of which have a dissolving effect on middle-ear structures.

In **suppurative** otitis media, the mucosa becomes filled with excessive amounts of blood, the superficial cells break down, and pus accumulates. Patients complain of pain in the ear, their pulse rates and body temperatures become elevated, and they are visibly ill. If pressure from the pus goes up, there will be compression of the small veins and capillaries in the middle ear, resulting in **necrosis** (death) of the mucosa, submucosa, and tympanic membrane. If the condition continues even further, the tympanic membrane may eventually rupture. Pus that cannot find its way out of the middle ear may invade the mastoid. The resulting **mastoiditis** causes a breakdown of the walls separating the air cells. Untreated mastoiditis can result in meningitis and sometimes death.

The general category of suppurative otitis media is frequently dichotomized by the terms **chronic** and **acute.** As a rule, the chronic form implies a condition of long standing. Symptoms of acute otitis media generally develop rapidly and include swelling, redness, and bleeding. Bleeding in the middle ear may also be caused by barotrauma, when there is a sudden pressure change, causing the blood vessels in the lining of the middle ear to rupture. Bleeding in the middle ear from any cause is called **hemotympanum.**

Audiometric Findings in Suppurative Otitis Media   Otitis media results in the typical audiogram of the conductive hearing loss (Figure 10.8). Generally, the amount of hearing loss is directly related to the accumulation of fluid in the middle ear. The audiometric contour is usually rather flat, showing approximately equal amounts of hearing loss across frequencies. Word-recognition scores are generally excellent, although proper masking must often be instituted to ensure against cross-hearing. Bone-conduction results are usually normal.

Measurements of static compliance show lower than normal values. The tympanometric function is a Type B (Figure 10.9), suggesting the presence of fluid behind the tympanic membrane. Acoustic reflexes cannot be elicited in either ear because the intensity of each reflex activating stimulus, even at maximum levels of the audiometer, is below the reflex threshold. Additionally,

SPEECH AND HEARING CENTER
The University of Texas at Austin 78712
AUDIOMETRIC EXAMINATION

NAME: Last - First - Middle	SEX	AGE	DATE	EXAMINER	RELIABILITY	AUDIOMETER

AIR CONDUCTION

MASKING TYPE	RIGHT									LEFT								
	250	500	1000	1500	2000	3000	4000	6000	8000	250	500	1000	1500	2000	3000	4000	6000	8000
NB	55	60	55/50	55	55	65	60	70	80	60	60	55/55	60	65	60	65	75	NR
	55	60				65				60	60	55	60	65	60	65	75	
EM Level in Opp. Ear	60	60				60				55	60	55	55	55	65	60	70	

BONE CONDUCTION

MASKING TYPE	RIGHT						FOREHEAD						LEFT					
	250	500	1000	2000	3000	4000	250	500	1000	2000	3000	4000	250	500	1000	2000	3000	4000
NB	10	15	15	20	20	25	5	10	15	20	20	25	5	10	15	20	20	25
EM Level in Opp. Ear	75	75	55	65	60	65							55	60	55	55	65	60

	2 Frequency	3 Frequency	WEBER							2 Frequency	3 Frequency
Pure Tone Average	53	55	M	M	M	M	M	M	Pure Tone Average	58	60

SPEECH AUDIOMETRY

MASKING TYPE	RIGHT				LEFT			
	SRT 1	SRT 2	Recognition 1	Recognition 2	SRT 1	SRT 2	Recognition 1	Recognition 2
WB	55	55	1A List 30 SL 100 %	List SL %	55	55	2A List 30 SL 96 %	List SL %
EM Level in Opp. Ear		55	90			55	85	

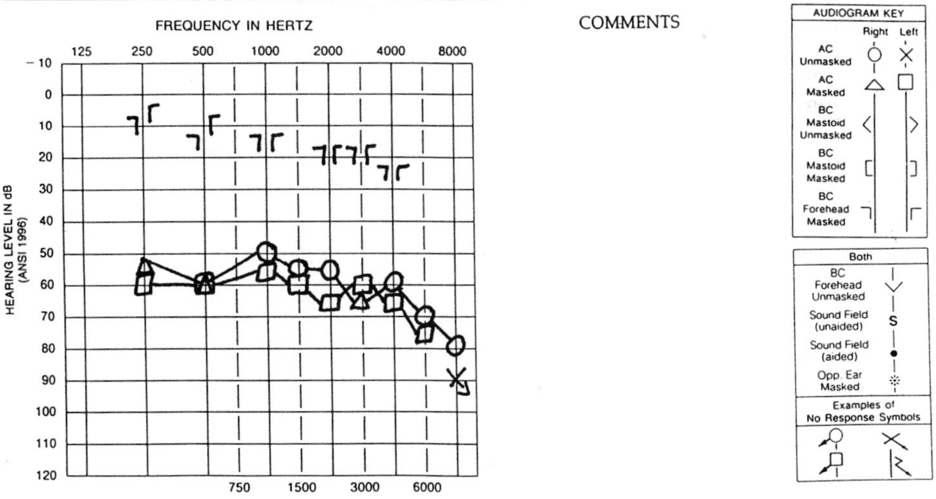

FREQUENCY IN HERTZ

COMMENTS

AUDIOGRAM KEY

FIGURE 10.8 Audiogram illustrating a moderate conductive hearing loss in both ears. The contour of the audiogram is relatively flat, and fairly typical of otitis media. Word-recognition scores are excellent. Note that masking is used for all tests. Because no cross-hearing was shown, interaural attenuation must exceed 50 dB for this case.

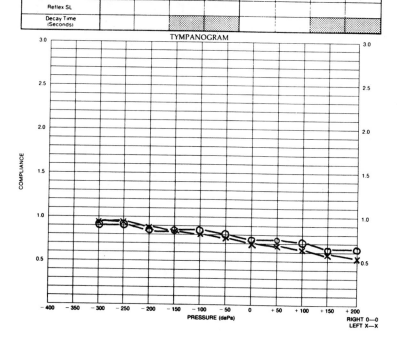

SPEECH AND HEARING CENTER
The University of Texas at Austin 78712
IMMITTANCE

NAME: Last - First - Middle		SEX	AGE	DATE	EXAMINER	INSTRUMENT

PRESSURE/COMPLIANCE FUNCTION

	-400	-350	-300	-250	-200	-150	-100	-50	0	+50	+100	+150	+200
Right			.90	.90	.85	.85	.85	.80	.74	.72	.70	.61	.61
Left			.91	.91	.89	.84	.80	.76	.70	.68	.62	.58	.53

STATIC COMPLIANCE $C_x = C_2 - C_1$

RIGHT					LEFT				
.61	c_1	.80	c_2	.19	c_x	.53	c_1	.70	c_2	.17	c_x

ACOUSTIC REFLEXES

Frequency (Hz)	RIGHT				LEFT			
	500	1000	2000	4000	500	1000	2000	4000
Ipsilateral (Probe same)		NR	NR			NR	NR	
Contralateral (Probe opposite)	NR	NR	NR	NR	NR	NR	NR	NR
Audiometric Threshold								
Reflex SL								
Decay Time (Seconds)								

TYMPANOGRAM

RIGHT 0—0
LEFT X—X

PRESSURE (daPa)

FIGURE 10.9   **Typical results on immittance tests performed on a patient with bilateral otitis media or serous effusion (see Figure 10.8). Note that the tympanogram is Type B, the static compliance is low, and acoustic reflexes are absent in both ears.**

abnormalities of the middle ear cause increased impedance of the ossicular chain, which resists movement in response to contraction of the stapedius muscle. Figures 10.10 and 10.11 show that the latencies of all the waves resulting from ABR testing are increased at all sensation levels. No otoacoustic emissions can be evoked. If measured, SISI scores would be expected to be low, and there would be little or no tone decay (Figure 10.12).

Many or all of the audiometric results that point so clearly to otitis media as the cause of the conductive hearing loss shown in Figures 10.8 through 10.12 may be unattainable in the infant or small child. However, with a minimal amount of patient cooperation, measurements of static compliance and tympanometry can be obtained and may suggest the presence of middle-ear infection.

Cholesteatoma

Whenever skin is introduced to the middle-ear cleft, the result may be a pseudotumor called **cholesteatoma.** Cholesteatomas form as a sac, with onion-like concentric rings made up of keratin (a very insoluble protein), mixed with squamous (scaly) epithelium, and with fats such as cholesterol. In patients with perforated tympanic membranes, the skin may enter the middle ear through the perforations. This invasion produces a secondary acquired cholesteatoma. A primary acquired cholesteatoma may occur without a history of otitis media if the epithelium of the attic of the middle ear becomes modified. This alteration may occur if the pars flaccida of the tympanic membrane becomes sucked into the middle ear through negative pressure and then opens, revealing the skin from the outer portion of the tympanic membrane to the middle ear.

Cholesteatomas may also enter the middle ear in several other ways. In any case they may be extremely dangerous: They have been known to occupy the entire middle ear and even pass down through the opening of the eustachian tube into the nasopharynx or up into the brain cavity. They are highly erosive and may cause destruction of bone and other tissue.

Although antibiotics may arrest otitis media, and even mastoiditis, the best treatment for cholesteatoma is still surgery. The condition spreads rapidly, and the surgeon must be absolutely certain that all the cholesteatomatous material has been removed, for if even a small amount remains the entire condition may flare up again in a short period of time. Most ears with cholesteatomas are secondarily infected, and produce foul-smelling discharges that drain from the ears (**otorrhea**).

Facial Palsy

In some cases of chronic otitis media, the bony covering of the fallopian canal becomes eroded, exposing the facial nerve to the disease process. Damage to the facial nerve may result in a flaccid paralysis of one side of the face. Appropriate treatment often involves middle-ear surgery.

At times, unilateral facial paralysis results when no other clinically demonstrable disease is present. Although there are several theories about why the paralysis, called **Bell's palsy,**[2] occurs, the reason is probably related to the blood supply to the nerve or to viral infection. A diagnosis of Bell's palsy is made by ruling out any other causative lesion in a patient with a flaccid facial paralysis. Bell's palsy resolves spontaneously in the majority of cases.

[2]For Sir Charles Bell, Scottish physiologist, 1774–1842.

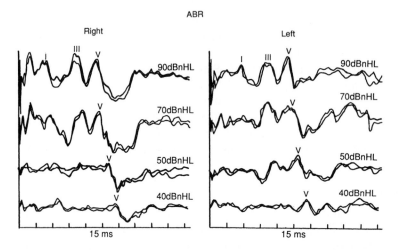

FIGURE 10.10   Results of auditory brainstem response testing on the patient with a bilateral conductive hearing loss, caused by otitis media (see Figure 10.8).

Antibiotic Treatment of Otitis Media

Bacterial infections, like those found in otitis media, survive by multiplication. Each bacterial cell forms a protective capsule around itself to ensure its survival. Some antibiotics kill the bacteria directly. Other antibiotics serve to inhibit the formation of the protective covering, thereby limiting the growth within the bacterial colony and allowing the white blood cells to surround and carry off the bacteria. When a substantial pocket of infection exists, as in suppurative otitis media, the mass of bacteria, by virtue of numbers alone, may resist a complete bacteria-killing action. Different drugs are specific to different organisms, and unless the appropriate drug is prescribed, the action may be less than useful. Modern laboratory facilities allow for culturing the organism causing the infection, so that the physician may take advantage of the specificity of a given antibiotic.

When the middle ear is filled with pus, produced by the body to carry cells to the area to ingest the bacteria, frequently the best procedure is to remove the pus, rather than to rely completely on the effects of antibiotics. As long as the tympanic membrane remains intact, drops in the external ear canal can have no therapeutic effect in cases of otitis media because the drops cannot reach the infection.

Dormant Otitis Media

The introduction of antibiotics at the close of World War II drastically altered the treatment of otitis media. Although antibiotics have dramatically decreased the number of serious effects of otitis media, they have also had some undesirable side effects. Unless the proper type and dosage of antibiotics are used, the disease may go not to resolution but to a state of quiescence. Because the overt symptoms may disappear, both the physician and patient may assume a complete cure. Several weeks later the patient may experience what seems like a whole new attack of otitis media, which is

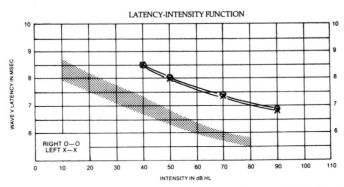

SPEECH AND HEARING CENTER
The University of Texas at Austin 78712

AUDITORY BRAINSTEM RESPONSE
(Adult Form)

NAME: Last - First - Middle	SEX	AGE	DATE	EXAMINER	RELIABILITY	INSTRUMENT

LATENCY-INTENSITY FUNCTION

RIGHT O—O
LEFT X—X

SHADED AREA REPRESENTS Normal Wave V Range for patients older than 16 mos. for 30 clicks per second.

	STIMULUS			WAVE LATENCY IN MSEC						
EAR	RATE	dB HL	FILTER	I	II	III	IV	V	VI	VII
R	33.1	90	150 - 1500	2.7		5.1		6.85		
L	33.1	90	150 - 1500	2.8		5.0		6.8		

SUMMARY OF RESULTS

INTERWAVE INTERVALS . . . . R __4.15__ L __4.0__
AMPLITUDE RATIO (V SAME OR > I) . . . . R __NORMAL__ L __NORMAL__
LATENCY CHANGE WITH INCREASED CLICK RATE . . . . R _____ L _____
INTERAURAL DIFFERENCES . . . . _____

ESTIMATED AIR CONDUCTION THRESHOLD IN dBHL (1-2 kHz) . . . . R __≤ 40__ L __≤ 40__
ESTIMATED BONE CONDUCTION THRESHOLD IN dB HL . . . . R _____ L _____

COMMENTS

FIGURE 10.11   Latency-intensity functions for wave V derived from the auditory brainstem response tracings shown in Figure 10.10 on the patient with a bilateral conductive hearing loss (see Figure 10.8). The latencies of all waves are increased at all levels tested.

in reality an exacerbation of the same condition experienced earlier, but allowed to lie dormant. Many patients discontinue their own antibiotic treatments when their symptoms abate, leaving some of the hardier bacteria alive. Then, when the condition flares up again, it is the result of a stronger strain, less susceptible to medication. Antibiotics, therefore, may lead to a false sense of security in the treatment of otitis media and mastoiditis.

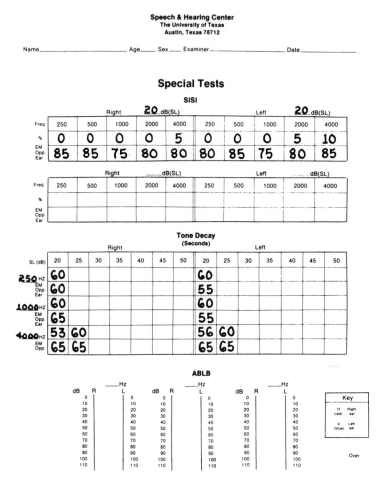

Speech & Hearing Center
The University of Texas
Austin, Texas 78712

Name_____ Age_____ Sex____ Examiner_____ Date _____

Special Tests

SISI

	Right				20 dB(SL)	Left			20 dB(SL)	
Freq	250	500	1000	2000	4000	250	500	1000	2000	4000
%	0	0	0	0	5	0	0	0	5	10
EM Opp Ear	85	85	75	80	80	80	85	75	80	85

	Right				____ dB(SL)	Left			____ dB(SL)	
Freq	250	500	1000	2000	4000	250	500	1000	2000	4000
%										
EM Opp Ear										

Tone Decay
(Seconds)

	Right							Left					
SL (dB)	20	25	30	35	40	45	50	20	25	30	35	40	45	50
250 HZ	60							60						
EM Opp Ear	60							55						
1000 HZ	60							60						
EM Opp Ear	65							55						
4000 HZ	53	60						56	60					
EM Opp.	65	65						65	65					

ABLB

	____ Hz			____ Hz			____ Hz	
dB	R	L	dB	R	L	dB	R	L
0		0	0		0	0		0
10		10	10		10	10		10
20		20	20		20	20		20
30		30	30		30	30		30
40		40	40		40	40		40
50		50	50		50	50		50
60		60	60		60	60		60
70		70	70		70	70		70
80		80	80		80	80		80
90		90	90		90	90		90
100		100	100		100	100		100
110		110	110		110	110		110

Key

O Right (red) ear

x Left (blue) ear

Over

FIGURE 10.12   Special site-of-lesion test results for the patient with a bilateral conductive hearing loss shown in Figure 10.8. Note the low SISI scores and absence of tone decay.

Surgical Treatment for Otitis Media

In the days predating antibiotics, therapy for otitis media was primarily surgical. Today surgery is still required in many cases. The primary purpose of surgery for patients with infection or destruction in the middle ear is to eliminate disease. Reconstructing a damaged hearing apparatus is an important, but secondary goal.

Myringotomy

When disease-laden fluids are present in the middle ear and must be removed, the surgical procedure is called **myringotomy.** Myringotomy is frequently performed as a simple office operation, but at times, especially with some small children, it requires brief hospitalization. An incision is made with a special knife, generally in the inferior-posterior quadrant of the tympanic membrane. The fluids are removed by a suction tip placed through the incision. If myringotomy is performed on small children while they are awake, they must be immobilized sufficiently so that any sudden movement does not redirect the action of the knife, which could possibly cause damage to the middle ear.

Mastoidectomy

Even with modern drug therapy, often the only treatment for mastoiditis is **mastoidectomy,** usually done under general anesthesia. In earlier days the incision was made behind the auricle and the bone in the mastoid process was scraped until all the infection was removed. This technique frequently resulted in a large concavity behind the ear. In addition, the surgically created mastoid bowl required cleaning for the rest of the patient's life, and was in itself a breeding ground for infection.

The modern surgical approach to mastoidectomy is to avoid creating a mastoid cavity whenever possible. When a mastoid cavity does exist, it can often be obliterated by using portions of the temporalis muscle and/or bone chips taken from the patient. The obliteration of the mastoid cavity may be done at the time of initial surgery, or it may be staged at a later date, depending on the disease process found in the mastoid. This procedure has been found to be very gratifying in recent years.

Tympanoplasty

Surgical reconstruction of the middle-ear auditory apparatus is called **tympanoplasty.** The simplest form of tympanoplasty is myringoplasty, repair of the tympanic membrane described in Chapter 9. Many surgical approaches have attempted to substitute metal or plastic prosthetic devices for damaged or missing ossicles. These attempts have met with limited success because the body tends to reject foreign materials. In recent years tympanoplasties have been performed by attaching existing middle-ear structures together. This attachment may mean the loss of the function of one or more ossicles. The surgeon may place the tympanic membrane directly on the head of the stapes to restore a remnant of ossicular chain function.

Hearing improvement following tympanoplasty varies considerably, depending on the preoperative condition of the middle ear and, to a great extent, on the function of the eustachian tube. If the tube fails to function properly, and the middle ear is not normally pressurized, the surgical procedure is almost certainly doomed to failure.

Sometimes, though rarely, a patient's hearing may be poorer following surgery. The surgeon may have found, for example, that the long process of the incus is necrosed, but instead of there being a hiatus between the main portion of the incus and the stapes, the gap has been closed by a bit of cholesteatoma. Removal of the cholesteatoma is necessary, even though the result is interruption of the ossicular chain and increased hearing loss. Patients to whom this has happened may be very difficult to console.

Audiograms of patients with interrupted ossicular chains show all the expected findings consistent with conductive hearing loss. The compliance of the tympanic membrane in such cases is unusually high because it has been decoupled from the stapes. The expected pressure-compliance function is a Type A_D (Figure 10.13).

Although static-compliance values may not in themselves determine the presence of a conductive problem in the middle ear, comparison of c_X in the right and left ears of the same patient may

SPEECH AND HEARING CENTER
The University of Texas at Austin 78712

IMMITTANCE

NAME: Last - First - Middle			SEX	AGE	DATE	EXAMINER		INSTRUMENT	

PRESSURE/COMPLIANCE FUNCTION

	– 400	– 350	– 300	– 250	– 200	– 150	– 100	– 50	0	+ 50	+ 100	+ 150	+ 200
Right					.52	.77	1.01	1.90	2.40	1.51	.99	.70	.48
Left					.42	.49	.52	.60	.82	.61	.53	.49	.41

STATIC COMPLIANCE

$$C_x = C_2 - C_1$$

RIGHT						LEFT					
.48	C_1	2.40	C_2	1.92	C_x	.41	C_1	.82	C_2	.41	C_x

ACOUSTIC REFLEXES

	RIGHT				LEFT			
Frequency (Hz)	500	1000	2000	4000	500	1000	2000	4000
Ipsilateral (Probe same)		NR	NR			95	85	
Contralateral (Probe opposite)	NR	NR	NR	NR	NR	NR	NR	NR
Audiometric Threshold								
Reflex SL								
Decay Time (Seconds)								

TYMPANOGRAM

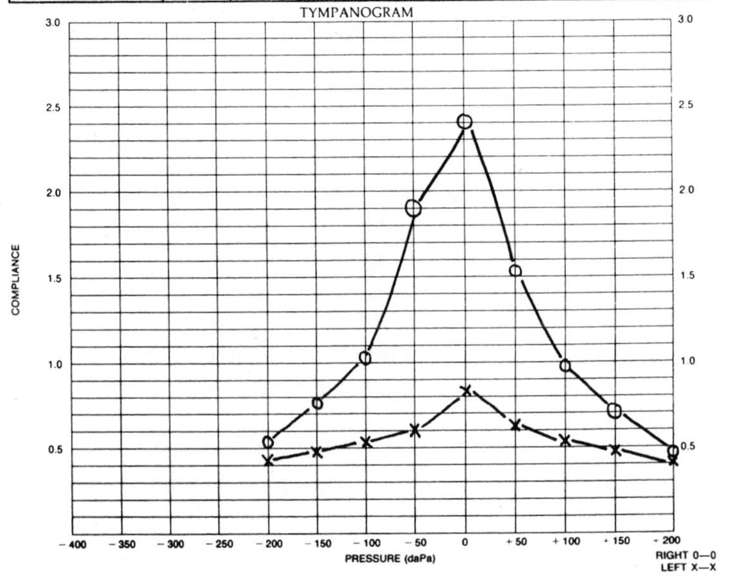

RIGHT 0—0
LEFT X—X

COMPLIANCE

PRESSURE (daPa)

FIGURE 10.13 Typical results on immittance tests performed on a patient with right ossicular chain discontinuity. Note that the tympanogram is Type A_D (normal middle-ear pressure but extremely compliant tympanic membrane), the static compliance is high, and reflex thresholds are absent in both ears. The left ear is normal in this case.

be extremely useful. De Jonge and Valente (1979) suggest that when the static-compliance difference between ears exceeds 0.22 cm³, a conductive problem may exist in one ear, even if both values fall within the normal range.

Anderson and Barr (1971) reported on high-frequency conductive hearing losses that may result from **subluxations** (partial dislocations) in the ossicular chain. When a portion of one of the ossicles is replaced by soft connective tissue, the elasticity of this connection, acting as an insulator against vibrations, transmits low frequencies more easily than high frequencies. Hearing losses caused by this condition are usually mild and result in an elevated acoustic reflex threshold.

Negative Middle-ear Pressure

Eustachian tube function may fail for a number of reasons. Two of the most common causes are edema of the eustachian tube secondary to infection or to allergy and blockage of the orifice of the eustachian tube by hypertrophied (overgrown) adenoids. Either infection or allergy may affect the adenoids, which further adds to the problem. Structural abnormalities of the mechanism responsible for opening the tube are sometimes also present.

Any condition that interferes with the eustachian tube's function of equating air pressure between the middle ear and outer ear may cause the air trapped within the middle ear to become absorbed by the tissues that line it, resulting in a drop in pressure. When this absorption occurs, the greater pressure in the external auditory canal causes the tympanic membrane to be retracted (Figure 10.14). The retraction from eustachian-tube dysfunction (ETD) interferes with the normal vibration of the tympanic membrane and may or may not produce a slight conductive hearing loss.

Another method has been developed to use the immittance meter to test eustachian tube function, if the eardrum membrane is intact, by using a pressure swallow technique (Williams, 1975). The patient is asked to swallow normally, after which a tympanogram is run. Then +400 daPa is applied to the membrane, and the patient is asked to swallow four times; a second tympanogram is then run on the same graph. Pressure is returned to 0 daPa and the patient swallows again to equalize middle-ear pressure. Finally, the patient is asked to swallow four times with –400 daPa in the external auditory canal, and a third tympanogram is run. If the eustachian tube is normal, the peaks

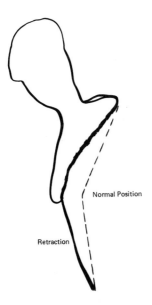

Normal Position

Retraction

FIGURE 10.14   Retracted tympanic membrane caused by negative middle-ear pressure.

of the three tympanograms will differ by at least 15 daPa. Differences smaller than this suggest dysfunction because the tube cannot equalize the middle-ear pressure.

When a retracted tympanic membrane is diagnosed, and no infectious fluids are present in the nose, the otologist may elect to pressurize the middle ear through a process called **politzerization.**[3] One nostril is held closed while an olive tip, connected to a tube or nebulizer, is held tightly in the other nostril. The patient elevates the soft palate by saying "k-k-k" and then swallows; the otologist, meanwhile, observes the movement of the tympanic membrane during this process. In this fashion, tympanic membrane perforation or eustachian tube failure may be diagnosed.

The patient may autoinflate the eustachian tube by increased pressure on forced expiration with the nostrils held shut, a maneuver called **Valsalva,**[4] which must be performed by divers as they descend or surface. Patients are often taught the Valsalva maneuver following middle-ear surgery. The **Toynbee maneuver**[5] accomplishes eustachian tube opening when the patient closes the jaw, holds the nose, and swallows.

Figure 10.15 illustrates a mild conductive hearing loss in the left ear. The bone-conduction results are essentially normal, as are word-recognition scores. Results on all site-of-lesion tests would be expected to suggest conductive hearing loss. Acoustic immittance measurements show normal compliance in both ears, with a Type C tympanometric function in the left ear typical of negative middle-ear pressure (Figure 10.16). All of these findings are produced by the partial vacuum set up within the left middle-ear space.

Patulous Eustachian Tube (PET)

There are some individuals in whom the eustachian tube is chronically patent (open), which often results in the sensation of **autophony,** the head-in-a-barrel feeling. As a result, their own voices are perceived as loud. Other annoying effects of patulous eustachian tube include the sound of breathing and noises during chewing as the sound travels up the tube. Causes ascribed to this condition include the hormonal changes brought on by pregnancy or the use of some birth control pills, sudden changes in body weight, the use of decongestant medications, temporomandibular joint syndrome, and stress (O'Conner & Shea, 1981).

The problem of patulous eustachian tubes is more widespread than many people realize, and the incidence may go as high as 30 percent of people with otherwise normal ears (Kumazawa, 1985). Ten percent of a group of women studied had patulous eustachian tubes during pregnancy (Plate, Johnsen, Pederson, & Thompsen, 1979). Misdiagnosis is common because patients' complaints often make the condition sound like serous effusion or blocked eustachian tube, resulting in completely inappropriate treatment.

If the patient suffers from a chronically patent eustachian tube and exhibits a Type A tympanogram, a simple test can verify the problem. Tympanic membrane compliance is observed during nasal breathing, oral breathing, and momentary cessation of breathing. If the tube is open, the compliance will increase during inhalation and decrease during exhalation. Interruption in breathing stops the changes in compliance. Henry and DiBartolomeo (1993) found tympanometry to be a useful tool in the diagnosis of patulous eustachian tube.

[3]For Adam Politzer, Hungarian otologist, 1835–1920.

[4]For Antonio Maria Valsalva, Italian anatomist, 1666–1723.

[5]For Joseph Toynbee, British otologist, 1815–1866.

SPEECH AND HEARING CENTER
The University of Texas at Austin 78712
AUDIOMETRIC EXAMINATION

NAME: Last - First - Middle	SEX	AGE	DATE	EXAMINER	RELIABILITY	AUDIOMETER

AIR CONDUCTION

MASKING TYPE	RIGHT									LEFT								
	250	500	1000	1500	2000	3000	4000	6000	8000	250	500	1000	1500	2000	3000	4000	6000	8000
	5	0	5/5	5	0	5	10	10	5	15	20	20/20	15	15	20	15	15	15
EM Level in Opp. Ear																		

BONE CONDUCTION

MASKING TYPE	RIGHT						FOREHEAD						LEFT					
	250	500	1000	2000	3000	4000	250	500	1000	2000	3000	4000	250	500	1000	2000	3000	4000
NB							0	5	0	0	0	5	5*	5*	5*	0*	0*	5*
EM Level in Opp. Ear																		

	2 Frequency	3 Frequency	WEBER							2 Frequency	3 Frequency
Pure Tone Average	0	2	∠	∠	∠	∠	∠	L	Pure Tone Average	20	18

SPEECH AUDIOMETRY

MASKING TYPE	RIGHT						LEFT				
	SRT 1	SRT 2	Recognition 1		Recognition 2		SRT 1	SRT 2	Recognition 1		Recognition 2
WB	0		1A List / SL 30	100 %	List / SL	%	15		2A List / SL 30	98 %	List / SL	%
EM Level in Opp. Ear									15		

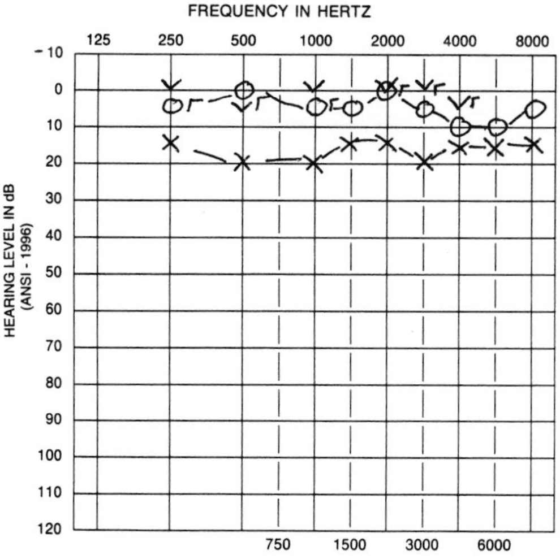

FREQUENCY IN HERTZ

COMMENTS

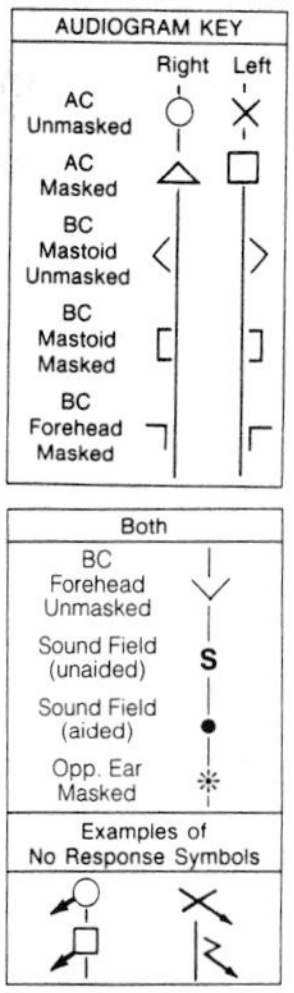

FIGURE 10.15 Audiogram illustrating a mild conductive hearing loss in the left ear produced by a retracted tympanic membrane. The right ear is normal. Masking was required for bone-conduction and word-recognition tests for the left ear. The Weber lateralizes to the left ear at all frequencies.

SPEECH AND HEARING CENTER
The University of Texas at Austin 78712
IMMITTANCE

NAME: Last - First - Middle		SEX	AGE	DATE	EXAMINER	INSTRUMENT

PRESSURE/COMPLIANCE FUNCTION

	−400	−350	−300	−250	−200	−150	−100	−50	0	+50	+100	+150	+200
Right						.65	.71	.77	.80	.99	.81	.70	.62	.55
Left				.75	.80	1.05	.87	.77	.72	.68	.64	.62	.60	.58

STATIC COMPLIANCE

$C_x = C_2 - C_1$

RIGHT					LEFT					
.55	c_1	.99	c_2	.44	c_x	.58	c_1	1.05	c_2	.47	c_x

ACOUSTIC REFLEXES

	RIGHT				LEFT			
Frequency (Hz)	500	1000	2000	4000	500	1000	2000	4000
Ipsilateral (Probe same)		90	85			NR	NR	
Contralateral (Probe opposite)	80	85	80	85	NR	NR	NR	NR
Audiometric Threshold	5	0	0	10				
Reflex SL	75	85	80	75				
Decay Time (Seconds)	10⁺	10⁺						

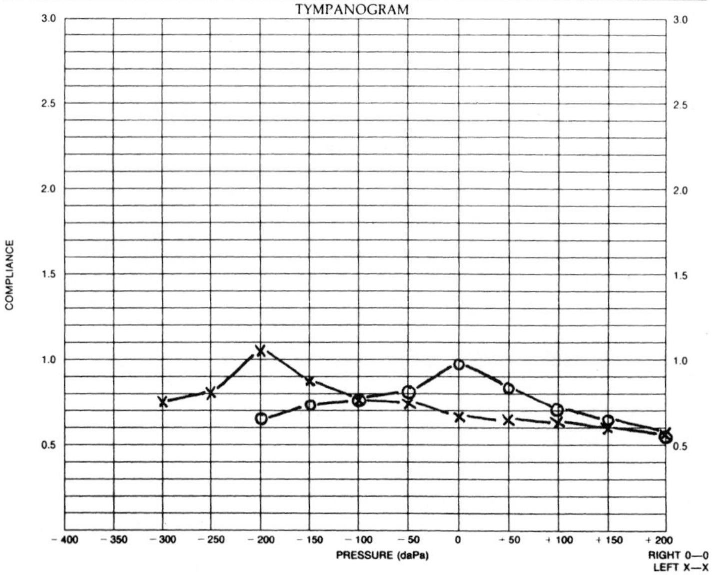

TYMPANOGRAM

FIGURE 10.16 Typical results on immittance tests performed on a patient with a normal right ear (Type A) and left negative middle-ear pressure (Type C). Static compliance is within the normal range for both ears. The right ipsilateral acoustic reflex threshold is normal and the left ipsilateral acoustic reflex is absent. When the reflex activating signal is introduced to the (normal) right ear (contralateral right stimulation), the acoustic reflex is shown here as present but may, in such cases, be absent. The hearing loss in the left ear causes the contralateral reflex to be absent when the RAS is presented to the left ear.

Serous Effusion of the Middle Ear

If a partial vacuum in the middle ear is allowed to continue, the fluids normally secreted by the mucous-membrane lining of the middle ear may literally be sucked into the middle-ear space, resulting in **serous effusion.** As the fluid level rises, otoscopic examination reveals the presence of a fluid line, called the **meniscus,** visible through the tympanic membrane. As the fluid pressure continues to increase, and the level rises, the tympanic membrane may return to its normal position when the meniscus rises above the superior margin of the tympanic membrane. At this stage the condition is sometimes difficult to diagnose visually.

When fluid fills the middle-ear space, a Type B tympanometric function results (Figure 10.9). This function occurs because no amount of air pressure delivered to the tympanic membrane from the pump of the immittance meter can match the pressure on the middle-ear side of the tympanic membrane. Because a serous accumulation in the middle ear affects the mass of the system, it is expected that the audiogram will initially show a greater loss for higher- than for lower-frequency sounds (Figure 10.17). It is likely that the slightly depressed bone-conduction thresholds in Figure 10.17 are artifacts produced by the fluid in the middle ear. Post-treatment audiograms would probably show a disappearance of the air-bone gap and some improvement in the bone-conduction thresholds.

Because serous effusion is often secondary to a poorly functioning eustachian tube, drug therapy, including decongestants or decongestant-antihistamine combinations, has long been used to restore normal middle-ear pressure and to help clear the tube of secretions. However, decongestants are now believed to be virtually useless for this purpose in infants and small children, whose eustachian tubes are less efficient than those of adults. As the middle ear may not be actively infected during serous effusion, antibiotics frequently are not indicated. However, some physicians prescribe antibiotics prophylactically because the fluid, though sterile, may serve as a culture base for bacterial infection. There is evidence that the three organisms most associated with otitis media in children have become resistant to the most commonly used antibiotics (Brooks, 1994), which, even if they destroy the organisms causing the condition, cannot eliminate the fluids that have formed in the middle-ear space.

If the fluid pressure continues to build within the middle ear, perforation of the tympanic membrane becomes a threat. If perforation appears imminent, the otologist may elect to perform a myringotomy to relieve the fluid pressure, suction out the remaining fluid, and place a plastic **pressure-equalizing (P.E.) tube** through the tympanic membrane. The tube allows for direct ventilation of the middle ear and functions as a sort of artificial eustachian tube to maintain normal middle-ear air pressure. The plastic tube provides a second vent to the middle ear, which acts much in the same way as the second hole punched in the top of a beer can. Air may enter the middle ear via the tube, allowing drainage down the eustachian tube. Figure 10.18 shows a myringotomy incision and a P.E. tube in position. A photograph of one kind of P.E. tube is shown in Figure 10.19. The tubes may remain in position from several weeks to several months, after which time some types extrude naturally and fall into the external auditory canal. In the interim, the eustachian tube problem should be appropriately handled through adenoidectomy, allergic desensitization, or whatever medical means seem to be indicated.

Some otologists have found that tubes remain in position longer if they are placed in the superior-anterior quadrant of the tympanic membrane because there is less migration of epithelium in this area than in the larger inferior quadrants. Positioning the tube in this superior area requires the use

SPEECH AND HEARING CENTER
The University of Texas at Austin 78712
AUDIOMETRIC EXAMINATION

NAME: Last - First - Middle	SEX	AGE	DATE	EXAMINER	RELIABILITY	AUDIOMETER

AIR CONDUCTION

MASKING TYPE	RIGHT									LEFT								
	250	500	1000	1500	2000	3000	4000	6000	8000	250	500	1000	1500	2000	3000	4000	6000	8000
NB	25	35	40/40	40	45	55	65 * 65	60	65	15	25	35/35	40	45	55	65 * 65	60	60
EM Level in Opp. Ear							70									70		

BONE CONDUCTION

MASKING TYPE	RIGHT						FOREHEAD						LEFT					
	250	500	1000	2000	3000	4000	250	500	1000	2000	3000	4000	250	500	1000	2000	3000	4000
NB	0*	5*	5*	15*	20*	25*	0	5	5	15	20	25	0*	5*	5*	15*	20*	25*
EM Level in Opp. Ear	15	25	35	45	55	65							25	35	40	40	45	60

	2 Frequency	3 Frequency	WEBER				2 Frequency	3 Frequency
Pure Tone Average	38	40				Pure Tone Average	30	35

SPEECH AUDIOMETRY

MASKING TYPE	RIGHT				LEFT			
	SRT 1	SRT 2	Recognition 1	Recognition 2	SRT 1	SRT 2	Recognition 1	Recognition 2
WB	40	40*	38 List/SL 30 96* %	List/SL %	40	40*	48 List/SL 30 98* %	List/SL %
EM Level in Opp. Ear		40	75			40	70	

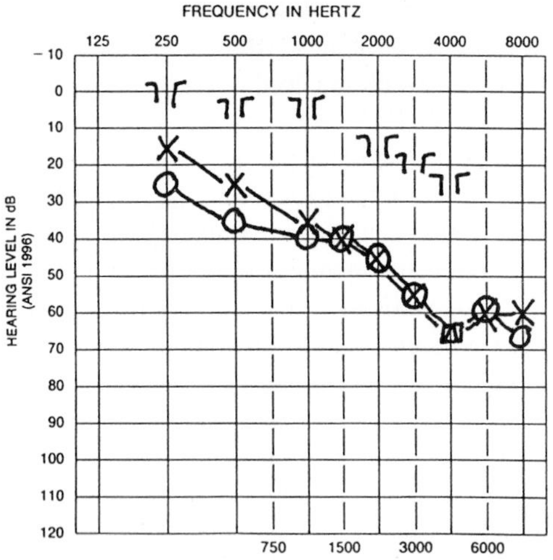

FREQUENCY IN HERTZ — HEARING LEVEL IN dB (ANSI 1996)

COMMENTS

AUDIOGRAM KEY

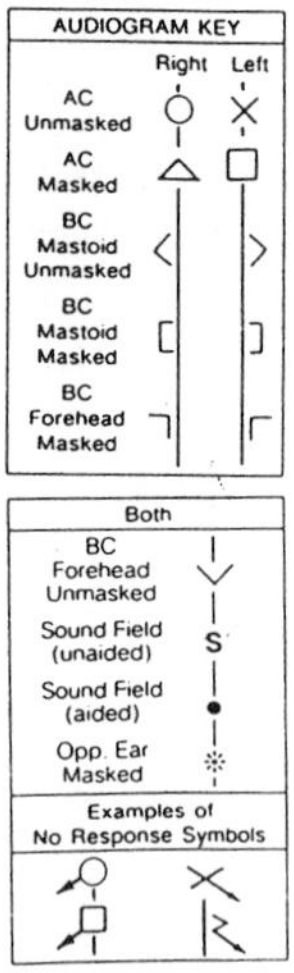

FIGURE 10.17 Audiogram illustrating conductive hearing loss in both ears produced by serous effusion. Note that masking was indicated for air-conduction tests in both ears only at 4000 Hz but that it was needed at all frequencies for bone conduction and word recognition. Word recognition is normal, the Weber does not lateralize, and the audiogram falls slightly in the higher frequencies.

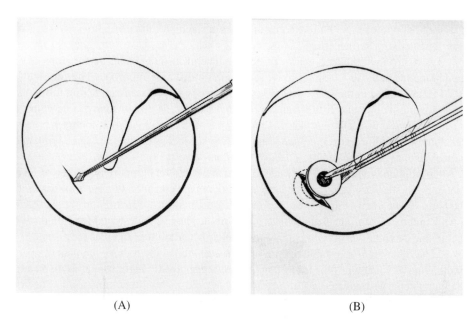

(A)   (B)

FIGURE 10.18   (A) A myringotomy incision. (B) A pressure-equalizing tube positioned through the tympanic membrane to allow for middle-ear ventilation. (Courtesy of James J. Pappas, M.D., Arkansas Otolaryngology Center)

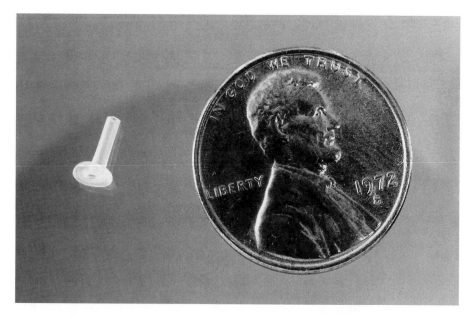

FIGURE 10.19   A pressure-equalizing tube for insertion through a myringotomy incision in a tympanic membrane to allow middle-ear drainage and ventilation. It is shown next to a penny to illustrate its small size.

of a surgical microscope. Failure to resolve the eustachian tube difficulty will frequently lead to a recurrent attack of serous effusion.

Acoustic immittance meters can be very useful in diagnosing perforations of the tympanic membrane, even those too small to be seen with an ordinary otoscope. The **physical-volume test (PVT)** can be used in the same way to test the patency of pressure-equalizing tubes placed through the tympanic membrane. If the clinician observes that c_1 is an unusually large value, in excess of 5 cm^3, he or she may assume that this measurement is of a cavity that includes both the outer-ear canal and the middle ear. Of course, many patients, especially children, have tympanic membrane perforations or open P.E. tubes and show less than 4 cm^3 as the c_1 value.

Immittance meters may be used to determine the very important matter of eustachian tube function. The tests are rapid and objective, and they take considerably less time than more elaborate methods. The patient is instructed to prevent eustachian tube opening during the test by not swallowing and by remaining as motionless as possible. The test is designed for patients with tympanic membrane perforations or with patent pressure-equalization tubes in place.

The first step is to establish a pressure of +200 daPa and to have the patient open the tube by swallowing or yawning. If the tube opens, pressure equalization will take place in the middle ear and the manometer will indicate a shift toward 0 daPa. Eustachian tube function has been qualified by Rock (1974) as "good," "fair," or "poor," depending on the degree to which the pressure is reduced by this maneuver. According to Gladstone (1984), the eustachian tube function test must be performed with positive air pressure in the external auditory canal because negative pressure could cause the tube to "lock" shut, rather than be forced open.

Mucous Otitis Media

At times, thick mucoid secretions, often blown through the eustachian tube, accumulate in the middle ear. If these secretions are allowed to remain, they may become dense and darken in color. This condition, which has been referred to as *glue ear,* produces the same kind of audiometric results as suppurative otitis media. After some period of time, however, the hearing loss is not reversible by simple myringotomy. Even after the inflammatory process has been removed, imperfect healing of the tissue may leave scars. The tissues forming these scars may be fibrous in nature, resulting in a network or web of adhesions. These adhesions cause particular difficulty because they may bind any or all of the ossicles. Besides adhesions in the middle ear, calcium deposits sometimes form on the tympanic membrane, resulting in a condition called **tympanosclerosis.** Surgical dissection of adhesions in the middle ear may be fruitless because they tend to recur, causing conductive hearing loss. According to Meyerhoff (1986), mucous otitis media is more common in younger children, whereas serous effusion is more common in older children.

Otosclerosis

Otosclerosis, a common cause of hearing loss in adults, is hereditary in at least 70 percent of all cases (Morrison & Bundey, 1970). The condition originates in the bony labyrinth of the inner ear and is recognized clinically when it affects the middle ear, causing conductive hearing loss. Otosclerosis is a progressive disorder, with a varying age of onset from mid-childhood to late middle-adult life. The great majority of patients begin to notice some loss of hearing soon after puberty, up to the age of 30. Otosclerosis is rare among children. It occurs primarily among members of the white race, with the incidence in women approximately twice that in men. Women frequently report increased hearing loss because of otosclerosis during pregnancy or menopause.

Otosclerosis appears as the formation of a new growth of spongy bone, usually over the stapedial footplate of one or both ears. Because the bone is not really sclerotic (hard), some clinicians call this condition (more appropriately) **otospongiosis.** When this growth occurs, the footplate becomes partially fixed in the oval window, limiting the amplitudes of vibrations transmitted to the inner ear. At times the growth appears on the stapedial crura or over the round window. Very rarely does it occur on other ossicles or occupy considerable space in the middle ear. Sometimes the abnormal bone, which replaces the normal bone of the middle ear, may completely obliterate the margins of the oval window.

Patients with otosclerosis often exhibit a bluish cast to the whites of their eyes, similar to that found with certain other bone diseases. They complain of difficulty hearing while chewing, probably a result of the increased loudness of the chewing sounds delivered to their inner ears by bone conduction. Frequently, they are also bothered by sounds called **tinnitus** in the affected ear(s). The hearing loss itself is usually slowly progressive. Physical examination of the ear shows normal structures and normal tympanic membrane landmarks. Occasionally the promontory becomes very vascular, resulting in a rosy glow that can be seen through the tympanic membrane. This glow is referred to as the **Schwartze sign.**

One interesting and peculiar symptom of otosclerosis is **paracusis willisii.** Most hard-of-hearing patients claim they hear and understand speech better in quiet surroundings. Patients with otosclerosis (and often those with other forms of conductive hearing loss) may find that speech is easier to understand in the presence of background noise. This phenomenon results from the fact that normal-hearing persons speak louder in noisy environments. This increase in vocal loudness, something we have all experienced, is called the **Lombard voice reflex.** Because these patients' hearing losses attenuate the background noise to some degree, such people are able to enjoy the increased loudness of speakers' voices with less distracting noise. Paracusis willisii is illustrated in Figure 10.20.

Audiometric Findings in Otosclerosis.   Carhart (1964) showed that the first symptom of otosclerosis is the appearance of a low-frequency air-bone gap. He also found that alterations in the inertia of the ossicular chain, produced by even partial fixation, alter the normal bone-conduction response. This artifact varies significantly from patient to patient, but on the average it causes the bone-conduction readings to appear poorer than the true sensorineural sensitivity by 5 dB at 500 Hz, 10 dB at 1000 Hz, 15 dB at 2000 Hz, and 5 dB at 4000 Hz. This anomaly of bone conduction is called the **Carhart notch,** and it probably occurs as a mechanical artifact because of a shift in the normal resonant frequency of the middle ear (about 2500 Hz) produced by the immobility of the oval window. The Carhart notch is also seen in some cases of middle-ear fluid.

Figure 10.21 illustrates an audiogram typical of early otosclerosis. Contrary to the typical audiometric contour in serous effusion, the otosclerotic shows a drop in sensitivity in the low-frequency areas first, which is consistent with what is known of the effects of stiffness on impedance. As the principal place of otosclerosis increases in size, the hearing loss becomes greater (Figure 10.22). Later in the disease, when the stapes has become completely fixed, the mass effect becomes apparent, causing a reduction of sensitivity in the high frequencies, thus flattening the audiogram. With complete fixation, the entire mass of the skull is in fact added to the stapes. All auditory tests for site of lesion remain consistent with conductive hearing loss.

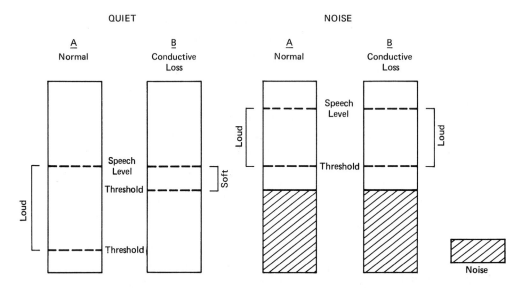

FIGURE 10.20   Illustration of paracusis willisii. The normal listener (A) has an advantage over the listener with a hearing loss (B) in the quiet situation because the speech is received for A at a higher sensation level, and is therefore louder. In the noisy situation, the thresholds are raised by the noise much more for A than for B. The speaker's voice is raised by the noise (the Lombard effect). Therefore, A and B both enjoy the same speech level above threshold (equal loudness), but B is much less aware of the background noise.

The pressure-compliance function remains normal in otosclerosis, except that the point of greatest compliance is not as great as normal on the tympanogram. Jerger (1970) has called this type of tympanogram (Figure 10.23) a Type A_S (stiffness). The A_S tympanogram appears in many, but not all, cases of otosclerosis. The acoustic reflex disappears early in otosclerosis, even in unilateral cases. When the tone is delivered to the involved ear, the hearing loss attenuates even a very intense sound, so that the reflex is not triggered. When a tone is delivered to a normal ear opposite the one with otosclerosis, the reflex does not register because the stapes is incapable of movement, even though it is pulled by the stapedius tendon. In otosclerosis the acoustic impedance may be expected to be high and the compliance low.

Treatment of Otosclerosis.   Interest in the surgical correction of otosclerosis dates back many years. Even in fairly recent times, surgical relief of otosclerotic hearing loss met with failure, primarily for two reasons. First, before the introduction of antibiotics, postoperative infection caused severe complications. Second, until the development of the operating microscope, middle-ear surgeons could not clearly see the very small operative field of the middle ear.

Because attempts to free the immobilized stapes resulted in failure, often in the form of fractured crura, attention was turned to bypassing the ossicular chain. A new window was created in the lateral semicircular (balance) canal of the inner ear so that sound waves could pass directly from the external ear canal to the new window. This procedure was conducted as a two-stage operation until the one-stage **fenestration** was developed by Lempert (1938).

SPEECH AND HEARING CENTER
The University of Texas at Austin 78712
AUDIOMETRIC EXAMINATION

NAME: Last - First - Middle	SEX	AGE	DATE	EXAMINER	RELIABILITY	AUDIOMETER

AIR CONDUCTION

MASKING TYPE	RIGHT									LEFT								
	250	500	1000	1500	2000	3000	4000	6000	8000	250	500	1000	1500	2000	3000	4000	6000	8000
	25	20	20/20	15	5	10	0	0	0	30	20	15/15	10	5	0	0	5	5
EM Level in Opp. Ear																		

BONE CONDUCTION

MASKING TYPE	RIGHT						FOREHEAD						LEFT					
	250	500	1000	2000	3000	4000	250	500	1000	2000	3000	4000	250	500	1000	2000	3000	4000
NB	0*	5*					-5	5	10	15	10	5	-5*	5*				
EM Level in Opp. Ear	60	50											60	55				

	2 Frequency	3 Frequency	WEBER							2 Frequency	3 Frequency
Pure Tone Average	13	15	M	M	M	M	M		Pure Tone Average	10	13

SPEECH AUDIOMETRY

MASKING TYPE	RIGHT				LEFT			
	SRT 1	SRT 2	Recognition 1	Recognition 2	SRT 1	SRT 2	Recognition 1	Recognition 2
WB	20		10 List 30 SL 96* %	List SL %	15		20 List 30 SL 94* %	List SL %
EM Level in Opp. Ear			50				30	

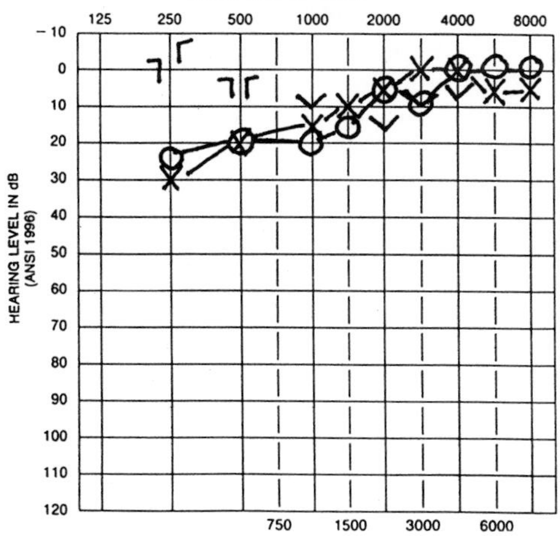

FREQUENCY IN HERTZ   COMMENTS

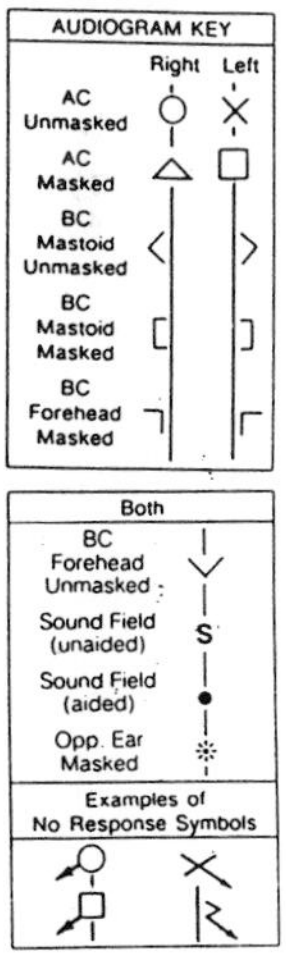

FIGURE 10.21 Audiogram illustrating early otosclerosis in both ears. The loss appears first in the low frequencies because of the increased stiffness of the ossicular chain. A small air-bone gap is present. Word-recognition scores are normal, and the Weber does not lateralize. Masking was used for bone conduction only at 250 and 500 Hz, and for word-recognition testing. Note the early appearance of the Carhart notch.

SPEECH AND HEARING CENTER
The University of Texas at Austin 78712
AUDIOMETRIC EXAMINATION

NAME: Last - First - Middle	SEX	AGE	DATE	EXAMINER	RELIABILITY	AUDIOMETER

AIR CONDUCTION

MASKING TYPE	RIGHT									LEFT								
	250	500	1000	1500	2000	3000	4000	6000	8000	250	500	1000	1500	2000	3000	4000	6000	8000
NB	45	50	40/40	40	40	35	40	40	35	50	50	45/45	40	40	40	45	45	40
	45*	50*								50*	50*					45*		
EM Level in Opp. Ear	50	50								45	50					40		

BONE CONDUCTION

MASKING TYPE	RIGHT						FOREHEAD						LEFT					
	250	500	1000	2000	3000	4000	250	500	1000	2000	3000	4000	250	500	1000	2000	3000	4000
NB	0*	10	15	20*	15	5*	0	10	15	20	15	5	0*	10*	15*	25*	15*	0*
EM Level in Opp. Ear	50	50	45	40	40	45							45	50	40	55	35	55

		2 Frequency	3 Frequency	WEBER							2 Frequency	3 Frequency
	Pure Tone Average	40	43	M	M	M	M	M		Pure Tone Average	43	45

SPEECH AUDIOMETRY

MASKING TYPE	RIGHT					LEFT				
	SRT 1	SRT 2	Recognition 1	Recognition 2		SRT 1	SRT 2	Recognition 1	Recognition 2	
WB	45	45*	1A List 30 SL / 100* %	List SL / %		45	45*	2A List 30 SL / 96* %	List SL / %	
EM Level in Opp. Ear		45	90				45	85		

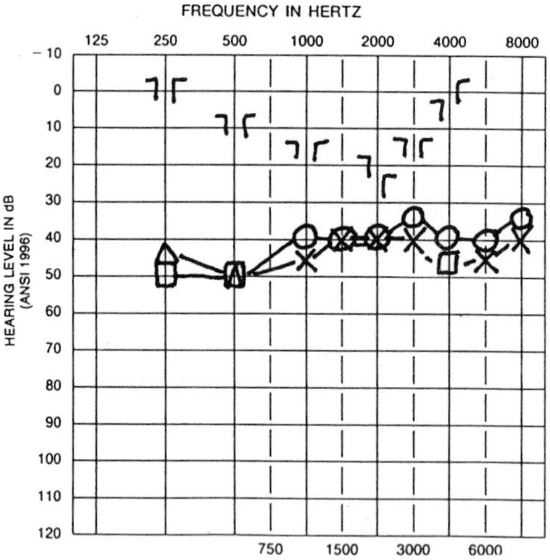

FREQUENCY IN HERTZ

COMMENTS

AUDIOGRAM KEY

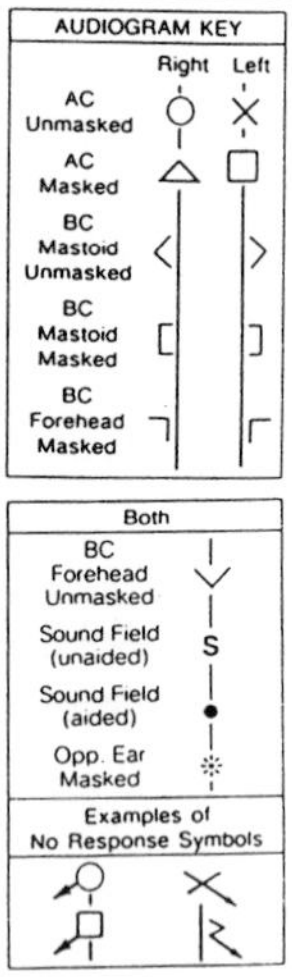

FIGURE 10.22 Audiogram showing a moderate loss of hearing in both ears caused by otosclerosis. The audiometric configuration is fairly flat, showing the combined effects of stiffness and mass. Bone conduction is normal except for the Carhart notch. Masking is required for air conduction at 250 and 500 Hz in both ears and for 4000 Hz in the left ear. All speech tests required masking.

SPEECH AND HEARING CENTER
The University of Texas at Austin 78712

IMMITTANCE

NAME: Last · First · Middle		SEX	AGE	DATE	EXAMINER		INSTRUMENT	

PRESSURE/COMPLIANCE FUNCTION

	-400	-350	-300	-250	-200	-150	-100	-50	0	+50	+100	+150	+200
Right					.60	.62	.65	.75	.84	.71	.76	.64	.62
Left					.76	.77	.79	.85	.95	.85	.80	.79	.77

STATIC COMPLIANCE

$c_x = c_2 - c_1$

RIGHT						LEFT					
.62	c_1	.84	c_2	.22	c_x	.77	c_1	.95	c_2	.18	c_x

ACOUSTIC REFLEXES

	RIGHT				LEFT			
Frequency (Hz)	500	1000	2000	4000	500	1000	2000	4000
Ipsilateral (Probe same)		NR	NR			NR	NR	
Contralateral (Probe opposite)	NR	NR	NR	NR	NR	NR	NR	NR
Audiometric Threshold								
Reflex SL								
Decay Time (Seconds)								

TYMPANOGRAM

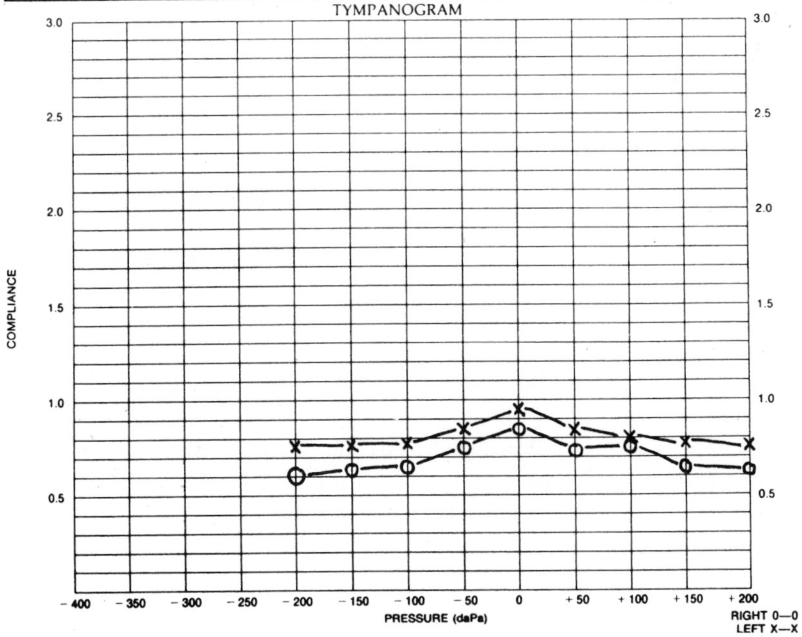

RIGHT 0—0
LEFT X—X

FIGURE 10.23 **Results on immittance test performed on a patient with bilateral otosclerosis (Figure 10.22). The tympanogram is Type A_S, the static compliance is low, and the acoustic reflexes are absent in both ears.**

Fenestration surgery resulted in considerable hearing improvements for many patients with otosclerosis. It was recognized early that complete closure of the preoperative air-bone gap was impossible, as a result of loss of the tympanic membrane and the ossicular chain. A 25 dB conductive hearing loss usually remained following even the best fenestration. The proper selection of candidates for surgery, based on their bone-conduction thresholds, was critical. Careful comparisons of preoperative and postoperative bone-conduction audiograms led to the discovery of the Carhart notch (1952).

Although many people were helped dramatically by fenestration surgery, numbers of others were less than satisfied with the results. Many people found no improvement in their hearing, and a number showed a considerable drop in their sensorineural sensitivity. Some individuals had total loss of hearing. Using Figure 10.22 as an example of a preoperative audiogram, Figure 10.24 shows the maximum improvement possible with fenestration surgery, and Figure 10.25 shows a poor result. Often, patients with poor fenestration results were bothered by vertigo and increased tinnitus, as well as by poorer word-recognition scores and occasional facial paralysis. Hearing-aid use was sometimes obviated in the operated ear by a combination of poor speech discrimination and the large ear cavity created during surgery. Even if some patients were happy with the hearing results of their surgery, they were bothered by the constant aftercare required to clean the cavity.

While palpating a stapes on a patient preparatory to performing a fenestration, Rosen (1953) managed to mobilize the stapes, breaking it free and restoring the sound vibrations into the inner ear. This happenstance led to a completely new introduction, the **stapes mobilization** procedure.

Advantages of the mobilization over the fenestration were manifold. Patients could be operated on using local anesthesia, eliminating some of the side effects of general anesthesia. Because the ossicular chain remained intact, the patient's potential for postoperative hearing could be fairly well predicted by the preoperative bone conduction. Of great importance was the fact that no aftercare was required for mobilizations because no mastoid cavity was created during surgery.

In stapes mobilization the ear canal is carefully cleansed and dried. The skin near the tympanic membrane is then injected to deaden the area. A triangular incision is made in the skin, and the tympanic membrane reflected, exposing the middle ear. The surgeon then places a right-angle hook against the neck of the stapes, determines that it is fixed, and then rocks it until it is freed.

A number of variations of Rosen's operation were introduced, and although many patients were initially helped, it was found that a great number of those patients whose hearing originally improved failed to retain this improvement after one year. The regression in hearing resulted from refixation of the stapes as new otosclerotic bone was laid down over the footplate. Refixation appears to be a greater problem for young patients, in whom the otosclerosis is more active, and for males.

Refixation following stapes mobilization led Shea (1958) to revive an operative procedure that had been described more than a half century earlier. This technique is called **stapedectomy,** which means "removal of the stapes." Stapedectomy is undoubtedly the procedure of choice for otosclerosis today.

The approaches to the middle ear for stapedectomy and mobilization are identical. After fixation has been determined, the incudostapedial joint is interrupted, the stapedius tendon is cut, and the superstructure of the stapes and remainder of the footplate are removed. In the original procedure a vein graft, taken from the patient's hand or arm, was placed over the open oval window, and draped on the promontory and over the facial ridge to obtain adequate blood supply. A hollow polyethylene strut was pulled onto the lenticular process of the incus, and the opposite end, which was beveled for a better fit, was placed in the oval window niche on the vein graft. In this way the polyethylene tube replaced the stapes.

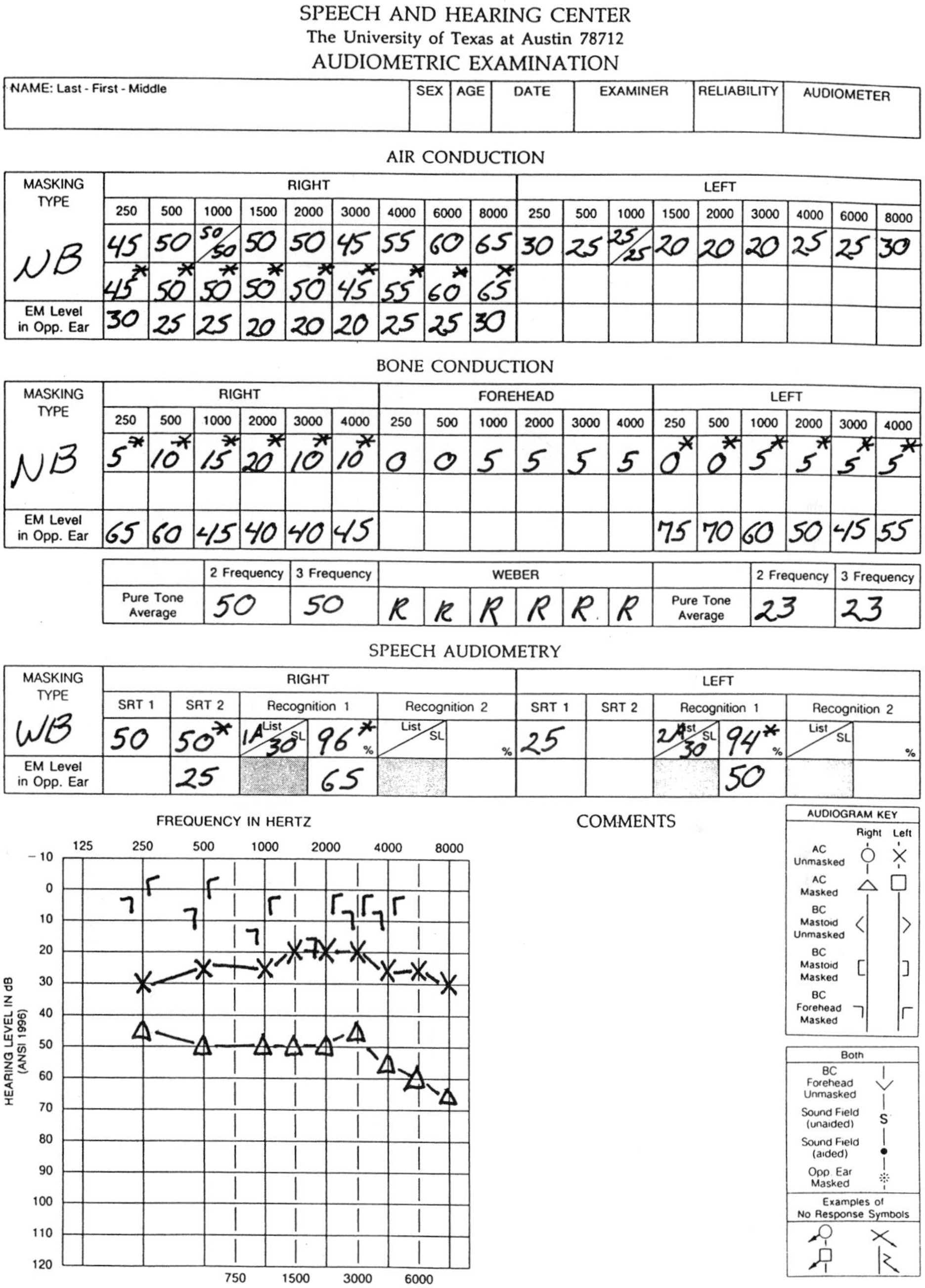

SPEECH AND HEARING CENTER
The University of Texas at Austin 78712
AUDIOMETRIC EXAMINATION

NAME: Last - First - Middle	SEX	AGE	DATE	EXAMINER	RELIABILITY	AUDIOMETER

AIR CONDUCTION

MASKING TYPE	RIGHT									LEFT								
	250	500	1000	1500	2000	3000	4000	6000	8000	250	500	1000	1500	2000	3000	4000	6000	8000
NB	45	50	50/50	50	50	45	55	60	65	30	25	25/25	20	20	20	25	25	30
	45*	50*	50*	50*	50*	45*	55	60*	65*									
EM Level in Opp. Ear	30	25	25	20	20	20	25	25	30									

BONE CONDUCTION

MASKING TYPE	RIGHT						FOREHEAD						LEFT					
	250	500	1000	2000	3000	4000	250	500	1000	2000	3000	4000	250	500	1000	2000	3000	4000
NB	5*	10*	15*	20*	10*	10*	0	0	5	5	5	5	0*	0*	5*	5*	5*	5*
EM Level in Opp. Ear	65	60	45	40	40	45							75	70	60	50	45	55

		2 Frequency	3 Frequency	WEBER							2 Frequency	3 Frequency
	Pure Tone Average	50	50	R	R	R	R	R	R	Pure Tone Average	23	23

SPEECH AUDIOMETRY

MASKING TYPE	RIGHT				LEFT			
	SRT 1	SRT 2	Recognition 1	Recognition 2	SRT 1	SRT 2	Recognition 1	Recognition 2
WB	50	50*	1A List 30 SL 96* %	List SL %	25	21 st 30 SL	List 94* %	List SL %
EM Level in Opp. Ear		25	65				50	

FREQUENCY IN HERTZ

COMMENTS

AUDIOGRAM KEY

FIGURE 10.24 **Audiogram showing a conductive hearing loss in both ears. The right ear shows a moderate loss caused by otosclerosis, and the left ear shows a postoperative fenestration. Note the presence of the Carhart notch in the right ear, and its absence in the left. The left ear shows the maximum obtainable result with fenestration surgery. Note the need for masking for most tests.**

SPEECH AND HEARING CENTER
The University of Texas at Austin 78712
AUDIOMETRIC EXAMINATION

NAME: Last - First - Middle	SEX	AGE	DATE	EXAMINER	RELIABILITY	AUDIOMETER

AIR CONDUCTION

MASKING TYPE	RIGHT									LEFT								
	250	500	1000	1500	2000	3000	4000	6000	8000	250	500	1000	1500	2000	3000	4000	6000	8000
NB	60	65	65/65	65	70	80	75	85	90	55	55	60/60	60	55	50	55	60	65
	70	75	75	75	80	90	85	90	NR	55	55	60	60	55	50	55	60	65
EM Level in Opp. Ear	75	75	75	80	80	75	75	80	80	70	75	75	80	80	90	85	90	90

BONE CONDUCTION

MASKING TYPE	RIGHT						FOREHEAD						LEFT					
	250	500	1000	2000	3000	4000	250	500	1000	2000	3000	4000	250	500	1000	2000	3000	4000
NB	NR	65	NR	NR	NR	NR	5	10	15	25	30	20	15	10	25	25	30	20
EM Level in Opp. Ear	80	90	90	90	85	90										80	90	90	80	95	85

	2 Frequency	3 Frequency	WEBER							2 Frequency	3 Frequency
Pure Tone Average	75	77	L	L	L	L	L	L	Pure Tone Average	55	57

SPEECH AUDIOMETRY

MASKING TYPE	RIGHT				LEFT			
	SRT 1	SRT 2	Recognition 1	Recognition 2	SRT 1	SRT 2	Recognition 1	Recognition 2
WB	65	80	44 list/30 SL 66 %	List/SL %	55		4B list/30 SL 96 %	List/SL %
EM Level in Opp. Ear		75	90					

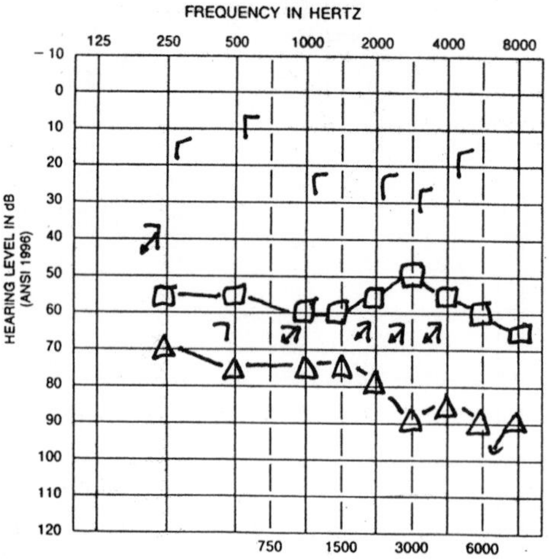

FREQUENCY IN HERTZ

COMMENTS

AUDIOGRAM KEY

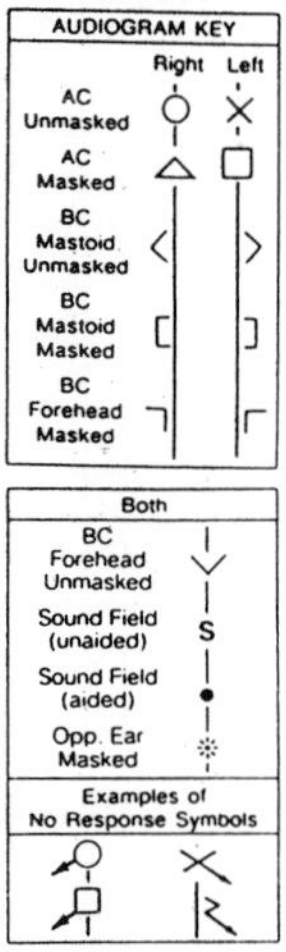

FIGURE 10.25   Audiogram illustrating a conductive hearing loss in the left ear caused by otosclerosis. The right ear shows a sensorineural hearing loss produced by unsuccessful middle-ear surgery to correct for otosclerosis. Note that masking is required to show the true bone-conduction thresholds for the right ear. Masked word-recognition tests show the right ear to be impaired. The Weber is lateralized to the left ear.

In some cases, the polyethylene with vein procedure, though very popular, resulted in **fistulas** (leaks of inner-ear fluids into the middle ear), perhaps as a result of the sharp end of the strut resting on the vein. Testing for a fistula can be accomplished with the pressure portion of an immittance meter and an electronystagmograph (ENG) (see Chapter 11). Positive pressure is delivered to the middle ear by increasing the output of air pressure from the meter to 300 or 400 daPa. This may be accomplished whether a perforation of the tympanic membrane exists or not. If a fistula is present, the increased pressure within the middle ear may result in vertigo and an increase in rapid eye movement, called *nystagmus,* which can be monitored on the ENG.

In recent years a number of modifications of the original Shea stapedectomy have been introduced. Different materials have been used as the prosthesis: stainless steel wire, stainless steel pistons, Teflon pistons, combinations of steel and plastic, and so on. Some surgeons have used fat plugs from the tragus of the pinna, or **fascia** (the tough protective cover over muscle), to cover the oval window and support the prosthesis. Although the success of stapedectomy has been substantial, and many patients with unsuccessful mobilizations have been reoperated on with great improvements in hearing, some adverse reactions can and do occur, including further loss of hearing and prolonged vertigo.

To reduce risk in stapedectomy, many middle-ear surgeons today prefer to use a small fenestra and avoid the trauma to the inner ear of complete removal of the stapedial footplate. Small fenestra stapedectomies have been referred to as *stapedotomies* (Bailey & Graham, 1984). One such procedure is illustrated in Figures 10.26 to 10.31. After the ear has been locally anesthetized, and the tympanic membrane elevated from its sulcus, exposing the middle ear, the stapedectomy is begun.

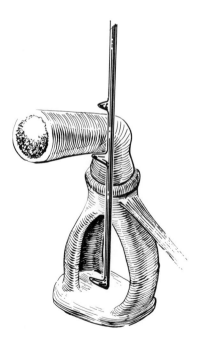

FIGURE 10.26   The proper length for the prosthesis is determined by measuring the distance from the undersurface of the incus to the footplate. A special measuring rod is used.

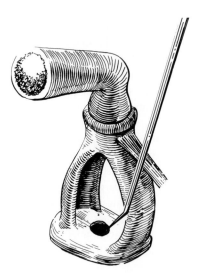

FIGURE 10.27   A small "control hole" is made in the center of the footplate; the hole is then enlarged with a pick or hand drill.

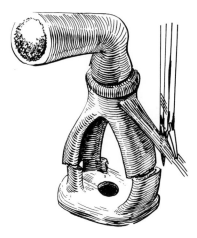

FIGURE 10.28   The crura are weakened and fractured, the incudostapedial joint is separated, and the stapedial tendon is severed with microscissors.

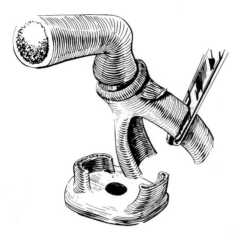

FIGURE 10.29   The superstructure of the stapes is removed.

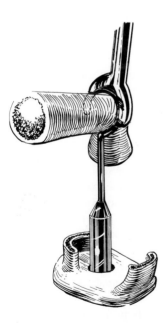

FIGURE 10.30   The prosthesis is carefully positioned, the wire hook is placed over the long process of the incus just above the lenticular process, and the hook is crimped snugly into position with a special crimping instrument.

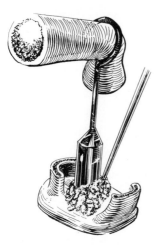

FIGURE 10.31   Superficial fascia from the temporalis muscle is placed around the end of the prosthesis, where it enters the footplate, to seal the inner ear. (Figures 10.26 through 10.31 courtesy of James Pappas, M.D., Arkansas Otolaryngology Center.)

As further modifications of the stapedectomy procedure continue to be perfected, such as the use of an argon laser, some form of stapedectomy will surely remain popular.

Other Causes of Middle-ear Hearing Loss

Numbers of middle-ear abnormalities occur in isolation or in association with other congenital anomalies. Some cases of stapedial fixation appear purely on a genetic basis. A number of congenital middle-ear disorders were found in the offspring of mothers who took the drug thalidomide during pregnancy. Such conditions as fixation of the incudomalleal joint have been associated with atresias of the external auditory canal and microtias of the auricle. Other ossicular abnormalities have been associated with syndromes of the cheek, jaw, and face. Congenital malformations of the middle and outer ears are often seen together because these areas arise from the same embryonic tissue. Meyerhoff (1986) recommends delaying surgical repair in these situations until the child is four to six years old to permit the mastoid air-cell system to enlarge, allowing better surgical access.

Skull fractures have been known to result coincidentally in fractures or interruptions of the ossicular chain. Ossicular interruption has been reported in cases of skull trauma, even without fracture. An ossicle may also be damaged by a foreign object during traumatic perforation of the tympanic membrane, as with a cotton swab or bobby pin.

Tumors, both benign and malignant, may form in the middle ear. They may take the form of polyps, vascular tumors, granulomas in response to middle-ear infections, or in rare cases, cancer of the squamous cells of the middle ear.

Summary

The middle ear is an air-filled space separating the external auditory canal from the inner ear. Its function is to increase sound energy through leverage, the step-down size ratio provided by the ossicular chain, and the area ratio between the tympanic membrane and the oval window.

Abnormalities of the structure or function of the middle ear result in conductive hearing losses, wherein the air-conduction thresholds are depressed in direct relationship with the amount of disease. Bone-conduction thresholds may deviate slightly from normal in conductive hearing losses, not because of abnormality of the sensorineural mechanism, but because of alterations in the middle ear's normal (inertial) contribution to bone-conduction. Alterations in the pressure-compliance functions give general information regarding the presence of fluid or negative air pressure in the middle ear, stiffness, or interruption of the ossicular chain. Measurements of static compliance may be higher or lower than normal, and acoustic reflex thresholds are either elevated or absent. Auditory brainstem responses show increased latencies for all waves and otoacoustic emissions are usually absent. Results on word recognition tests and behavioral site of lesion tests such as SISI and tone decay are identical to those of normal hearers.

Remediation of middle-ear disorders should first be concerned with medical or surgical reversal of the problems. When this fails, must be postponed, or is not available, careful audiological counseling should be undertaken and therapeutic avenues, such as the use of hearing aids, investigated. Patients with conductive hearing losses are excellent candidates for hearing aids because of their relatively flat audiometric contours, good word recognition, and tolerance for loud sounds.

STUDY QUESTIONS

1. List as many parts of the middle ear as you can. Consider their functions. Compare your list to the diagram of the ear in Figure 10.1.

2. Make a list of disorders of the middle ear that produce conductive hearing loss. Next to each item, name an appropriate treatment.

3. For each of the disorders just listed, sketch a pure-tone audiogram. What would the probable results be on the following tests: SRT, word recognition, acoustic immittance, ABR, OAE, ABLB, SISI, and tone decay?

GLOSSARY

Acute A condition characterized by rapid onset, frequently of short duration.

Aditus ad antrum A space in the middle ear containing the head of the malleus and the greater part of the incus. It communicates upward and backward with the mastoid antrum.

Autophony A condition produced by some middle-ear or eustachian tube abnormalities, in which individuals' voices seem louder than normal to themselves.

Barotrauma Damage to the ear by sudden changes in pressure, as in flying or diving.

Bell's palsy Paralysis of the peripheral branch of the facial nerve.

Carhart notch An artifactual depression in the bone-conduction audiogram of patients with otosclerosis. It is most evident at 2000 Hz and disappears following corrective surgery.

Carotid artery The main large artery on either side of the neck. It passes beneath the anterior wall of the middle ear.

Cholesteatoma A tumor, usually occurring in the middle ear and mastoid, that combines fats and epithelium from outside the middle-ear space.

Chorda tympani nerve A branch of the facial nerve that passes through the middle ear. It conveys information about taste from the anterior two-thirds of one side of the tongue.

Chronic A condition characterized by long duration.

Cilia Eyelash-like projections of some cells that beat rhythmically to move certain substances over their surfaces.

Crura Legs, as of the stapes.

Crus Singular of *Crura*.

Epitympanic recess That part of the middle ear above the upper level of the tympanic membrane. Also called the *attic* of the middle ear.

Eustachian tube The channel connecting the middle ear with the nasopharynx on each side. It is lined with mucous membrane and is sometimes called the auditory tube.

Facial nerve The VIIth cranial nerve. It innervates the muscles of the face and the stapedius muscle.

Fallopian canal A bony channel, on the medial wall of the middle ear, through which the facial nerve passes. It is covered with mucous membrane.

Fascia Layers of tissue that form the sheaths of muscles.

Fenestration An early operation designed to correct hearing loss from otosclerosis. A new window is created in the lateral balance canal of the inner ear, and the ossicular chain is bypassed.

Fistula An abnormal opening, as by incomplete closure of a wound, that allows fluid to leak out.

Footplate The base of the stapes, which occupies the oval window.

Hemotympanum Bleeding in the middle ear.

Incus The second bone in the ossicular chain, connecting the malleus to the stapes. It is named for its resemblance to an anvil.

Jugular bulb The bulbous protrusion of the jugular vein in the floor of the middle ear.

Lombard voice reflex The normal elevation of vocal intensity when the speaker listens to a loud noise.

Malleus The first and largest bone in the ossicular chain of the middle ear, connected to the tympanic membrane and the incus; so named because of its resemblance to a hammer.

Manubrium A process of the malleus embedded in the fibrous layer of the tympanic membrane.

Mastoidectomy An operation to remove infected cells of the mastoid. Mastoidectomies are termed as simple, radical, and modified radical, depending on the extent of surgery.

Mastoiditis Infection of the mastoid.

Mastoid process A protrusion of the temporal bone, one portion of which is pneumatized (filled with air cells).

Meniscus The curved surface of a column of fluid. A meniscus is sometimes seen through the tympanic membrane when fluids are present in the middle ear.

Middle-ear cleft The space made up of the middle ear and the eustachian tube.

Mucous membrane A form of epithelium found in many parts of the body, including the mouth, nose, paranasal sinuses, eustachian tube, and middle ear. Its cells contain fluid-producing glands.

Myringotomy Incision of the tympanic membrane.

Nasopharynx The area where the back of the nose and the throat communicate.

Necrosis The death of living cells.

Ossicles The chain of three tiny bones found in each middle ear (malleus, incus, and stapes).

Otitis media Any infection of the middle ear.

Otorrhea Any discharge from the external auditory canal or from the middle ear.

Otosclerosis The laying down of new bone in the middle ear, usually around the footplate of the stapes. When it interferes with stapedial vibration, it produces a progressive conductive hearing loss.

Otospongiosis See *Otosclerosis*.

Oval window A tiny, oval-shaped aperture beneath the footplate of the stapes. The oval window separates the middle ear from the inner ear.

Paracusis willisii A condition found among patients with conductive hearing loss in which they understand speech better in noisy than in quiet surroundings.

Physical-volume test (PVT) A high sound intensity, suggesting a large volume of air (greater than 5 cm^3) may be observed on c_1 during immittance measures. This indicates that a patent P.E. tube or tympanic membrane perforation is present.

Politzerization Inflation of the middle ear via the eustachian tube by forcing air through the nose.

Pressure-equalizing (P.E.) tube A short tube or grommet placed through a myringotomy incision in a tympanic membrane to allow for middle-ear ventilation.

Promontory A protrusion into the middle ear, at its labyrinthine wall, produced by the basal turn of the cochlea.

Purulent Related to the formation of pus.

Round window A small, round aperture containing a thin but tough membrane. The round window separates the middle ear from the inner ear.

Schwartze sign A red glow seen through the tympanic membrane and produced by increased vascularity of the promontory in some cases of otosclerosis.

Serous effusion The collection of fluid in the middle-ear space, with possible drainage into the external ear canal. Often called *serous otitis media.*

Stapedectomy An operation designed to improve hearing in cases of otosclerosis by removing the affected stapes and replacing it with a prosthesis.

Stapedius muscle A tiny muscle, innervated by the facial nerve, and connected to the stapes in the middle ear by the stapedius tendon.

Stapes The third and smallest bone in the ossicular chain of the middle ear, connected to the incus and standing in the oval window; so named because of its resemblance to a stirrup.

Stapes mobilization An operation to improve hearing in cases of otosclerosis by breaking the stapes free of its fixation in the oval window and allowing normal vibration.

Subluxation An incomplete dislocation or sprain.

Suppurative Producing pus.

Tensor tympani muscle A small muscle, innervated by the trigeminal nerve, and inserted into the malleus in the middle ear.

Tinnitus Ear or head noises, usually described as ringing, roaring, or hissing.

Toynbee maneuver A method for forcing the eustachian tube open by swallowing with the nostrils and jaw closed.

Trigeminal nerve The Vth cranial nerve, which innervates the tensor tympani and also some of the palatal muscles.

Tympanoplasty A surgical procedure designed to restore the hearing function to a middle ear that has been partially destroyed (as by otitis media).

Tympanosclerosis New calcium formations in the middle ear or on the tympanic membrane secondary to otitis media. The result is loss of mobility of the conductive mechanism.

Umbo A slight projection at the approximate center of the tympanic membrane.

Valsalva Autoinflation of the middle ear by closing off the mouth and nose and forcing air up the eustachian tube.

REFERENCES

Anderson, E. E., & Barr, B. (1971). Conductive high-tone hearing loss. *Archives of Otolaryngology, 93,* 599–605.

Bailey, H. A. T., & Graham, S. S. (1984). Reducing risk in stapedectomy: The small fenestra stapedectomy technique. *Audiology: A Journal for Continuing Education, 9,* 1–3.

Brooks, A. C. (1994). Middle ear infections in children. *Science News, 146,* 332–333.

Carhart, R. (1952). Bone conduction advances following fenestration surgery. *Transactions of the American Academy of Ophthalmology and Otolaryngology, 56,* 621–629.

———. (1964). Audiometric manifestations of preclinical stapes fixation. *Annals of Otology, Rhinology and Laryngology, 3,* 740–755.

De Jonge, R. R., & Valente, M. (1979). Interpreting ear differences in static compliance measurements. *Journal of Speech and Hearing Disorders, 44,* 209–213.

Giebink, G. S. (1984). Epidemiology and natural history of otitis media. In D. Lim, C. Bluestone, J. Klein, & J. Nelson (Eds.), *Recent advances in otitis media.* Philadelphia: B. C. Decker.

Gladstone, V. S. (1984). Advanced acoustic immittance considerations. In H. Kaplan, V. S. Gladstone, & J. Katz (Eds.), *Site of lesion testing: Audiometric interpretation* (Vol. 2, pp. 59–79). Baltimore: University Park Press.

Henry, D. F., & DiBartolomeo, J. R. (1993). Patulous eustachian tube identification using tympanometry. *Journal of the American Academy of Audiology, 4,* 53–57.

Jerger, J. (1970). Clinical experience with impedance audiometry. *Archives of Otolaryngology, 92,* 311–324.

Kraemer, M. J., Richardson, M. A., Weiss, N. S., Furukawa, C. T., Shapiro, G. G., Pierson, W. E., & Bierman, C. W. (1983). Risk factors for persistent middle-ear effusions. *Journal of the American Medical Association, 249,* 1022–1025.

Kumazawa, T. (1985). Three acoustic impedance recording methods. *Annals of Otology, Rhinology and Laryngology, 94,* 25–26.

Lempert, J. (1938). Improvement of hearing in cases of otosclerosis: A new one-stage surgical technique. *Archives of Otolaryngology, 28,* 42–97.

Meyerhoff, W. L. (1986). *Disorders of hearing.* Austin, TX: Pro-Ed.

Morrison, A. W., & Bundey, S. E. (1970). The inheritance of otosclerosis. *Journal of Laryngology and Otology, 84,* 921–932.

O'Conner, A. F., & Shea, J. J. (1981). Autophony and the patulous eustachian tube. *Laryngoscope, 91,* 1427–1435.

Orchik, D. J., Schumaier, D. R., Shea, J. J., Xianxi, G. (1995), Middle ear and inner ear effects on clinical bone-conduction threshold. *Journal of the American Academy of Audiology, 6,* 256–260.

Plate, S., Johnsen, M. N. J., Pederson, N., & Thompsen, K. A.. (1979). The frequency of patulous eustachian tubes in pregnancy. *Clinical Otolaryngology, 4,* 393–400.

Rock, E. H. (1974). Practical otologic applications and considerations in impedance audiometry. *Impedance newsletter supplement* (Vol. 3). New York: American Electromedics Corporation.

Rosen, S. (1953). Mobilization of the stapes to restore hearing in otosclerosis. *New York Journal of Medicine, 53,* 2650–2653.

Shea, J. J. (1958). Fenestration of the oval window. *Annals of Otology, Rhinology and Laryngology, 67,* 932–951.

Williams, P. S. (1975). A tympanometry pressure swallow test for assessment of eustachian tube function. *Annals of Otology, Rhinology and Laryngology, 84,* 339–343.

SUGGESTED READINGS

Clark, J. G., & Jaindl, M. (1996). Conductive hearing loss in children: Etiology and Pathology. In F. N. Martin & J. G. Clark (Eds.), *Hearing care for children* (pp. 45–72). Boston: Allyn & Bacon.

Kenna, M. A. (1996). Embryology and developmental anatomy of the ear. In C. D. Bluestone, S. E. Stool, & M. A. Kenna (Eds.), *Pediatric otolaryngology* (Vol. I, pp. 113–126). Philadelphia: W. B. Saunders.

Lipscomb, D. M. (1996). The external and middle ear. In J. L. Northern (Ed.), *Hearing disorders* (pp. 1–13). Boston: Allyn & Bacon.

REVIEW TABLE 10.1 Conductive Hearing Loss in the Middle Ear

Etiology	Degree of Loss	Audiometric Configuration	Static Compliance	Tympanogram Type
Suppurative otitis media	Mild-to-moderately severe	Flat	Normal to low	B
Tympanic membrane perforation	Mild	Flat	Not testable Large equivalent volume .	Not testable
Ossicular chain discontinuity	Moderate	Flat	High	A_D
Serous effusion	Mild-to-moderate	Flat or poorer in high frequencies	Normal-to-low	B
Negative middle-ear pressure	Mild	Flat	Normal	C
Otosclerosis	Mild-to-moderately severe	Flat or poorer in low frequencies	Low	A_S
Congenital disorders	Mild-to-moderately severe	Varies	Varies	Varies

11 The Inner Ear

Since the animal brain cannot use sound vibrations in the form described in Chapter 3, the function of the inner ear is to **transduce** the mechanical energy delivered from the middle ear into a form of energy that can be interpreted by the brain. In addition to hearing information, the inner ear also converts information regarding the body's position and movement into a bioelectrical code. Because of its similarity to an intricately winding cave, the inner ear has been called a **labyrinth.** The inner ear is extremely complicated, with literally thousands of moving parts, but it is so tiny that it has been compared to the size of a small pea.

Chapter Objectives

This chapter describes the inner ear as a device that provides the brain with information about sound and the body's position in space. The reader is exposed first to the anatomy and physiology of the inner ear, along with a number of disorders that affect it and their causes. Probable results on the auditory tests, described earlier in this volume, should be understood in terms of inner-ear disorders.

Anatomy and Physiology of the Inner Ear

The footplate of the stapes fits neatly into the oval window, so called because of its shape. The oval window is the separation between the middle ear and the inner ear. The immediate entryway is called the **vestibule;** it is an area through which access may be gained to various chambers of the inner ear, just as the vestibule in a house is a space that may communicate with several different rooms. The vestibule is filled with a fluid called **perilymph.** It is within the vestibular portion of the inner ear that the organs of equilibrium are housed. The connections between the balance (vestibular) and auditory (cochlear) portions of the inner ear are considered separately here for ease of learning, but they are intricately connected both anatomically and physiologically (Figure 11.1).

The Vestibular Mechanism

As in many animals, the human ability to maintain balance depends on information from several body systems, whose interactions are controlled in the **cerebellum.** These systems include visual, proprioceptive, and vestibular input. The visual system provides direct information from surrounding objects on the orientation of the body and depends on the ability of the eyes to see and the pres-

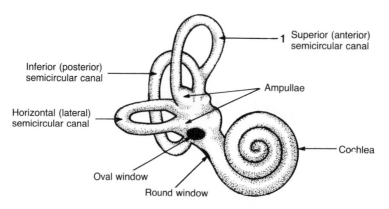

Inferior (posterior) semicircular canal

Horizontal (lateral) semicircular canal

1 Superior (anterior) semicircular canal

Ampullae

Cochlea

Oval window

Round window

FIGURE 11.1   **Anatomy of the human inner ear.**

ence of sufficient light to make surroundings visible. Proprioception concerns **somatosensory** stimuli received in tissue from supporting structures, such as the muscles and tendons of the body. These stimuli allow the perception of body-part positioning. The vestibular system relies on the forces of gravity and inertia.

Within the vestibule are membranous sacs called the **utricle** and the **saccule.** Both sacs are surrounded by perilymph and contain another fluid, very similar in constitution, called **endolymph.** The saccule is slightly smaller than the utricle. The end organ for balance within the utricle (*macula acoustica utriculi*) is located at the bottom, and the end organ within the saccule (*macula acoustica sacculi*) is located on the side.

Arising from the utricle are the superior, lateral, and posterior **semicircular canals,** which are also membranous, containing endolymph and surrounded in a larger bony cavern by perilymph. Each of the three canals returns to the utricle through enlarged areas called *ampullae*. Each **ampulla** contains an end organ (*crista*) for the sense of equilibrium. The semicircular canals are arranged perpendicular to one another to cover all dimensions in space. With any angular acceleration at least one semicircular canal is stimulated.

When the head is moved, the fluids in the vestibule tend to lag behind because of their inertia. In this way the fluids are set into motion, which stimulates the vestibular mechanism. The utriculosaccular mechanism is responsible for interpreting *linear acceleration,* and it is through this mechanism that we perceive when an elevator or automobile is picking up speed or slowing down. The utricle and saccule are stimulated by the rate of change of linear velocity, which can be measured in centimeters per second squared. The semicircular canals provide for the perception of motion. Therefore, they are the receptors for *angular acceleration,* or the rate of change of angular velocity. These receptors report, for example, the increase or decrease in the number of revolutions per minute that the body is turning. Thus, angular acceleration can be measured in degrees per second squared.

When the vestibular mechanisms become damaged or diseased, a common symptom called **vertigo** results. Patients with vertigo are truly ill because they experience the sensation of whirling or spinning. Because of connections in the brain between the vestibular portion of the auditory nerve and the oculomotor nerve, a rapid rocking movement of the eyes, called **nystagmus,** sometimes occurs. Nystagmus always occurs with vertigo, whether one can see it or not, and it may occur spontaneously in cases of vestibular upset. It is important to differentiate true vertigo from dizziness, light-headedness, or falling tendencies, which do not result in the sensation of true turning.

Tests for Vestibular Abnormality. For some time, attempts to determine the normality of the vestibular system have centered around artificial stimulation. In one test the patient is placed in a chair capable of mechanically controlled rotation. Following a period of rotation, the eyes are examined for nystagmus. The presence, degree, and type of nystagmus are compared to the examiner's concept of "normal."

A considerably easier test to administer in the otologist's or audiologist's office is the **caloric test.** Stimulation of the labyrinth is accomplished by "washing" cold or warm water or air against the tympanic membrane, with temperatures actually varying only slightly below or above normal body temperatures. In patients with normal vestibular systems, the result when cold water or air is used is a nystagmus with rapid movement away from the irrigated ear and slow movement back. When warm is used, the direction of nystagmus is reversed. The acronym COWS (cold-opposite, warm-same) is a useful mnemonic. Interpretations of responses as normal, hyperactive, or hypoactive are highly subjective and vary considerably among administrators of this test.

There is a difference in electrical potential between the cornea (positive charge) and the retina (negative charge) of the eye. Knowledge of this fact led to the development of a device called the **electronystagmograph (ENG)** to measure the changes in potential produced by nystagmus and to increase the objectivity of vestibular testing. Electrodes are placed on the bony ridge of the outer angle of each eye, and a ground electrode is placed in the center of the forehead above the eyes. This equipment allows for measurement of the rate and direction of nystagmus, which can be displayed on a paper chart as a permanent recording or displayed on a computer terminal and saved or printed. Most commercial ENGs heat and cool the water for irrigation to precise temperatures (30° and 44°C) and eject the proper amount (250 milliliters) over a prescribed period of time (40 seconds). A slightly longer irrigation is required for air calorics. All this automaticity has considerable advantage over manual methods of testing, but most important is the fact that a permanent and accurate result is available. A photograph of an electronystagmograph is shown in Figure 11.2. A patient with electrodes placed for ENG is shown in Figure 11.3.

Until recently, vestibulography was limited to the vestibulo-ocular reflexes, the connections between the balance and visual systems in the brain. There are new pursuits of other central nervous system interactions, including posturography, the assessment of the ability to coordinate movement by measuring vestibulospinal reflexes. Many of the tests now available are directly related to the introduction of computers to the measurement of vestibular function.

The use of microcomputers in vestibulography allows for better quantification of the eyebeats resulting from caloric testing through better control of the stimuli and resolution of the responses. A variety of tests is currently available, and software is constantly being upgraded. Also significant are the ways in which data can be stored and retrieved without the need for searching, cutting, and pasting long paper readouts. Computers have allowed for the reintroduction of rotary chairs as a means of assessing the functions of the vestibular system, including measurements on children.

A new system of electronystagmography has been developed that does away with the need for electrodes with all of their calibration, physiologic noise, and other problems. An infrared video system uses tiny video cameras to track eye movements in response to vestibular tests (Figure 11.4). The area inside the goggles is dark, allowing patients to keep their eyes open during testing as the

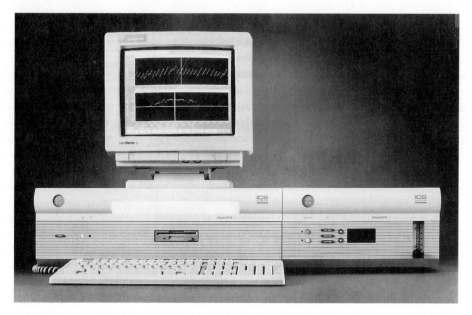

(A)

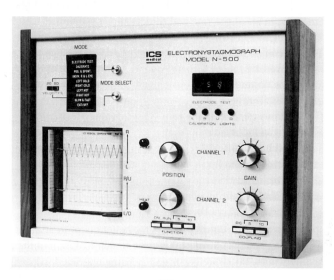

(B)

FIGURE 11.2   (A) Computerized electronystagmography (ENG) system—House Infrared/Video ENG system. (B) Strip chart ENG recorder. (Courtesy of Eye Dynamics, Inc., and JEDMED Instrument Company)

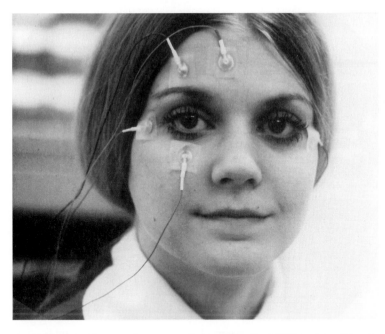

FIGURE 11.3   Proper placement of electrodes for ENG testing. (Courtesy of Tracoustics)

infrared light is invisible to them. The absence of electrodes makes testing easier and eye movements can be viewed on a video monitor or videotaped for later review.

Before the advent of computerized vestibulography, ENG testing on infants and small children was difficult, if not impossible. Cyr and Møller (1988) recommend that children be tested for vestibular dysfunction if (1) they show delayed or abnormal motor function, (2) they take ototoxic drugs, (3) they have a spontaneous nystagmus, or (4) there is suspected neurological disease. It would probably be advisable to carry out vestibular testing on children with sensorineural hearing loss whenever possible because many of them apparently suffer from significant vestibular abnormalities (Brookhouser, Cyr, & Beauchaine, 1982).

The diagnosis of patients with balance disorders is enhanced through the inclusion of **computerized dynamic posturography (CDP).** While measuring patients' postural compensations as the platform on which they are standing is rotated at various angles, this procedure provides a quantitative assessment of upright balance through simulation of conditions encountered in daily life. By isolating the sensory, motor, and biochemical components that contribute to balance, CDP analyzes a patient's ability to use these components individually, and in combination to maintain balance.

While some of the test protocols within CDP provide insights on a patient's functional capacity for a variety of daily life tasks, others help to localize the cause of a balance disorder (Nashner, 1993). CDP test results can aid in the diagnosis of specific underlying disease processes.

Although computerized vestibulography is lending innovative and exciting aspects to the diagnosis of diseases of the inner ear and central nervous system, it should be regarded as just one of many tools to be used. Vestibular function tests must be considered along with the medical history, medical examination, and audiometric findings, and the extent to which audiologists should be clinically involved in such procedures continues to be debated.

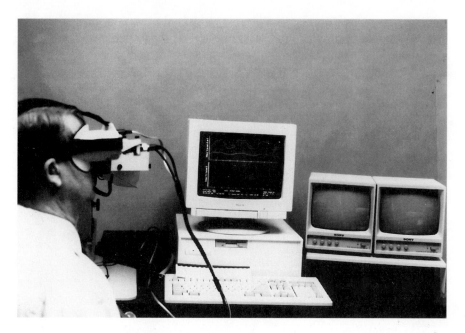

FIGURE 11.4   Infrared video electronystagmography system with goggle assembly on patient during positional testing. (Photo courtesy of Eye Dynamics, Inc. and JEDMED Instrument Company)

The Auditory Mechanism

The vestibular portions of the inner ear were shown in Figure 11.1, along with the auditory portions. Notice that the vestibule also communicates with a snail-like shell called the **cochlea.** For clarification, teachers are fond of "unrolling" the cochlea (Figure 11.5), an act that is graphically advantageous but physically impossible because the cochlea is made up of a twisting bony shell about 1 cm wide and 5 mm from base to apex (in humans).

Beyond the oval window within the cochlea lies the **scala vestibuli,** so named because of its proximity to the vestibule and its resemblance to a long hall. At the bottom of the cochlea, the **scala tympani** is visible, beginning at the round window. Both of these canals contain perilymph, which is continuous through a small passageway at the apex of the cochlea called the **helicotrema.** For frequencies above about 60 Hz, there is little fluid movement through the helicotrema, as energy is transmitted through the fluid levels of the cochlea by the movement of the membranes.

Between the two canals just described lies the **scala media,** or **cochlear duct.** This third canal is filled with endolymph, which is continuous through the **ductus reuniens** with the endolymph contained in the saccule, utricle, and semicircular canals. The scala media is separated from the scala vestibuli by **Reissner's membrane**[1] and from the scala tympani by the **basilar membrane.** When the cochlea, which curls about two and a half turns, is seen from the middle ear, the large turn at the base forms the protrusion into the middle ear called the promontory.

---

[1] For Ernst Reissner, German anatomist, 1824–1878.

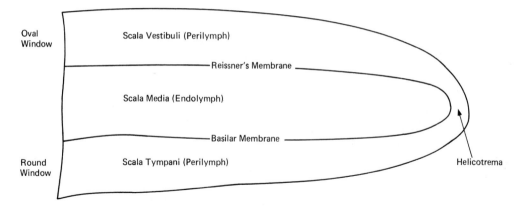

FIGURE 11.5   Diagram of an "unrolled" cochlea, showing the relationships among the three scalae.

Along the full length of the scala media lies the end organ of hearing—the **organ of Corti,**[2] which resides on the basilar membrane, one of the three walls of the scala media. The other two walls are made up of Reissner's membrane and a bony shelf formed by a portion of the bony labyrinth. From this shelf extends the **spiral ligament,** support for the scala media, and also the **stria vascularis,** which produces the endolymph and supplies oxygen and other nutrients to the cochlea. The blood supply and nerve supply enter the organ of Corti by way of the **modiolus,** the central core of the cochlea around which it is wound.

A cross section of the cochlea is shown in Figure 11.6. Much of what is known of the anatomy and physiology of the inner ear has been advanced in recent years with the introduction of electron microscopy.

Basilar Membrane

The basilar membrane is about 35 mm long and varies in width from less than 0.1 mm at the basal turn to about 0.5 mm at the apical turn, quite the reverse of the cochlear duct, which is broad at the basal end and narrow at the apex. Situated on the fibrous basilar membrane are three to five parallel rows of 12,000 to 15,000 outer hair cells and one row of 3,000 inner hair cells. The outer and inner hair cells are separated from each other by **Corti's arch.** The auditory nerve endings are located on the basilar membrane. Some of these nerve fibers connect to the hair cells in a one-to-one relationship, while others make contact with many hair cells. The hair cells themselves are about 0.01 mm long and 0.001 mm in diameter. Located on top of each hair cell are hairlike projections called **stereocilia.** The direction in which they are bent during stimulation is of great importance. If the cilia bend in one direction, the nerve cells are stimulated; if they bend the other way, the nerve impulses are inhibited; and if they bend to the side, there is no stimulation at all. A flow diagram showing a model of cochlear function is shown in Figure 11.7.

[2]For Alfonso Corti, Italian anatomist, 1822–1888.

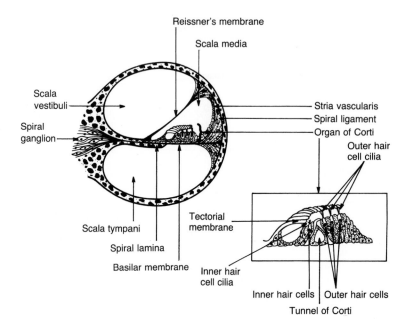

FIGURE 11.6   Cross section of the cochlea.

Physiology of the Cochlea

When the oval window is moved in by the stapes, the annular ligament around the footplate stretches and displaces the perilymph at the basal end of the cochlea, propagating a wave toward the apex of the cochlea. Because the fluids of the inner ear are noncompressible, when they are displaced inward the round window membrane must yield, moving into the middle ear. It may be said, therefore, that the two windows are out of phase. It is obvious that if they were in phase, a great deal of cancellation of sound waves would take place within the cochlea, just the opposite of the desired effect.

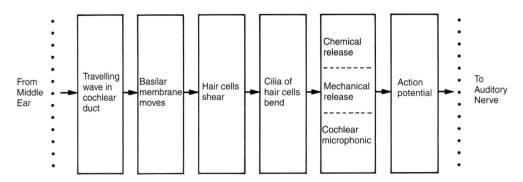

FIGURE 11.7   The functions of the cochlea.

Sound vibrations that are introduced to the scala vestibuli are conducted into the cochlear duct by the yielding of Reissner's membrane. The endolymph is thereby disturbed, and so the vibrations continue and the basilar membrane is similarly displaced, resulting in the release of the round window membrane. Therefore, sounds introduced to the inner ear cause a wavelike motion, which always moves from the base of the cochlea to the apex. This is true of either air- or bone-conducted sounds. Given areas along the basilar membrane show greater displacement for some frequencies than for others. Tones of low frequency with longer wavelengths show maximum displacement near the apical end, whereas tones of high frequency with shorter wavelengths show maximum displacement near the basal end.

The basilar membrane reacts more to vibrations of the inner ear than do most of the other structures. Because the organ of Corti resides on this membrane, the vibrations are readily transmitted to it. The stereocila on the tips of the outer hair cells are embedded in the **tectorial membrane,** a gelatinous flap that is fixed on its inner edge and, according to some researchers, on its outer edge as well. When the basilar membrane moves up and down in response to fluid displacement caused by the in-and-out movement of the stapes, the hair cells are sheared (twisted) in a complex manner. Part of this shearing is facilitated by the fact that the basilar membrane and the tectorial membrane have slightly different axes of rotation and slide in opposite directions as they are moved up and down. There is some debate over whether the cilia of the inner hair cells are actually embedded in the tectorial membrane, leaving uncertain the precise manner in which they are stimulated. It appears likely that although stimulation of outer hair cells takes place because of the magnitude of basilar membrane *displacement,* stimulation of the inner hair cells is due to the *velocity* of the membrane's movement—that is, the rate at which the displacement of the membrane changes.

The mechanics of the organ of Corti are very complex, resulting from motion of the basilar membrane in directions up and down, side to side, and lengthwise. The size of electrical response of the cochlea is directly related to the extent to which the hair cells, or the ciliary projections at their tops, are sheared. The source of the electrical charge is derived from within the hair cell. When the cilia are sheared, a chemical is released at the base of the hair cell.

Each inner hair cell of the cochlea is supplied by about twenty nerve fibers, each nerve fiber contacting only one hair cell. This is not true of the outer hair cells, where the neuron/hair cell ratio is 1:10. Each outer hair cell may be innervated by many different nerve fibers, and a given nerve fiber goes to several outer hair cells. The nerve fibers exit the cochlea and extend centrally toward the modiolus, where their cell bodies group together to form the spiral ganglion. The nerve fibers pass from the modiolus to form the cochlear branch of the auditory (VIIIth cranial) nerve.

The Auditory Neuron

The human cochlea contains about 30,000 afferent (sensory) **neurons** and about 1800 efferent neurons. A neuron is a specialized cell designed as a conductor of nerve impulses. It comprises a **cell body,** an **axon,** and **dendrites** (Figure 11.8). The axon and dendrites are branching systems. The dendrites, which consist of many small branches, receive nerve impulses from other nerve cells. The axon transmits the impulses along the neurons, which vary dramatically in length. The afferent neurons carry impulses from the cochlea to the central auditory nervous system and have their cell bodies in the spiral ganglion in the modiolus. As Figure 11.8 shows, auditory neurons are bipolar, in this case having one dendritic projection to the hair cells and another axon projecting to the sensory cells

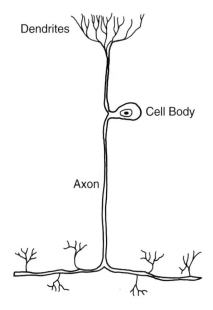

FIGURE 11.8   Diagram of a bipolar sensory neuron, such as are seen in the cochlea.

in the brainstem. The efferent axons project from the superior olivary complex in the brainstem and contact the hair cells both directly and indirectly, as well as in a variety of proportions.

Electrical impulses travel along the entire length of the axon. The stimulus is received by the dendrites, which conduct it to the cell body and then to the axon. The electrical power of the neuron is derived from the axon, which generates its voltage chemically from its surroundings. Connections between neurons are called **synapses.** Once the threshold has been reached, a neuron always responds with its maximum charge, regardless of the stimulus intensity. This has been called the *all-or-none* principle.

The act of conveying information between neurons is called **neurotransmission.** At one end of each nerve cell connections are made with other nerve cells, either through their dendrites, or directly with their cell bodies. Chemical substances, called **neurotransmitters,** that cause activation or inhibition of adjacent neurons, are released at these junctions.

The Fluids of the Cochlea

Though similar, the constituents of the perilymph and endolymph are different in ways essential to the physiology of hearing. Endolymph is high in its concentration of potassium ions and low in sodium, whereas the reverse is true of perilymph. Another way in which the two fluids are dissimilar is in their DC (direct current) potentials (voltages). Endolymph exhibits a strong positive potential, averaging about 80 millivolts (mV), caused by its high potassium concentration, compared to the perilymph of the scala tympani. The perilymph in the scala vestibuli demonstrates a positive, but much smaller, potential of about 3 mV when compared to the perilymph of the scala tympani. The remainder of the cochlear structures exhibit a negative DC potential. All of these potentials fluctuate.

The Cochlear Microphonic

The cochlea is the transducer that converts sound waves into an energy form useful to the auditory nerve. Because of this resemblance to the action of a microphone, which converts the pressure waves issuing from a speaker's mouth into an alternating electrical current, this action has been named the **cochlear microphonic (CM).** The cochlear microphonic is probably the result of changes in polarization caused by the bending back and forth of the hair cell cilia. For every up-and-down cycle of the basilar membrane, there is one in-and-out cycle of the stereocilia of the outer hair cells, causing them to become alternately depolarized and hyperpolarized. The size of the cochlear microphonic has been measured by placing pickup electrodes over the round window and, in some cases, within the cochlea.

The Action Potential

At the moment that auditory neurons are stimulated by the hair cells that rest on them, a change in the electrical potential occurs on the surface of each neuron. This is called the **action potential (AP).** Increases in the intensity of the auditory input signal to the cochlea result in increased electrical output from the hair cells. This stimulation causes increased electrical activity in the neuron, although each individual neuron continues to follow the all-or-none rule.

The Efferent System of the Cochlea

We tend to think of our sensory systems as being entirely **afferent,** carrying messages only from the sense organs, like the ear, to the brain for analysis. However, it is clear that the cochlea contains an efficient **efferent** system, receiving impulses from the brain. The relationship between afferent and efferent fibers is delicately balanced to provide a feedback, or monitoring system for the cochlea.

Theories of Hearing

The precise means by which we hear remains unknown. Most of the theories that attempt to explain how the ear utilizes the mechanical energy delivered to the cochlea from the middle ear are largely theories of how we perceive pitch.

Helmholtz's[3] **resonance theory of hearing** stated that the structures within the cochlea consist of many tiny resonators, each tuned to a specific frequency. He postulated that when a complex tone is introduced to the cochlea, each resonator responds to the frequency at which it is tuned, and that the ear performs a Fourier analysis, breaking each complex sound into its components. It is probable that Helmholtz mistook the transverse fibers of the basilar membrane for these small resonators. He believed that each resonator responded most vigorously to its tuned frequency and with less amplitude to adjacent frequencies. It was Helmholtz who described the placement of the higher frequency fibers at the basal end of the cochlea and the lower frequencies near the apex.

A logical early belief was that every tone that could be heard was assigned to its own specific place within the cochlea, much as the keys of a piano are laid out with specific representation.

[3]Hermann Ludwig Ferdinand Helmholtz, German physicist and physiologist, 1821–1894.

Therefore, the **place theory of hearing** is largely mechanical in nature and assumes that there is neural representation for every place on the basilar membrane. Place theories are handy for explaining some hearing phenomena, such as masking and the sharp pitch discriminations the human ear can make. The theory begins to break down when it attempts to explain why pitch discrimination is so poor close to auditory threshold. The place theory, therefore, is unacceptable as a theory of hearing, although its consideration as an incomplete theory of pitch perception may be viable.

Békésy[4] (1960) described what he called the **traveling wave theory.** For each inward and outward movement of the footplate of the stapes, there is a downward and upward movement of the basilar membrane, produced by disturbance of the endolymph. The wave moves down the cochlear duct from base to apex, with the maximum amplitude for high-frequency tones occurring at the basal end and that for the low frequencies at the apical end. Although high frequencies excite only the fibers in the basal turn of the cochlea, the low frequencies excite fibers all along the length of the basilar membrane. The input frequency, then, determines not only the *distance* the traveling wave moves before it peaks, but also the *rate* of basilar membrane vibration. The frequency of basilar membrane vibration is directly related to frequency and inversely related to period.

The place theories attributed analysis of pitch to the cochlea, but the **frequency theories of hearing,** of which there were several, considered that this analysis was accomplished in a **retro-cochlear** area. The frequency theories had in common the belief that the auditory nerve transmits a pattern that corresponds directly with the input signal; that is, if a 100 Hz tone is introduced, the auditory nerve would fire 100 times in a second. Because the auditory nerve is only capable of firing up to about 400 times per second, the frequency theory does not explain the perception of tones above this frequency. It was suggested by Wever (1949) that a series of impulses is sent along the auditory nerve, and that the sum of these impulses represents a reproduction of the vibrations of the basilar membrane. Basically, this **volley theory of hearing** suggests that during the refractory (rest) period of one set of neurons, another set is actively firing. Experimental evidence suggests that only frequencies up to 4000 Hz may be accounted for by volley theory alone.

The **resonance-volley theory of hearing** combines the spatial representation suggested by the place theories plus the temporal dimension of the volley theories. In this way, place explains high-frequency perception, and volley explains low-frequency interpretation, with some overlapping no doubt taking place.

The place theories explain loudness in terms of the amplitude of movement of the basilar membrane; that is, a louder sound creates a greater amplitude than a softer sound. This greater amplitude increases the number of impulses transmitted by the nerve fibers. The frequency theories explain loudness in terms of the amount of spread along the basilar membrane. The greater the amplitude of the input signal, the larger the surface area of the basilar membrane stimulated, and the greater the number of nerve fibers firing, both at the peak of the traveling wave and on both sides of it. Although intensity coding is extremely complicated and poorly understood, it is generally agreed that as the intensity of a signal is increased, neurons in the brainstem fire at higher rates (Musiek & Baran, 1986), resulting in greater loudness of the signal.

---

[4]Georg von Békésy, Hungarian physicist and Nobel Prize winner, 1899–1972.

Hypotheses for Hair Cell Transduction

It is still not entirely understood how the mechanical motion of the hair cells (shearing) converts a sound source into a form of energy that can be transmitted by the auditory nerve. The *mechanical hypothesis* assumes that the pressure that moves the hair cells stimulates the nerve endings directly. The *chemical hypothesis* assumes that when the hair cells are deformed, a neurotransmitter substance is released that stimulates the nerve endings. The *electrical hypothesis* assumes that the cochlear potential stimulates the nerve endings.

Otoacoustic Emissions

A great deal of thinking about the way the inner ear works has changed because of the remarkable discovery by Kemp (1978) that the cochlea, previously believed to be an organ that responds only to sounds entering the inner ear from the middle ear, in fact generates sounds of its own. Acoustic emissions had been observed in previous research, but were ignored and considered to be experimental artifacts. What Kemp discovered, through miniature microphones sealed in the external ear canals of human subjects, was an actual, weak acoustic signal, probably generated by the motility of the outer hair cells. These **otoacoustic emissions (OAEs)** now allow for study of cochlear function in animals and humans alike (Allen & Lonsbury-Martin, 1993) and add credence to the theory of the cochlear amplifier.

Spontaneous otoacoustic emissions (SOAEs), which can be detected without external stimulation, occur in 40 to 60 percent of normal ears (DeVries & Decker, 1992; Probst, Lonsbury-Martin, & Martin, 1991). In some cases they are audible to the subjects themselves at very low sensation levels. SOAEs may be understood on the basis of several generally accepted facts about the cochlea, specifically that the normal cochlea is very sharply tuned and processes sound nonlinearly. Damage to outer hair cells usually causes the emission to disappear.

Outer hair cell movement appears to generate waves that are conducted along the basilar membrane, through the intracochlear fluids, toward the basal end of the cochlea, then via the ossicular chain to the tympanic membrane, which acts as a loudspeaker in delivering a weak sound into the external auditory canal. It is known that the emissions are present in one or both ears of some humans (more often in right ears than in left ears, and more often in females than in males), but not of others, and that they are often absent in people with cochlear hearing loss. Any conductive hearing loss will attenuate the intensity of the sound traveling outward from the cochlea and will generally make the emissions unrecordable (Whitehead, Lonsbury-Martin, & Martin, 1992).

Arguments that the phenomenon of OAEs arises from something other than a cochlear event (such as a muscular contraction, or a sound generated in the middle ear) have been systematically eliminated. The relationship between these emissions and cochlear tinnitus (ringing, roaring, or noises in the ears) has been studied (e.g., Kemp, 1981), but at present, emission behavior cannot explain this symptom in most patients with cochlear impairments.

A signal is now known to emanate from the cochlea between 5 and 20 milliseconds after the presentation of a stimulus introduced into the external ear, and it typically does not exceed 30 dB SPL, regardless of the intensity of the evoking stimulus (Whitehead et al., 1992). This signal is called the *transient-evoked otoacoustic emission (TEOAE)*. These so-called "Kemp echoes" are generally described as being in the frequency range between 500 and 4000 Hz. Additionally, when brief pure tones are used as stimuli the emissions are close to the frequency of the evoking stimulus. To separate the TEOAE from ambient noise in the ear, a number of stimuli are presented and the response waveforms are computer averaged.

The discovery of OAEs is providing a new way of understanding how the auditory system functions, a new means of identifying hearing loss, and another method for determining site of lesion. Some of the clinical applications of OAEs are discussed in Chapter 6.

Frequency Analysis in the Cochlea

The frequency response of the nerve cells of the cochlea is laid out in an orderly fashion, with the lowest frequencies to which the ear responds (about 20 Hz) at the apical end. The spacing between the nerve fibers is not equal all along the basilar membrane. Fibers for the frequencies between 2000 and 20,000 Hz (the highest frequency to which the ear responds to air-conducted sounds) lie from the midpoint of the basilar membrane to the basal end of the cochlea near the oval window. Fibers for frequencies below 2000 Hz are contained on the other half of the basilar membrane.

Humans are capable of excellent frequency discrimination, in part because auditory nerve fibers are sharply tuned to specific frequencies. The frequency that can increase the firing rate of a neuron above its spontaneous firing rate is called its *characteristic frequency* or *best frequency*. Békésy (1960), who was among the first to study the tuning mechanism of the cochlea, observed that the tuning becomes sharper (narrower bandwidth) as frequency is increased (traveling wave peak closer to the basal end of the cochlea), although it is less sharply tuned than the auditory nerve. The slope of the tuning curve is much steeper above the stimulating frequency than below it.

The concept of the **psychophysical tuning curve (PTC)** (e.g., Pick, 1980) has been used to attempt measurements of the cochlea's frequency-resolving abilities. It seems apparent that when the cochlea becomes damaged, its frequency-resolving power may become poorer, but this is not evident in all cases. Preservation of the normal psychophysical tuning curve contributes to the ear's ability to resolve complex auditory signals, such as speech. Conversely, widening the PTC in damaged ears may help to explain the kinds of speech-discrimination difficulties characteristic of patients with cochlear impairment.

Development of the Inner Ear

Differentiation of the inner ear begins during the third week of gestation, and it reaches adult size and configuration by the sixth month. Placodes form early in embryonic life as thickened epidermal plates. The **auditory placode** infolds to form a pit, which closes off to form a capsule. This capsule divides to form a saccular division, from which the cochlea arises, and a utricular division, which forms the semicircular canals and probably the endolymphatic duct and sac. The vestibular portions of the inner ear develop earlier than the auditory portions. The fact that development takes place so rapidly probably accounts for the observation that interruption of normal development, as by a maternal disease in early pregnancy, can have such dire consequences for the inner ear.

The inner ear springs primarily from entoderm, although the membranous labyrinth is ectodermal in origin. The structure forms initially as cartilage and then changes to bone, usually by the twenty-third gestational week. The cochlea and vestibule reach full size in their primitive form by the twentieth week.

The cochlear turns begin to develop at about the sixth week, and are complete by the ninth or tenth week. This is a particularly active time of embryogenesis of the inner ear because the endolymphatic sac and duct and the semicircular canals are also forming, and the utricle and saccule are clearly separated. The utricle, saccule, and endolymphatic duct form from the **otocyst,** the auditory vesicle, or sac, that begins its formation at the end of the first month of gestational age.

By the middle of the eighth week the scalae are forming, and the semicircular canals reach adult configuration, including the ampullae with the cristae forming inside. The maculae are also forming within the utricle and saccule, as are the ducts that connect the saccule with the utricle and cochlear duct.

Between the tenth and twelfth weeks the organ of Corti has begun to form. By the eighteenth week adult configuration of the membranous labyrinth has been reached, and by twenty-five weeks the inner ear has fully formed.

Hearing Loss and the Inner Ear

Because the inner ear contains both sensory cells and nerve cells, **sensorineural hearing loss** is the expected result of abnormality of the cochlea. In such cases air- and bone-conduction sensitivity should be equally depressed in direct relationship to the severity of the disorder. The reasons that air-conduction and bone-conduction results may not be identical in cases of pure sensorineural hearing loss were discussed in Chapter 4, and some variations should be expected, even though the inner ear theoretically contributes the pure distortional mode of bone conduction.

Disorders of the Cochlea

Disorders of hearing produced by abnormality or disease of the cochlea probably constitute the largest group of hearing losses, called sensorineural. One fact generally agreed on is that as damage or abnormality occurs in the cochlea, loss of hearing sensitivity is not the only symptom. Indeed, a common complaint of patients with sensorineural hearing loss is not that they cannot hear, but that they have difficulty understanding speech. This speech-discrimination problem has been called **dysacusis,** to differentiate it from **hypacusis,** which suggests merely a loss of sensitivity to sound. Dysacusis probably results from a combination of frequency and harmonic distortion in the cochlea. As a general rule, patients with greater cochlear hearing losses have more dysacusis.

Many patients with unilateral hearing losses indicate that a pure tone of a given frequency has a different pitch in each ear. This is often noted during performance of the alternate binaural loudness balance test and is called **diplacusis binauralis.** At times patients perceive that a pure tone lacks the musical quality we associate with it and that it sounds like a musical chord or a noise instead. This has been described as sounding like "bacon frying." Such a lack of perception of tonal quality for a pure tone is called **diplacusis monauralis.**

Causes of Inner-ear Disorders

Alterations in the structure and function of the cochlea produce more hearing losses than do abnormalities in other areas of the sensorineural system. Hearing losses may result from either **endogenous** or **exogenous** causes. For purely arbitrary reasons, this chapter examines cochlear hearing losses as they relate generally to the patient's age at onset.

Prenatal Causes

Prenatal causes are those that have an adverse effect on the normal development of the cochlea. It is difficult to know, in cases of congenital hearing loss, the extent of genetic versus environmental factors, or their possible interrelationships in a given patient. For some time it has been known that some forms of hearing loss tend to run in families. Some patients are born with the hearing loss, and others inherit the tendency for abnormalities to occur later in life. This latter form has been called **hereditodegenerative hearing loss.**

All hereditary information is incorporated in a molecule called **DNA** and is contained in **genes,** which are the blueprints for the hereditary code. The physical manifestation of a trait is called a **phenotype,** and the actual genetic makeup that results in that trait is called a **genotype.** All 50,000 to 100,000 genes are strung in a beadlike fashion along **chromosomes,** of which there are 23 pairs, 22 pairs of **autosomes** (nonsex chromosomes) and one pair of sex chromosomes. One chromosome from each pair is inherited from each parent and is randomly selected. Different forms of a gene are called **alleles.** If an allele is inherited from both parents, that trait is said to be **homozygous** (pure); if the alleles are different, this is called **heterozygous** (mixed).

Hereditary disorders can take a variety of forms. When a gene from only one parent is required for a trait to be shown, that allele is said to be dominant. If the allele from both parents is required for a trait to be shown, it is called recessive. **Autosomal dominant** hearing losses are relatively obvious, since each child has a 50 percent chance of inheriting the disorder, and a family pattern can be observed. In some cases, the dominant gene is not penetrant; that is, it does not show up phenotypically, and the hearing loss appears to skip one or more generations. Further complicating this matter is the factor of **variable expressivity,** which means that not all the signs of a hereditary condition may appear phenotypically.

Autosomal recessive inheritance accounts for about 80 percent of profound genetic hearing impairments (Smith, 1994), about half of which are associated with syndromes. Children with autosomal recessive hearing loss usually have two parents with normal hearing who are **carriers** of the recessive gene, resulting in a 25 percent chance of that gene being passed on with each pregnancy to the child who will manifest the hearing loss, and each normal-hearing child having a two in three chance of being a carrier.

Although both of a female's sex chromosomes (labeled X) carry considerable genetic information, called **X-linked,** the male sex chromosome (which is smaller and labeled Y) contains only the information required to produce the male sex. Many recessive alleles for hearing loss are X-linked, so that a female child receiving an allele for hearing loss from one parent will not show the trait; but a male child, not having the corresponding normal gene, will probably develop the hearing loss. A female who is heterozygous for an X-linked recessive hearing loss will not have a genetic hearing loss but will be a carrier and produce sons, each of whom will have a 50 percent chance of having the hearing loss, and daughters, each of whom will have a 50 percent chance of being a carrier. Males with X-linked hearing loss have sons who do not show the trait and daughters who would be carriers. **Multifactorial** hereditary disorders are the result of combinations of hereditary and environmental factors.

Cases of hereditary hearing loss have been documented in patients with no associated abnormalities, as well as in association with external ear, skull, and facial deformities; cleft palate; optic disorders; changes in eye, hair, and skin pigmentation; thyroid disease; disorders of the heart; musculoskeletal anomalies; mental retardation; difficulty with balance and coordination; and other sensory and motor deficits. Whenever a group of symptoms is considered together for the diagnosis of a particular disorder, such a combination of signs is called a **syndrome.**

At times, portions of the chromosomes are missing, or extra material is found. In some cases an extra (third) chromosome is present; this is called **trisomy.** In cases of chromosomal disorders, the parents may be perfectly normal, but the fetus may have difficulty in surviving the pregnancy or may be severely impaired. For reasons not entirely understood, women above the age of 40 show an increased risk of bearing children with trisomic chromosomal disorders, such as Down syndrome.

It is unknown how many disorders are determined entirely by heredity, but it is likely that genetics plays a major role in many conditions. As researchers perfect the science of gene mapping, the potential for altering the course of future diseases of all kinds brings an understandable excitement. Nevertheless, some medical ethicists fear that knowledge of an individual's susceptibility to a variety of conditions may carry with it a number of sociological dilemmas.

Different audiometric configurations have been suggested as *typical* of a given cause. There is, however, no unanimity on hereditary hearing loss, and clearly some cases may be moderate to severe bilateral losses with flat audiograms (Figure 11.9) or predominantly high-frequency or low-frequency patterns. Some losses have been described as typically unilateral.

Problems associated with the Rh baby have become fewer in recent years as physicians have learned to predict and prevent the disorders with maternal immunization and infant blood transfusion immediately after birth. The danger presents itself when a fetus whose blood contains the protein molecule called the **Rh factor** is conceived by a mother in whom the factor is absent. The mother's body produces antibodies for protection against the harmful effects of the Rh factor, and this antibody count is increased with succeeding pregnancies. Usually by the third pregnancy there is a sufficient number of antibodies so that the developing red blood cells of the fetus are damaged to the extent that they cannot properly carry oxygen to essential body parts, including the cochlea. In addition, the blood of the newborn child may carry bilirubin (a component of liver bile) in increased concentration, so that it may become deposited in the cochlea and produce a sensorineural hearing loss.

In addition to hearing loss, Rh incompatibility can result in a number of abnormalities in the newborn, including **cerebral palsy.** Cerebral palsy may be defined as damage to the brain, usually congenital, that affects the motor and frequently the sensory systems of the body. There are a number of causes of cerebral palsy, including the Rh factor, many of which are associated with sensorineural hearing loss. Athetotic cerebral palsy, or **athetosis,** wherein the patient exhibits an uncontrolled writhing or squirming motion, has long been associated with hearing loss. Until fairly recently it was assumed that because cerebral palsy is the result of brain damage, the hearing loss is also produced by damage in the central auditory nervous system. There is evidence that in many cases the damage may be cochlear. Because the hearing loss that accompanies athetotic cerebral palsy is often in the high frequencies, it may escape detection for years, masked by the more dramatic motor symptoms.

In the 1960s, thalidomide, a tranquilizing drug first used in Europe, was introduced to pregnant women. The drug was allegedly free from unwanted complications, but this lack of side effects was more apparent than real, as evidenced over time by the number of children born with horrible birth deformities to mothers who had taken the drug. The most dramatic symptom was missing or malformed arms and legs; in addition, although it was not generally known, disorders of hearing also afflicted a large number of the thalidomide babies. Because large quantities of drugs, both legal and illegal, are being consumed by women of child-bearing age, it is probable that future research will disclose that many of these also contribute to congenital hearing loss.

SPEECH AND HEARING CENTER
The University of Texas at Austin 78712
AUDIOMETRIC EXAMINATION

NAME: Last - First - Middle	SEX	AGE	DATE	EXAMINER	RELIABILITY	AUDIOMETER

AIR CONDUCTION

MASKING TYPE	RIGHT									LEFT								
	250	500	1000	1500	2000	3000	4000	6000	8000	250	500	1000	1500	2000	3000	4000	6000	8000
	40	45	50/50	50	55	60	60	60	65	40	40	50/50	55	60	60	65	65	65
EM Level in Opp. Ear																		

BONE CONDUCTION

MASKING TYPE	RIGHT						FOREHEAD						LEFT					
	250	500	1000	2000	3000	4000	250	500	1000	2000	3000	4000	250	500	1000	2000	3000	4000
							40	40	50	60	60	60						
EM Level in Opp. Ear																		

	2 Frequency	3 Frequency	WEBER		2 Frequency	3 Frequency
Pure Tone Average	48	50	M M M M M	Pure Tone Average	45	50

SPEECH AUDIOMETRY

MASKING TYPE	RIGHT				LEFT			
	SRT 1	SRT 2	Recognition 1	Recognition 2	SRT 1	SRT 2	Recognition 1	Recognition 2
	50		1A List 30 SL 84 %	List SL %	45		2A List 30 SL 78 %	List SL %
EM Level in Opp. Ear								

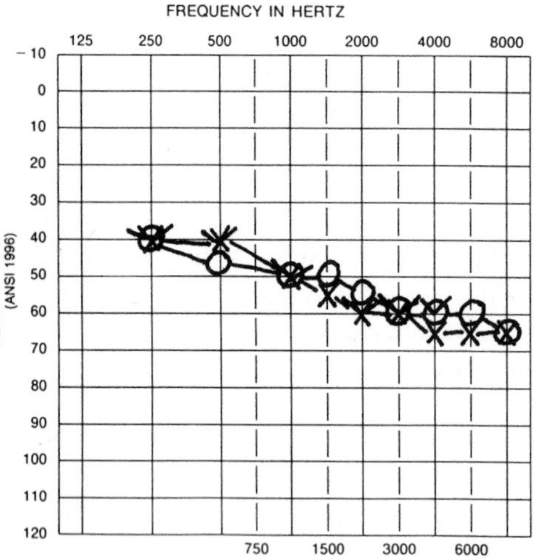

FREQUENCY IN HERTZ   COMMENTS

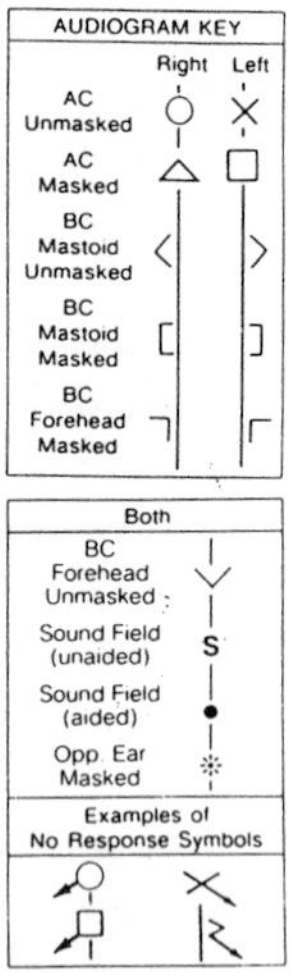

FIGURE 11.9 Audiogram showing a moderate sensorineural hearing loss in both ears. The contour of the audiogram is relatively flat, which suggests approximately equal hearing loss at all frequencies. The SRTs and pure-tone averages are in close agreement, and the word-recognition scores show some difficulty in understanding speech. Masking is not required for any of the tests.

Although a pregnant woman must always be fearful of contracting a viral disease, the fear is greatest during the first trimester (three months) of pregnancy, when the cells of the inner ear and central nervous system are differentiating most rapidly. For many years probably the most dreaded viral infection was rubella, or German measles, as it is one of the few viruses that cross the placental barrier. Although this disease was known to be mild, or even asymptomatic in the patient, the effects on the fetus may be devastating.

Epidemics of rubella were seen to occur every six to nine years, the latest one being in 1964–1965, with a reported 12.5 million cases and 20,000 infants born with Congenital Rubella Syndrome (CRS). The introduction of a vaccine in 1969 reduced the number of reported cases drastically, although there have been several resurgences through the years, mostly among the poor and religious groups that forbid vaccination. Statistics in developing countries are not readily available, so CRS continues to be a health threat.

Rubella babies tend to be smaller at birth and to develop more slowly than normal infants. They are shorter, weigh less, and have head circumferences that are less than normal. Common results of maternal rubella are brain damage, blindness, heart defects, mental retardation, and sensorineural hearing loss. The rubella hearing-impaired child presents special difficulties in habilitation and education because of the probability of multiple disorders.

Viral infections may actually kill or destroy cells, or they may slow down the rate at which each cell can divide and reproduce by mitosis. The rubella baby has normal-sized cells, but fewer of them. It is not always clear whether the virus has affected the fetus by crossing the placental barrier, or by contagion during the birth process. As the maternal body temperature increases in response to a viral or other infection, the oxygen requirement of the fetus increases dramatically. Oxygen deprivation is called **anoxia,** and may result in damage to important cells of the cochlea.

Of all the congenital abnormalities produced by maternal rubella in the first trimester of pregnancy, hearing loss is the most common (Karmody, 1969). The main development of the cochlea occurs during the sixth fetal week and of the organ of Corti at the twelfth week, making these critically susceptible times.

It is highly likely that the virus enters the inner ear through the stria vascularis, which would explain why the cochlea, rather than the vestibular apparatus, is usually affected. Alford (1968) has suggested that the rubella virus remains in the tissues of the cochlea even after birth. If destruction of cochlear tissue continues, the child may experience a form of progressive hearing loss that might not be associated with a prenatal cause.

In recent years there has been a major focus on the **acquired immune deficiency syndrome (AIDS)** and on the **human immunodeficiency virus (HIV)** found in those with AIDS. Mothers with HIV have a 50 percent chance of delivering a baby with the disease (Lawrence, 1987). How HIV affects the cochlea and the incidence with which this occurs are not known, although long-term treatment with corticosteroids has resulted in the reversal of some hearing losses and arrest in the progression of others. Viral infections in the unborn are far more likely to occur when the mother suffers from a disease causing deficiency in her immune system.

Probably a major cause of prenatal sensorineural hearing loss is **cytomegalovirus (CMV),** a seemingly harmless, and often asymptomatic illness, which is a member of the herpes group of viruses. The cause of the problem is an infection called cytomegalic inclusion disease (CID). When the developing fetus is infected, a variety of physical symptoms may be present, in addition to hearing loss. About 31 percent of infants infected with CMV have a serious hearing loss (Johnson, Hosford-Dunn, Paryani, Yeager, & Malachowski, 1986).

Cytomegalovirus maybe transmitted from mother to child in several ways:

1. *Prenatally:* It may be transmitted through the placenta.
2. *Perinatally:* The infant may contract the virus from the cervix of an infected mother during the birth process.
3. *Postnatally:* The virus may be transmitted in infected mother's milk.

When CMV is acquired perinatally or postnatally, there are usually no serious side effects in the child. Unlike rubella, CMV does not warn an expectant mother with a telltale rash or other symptoms. Another difference is that at present there is no vaccine to prevent CMV.

Perinatal Causes

Perinatal causes of hearing loss are those that occur during the process of birth itself. Such causes frequently produce multiple handicaps.

A common cause of damage both to the cochlea and to the central nervous system is anoxia, deprivation of oxygen to important cells, which alters their metabolism and results in damage or destruction. In the newborn, anoxia may result from prolapse of the umbilical cord, which cuts off the blood supply to the head; from premature separation of the placenta; or from a wide variety of other factors.

Accumulations of toxic substances in the mother's bloodstream may reduce the passage of oxygen across the placenta, which also results in anoxia. The fetus may also suffer from damage produced by the toxic substances themselves. For this reason, pregnant women should cautiously avoid exposure to contagious diseases, such as hepatitis.

Prematurity is determined by the weight of the child at the time of birth, and not necessarily by the length of the pregnancy, as the word itself suggests. When infants weigh less than 1500 grams (3.5 pounds) at birth, they are considered premature. Prematurity is often associated with multiple births, and both are associated with sensorineural hearing loss.

It is common practice to place premature infants in incubators so that, at least for the early days of life, their environments can be carefully controlled. Care must be taken not to overadminister oxygen because this produces retinal defects. Some motors operating incubators have been found to produce extremely high noise levels (up to 95 dB SPL). Hearing losses in children thus treated may have been produced by noise, rather than, or in addition to, the results and causes of prematurity.

Trauma to the fetal head, either by violent uterine contractions or by the use of "high forceps" during delivery, may also result in damage to the brain and to the cochlea. It is possible that the head trauma itself does not produce the damage; instead, the initial cause of the difficulty in delivery may be the cause of the hearing loss.

Postnatal Causes

Postnatal causes of cochlear hearing loss are any factors occurring after birth. An often-named cause is otitis media. The toxins from the bacteria in the middle ear may enter the inner ear by way of the round or oval window, or pus may enter the labyrinth from the middle ear or from the meninges, the protective covers of the brain and spinal cord. **Meningitis,** inflammation of the meninges, may cause total deafness, because if the labyrinth fills with pus, as healing takes place, the membranes and other loosely attached structures of the labyrinth are replaced by bone. Early treatment with corticosteroids may arrest the hearing loss before it becomes severe. If the enzymes produced by the infectious process enter the cochlea by diffusion through the round window, a hearing loss will surely result. Often, patients with primarily conductive hearing losses produced by otitis media begin to show additional cochlear degeneration, resulting in **mixed hearing loss** (Figure 11.10).

Some viral infections have definitely been identified as the causative factors in cochlear hearing loss. These infections include measles, mumps, chicken pox, influenza, and viral pneumonia, among others. The two most common are measles and mumps. Rubeola, the 10-day variety of measles, carries a significantly greater threat to the patient than does rubella. Rubeola may cause a sudden hearing loss that may not begin until some time after the other symptoms disappear.

Most virus-produced hearing losses are bilateral, but some viral infections, notably mumps, are associated with unilateral losses as well. Everberg (1957) estimates an incidence of hearing loss from mumps at 0.05 per 1000 in the general population. Although the precise mechanism producing hearing loss from mumps is not clear, it seems likely that the route of infection is the bloodstream. Other theories, such as general infection of the labyrinth, would not explain why vestibular symptoms are frequently absent.

A disease once thought to be on the decrease, but now recognized as quite the opposite, is syphilis. This disease may be prenatal or acquired, and it often goes through three distinct but overlapping stages. Because its symptoms may resemble those of a number of different systemic diseases, it has been called the "great imitator." Brain damage is a frequent sequela of syphilis, but the cochlea may also be involved. A number of bizarre audiometric patterns have been associated with syphilis, and the variations are so great that a typical pattern does not emerge.

Infections of the labyrinth are called **labyrinthitis,** and may affect both the auditory and vestibular mechanisms, producing symptoms of hearing loss and vertigo. The causes of labyrinthitis are not always known, and the condition is frequently confused with other causes of hearing loss; however, tuberculosis, syphilis, cholesteatoma, or viral infection may be the cause.

The body's natural response to infection is elevation of temperature. When the fevers become excessive, however, cells, including those of the cochlea, may become damaged. Sometimes children run high fevers with no apparent cause, but with ensuing hearing loss. When such histories are clear-cut, it is tempting to blame the fever, even when it would be logical to suspect the initial cause of the fever, such as a viral infection, as the real cause. In many cases, diagnosis of the primary cause of a hearing loss is mere speculation.

Infections of the kidneys may result in the deposit of toxic substances in the inner ear. Kidney disease may prevent medications from being excreted, thereby raising their levels in the blood abnormally high and introducing ototoxicity. Other illnesses, including diabetes, have also been directly linked to cochlear damage.

Toxic Causes of Cochlear Hearing Loss

It has been said that progress has its side effects. This is notably true of the side effects of antibiotics, the wonder drugs that have saved many lives in the last six decades. Most noted among the drugs that are cochleotoxic (i.e., cause hearing loss) are dihydrostreptomycin, viomycin, neomycin, and kanamycin. Because hearing losses ranging from mild to profound may result from the use of these drugs, it is hoped that they are not prescribed unless it is fairly certain that other drugs, with fewer or less severe side effects, will not be just as efficacious. Vestibulotoxic drugs (those that are known to affect the vestibular organs) include streptomycin and gentamycin.

SPEECH AND HEARING CENTER
The University of Texas at Austin 78712
AUDIOMETRIC EXAMINATION

NAME: Last - First - Middle	SEX	AGE	DATE	EXAMINER	RELIABILITY	AUDIOMETER

AIR CONDUCTION

MASKING TYPE	RIGHT									LEFT								
	250	500	1000	1500	2000	3000	4000	6000	8000	250	500	1000	1500	2000	3000	4000	6000	8000
N B	60	65	70/70	70	75	80	80	85	85	55	55	60/60	60	60	70	75	75	70
	60*									55*								
EM Level in Opp. Ear	55									60								

BONE CONDUCTION

MASKING TYPE	RIGHT						FOREHEAD						LEFT					
	250	500	1000	2000	3000	4000	250	500	1000	2000	3000	4000	250	500	1000	2000	3000	4000
N B	15	25	35	50	55	55	15	25	35	50	55	55	20	35	45	50	55	55
EM Level in Opp. Ear	55	55	60	60	70	75							75	85	90	75	80	80

		2 Frequency	3 Frequency	WEBER					2 Frequency	3 Frequency
	Pure Tone Average	68	70					Pure Tone Average	57	58

SPEECH AUDIOMETRY

MASKING TYPE	RIGHT					LEFT				
	SRT 1	SRT 2	Recognition 1	Recognition 2		SRT 1	SRT 2	Recognition 1	Recognition 2	
			List SL	List SL				List SL	List SL	
W B	70	70*	1A 30 / 80* %	/ %		60	60*	2A 30 / 76 %	/ %	
EM Level in Opp. Ear		60	85				70	85		

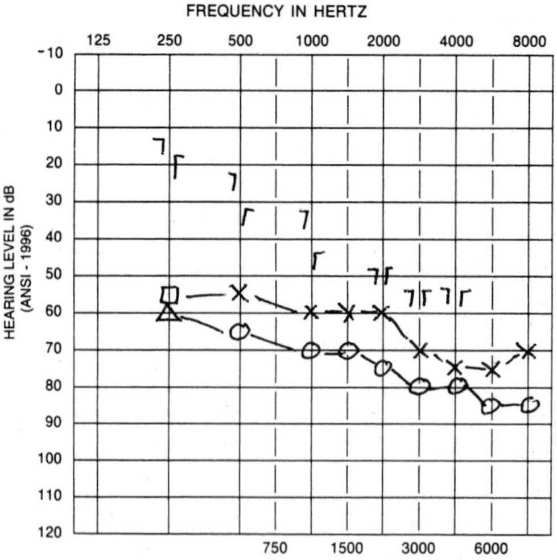

FREQUENCY IN HERTZ   COMMENTS

AUDIOGRAM KEY

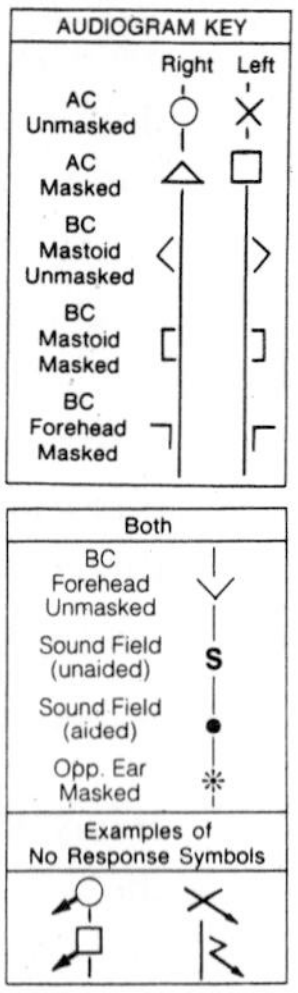

FIGURE 11.10 Audiogram showing a mixed hearing loss in both ears. Repeating bone conduction with masking was indicated because of the air-bone gaps. The sensorineural component of the loss is reflected by the impaired word recognition.

Tuberculosis, which only a short time ago was declining in frequency, is experiencing a resurgence. Not only does this disease cause cochlear hearing loss, but when the prolonged use of **ototoxic** drugs is mandatory, such as in tuberculosis sanitaria, the patient's hearing should be monitored frequently so that any loss of hearing, or its progression, may be noted. In such cases, decisions regarding continued use of the medication must be made on the basis of the specific needs of the patient. Although the final decision on drug use is always made by a physician, it is within the purview of audiologists to make their concerns over hearing loss known.

Quinine is a drug that has long been used to combat malaria and to fight fever and reduce the pain of the common cold. Many patients who have taken this drug have complained of annoying tinnitus and hearing loss. Although with less frequency, quinine is still prescribed for certain disorders and continues to be marketed as an over-the-counter medication.

Other drugs that have been associated with hearing loss include aspirin, certain diuretics, nicotine, and alcohol. It is usually expected that these drugs will not affect hearing unless they are taken in large amounts and over prolonged periods of time. Certainly there are many individuals who appear to consume these substances in what might be considered excess with no side effects. The individual's own constitutional predispositions must surely be a factor here.

For some time it has been recognized that hearing loss from ototoxic drugs initially occurs, in most cases, in the high-frequency range (Jacobson, Downs, & Fletcher, 1969). Thus, physicians prescribing potentially ototoxic drugs often have time to consider alternate medications before the hearing loss encroaches on the frequencies that are more essential to discriminating speech. One of the difficulties in testing ultra-audiometric frequencies (above 8000 Hz) has been the interference patterns that are set up when pure tones with short wavelengths are presented to the external auditory canal. Even slight differences in placement of the earphone may cause difficulty. That problem has been lessened with the use of insert earphones (Valente, Valente, & Goebel, 1992). Using extended high-frequency audiometry can detect early hearing loss from noise, chemotherapy, kidney disease, otitis media, as well as ototoxicity, and can be helpful in understanding some causes of tinnitus in patients who have normal hearing through the normal frequency range.

ASHA (1994) has published guidelines for monitoring patients who receive cochleotoxic drugs. Elements of these guidelines include:

1. Specific criteria for identification of toxicity
2. Timely identification of at-risk patients
3. Pretreatment counseling regarding potential cochleotoxic effects
4. Valid baseline measures (hearing tests) performed before treatment or shortly after treatment begins
5. Periodic monitoring evaluations at intervals timed to document progression of hearing loss
6. Follow-up evaluations to determine post-treatment effects.

Otosclerosis

As mentioned in Chapter 10, otosclerosis is a disease of the bony labyrinth that causes a conductive hearing loss when the new bone growth affects either the oval window or the round window. If the otosclerosis involves the cochlea, sensorineural hearing loss results, which may be either bilateral or unilateral. Although there are no binding rules, the audiometric configuration is generally flat, and word recognition is not severely affected. Attempts have been made to arrest the progression of cochlear otosclerosis with sodium fluoride, but the effectiveness of this treatment has not been proved.

Barotrauma

Barotrauma was mentioned as a cause of conductive hearing loss. In addition, sudden changes in middle-ear pressure, as from diving, flying, or even violent sneezing, may cause a rupture in the round window, or a tearing of the annulus of the oval window. The resulting fistula (perilymph leak) can often be surgically repaired, and may reverse a permanent or fluctuating cochlear hearing loss and/or vertigo. Barotrauma may produce a mild-to-profound hearing loss.

Noise-induced Hearing Loss

The Industrial Revolution's introduction of high levels of noise brought a greater threat to the human auditory system than evolution had prepared for. Documented cases of noise-induced hearing loss go back more than 200 years. Hearing losses from intense noise may be the result of brief exposure to high-level sounds, with subsequent partial or complete hearing recovery, or repeated exposure to high-level sounds, with permanent impairment. Cases in which hearing thresholds improve after an initial impairment following noise are said to be the result of **temporary threshold shift (TTS);** irreversible losses are called **permanent threshold shift (PTS).**

A number of agents may interact with noise to increase the danger to hearing sensitivity. Research has shown that aspirin, which has been known to produce reversible hearing loss after ingestion, synergizes with noise to produce a greater temporary threshold shift than would otherwise be observed (McFadden & Plattsmier, 1983). Although the effects of aspirin on permanent hearing loss have not been demonstrated, it certainly seems prudent for audiologists to advise that people who must be exposed to high levels of noise should refrain from taking this drug, at least at times closely related to exposure.

Although controversy continues over many aspects of noise-induced hearing loss, certain facts are generally agreed on. Men appear to have a higher incidence of hearing loss from noise than do women (Ewertson, 1973), perhaps because as a group they have greater noise exposure, both on the job and during leisure activities. There is evidence that children are suffering increased amounts of hearing loss from such objects as toy phones, musical instruments, firecrackers, stereo systems, and firearm toys, some of which produce noise levels up to 155 dBA (Nadler, 1997). The fact that children's arms are shorter than adults' results in anything noisy held in the hand being closer to the ear.

Postmortem electron microscope studies have shown loss of hair cells and their supporting structures in the basal end of the cochlea and nerve degeneration in the osseous lamina (Johnson & Hawkins, 1976) in patients with noise-induced hearing loss. The hearing loss may be due to biological changes in the sensory cells, physical dislodging of hair cells during hyperacoustic stimulation, changes in the cochlear blood supply with consequent alterations in the function of the stria vascularis, loss of the outer hair cells, rupture of Reissner's membrane, detachment of the organ of Corti from the basilar membrane, or a variety of other causes.

Acoustic trauma is the term often used to describe noise-induced hearing loss from impulsive sounds, such as explosions. A typical audiometric configuration has emerged, shown in Figure 11.11, depicting what has been called the **acoustic trauma notch.** Characteristically, the hearing is poorest in the range between 3000 and 6000 Hz, with recovery at 8000 Hz, suggesting damage to the

SPEECH AND HEARING CENTER
The University of Texas at Austin 78712
AUDIOMETRIC EXAMINATION

NAME: Last - First - Middle		SEX	AGE	DATE	EXAMINER	RELIABILITY	AUDIOMETER

AIR CONDUCTION

MASKING TYPE	RIGHT									LEFT								
	250	500	1000	1500	2000	3000	4000	6000	8000	250	500	1000	1500	2000	3000	4000	6000	8000
	5	0	5/5	5	10	25	60	35	20	0	0	5/5	10	20	40	70	55	25
EM Level in Opp. Ear																		

BONE CONDUCTION

MASKING TYPE	RIGHT						FOREHEAD						LEFT					
	250	500	1000	2000	3000	4000	250	500	1000	2000	3000	4000	250	500	1000	2000	3000	4000
							0	5	5	15	35	65						
EM Level in Opp. Ear																		

	2 Frequency	3 Frequency		WEBER				2 Frequency	3 Frequency
Pure Tone Average	3	5					Pure Tone Average	3	8

SPEECH AUDIOMETRY

MASKING TYPE	RIGHT				LEFT			
	SRT 1	SRT 2	Recognition 1	Recognition 2	SRT 1	SRT 2	Recognition 1	Recognition 2
	5		4C List 30 SL 96 %	List SL %	5		5C List 30 SL 94 %	List SL %
EM Level in Opp. Ear								

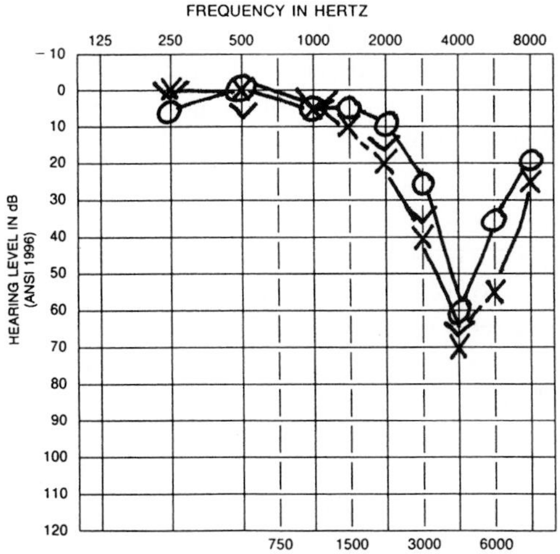

FREQUENCY IN HERTZ

COMMENTS

AUDIOGRAM KEY

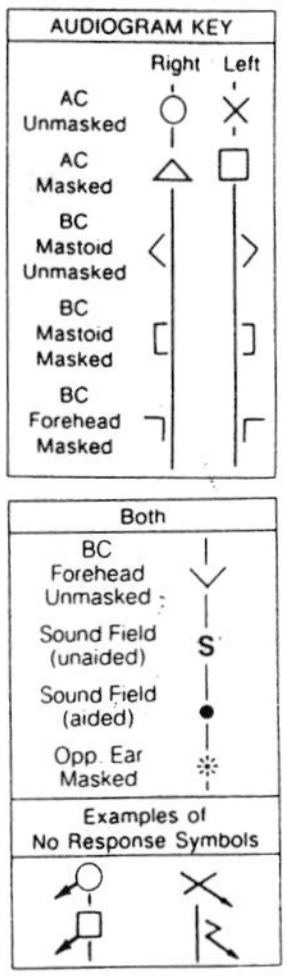

FIGURE 11.11 Audiogram showing a typical acoustic trauma notch at 4000 Hz. SRTs and WRSs are normal showing little difficulty in quiet because the hearing loss is primarily above the critical frequency range for hearing and understanding speech. It can be expected that the patient experiences considerable difficulty in understanding speech in the presence of background noise.

portion of the basal turn of the cochlea related to that frequency range. As a rule, the amounts of hearing loss are similar in both ears when individuals acquire noise-induced hearing losses in the workplace. Rifle shooters generally show more hearing loss in the ear opposite the shoulder to which the rifle stock is held; that is, right-handed shooters will have more hearing loss in the left ear. A survey in Canada on noise-induced hearing loss in truck drivers revealed greater loss in the left ear, probably produced by the rush of air past the open window on the driver's side (Dufresne, Alleyne, & Reesal, 1988).

The acoustic trauma notch is not found in all cases of noise-induced hearing loss, nor is it restricted to this cause. It is, however, strongly suggestive of noise and should be corroborated with supporting evidence, such as the clinical history. If noise-induced hearing loss is suspected, hearing should always be tested at 3000 and 6000 Hz, even if sensitivity at adjacent octave and midoctave frequencies is normal.

Industrial noise is a factor long recognized as a cause of hearing loss. The term *boilermaker's disease* was coined many years ago to describe the hearing losses sustained by men working in the noisy environs of that industry. Although boilermakers may be fewer in number today, modern technology has produced new and even noisier industries. Exposure to jet engines, drop forges, pneumatic hammers, subways, loud music, and even computers, has been documented as causing hearing loss. A study of the effects of noise on hearing (Rosen, Bergman, Plester, El-Mofty, & Hammed, 1962) has shown that older populations in societies that have lower noise-exposure levels, exhibit better hearing sensitivity than do those populations in other societies. Of course, differences in diet, lifestyle, and so on may also account for the better hearing sensitivity of the older members of more primitive societies.

Noise in society is an ever-increasing problem. Millions of dollars are paid to military veterans in compensation for hearing loss. Insurance companies, whose coverage includes noisy industries, have been forced to become increasingly concerned with the effects of noise on hearing. Aside from the psychological, social, and vocational handicaps imposed on patients with noise-induced hearing loss, the financial figures have led to concern on the part of government and industry alike.

After a number of proposals, lawsuits, and reversals, the Occupational Safety and Health Administration (OSHA) (1983) has recommended a scale on which the time that a worker may be safely exposed to intense sounds is decreased, as the intensity of the noise is increased. Under this rule, the maximum exposure level is 85 dBA for an eight-hour work day. For every 5 dB increase in noise, half the time is allowed—for example, four hours for 90 dBA, two hours for 95 dBA, one hour for 100 dBA, 30 minutes for 105 dBA, and so on.

Sound-level meters, or individually worn noise dosimeters, are used to measure the intensity of sound in noisy areas, such as in factories and around aircraft, to determine whether the noise levels fall within or exceed the **damage-risk criteria** set up by OSHA (1983). Lipscomb (1992) points out that readings from noise dosimeters can be misleading and can appear substantially different, depending on how the instrument is set. Hearing conservation is really not an area in which audiologists can merely dabble without the proper background and knowledge.

Because of the increasing interest in noise-induced hearing loss in industry, numbers of hearing-conservation programs have developed in the United States and around the world. Lipscomb (1992) defines a comprehensive hearing conservation program (HCP) as one that (1) identifies people who are at risk for noise-induced hearing loss, (2) abates dangerous noise levels as economically as possible, and (3) protects employees who are at risk for noise-induced hearing loss.

Workers are being advised about the dangers of noise and are encouraged to wear hearing protectors, such as those shown in Figures 11.12 and 11.13. It is likely that hearing protectors may pro-

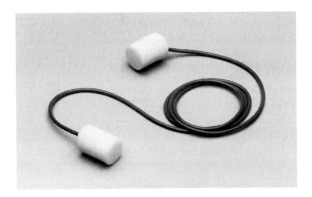

FIGURE 11.12   Commercial ear plugs designed to attenuate high noise levels. (Courtesy of E.A.R. Division of Cabot Corp.)

vide a false sense of security, assuring wearers that they are "safe" from noise damage. However, many problems are associated with fitting and wearing hearing protectors, and the amount of sound attenuation found in the laboratory may be considerably more than that actually obtained on the job (Berger, 1988). The more experience individuals have in fitting earplugs in their own ears, the greater the sound attenuation provided (Merry, Sizemore, & Franks, 1992). Audiologists should warn hearing aid users that the hollow shell of a turned-off hearing aid provides little effective protection.

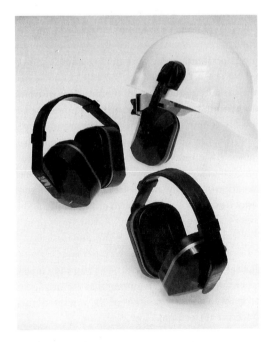

FIGURE 11.13   Commercial ear muffs designed to be worn in areas of intense noise. (Courtesy of E.A.R. Division of Cabot Corp.)

Many preemployment physical examinations now include pure-tone audiometry, but OSHA (1983) requires the first test to be carried out within six months of employment. After that, annual tests (defined as no further apart than 15 months) must be made. Routine tests may be contaminated by recent noise exposure, and the amount of temporary threshold shift and time to recovery is determined, in large part, by the intensity of the previous exposure. According to Melnick (1984), some TTS does not recover for a week or even longer.

The amount of hearing loss shown by a person exposed to high noise levels in the workplace can vary for many reasons. Genetic factors are always a consideration, as are disease, aging, and noise exposure off the job site. The insidious nature of noise-induced hearing loss often results in long delays before the onset of hearing problems and consultation with a hearing specialist.

A surprising amount of the noise-induced hearing loss seen today is caused by other than work-related activities. Many millions of people are engaged in hobbies involving motor boats, snowmobiles, motor bikes, and race cars, in addition to the use of guns. The term "recreational audiology" has been coined to describe the activities of professionals involved in finding these hearing losses and taking appropriate precautionary steps. Exposure to intense sounds by professional musicians has caused a special concern for this group. Musicians generally rely more on the sense of hearing than many others who suffer from noise-induced hearing loss and may spend many hours a day exposed to intense sounds. Data are only beginning to appear in the literature about hearing loss that may have been caused by deploying air bags in automobiles. More research is required in this area.

A patient with apparent noise-induced hearing loss should be advised to limit exposure to loud noise and to use protective earplugs or muffs whenever exposure is necessary. Periodic hearing examinations to monitor progression should also be encouraged. Hunters, target shooters, and snow-mobile drivers are often a particularly difficult group to work with because of their reluctance either to wear hearing protectors or to limit their sport. Music enthusiasts who use stereo headphones or portable stereo systems are often at risk for hearing loss because of the high levels of sound delivered directly to their ears. Special hearing protection that does not distort sound quality is available for musicians.

Often, initial examination of hearing is made on the basis of a complaint of tinnitus alone. In patients with an acoustic trauma notch, the tinnitus is often described as a pure tone and can be matched to frequencies in the 3000 to 6000 Hz range. Many such patients are unaware of the existence of hearing loss and may even deny it. By the time progression of the impairment has been demonstrated to patients, their communicative difficulties have worsened considerably. The persuasiveness and tact of the audiologist in counseling such patients is of paramount importance.

There is increasing evidence that in addition to hearing loss, noise has other adverse effects. Noise may play a role in increased anxiety levels, loss of the ability to concentrate, and loss of sleep.

Cochlear Hearing Loss Following Surgical Complications

There are times when even the best middle-ear surgeon not only fails to improve hearing with corrective surgery but, in fact, makes it worse. Many otologists estimate that the chance of a cochlear hearing loss following stapedectomy is probable in 1 or 2 percent of the operated population. The odds appear very good, except, of course, for the unfortunate few.

Postoperative infections are rare today, although they may occur. An early practice during stapedectomy was to move the ossicular chain following stapedectomy to check for a light reflex on the round window to ensure mobility. This is no longer done because it has been found to generate traveling waves of an amplitude greater than most environmental sounds that can cause cochlear damage.

Excessive bleeding, or other surgical complications, may account for some cases of cochlear hearing loss following middle-ear surgery, but some cases of even total hearing loss in the ear operated on cannot be related to any specific cause. A number of technically perfect operations are also followed by total deafness of the operated ear. Evidently, for specific physiological reasons, some patients do not tolerate the surgery well. It is to this group that the term *fragile ears* has been assigned, and it is unfortunate that these cases cannot be predicted preoperatively. Common complications of middle-ear surgery include transitory vertigo and alterations in the sense of taste.

Vasospasm of the Internal Auditory Artery

The nutrition of the cochlea is supplied by the stria vascularis, which is fed by the internal auditory artery, with no collateral blood supply. If a spasm occurs in that artery, total unilateral deafness may result. For this reason, sudden loss of hearing in one ear should be treated as a medical emergency, with therapy directed at vasodilation. Naturally, the sooner therapy is instituted following the onset of symptoms, the better is the prognosis for complete recovery. Such treatment of **vasospasm** often includes hospitalization, with intravenous administration of the appropriate medications. At times, hearing recovery is complete. Vestibular symptoms, such as vertigo and nausea as well as the often-accompanying tinnitus, may also abate. In some patients symptoms disappear spontaneously, whereas in others symptoms persist in the form of severe or total unilateral hearing loss.

Méniére Disease

Another cause of sudden unilateral hearing loss is **Méniére disease.**[5] The seat of the difficulty lies within the labyrinth. The disorder is characterized by sudden attacks of vertigo, tinnitus, vomiting, and unilateral hearing loss. Bilateral Méniére disease has been observed in 5 to 10 percent of the cases of aural vertigo studied.

The onset of symptoms is described by many patients in the same way. The difficulty may begin with a sensation of fullness in one ear, followed by a low-frequency roaring tinnitus, hearing loss, with great difficulty in speech recognition, the sensation of violent turning or whirling in space, and vomiting.

Many authorities believe that Méniére disease is caused by endolymphatic hydrops, the oversecretion or underabsorption of endolymph. As the fluid pressure builds in the cochlear duct, the pressure on the hair cells produces the tinnitus and hearing loss. If the pressure builds sufficiently, the vestibular apparatus becomes overstimulated, and vertigo ensues. One excellent procedure for diagnosing Méniére disease is the **glycerol test.** Pure-tone thresholds and word-recognition scores are measured, after which the patient is asked to drink six ounces of a mixture of 50 percent glucose and water. These audiometric procedures are repeated after a three-hour wait. Because glycerol acts as a diuretic, increasing urinary output, the fluid pressure in the labyrinth is expected to drop temporarily, resulting in improved pure-tone thresholds of at least 10 dB at three frequencies in the 250 to 4000 Hz range and an improvement of at least 12 percent in word-recognition scores (Klockhoff, 1976).

---

[5]Named for Prosper Méniére, French physician, 1799–1862, who first described this syndrome.

According to Lawrence (1969), excessive endolymphatic pressure alone could not alter the function of the inner ear unless the metabolic or ionic balances were disturbed, as by a rupture of Reissner's membrane. Treatment is usually designed to limit fluid retention through diuretic drugs and the decrease of sodium intake in the diet. Sedatives, tranquilizers, and vestibular suppressants have all been used. Reports on the success rates of different therapies vary in the medical literature; some have even been ascribed as placebo effects. Anxiety and allergic factors have been considered as causes of Méniére disease, which affects more men than women and rarely affects children. Other causes may be trauma, surgery, syphilis, hypothyroidism, and low blood sugar.

Méniére disease may be extremely handicapping. The paroxysmal (sudden, without warning) attacks of vertigo may interfere with driving an automobile, or even with performing one's job. Cases of bilateral hearing loss due to Méniére disease are helped best with multi-memory hearing aids, which offer more than one pattern of amplification to address fluctuating hearing loss. The disease has been called the "labyrinthine storm," because of the sudden and dramatic appearance of symptoms; it is characterized by remissions and exacerbations.

Surgical approaches to Méniére disease are often aimed at decompressing the endolymphatic sac or draining the excessive endolymph by inserting a shunt into spaces in the skull so that the fluid can be excreted along with cerebrospinal fluid. Ultrasonic and freezing procedures have also been used. In extreme cases, the entire labyrinth has been surgically destroyed or the auditory nerve cut to alleviate the vertigo and tinnitus. Even such dramatic steps as these are not always entirely successful. Audiometric findings in Méniére disease are shown in Figures 11.14 through 11.18. Absent otoacoustic emissions are typical of cochlear lesions as well. Specific diagnosis of this condition can often be accomplished with electrocochleography (Ferraro, 1992).

Head Trauma

Often when a hearing loss is directly related to a head injury, the audiogram is quite similar to those typical of acoustic trauma, showing a "notch" in the 3000 to 4000 Hz range.

In addition to damage to the tympanic membrane and middle-ear mechanism, the structures of the inner ear may be torn, stretched, or deteriorated from the loss of oxygen following hemorrhage. If a fracture line runs through the cochlea, the resulting hearing loss will be severe to profound, and may be total. External and/or internal hair cells may be lost, and the organ of Corti may be flattened or destroyed. Trauma to the skull may also result in complications such as otitis media or meningitis, which may themselves be the cause of a hearing loss. Hearing loss may result from head trauma, even without fracture, if there is a contusion of the cochlea, or if a strong pressure wave is conducted through the skull to the cochlea (Schuknecht, 1993). This may be ipsilateral or contralateral to the skull insult.

Head injuries, acoustic trauma, diving accidents, or overexertion may cause rupture of the round window membrane, or a fistula of the oval window with a perilymph leak into the middle ear. When there is the possibility of a fluid leak, the fistula test, using an immittance meter as described in Chapter 6, can be of great assistance in medical diagnosis.

Presbycusis

The caseload of any audiology clinic will include a large number of patients who have no contributing etiological factors to hearing loss except advancing age. It would be inaccurate to assume

SPEECH AND HEARING CENTER
The University of Texas at Austin 78712
AUDIOMETRIC EXAMINATION

NAME: Last - First - Middle	SEX	AGE	DATE	EXAMINER	RELIABILITY	AUDIOMETER

AIR CONDUCTION

MASKING TYPE	RIGHT									LEFT								
	250	500	1000	1500	2000	3000	4000	6000	8000	250	500	1000	1500	2000	3000	4000	6000	8000
NB	45	50	45/45	50	55	55	60	65	60	10	5	5/5	5	0	5	10	16	5
	45	50	45	50	55	55	60	65	60									
EM Level in Opp. Ear	30	25	20	20	20	20	25	25	25									

BONE CONDUCTION

MASKING TYPE	RIGHT						FOREHEAD						LEFT					
	250	500	1000	2000	3000	4000	250	500	1000	2000	3000	4000	250	500	1000	2000	3000	4000
NB	45	45	45	55	55	60	10	5	5	0	5	15						
EM Level in Opp. Ear	55	40	30	15	20	25												

	2 Frequency	3 Frequency	WEBER							2 Frequency	3 Frequency
Pure Tone Average	48	50	∠	∠	∠	∠	∠	∠	Pure Tone Average	3	3

SPEECH AUDIOMETRY

MASKING TYPE	RIGHT				LEFT			
	SRT 1	SRT 2	Recognition 1	Recognition 2	SRT 1	SRT 2	Recognition 1	Recognition 2
WB	50	50*	List 1A SL 30 / 70 %	List SL / %	5		List 2A SL 30 / 100 %	List SL / %
EM Level in Opp. Ear		5	35					

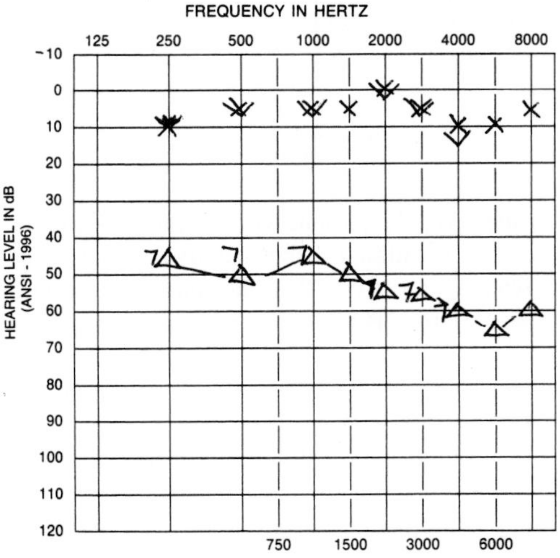

FREQUENCY IN HERTZ

COMMENTS

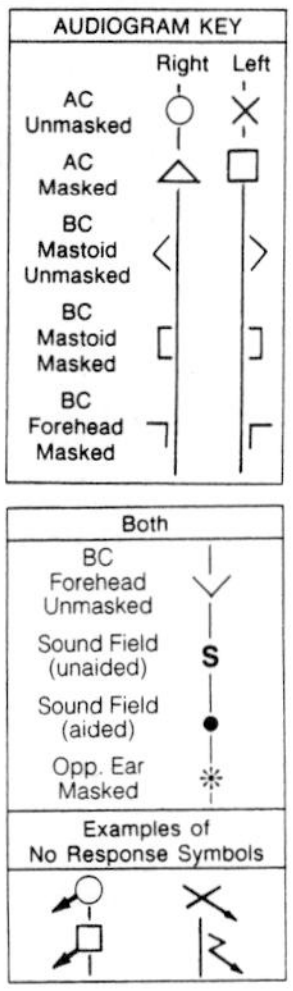

FIGURE 11.14 Audiogram showing a unilateral (right) sensorineural hearing loss observed in a patient with Méniére disease. Word recognition is impaired in the right ear. This case points up the great need for proper masking on all tests performed on the right ear.

SPEECH AND HEARING CENTER
The University of Texas at Austin 78712

IMMITTANCE

NAME: Last - First - Middle		SEX	AGE	DATE	EXAMINER	INSTRUMENT

PRESSURE/COMPLIANCE FUNCTION

	– 400	– 350	– 300	– 250	– 200	– 150	– 100	– 50	0	+ 50	+ 100	+ 150	+ 200
Right					.44	.48	.50	.72	.80	.71	.50	.44	.40
Left					.55	.59	.68	.87	.96	.86	.64	.52	.45

STATIC COMPLIANCE $C_x = C_2 - C_1$

RIGHT					LEFT			
.40	C_1	.80	C_2	.40	C_x	.45	C_1	.96	C_2	.51	C_x

ACOUSTIC REFLEXES

	RIGHT				LEFT			
Frequency (Hz)	500	1000	2000	4000	500	1000	2000	4000
Ipsilateral (Probe same)		90	90			95	100	
Contralateral (Probe opposite)	95	90	100	100	85	85	90	95
Audiometric Threshold	50	45	55	60	5	5	0	10
Reflex SL	45	45	45	40	80	80	90	85
Decay Time (Seconds)	10^+	10^+			10^+	10^+		

TYMPANOGRAM

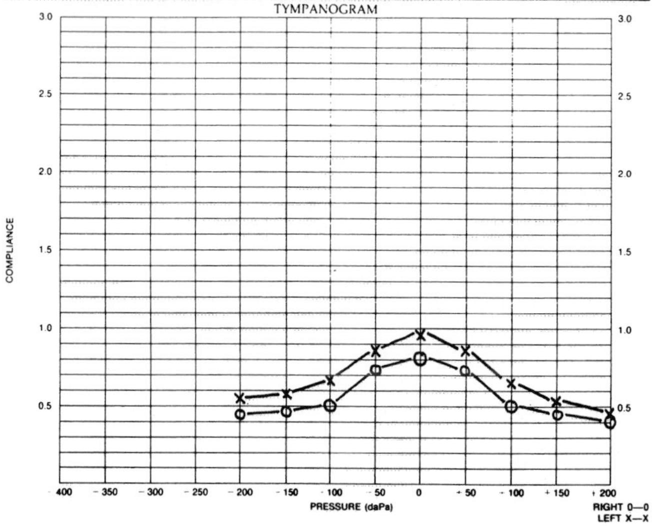

RIGHT 0—0
LEFT X—X
PRESSURE (daPa)

FIGURE 11.15   Results on immittance measures for the patient with Méniére disease, illustrated in Figure 11.14. The tympanogram in the left ear is normal, but shows a lower point of maximum compliance on the right ear because of increased pressure in the inner ear. Static compliance is lower in the right ear than in the left. The sensation level of the acoustic reflex is reduced in the right ear, suggesting a lesion of the cochlea.

that lesions in **presbycusis** (hearing loss due to aging) are restricted to the cochlea, regardless of the relationship to noise exposure mentioned earlier. The aging process undoubtedly produces alterations in many areas of the auditory system, including the tympanic membrane, ossicular chain, cochlear windows, and central auditory nervous system. There is probably some relationship to general oxygen deficiency caused by arteriosclerosis. A definition of the age at which presbycusis begins is lacking in the literature, but it should be expected in men by the early 60s and women by the late 60s, all other factors being equal. It is possible that the hearing mechanism begins to deteriorate slowly at birth.

Speech & Hearing Center
The University of Texas
Austin, Texas 78712

Name_____ Age_____ Sex_____ Examiner_____ Date_____

Special Tests

SISI

	Right		20 dB(SL)			Left		20 dB(SL)	
Freq	250	500	1000	2000	4000	250	500	1000	2000	4000
%	40*	60*	100*	100*	100*	O	5	O	10	O
EM Opp. Ear	30	35	35	40	45					

	Right		___dB(SL)			Left		___dB(SL)	
Freq	250	500	1000	2000	4000	250	500	1000	2000	4000
%										
EM Opp. Ear										

Tone Decay
(Seconds)

SL (dB)	Right							Left						
	20	25	30	35	40	45	50	20	25	30	35	40	45	50
250 Hz	60*							60						
EM Opp. Ear	80													
1000 Hz	60*							60						
EM Opp. Ear	80													
4000 Hz	48*	60*						60						
EM Opp.	95													

ABLB

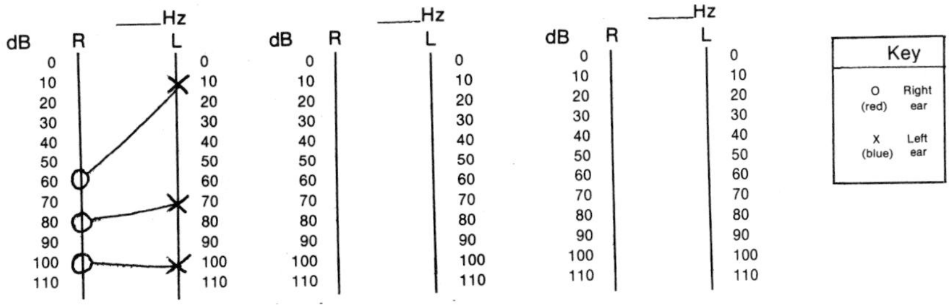

Key	
O (red)	Right ear
X (blue)	Left ear

FIGURE 11.16 Behavioral site-of-lesion test results shown for the patient with Méniére disease (Figure 11.14). Note the high SISI scores in the higher frequencies and the presence of loudness recruitment in the right (impaired) ear. The moderate amount of tone decay is consistent with a cochlear lesion in the right ear.

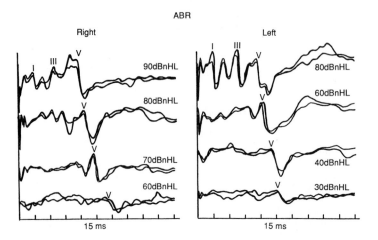

FIGURE 11.17   Results of auditory brainstem response testing on the patient with a cochlear hearing loss (Méniére disease) in the right ear (see Figure 11.14). Absolute latencies are shown in Figure 11.18.

A common characteristic of presbycusis is significant difficulty in word recognition, which Gaeth (1948) has called **phonemic regression.** Many older people report that they often understand speech better when people speak slowly than when they speak loudly. A number of "typical" presbycusic audiometric contours have been suggested.

The classical work on presbycusis is by Schuknecht (1993), who defined four different, but overlapping, causes of this hearing loss:

1. *Sensory presbycusis.* This sensory loss is produced by a loss of outer hair cells and supporting cells in the basal turn of the cochlea. The audiogram shows a greater hearing loss in the higher frequencies.
2. *Neural presbycusis.* Loss of neurons in the cochlea causes poor word recognition. The audiogram may be generally flat or slightly poorer in the higher frequencies.
3. *Strial presbycusis.* Atrophy of the stria vascularis in the middle and apical turns of the cochlea produce a fairly flat audiogram. Word recognition is reasonably good.
4. *Cochlear conductive presbycusis.* Impaired mobility of the cochlear partitions produces a sensorineural hearing loss that is primarily mechanical in nature.

Some gender effects have been noted regarding the audiometric configuration of presbycusic patients. Jerger, Chmiel, Stach, and Spretnjak (1993) surveyed a large number of audiograms over a fifty-year period and found that elderly males tend to show greater hearing loss above 1000 Hz, whereas elderly females have poorer sensitivity below 1000 Hz, even when accounting for such environmental factors as noise exposure. A possible explanation for this difference is the greater presence of cardiovascular disease in elderly females.

Approximately 25 percent of adults in the age range from 45 to 64 years and 40 percent of those over 65 have some degree of hearing loss (Glass, 1990). Hearing loss in this context is defined as a handicap in social, emotional, vocational, and psychological areas (ASHA, 1992). Efforts are

SPEECH AND HEARING CENTER
The University of Texas at Austin 78712

AUDITORY BRAINSTEM RESPONSE
(Adult Form)

NAME: Last - First - Middle	SEX	AGE	DATE	EXAMINER	RELIABILITY	INSTRUMENT

LATENCY-INTENSITY FUNCTION

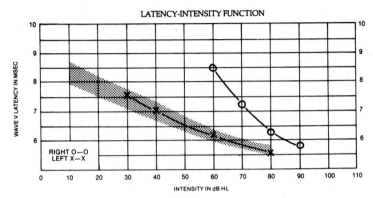

SHADED AREA REPRESENTS Normal Wave V Range for patients older than 16 mos. for 30 clicks per second.

	STIMULUS			WAVE LATENCY IN MSEC						
EAR	RATE	dB HL	FILTER	I	II	III	IV	V	VI	VII
R	33.1	90	150-1500	1.6		3.75		5.8		
L	33.1	80	150-1500	1.52		3.7		5.6		

SUMMARY OF RESULTS

INTERWAVE INTERVALS . . . . R __4.2__ L __4.08__

AMPLITUDE RATIO (V SAME OR > I) . . . . R __NORMAL__ L __NORMAL__

LATENCY CHANGE WITH INCREASED CLICK RATE . . . . R _____ L _____

INTERAURAL DIFFERENCES . . . . _____

ESTIMATED AIR CONDUCTION THRESHOLD IN dBHL (1 - 2 kHz) . . . . R __≤ 60__ L __≤ 30__

ESTIMATED BONE CONDUCTION THRESHOLD IN dB HL . . . . R _____ L _____

COMMENTS

FIGURE 11.18 Latency-intensity functions for wave V derived from the auditory brainstem response tracings shown in Figure 11.17 on the patient with a unilateral (right) cochlear hearing loss (see Figure 11.14). The latencies are normal for the left ear and increased for the right ear, primarily at lower intensities.

being made to screen elderly citizens for hearing loss, in ways similar to screening infants and schoolchildren, in order to identify problems and seek solutions as early as possible. Such screening tests must be effective, high in sensitivity and specificity, and yield a high predictive value.

Screening instruments are available that can be used effectively by primary-care physicians to identify their patients with sufficient hearing loss to consider amplification with hearing aids. These instruments can deliver pure tones at 500, 1000, 2000, and 4000 Hz at 40 dB HL. Since the devices are easy to use and quickly become cost effective, it may soon be possible for audiologists to receive referrals so that they may serve adults earlier in the development of their hearing problems. Widespread definitive programs for screening elderly adults may be on the horizon.

Summary

The inner ear is a fluid-filled space, interfaced between the middle ear and the auditory nerve. It acts as a device to convert sound into a form of electrochemical energy that transmits information to the brain about the frequency, intensity, and phase of sound waves. The vestibular portion of the inner ear provides the brain with data concerning the position and movement of the body.

When the cochlear portion of the inner ear becomes abnormal, the result is a combination of sensorineural hearing loss and dysacusis. Bone-conduction and air-conduction results essentially interweave on the audiogram, and word recognition generally becomes poorer in direct relation to the amount of hearing loss. Results on tympanometry and static immittance in the plane of the tympanic membrane are usually within normal limits, unless the sensorineural loss has a superimposed conductive component, resulting in a mixed hearing loss. Acoustic reflex thresholds are expected at low sensation levels. In pure cochlear hearing losses the latency-intensity functions obtained from ABR testing are rather steep, showing longer latencies close to threshold. If the outer hair cells are damaged causing more than a mild hearing loss otoacoustic emissions will be absent.

If behavioral site-of-lesion tests are performed, patients with cochlear hearing loss are expected to show high SISI scores and moderate amounts of tone decay (especially in the higher frequencies). Recruitment of loudness can usually be found, which often complicates auditory rehabilitation.

Habilitation or rehabilitation of patients with sensorineural hearing losses of cochlear origin is considerably more difficult than for patients with conductive lesions. Medical or surgical correction is usually obviated by the very nature of the disorder; however, there are several important exceptions to this. Combinations of harmonic and frequency distortion and loudness recruitment often make the use of hearing aids difficult but not impossible. Auditory rehabilitation of patients with cochlear disorders is of special concern to audiologists.

STUDY QUESTIONS

1. List from memory as many parts of the inner ear as you can, separating them into auditory and vestibular categories.

2. List some disorders of the inner ear. Break them down according to age of onset.

3. Draw typical audiograms from the preceding list. Hypothesize the results on such tests as: SRT, WRS, ABR, OAE, acoustic immittance, ABLB, SISI, and tone decay.

GLOSSARY

Acoustic trauma notch A precipitous increase in hearing loss in the 3000 to 6000 Hz range, with recovery of hearing function at higher frequencies. It is usually, but not exclusively, associated with patients with noise-induced hearing loss.

Acquired immune deficiency syndrome (AIDS) See *Human immunodeficiency virus*.

Action potential (AP) A change in voltage measured on the surface of a neuron when it fires.

Afferent Nerves that carry impulses from the periphery toward the brain.

Allele One of two or more forms of a gene occupying corresponding locations on corresponding chromosomes.

Ampulla The widened end of each of the three semicircular canals where they return to the utricle. Each ampulla contains an end organ for the sense of equilibrium.

Anoxia Deprivation of oxygen to specific cells of the body affecting their normal metabolism.

Athetosis One of the three major categories of cerebral palsy, characterized by squirming or writhing movements.

Auditory placode A thickened plate, near the hindbrain in the human embryo, that develops into the inner ear.

Autosomal dominant The capacity of a gene to express itself when carried by only one of a pair of homologous chromosomes.

Autosomal recessive The inability of a gene to express a trait unless it is carried by both members of a pair of homologous chromosomes.

Autosome Any chromosome other than a sex chromosome. There are 22 pairs in humans.

Axon The efferent portion of a neuron.

Basilar membrane A membrane extending the entire length of the cochlea, separating the scala tympani from the scala media, and supporting the organ of Corti.

Caloric test Irrigation of the external auditory canal with warm or cold water to stimulate the vestibular labyrinth. In normal patients the result is nystagmus with some sensation of vertigo.

Carrier A phenotypically normal individual, whose body contains a recessive gene for an abnormal trait, along with its normal allele.

Cell body The central portion of a nerve cell.

Cerebellum The area in the base of the skull behind the brainstem that is concerned with coordination of movement.

Cerebral palsy A motor disorder produced by damage to the brain; it usually occurs prenatally, perinatally, or in early infant life.

Chromosome A structure in every animal cell nucleus that bears the genetic information.

Cochlea A cavity in the inner ear resembling a snail shell and containing the essential end organs for hearing.

Cochlear duct See *Scala media*.

Cochlear microphonic (CM) The measurable electrical response of the hair cells of the cochlea.

Computerized dynamic posturography (CDP) A quantitative assessment of balance function for postural stability, performed by a computer-based moving platform and motion transducers.

Corti's arch A series of arches made up of the rods of Corti in the cochlear duct.

Cytomegalovirus (CMV) A common virus that is a member of the herpes family of viruses and can cause congenital hearing loss when contracted by a pregnant woman.

Damage-risk criteria The maximum safe allowable noise levels for different bandwidths.

Dendrite The branched portion of a neuron that carries the nerve impulse to the cell body.

Diplacusis binauralis Hearing a tone of single frequency as different pitches in the two ears.

Diplacusis monauralis Hearing a single frequency in one ear as a chord or noise.

DNA Deoxyribonucleic acid, the fundamental molecular material that carries the genetic code.

Ductus reuniens A tube connecting the saccule with the scala media that carries endolymph to the cochlea.

Dysacusis Distortion of an auditory signal that is associated with loss of auditory sensitivity. Evidenced by poor word recognition.

Efferent Nerves that carry impulses from the brain toward the periphery.

Electronystagmograph (ENG) A device used to monitor electrically the amount of nystagmus occurring spontaneously or from vestibular stimulation.

Endogenous Produced or originating within the organism.

Endolymph The fluid contained within the membranous labyrinth of the inner ear in both the auditory and vestibular portions.

Exogenous Produced or originating outside the organism.

Frequency theory of hearing The explanation for pitch perception based on the frequency of neural impulses in the auditory nerve.

Gene The unit of heredity, composed of a sequence of DNA, that is located in a specific position on a chromosome.

Genotype The genetic constitution of an individual.

Glycerol test A test for Méniére disease in which pure-tone thresholds and word-recognition scores are measured before, and several hours after, a patient ingests concentrated glucose and water. Improvements in threshold and word recognition suggest that the diuretic action of the glucose solution results in decreased endolymphatic pressure, making the test positive for Méniére disease.

Helicotrema A passage at the apical end of the cochlea connecting the scala vestibuli with the scala tympani.

Hereditodegenerative hearing loss Hearing loss that has its onset after birth but is nonetheless hereditary.

Heterozygous Possessing different genes at a specific site between paired chromosomes.

Homozygous Possessing identical genes at a specific site between paired chromosomes.

Human immunodeficiency virus (HIV) A virus transmitted through body fluids that first appeared in the United States in the early 1980s. The virus affects the immune system and creates the possibilities of conductive, sensory, and neural hearing loss.

Hypacusis Loss of hearing sensitivity.

Labyrinth The system of interconnecting canals of the inner ear, composed of the bony labyrinth (filled with perilymph), that contains the membranous labyrinth (filled with endolymph).

Labyrinthitis Inflammation of the labyrinth, resulting in hearing loss and vertigo.

Méniére disease A disease of the inner ear, the symptoms of which include tinnitus, vertigo, and hearing loss (usually fluctuating and unilateral).

Meningitis Inflammation of the meninges, the three protective coverings of the brain and spinal cord.

Mixed hearing loss A sensorineural hearing loss with superimposed conductive hearing loss. The air-conduction level shows the entire loss; the bone-conduction level, the sensorineural portion; and the air-bone gap, the conductive portion.

Modiolus The central pillar of the cochlea.

Multifactorial genetic considerations Arising from the interaction of several genes and environmental factors.

Neuron A cell specialized as a conductor of nerve impulses.

Neurotransmission The manner in which neurons communicate with one another neurochemically.

Neurotransmitter A chemical substance that is released to bridge the gap between neurons so that neurotransmission can be facilitated.

Nystagmus An oscillatory motion of the eyes.

Organ of Corti The end organ of hearing found within the scala media of the cochlea.

Otoacoustic emissions (OAEs) Sounds emanating from the cochlea that can be detected in the external auditory canal with probe-tube microphones.

Otocyst The auditory vesicle (sac) of the human embryo.

Ototoxic Poisonous to the ear.

Perilymph The fluid contained in both the auditory and vestibular portions of the bony labyrinth of the inner ear.

Permanent threshold shift (PTS) Permanent sensorineural loss of hearing, usually associated with exposure to intense noise.

Phenotype The observable makeup of an individual, which is determined by genetic or a combination of genetic and environmental factors.

Phonemic regression A slowness in auditory comprehension associated with advanced age.

Place theory of hearing The explanation for pitch perception based on a precise place on the organ of Corti, which when stimulated results in the perception of a specific pitch.

Presbycusis Hearing loss associated with old age.

Psychophysical tuning curve (PTC) The measurable response in the cochlea to specific frequencies introduced into the ear.

Reissner's membrane A membrane extending the entire length of the cochlea, separating the scala media from the scala vestibuli.

Resonance theory of hearing A nineteenth-century theory of pitch perception that suggested that the cochlea consisted of a series of resonating tubes, each tuned to a specific frequency.

Resonance-volley theory of hearing A combination of the place and frequency theories of hearing, which suggests that nerve units in the auditory nerve fire in volleys, allowing pitch perception up to about 4000 Hz. Perception of pitch above 4000 Hz is determined by the point of greatest excitation on the basilar membrane.

Retrocochlear Located behind the cochlea.

Rh factor Pertaining to the protein factor found on the surface of the red blood cells in most humans. Named for the Rhesus monkey, in which it was first observed.

Saccule The smaller of the two sacs found in the membranous vestibular labyrinth; it contains an end organ of equilibrium.

Scala media The duct in the cochlea separating the scala vestibuli from the scala tympani. It is filled with endolymph and contains the organ of Corti.

Scala tympani The duct in the cochlea below the scala media, filled with perilymph.

Scala vestibuli The duct in the cochlea above the scala media, filled with perilymph.

Semicircular canals Three loops in the vestibular portion of the inner ear responsible for the sensation of turning.

Sensorineural hearing loss Formerly called *perceptive loss* or *nerve loss,* this term refers to loss of hearing sensitivity produced by damage or alteration of the sensory mechanism of the cochlea or the neural structures that lie beyond.

Somatosensory Spatial orientation provided by proprioceptive input, as by the support the body receives on a surface.

Spiral ligament The thickened outer portion of the periosteum of the cochlear duct, which forms a spiral band and attaches to the basilar membrane.

Spontaneous otoacoustic emissions (SOAEs) Those sounds, produced in the cochlea, that are detectable in the external auditory canal and occur normally in persons with no hearing loss.

Stereocilia A protoplasmic filament on the surface of a cell (e.g., a hair cell).

Stria vascularis A vascular strip that lies along the outer wall of the scala media. It is responsible for the secretion and absorption of endolymph, it supplies oxygen and nutrients to the organ of Corti, and it affects the positive DC potential of the endolymph.

Synapse The area of communication between neurons where a nerve impulse passes from an axon of one neuron to the cell body or dendrite of another.

Syndrome A set of symptoms that appear together to indicate a specific pathological condition.

Tectorial membrane A gossamer membrane above the organ of Corti in the scala media, in which the tips of the cilia of the hair cells are imbedded.

Temporary threshold shift (TTS) Temporary sensorineural hearing loss, usually associated with exposure to intense noise.

Transduce To convert one form of power to another (e.g., pressure waves to electricity, as in a microphone).

Traveling wave theory The theory that sound waves move in the cochlea from its base to its apex along the basilar membrane. The crest of the wave resonates at a particular point on the basilar membrane, resulting in the perception of a specific pitch.

Trisomy The presence of an additional (third) chromosome.

Utricle The larger of the two sacs found in the membranous vestibular labyrinth; it contains an end organ of equilibrium.

Variable expressivity The extent to which an inheritable trait is manifested.

Vasospasm The violent constriction of a blood vessel, usually an artery.

Vertigo The sensation that a person (or his or her surroundings) is whirling or spinning.

Vestibule The cavity of the inner ear containing the organs of equilibrium and giving access to the cochlea.

Volley theory of hearing A variation of the frequency theory in which some neurons fire during the refractory periods of other neurons.

X-linked Characteristics transmitted by genes on the X chromosome (sex-linked).

REFERENCES

Alford, B. (1968). Rubella: A challenge for modern medical science. *Archives of Otolaryngology, 88,* 27–28.

Allen, J. B., & Lonsbury-Martin, B. L. (1993). Otoacoustic emissions. *Journal of the Acoustical Society of America, 93,* 568–569.

American Speech-Language-Hearing Association (ASHA). (1992). Considerations in screening adults/older persons for handicapping hearing impairments. *Asha, 34,* 81–87.

———. (1994). Guidelines for the audiologic management of individuals receiving cochleotoxic drug therapy. *Asha, 36,* 11–19.

Békésy, G. v. (1960). Wave motion in the cochlea. In E. G. Wever (Ed.), *Experiments in hearing* (pp. 485–534). New York: McGraw-Hill.

Berger, E. H. (1988). Hearing protectors: Specification, fitting, use and performance. In D. Lipscomb (Ed.), *Hearing conservation in industry, schools and the military* (pp. 145–191). Boston: Little, Brown and Company.

Brookhouser, P. E., Cyr, D. G., & Beauchaine, K. (1982). Vestibular findings in the deaf and hard of hearing. *Otolaryngology, Head and Neck Surgery, 90,* 773–777.

Cyr, D. G., & Møller, C. G. (1988). Rationale for the assessment of vestibular function in children. *The Hearing Journal, 41,* 38–39, 45–46, 48–49.

DeVries, S. M., & Decker, T. N. (1992). Otoacoustic emissions: Overview of measurement methodologies. *Seminars in Hearing, 13,* 15–22.

Dufresne, R. M., Alleyne, B. C., & Reesal, M. R. (1988). Asymmetric hearing loss in truck drivers. *Ear and Hearing, 9,* 41–42.

Everberg, G. (1957). Deafness following mumps. *Acta Otolaryngologica, 48,* 397–403.

Ewertson, H. W. (1973). Epidemiology of professional noise-induced hearing loss. *Audiology, 12,* 453–458.

Ferraro, J. A. (1992). Electrocochleography: What and why. *Audiology Today, 4,* 25–27.

Gaeth, J. H. (1948). *A study of phonemic regression in relation to hearing loss.* Doctoral dissertation, Northwestern University, Evanston, IL.

Glass, L. (1990). Hearing impairment in geriatrics. *Geriatric rehabilitation.* Boston: College Hill Press.

Jacobson, E., Downs, M., & Fletcher, J. (1969). Clinical findings in high-frequency thresholds during known ototoxic drug usage. *Journal of Auditory Research, 81,* 379–385.

Jerger, J., Chmiel, R., Stach, B., & Spretnjak, M. (1993). Gender affects audiometric shape in presbyacusis. *Journal of the American Academy of Audiology, 4,* 42–49.

Johnson, L. G., & Hawkins, J. E. (1976). Degeneration patterns in human ears exposed to noise. *Annals of Otology, 85,* 725–739.

Johnson, S. J., Hosford-Dunn, H., Paryani, S., Yeager, A. S., & Malachowski, N. (1986). Prevalence of sensorineural hearing loss in premature and sick term infants with perinatally acquired cytomegalovirus infection. *Ear and Hearing, 7,* 325–327.

Karmody, C. (1969). Asymptomatic maternal rubella and congenital deafness. *Archives of Otolaryngology, 89,* 720–726.

Kemp, D. T. (1978). Stimulated acoustic emissions from within the human auditory system. *Journal of the Acoustical Society of America, 65,* 1386–1391.

———. (1981). Physiologically active cochlear micromechanics—one source of tinnitus. In D. Evered & G. Lawrenson (Eds.), *Tinnitus, Ciba Foundation Symposium* (Vol. 85, pp. 54–81). Bath, England: Pittman Books.

Klockhoff, I. (1976). Diagnosis of Méniére disease. *Archives of Otolaryngology, 212,* 309–312.

Lawrence, J. (1987). HIV infections in infants and children. *Infections in Surgery, 8,* 249–255.

Lawrence, M. (1969). Labyrinthine fluids. *Archives of Otolaryngology, 89,* 85–89.

Lipscomb, D. M. (1992). Fallacies and foibles in hearing conservation. *Audiology Today, 4,* 29–33.

McFadden, D., & Plattsmier, H. S. (1983). Aspirin can potentiate the temporary hearing loss induced by noise. *Hearing Research, 9,* 295–316.

Melnick, W. (1984). Auditory effects of noise exposure. In M. Miller & C. Silverman (Eds.), *Occupational hearing conservation* (pp. 100–132). Englewood Cliffs, NJ: Prentice-Hall.

Merry, C. J., Sizemore, C. W., & Franks, J. R. (1992). The effect of fitting procedure on hearing protector attenuation. *Ear and Hearing, 13,* 11–18.

Musiek, F. E., & Baran, J. A. (1986). Neuroanatomy, neurophysiology, and central auditory assessment: Part I. Brain stem. *Ear and Hearing, 7,* 207–219.

Nadler, N. (1997). Noisy toys: Hidden hazards. *Hearing Health,* November–December, 18–21.

Nashner, L. M. (1993). Computerized dynamic posturography. In G. P. Jacobson, C. W. Newman, & J. M. Kartush, *Handbook of balance function testing* (pp. 280–307). St. Louis, MO: Mosby.

Occupational Safety and Health Administration (OSHA). (1983, March 8). Occupational noise exposure: Hearing conservation amendment; final rule. *Federal Register, 46,* 9738–9785.

Pick, G. F. (1980). Level dependence of psychological frequency resolution and auditory filter shape. *Journal of the Acoustical Society of America, 68,* 1085–1095.

Probst, R., Lonsbury-Martin, B. L., & Martin, G. K. (1991). A review of otoacoustic emissions. *Journal of the Acoustical Society of America, 89,* 2027–2067.

Rosen, S., Bergman, M., Plester, D., El-Mofty, A., & Hammed, H. (1962). Presbycusis study of a relatively noise-free population in the Sudan. *Annals of Otology, Rhinology and Laryngology, 71,* 727–743.

Schuknecht, H. F. (1993). *Pathology of the ear* (2nd ed.). Philadelphia: Lea & Febiger.

Smith, S. D. (1994). Genetic counseling. In J. G. Clark & F. N. Martin (Eds.), *Counseling hearing-impaired individuals and their families* (pp. 70–91). Englewood Cliffs, NJ: Prentice Hall.

Valente, M., Valente, M., & Goebel, J. (1992). High-frequency thresholds: Circumaural earphone versus insert earphone. *Journal of the American Academy of Audiology, 3,* 410–418.

Wever, G. (1949). *Theory of hearing.* New York: Wiley.

Whitehead, M. L., Lonsbury-Martin, B. L., & Martin, G. K. (1992). Relevance of animal models to the clinical application of otoacoustic emissions. *Seminars in Hearing, 13,* 81–101.

SUGGESTED READINGS

Evans, E. F. (1983). Pathophysiology of the peripheral hearing mechanism. In M. E. Lutman & M. P. Haggard (Eds.), *Hearing science and hearing disorders* (pp. 61–80). New York: Academic Press.

Gans, R. E. (1996). *Vestibular rehabilitation: Protocols and programs.* San Diego: Singular.

Lipscomb, D. M. (Ed.). (1992). *Hearing conservation in industry, schools and the military.* Boston: College-Hill Press.

Moore, B. C. J. (1982). *An introduction to the psychology of hearing.* New York: Academic Press.

Pickles, J. O. (1982). *An introduction to the physiology of hearing.* New York: Academic Press.

REVIEW TABLE 11.1   Common Causes of Cochlear Hearing Loss According to Age at Onset

Prenatal	Childhood	Adulthood
Anoxia	Birth trauma	(All of column 2 plus)
Heredity	Drugs	Labyrinthitis
Prematurity	Head trauma	Otosclerosis
Rh Factor	High fevers	Méniére disease
Toxemia of pregnancy	Kidney infection	Presbycusis
Trauma	Noise	Vasospasm
Viral infection (maternal)	Otitis media	
	Surgery (middle ear)	
	Systemic illness	
	Venereal disease	
	Viral infections	

12 The Auditory Nerve and Central Auditory Pathways

The previous three chapters have been concerned with the propagation and conduction of sound waves through the outer and middle ears and the transduction in the cochlea of these pressure waves into neural activity to be processed by the central auditory system. Because sound is meaningful only if it is perceived, understanding of its transmission to, and perception by, the brain is essential to the audiologist. Much remains to be learned about how the nervous system receives, processes, and transmits information related to sound. This chapter's treatment of the anatomy and physiology of the central auditory system is designed mainly to introduce the reader to these processes, and it is therefore far from complete.

Diagnosis of disorders of the auditory system from the outer ear through the auditory nerve is best made through the test battery. This battery includes pure-tone and speech audiometry, measurements of acoustic immittance at the tympanic membrane, the possible administration of such behavioral site-of-lesion measures as SISI, tone decay, and loudness-balance tests, and the objective measures of ABR and OAE. The special tests described in this chapter for site-of-lesion diagnosis in the brain have met with varying degrees of clinical acceptance and are offered to the new student in diagnostic audiology because they seem to be the most appropriate ones at the time of this writing.

Chapter Objectives

As in the previous chapter, this presentation relies heavily on what has been learned in the foregoing sections of this book. The reader should gain an appreciation of the complexity of the central auditory system and the difficulties of diagnosing disorders in the brain to be able to institute and interpret test procedures for proper diagnosis. The purpose of any diagnostic measure is to guide the clinician in the management of the revealed disorder. Management considerations for disorders of the auditory nerve and central auditory nervous system are reviewed. For a deeper understanding of these issues the reader is encouraged to pursue the suggested readings.

Anatomy and Physiology of the Auditory Nerve and Ascending Auditory Pathways

Almost without exception, every anatomical structure on one side of the brain has an identical structure on the opposite side of the brain. For clarity, a block diagram (Figure 12.1), rather than a realistic drawing, is shown to illustrate the auditory pathways. This diagram represents the anatomical

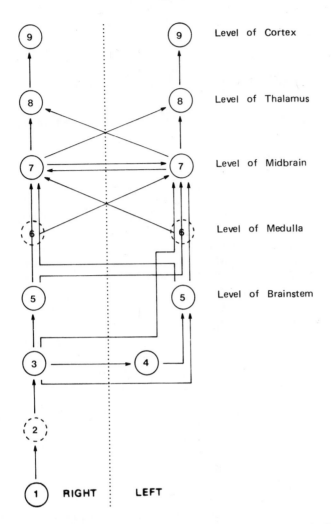

FIGURE 12.1   Block diagram of the auditory pathways. (1) Cochlea (hair cells). (2) Auditory nerve fibers. (3) Cochlear nucleus. (4) Trapezoid body. (5) Superior olivary complex. (6) Lateral lemniscus. (7) Inferior coliculus. (8) Medial geniculate body. (9) Auditory cortex.

arrangement in the system and illustrates the directions of neural impulses and the primary waystations from cochlea to auditory cortex.

The Auditory Nerve

Nerve fibers pass from the modiolus of the cochlea through the **internal auditory canal,** which begins at the modiolus and terminates at the base of the brain. The internal auditory canal also carries the vestibular portion of the VIIIth nerve, whose fibers are innervated by the utricle, saccule, and semicircular canals. There are approximately 30,000 nerve fibers in the cochlear portion and 20,000 in the vestibular portion. The auditory portion of the VIIIth nerve actually spirals through the internal auditory canal. The nerve fibers form a cylindrically arranged bundle, or "cable," with fibers that arise from the basal (high frequencies) turn of the cochlea forming the outer portion and fibers from the apical (low frequencies) areas forming the center, together creating the nerve trunk. In addition to the VIIIth nerve, the internal auditory canal, which runs a distance of approximately 10 mm in adults, also carries the internal auditory artery and fibers of the VIIth (facial) nerve.

The **auditory nerve** extends 17 to 19 mm beyond the internal auditory canal, where it attaches to the brainstem where the **cerebellum, medulla oblongata,** and **pons** join to form the **cerebello-pontine angle (CPA).** At this level the auditory and vestibular portions of the VIIIth nerve separate. One part of the cochlear bundle descends to the **dorsal cochlear nucleus,** and the other ascends to the **ventral cochlear nucleus.**

The Cochlear Nucleus

As previously mentioned, neurons from the cochlea are arranged in an orderly fashion in the cochlear bundle according to frequency. The arrangement of fibers in the cochlea and auditory nerve is repeated in the cochlear nuclei and is said to represent **tonotopic** organization. The auditory nerve fibers terminate in the cochlear nuclei—basal turn fibers in one area, apical turn fibers in other areas, and so on.

Each cochlear nucleus is divided into three portions: anteroventral, posteroventral, and dorsal, with each division organized tonotopically. The cochlear nucleus is made up of a variety of different cell types. These different cells react differently to the incoming auditory nerve impulses, thus modifying input to the brain. It is probable that the cochlear nucleus preserves, but does not necessarily enhance, information it receives from the auditory nerve.

The brain is characterized by many **decussations,** or crossover points, that unite symmetrical portions of its two halves. Specialized nerve fiber bundles called **commissures** unite similar structures on both sides of the brain or spinal cord. The first decussation in the auditory pathways occurs after the cochlear nucleus at the level of the **trapezoid body** of the pons.

Some fibers terminate in the contralateral trapezoid body, but other fibers begin their ascent in the brain on both the same and opposite sides. This is the beginning of bilateral representation from a signal presented to just one ear. The fibers from the ventral cochlear nucleus proceed to the ipsilateral and contralateral **superior olivary complexes (SOCs).** Some fibers from the dorsal cochlear nucleus extend to the contralateral **inferior colliculus.** The ascending pathway is along the **lateral lemniscus,** which is an extension of the olivary complex on both sides of the brain. Fibers also pass from the ventral cochlear nucleus to the reticular formation.

The Reticular Formation

The **reticular formation** resides in the center of the brainstem and communicates with virtually all areas of the brain, including the cortex and the spinal cord. It plays a major role in auditory alertness, reflexes, and habituation. Sometimes called the reticular activating system, the reticular formation may be the primary control center for the central nervous system.

The Superior Olivary Complex

Most of the fibers from the cochlear nucleus project to the superior olivary complex. The lateral superior olivary nucleus, the largest area, and the medial superior olivary complex receive input from both the ipsilateral and contralateral cochlear nuclei. The large number of ipsilateral and contralateral neural inputs allows the superior olivary complex to sense the direction of a sound source by analyzing small differences in the time or intensity of sounds arriving at the two ears.

In addition to its major function as a relay station for neural activity on the way to the cerebral cortex, the superior olivary complex also mediates the reflex activity of the tensor tympani and stapedius muscles of the middle ear. Some of the cells of the superior olive interact with some neurons of the facial nerve. Intense sounds produce activation of certain motor fibers of the facial (VIIth) nerve, which innervate the stapedial branch of this nerve. The decussations at this anatomical point explain the contraction of the stapedius muscles in both middle ears when sound is presented to just one ear.

The Lateral Lemniscus

The lateral lemniscus provides a major pathway for the transmission of impulses from the ipsilateral lower brainstem. Some fibers terminate in the nucleus of the lateral lemniscus, others course to the contralateral lemniscus, and still others continue to the inferior colliculus. As in the cochlear nucleus and the superior olivary complex, definite tonotopic organization can be found within the lateral lemniscus.

The Inferior Colliculus

The inferior colliculus receives afferent stimulation from both superior olivary complexes. This is the first waystation at which a 1:1 ratio of entering and departing fibers is found. Most fibers from the lower centers at each cochlear nucleus and superior olive reach the higher centers by way of the inferior colliculus of the midbrain. Neurons that connect the inferior colliculus with the next relay station, the **medial geniculate body,** represent the third or fourth link in the ascending auditory system. A few fibers bypass the inferior colliculus to reach the medial geniculate body directly from the lateral lemniscus.

The Medial Geniculate Body

The medial geniculate body, located in the **thalamus,** is the last subcortical relay station for auditory impulses. Only one of its three main areas, the ventral division, is responsible specifically for auditory information. There is some spiral organization in this area, but tonotopicity is uncertain. Most of the fibers come from the ipsilateral inferior colliculus, and a few fibers come from the lateral lemniscus. After this point, nerve fibers fan out as the **auditory radiations** and then ascend to the auditory cortex. Because there are no commissural neurons at the level of the medial geniculate body, no decussations exist there.

The Auditory Cortex

The areas of auditory reception are in the **temporal lobes** on both sides of the cerebral cortex in an area called the **superior temporal gyrus** or **Heschl's gyrus.** Because there are many interconnections among parts of the cortex through association areas, a part of the cortex is involved in the process of hearing.

There is evidence that the selective representation of frequency, observed at specific places in the cochlea, is repeated in the auditory cortex, though to a lesser degree. Apparently the **temporal** area is concerned primarily with the frequency characteristics of sound, the **insular** area with temporal aspects of sound, the **parietal** area with association of sound with past experiences (and because this area has inputs from all sensory modalities, the auditory stimulus is compared or matched with input from other senses), and the frontal area with the memory of sounds.

At one time it was believed that the auditory cortex was the only center of auditory discrimination. It is now known that many discriminations may be mediated subcortically. Perceptions of pitch and loudness can be maintained in animals whose cortices have been surgically removed. Although discrimination of some simple sounds may be retained, the understanding of speech requires at least minimal integrity of the auditory cortex.

The Descending Auditory Pathways

The auditory system is generally considered to be a sensory system (like the skin or the eyes) that provides the brain with information conducted to the cochlea, in the form of pressure waves, and transduced by the cochlea into neural activity. Rasmussen (1960, 1964) has shown that in addition to the afferent pathways, the auditory system contains a complex efferent system of descending fibers. These descending fibers correspond closely with the ascending fibers and connect the auditory cortex with lower centers and with the cochlea. One purpose of this descending system is to provide inhibitory feedback by elevating the thresholds of neurons at lower stations in the auditory tract. It is true, however, that some descending connections have an excitatory function, but its purpose is not clearly understood.

The Efferent Tract

Descending fibers appear to originate in all auditory areas of the cerebral cortex and descend first in the auditory radiations. Some of these fibers terminate in the medial geniculate body, and some continue to the inferior colliculus and lateral lemniscus. These fibers terminate on both sides of the brain in the **olivocochlear bundle (OCB)** in the pons, which consists largely of efferent neurons. The olivocochlear bundle originates in the superior olivary complex and terminates in the hair cells of both the ipsilateral and contralateral cochleas. The ability of animals to detect signals in the presence of background noise is improved when the olivocochlear bundle is activated (Musiek, 1992).

A second efferent pathway also arises from the auditory cortex. Although some fibers terminate in various areas of the brain, most continue down to the inferior colliculus. Fibers from this area pass to the ipsilateral dorsal cochlear nucleus. Other fibers pass from the superior olive to the ventral cochlear nucleus. The ventral cochlear nucleus also receives fibers from the olivocochlear bundle.

Development of the Auditory Nerve and Central Auditory Nervous System

Relatively little information is available on the prenatal development of the VIIIth nerve and central auditory nervous system. Development of the nervous system (neurogenesis) in general is still poorly understood. In humans, the VIIIth nerve begins to form at about the twenty-fifth gestational day, and appears almost complete at about 45 days. It is probable that the efferent fibers develop later than the afferent fibers. The cochlear and vestibular ganglia appear by the fifth week.

Improved understanding of the embryogenesis and fetogenesis of the central auditory pathways would undoubtedly provide insights into the causes of some types of lesions of the auditory nervous system. It is generally agreed that the entire nervous system forms from the ectoderm.

Summary of the Auditory Pathways

The auditory nerve and central pathways are tremendously complex. The ascending (afferent) system provides stimulation from one ear to both sides of the brain, including the temporal cortex. Descending efferent fibers from each side of the brain provide inhibition to both cochleas.

The waystations in the auditory system perform the complex processing of the incoming nerve impulses. The series of cochlear nucleus, superior olivary complex, lateral lemniscus, inferior colliculus, and medial geniculate body are not simply parts of an elaborate transmission line, whereby the coded information of the VIIIth nerve is relayed to the cortex. Recoding and processing of information take place all the way up through the system.

Hearing Loss and the Auditory Nerve and Central Auditory Pathways

Because there are many collateral nerve fibers and so much analysis and reanalysis of an acoustic message as it travels to the higher brain centers, it is said that the auditory pathways provide considerable *intrinsic redundancy*. There are also many forms of *extrinsic redundancy* in speech messages themselves, such as the usual inclusion of more words than necessary to round out acceptable grammar and syntax. Also, the acoustics of speech offer more frequency information than is absolutely essential for understanding. People with normal auditory systems rarely appreciate the ease these factors provide in understanding spoken language. Those who are deprived of some intrinsic redundancy may not show difficulty in discrimination until the speech message has been degraded by noise, distortion, or distraction.

Lesions in the conductive portions of the outer and middle ears, and the sensory cells of the cochlea, result in the loss of hearing sensitivity. The extent of the hearing loss is in direct proportion to the degree of damage. Loss of hearing sensitivity, such as for pure tones, becomes less obvious as disorders occur in the higher centers of the brain. For these reasons, even though site-of-lesion tests may be extremely useful in diagnosing disorders in the more peripheral areas of the central auditory pathways, such as the auditory nerve and cochlear nuclei, these tests frequently fail to identify disease in the higher centers.

Disorders of the Auditory Nerve

Lesions of the auditory nerve result in hearing losses that are classified as sensorineural. Bone conduction and air conduction interweave on the audiogram, and there is usually nothing in the general audiometric configuration that differentiates cochlear from VIIIth nerve disorders. Johnson (1977) points out that in more than 50 percent of a series of patients with acoustic tumors, consistent audiometric configurations appeared but could not be differentiated from cochlear lesions according to audiometric patterns. In fact, a small percentage of patients with acoustic neuromas will have normal pure-tone audiograms and normal ABR findings (Telian, Kileny, Niparko, Kemink, & Graham,

1989). Two common early symptoms of auditory nerve disorders are tinnitus and high-frequency sensorineural hearing loss. Whenever cases of unilateral or bilateral sensorineural hearing loss with different degrees of impairment in each ear occur, alert audiologists suspect the possibility of neural lesions. The philosophy that all unilateral sensorineural hearing losses are of neural origin until proved otherwise is a good one to adopt.

A second symptom of auditory nerve disorders is apparent when there is a discrepancy between the amount of hearing loss and the scores on word-recognition tests. In most cochlear disorders, as the hearing loss increases, the amount of dysacusis also increases. When difficulties in word recognition are excessive for the amount of hearing loss for pure tones, a neural lesion is suggested. In some cases of VIIIth nerve disorder, hearing for pure tones is normal in the presence of word-recognition difficulty. Despite these statements, it must be remembered that even in cases of neural lesions, patients' word-recognition scores may be perfectly normal.

Causes of Auditory Nerve Disorders

Lesions of the VIIIth nerve may occur as a result of disease, irritation, or pressure on the nerve trunk. Because the cochlear nerve extends into the brain for a short distance beyond the end of the internal auditory canal, some lesions of the nerve may occur in the canal and some in the cerebellopontine angle.

Tumor of the Auditory Nerve

Most tumors of the auditory nerve are benign, and vary in size depending on the age of the patient and the growth characteristics of the **neoplasm.** Usually these tumors arise from sheaths that cover the vestibular branch of the VIIIth nerve. The term usually applied to these tumors is **acoustic neuroma,** although some neuro-otologists believe that the term *acoustic neurinoma* is more descriptive of some growths that arise from the peripheral cells of the nerve. Since most acoustic neuromas arise from the Schwann cells that form the sheath of the vestibular branch of the VIIIth nerve, it has been suggested that the term *vestibular schwannoma* would be most descriptive.

An acoustic neuroma is considered small if it is contained within the internal auditory canal, medium-sized if it extends up to 1 centimeter into the cerebellopontine angle, and large if it extends any further (Pool, Pava, & Greenfield, 1970). The larger the tumor within the canal, the greater the probability that pressure will cause alterations in the function of the cochlear, vestibular, and facial nerves, as well as the internal auditory artery. The larger the tumor extending into the cerebellopontine angle, the greater the likelihood that the pressure will involve other cranial nerves and the cerebellum, which is the seat of balance and equilibrium in the brain. It is difficult to predict the growth rate of acoustic neuromas but most increase slowly in size, on the average of 0.11 cm per year (Strasnick, Glasscock, Haynes, McMenomey, & Minor, 1994).

Acoustic neuromas occur in the United States at the rate of about 1 per 100,000 each year. Most cases occur in adults over the age of 30, although naturally there are exceptions. About 95 percent of these tumors are unilateral, and all are thought to be the result of the absence of a tumor-suppresser gene (NIH Consensus Statement, 1991). Acoustic neuromas have been known to occur in both ears, either simultaneously or successively. One disease, **neurofibromatosis (NF),** or von Recklinghausen disease,[1] may cause dozens or even hundreds of neuromas in different parts of the body, including the internal auditory canal.

---

[1]For Friedrich Daniel von Recklinghausen, German pathologist, 1833–1910.

The earlier in their development acoustic neuromas are discovered, the better the chance for successful surgical removal. Audiological examination is very helpful in making an early diagnosis. Most hearing clinics, however, do not see patients with early acoustic neuromas because hearing loss is not a primary concern in the initial stages. As the tumor increases in size, VIIIth nerve symptoms, such as tinnitus, dizziness, hearing loss, and word-recognition difficulties, become apparent. Valente, Peterein, Goebel, and Neely (1995) reported on four cases of acoustic neuroma in whom hearing was normal and the only symptom present was tinnitus.

Although acoustic neuromas usually result in gradually progressive hearing loss, pressure on the internal auditory artery may result in interference with the blood supply to the cochlea and cause sudden hearing loss and/or progressive sensory hearing loss as a result of damage in the cochlea. Changes in blood supply to the cochlea may cause cochlear symptoms to appear, such as misleading ABR patterns, loudness recruitment, and high SISI scores, and may result in the misdiagnosis of cochlear disease as the primary disorder.

Cranial nerves other than number VIII may be affected as an acoustic tumor increases in size. Symptoms of Vth (trigeminal) nerve involvement include pain and numbness in the face. Occasionally nerve VI (abducens) becomes compressed, causing double vision (diplopia). VIIth (facial) nerve symptoms include the formation of tears in the eyes; alterations in the sense of taste; and development of facial weakness, spasm, or paralysis. Abnormalities of the facial nerve often result in the loss of the corneal reflex; that is, the patient's eyes may not show the expected reflexive blink when a wisp of cotton is touched to the cornea. Dizziness and blurred vision may also occur. The loss of both ipsilateral and contralateral acoustic reflexes may result when measurement is taken with the probe in the ear on the same side as an impaired facial nerve (Figure 6.7H). As the IXth (glossopharyngeal), Xth (vagus), or XIIth (hypoglossal) cranial nerves become involved, difficulty in swallowing (dysphagia) and speaking (dysarthria) may ensue. When the brainstem is compressed as a tumor increases in size, symptoms include coma and eventually death. Audiologists should always consider the possibility of an intracranial tumor when patients present symptoms that include headache, vomiting, lethargy, respiratory distress, and unilateral hearing loss. Figure 12.2 shows an audiogram illustrating a high-frequency hearing loss. The findings of special tests for the patient illustrated are typical of acoustic neuroma, but in any given case one or more of these results may differ from what is expected. Auditory nerve lesions cannot be diagnosed on the bases of a "typical" audiometric configuration.

Proper audiological diagnosis consists of applying the entire test battery. As shown in Figure 12.2, word-recognition scores are poor in the impaired ear. Acoustic reflexes are absent in many cases (Figure 12.3), even at very high stimulus levels (Anderson, Barr, & Wedenberg, 1969). If an acoustic reflex can be obtained, the time required for its amplitude to decay by 50 percent is markedly reduced in the low frequencies (less than 10 seconds). In ten cases of acoustic neuroma described by Anderson and colleagues, the acoustic reflex half-life was less than 3 seconds for frequencies at and below 1000 Hz. Jerger, Oliver, and Jenkins (1987) reported on several cases of acoustic tumors in which the most dramatic finding was the decrease in acoustic reflex amplitude when the eliciting stimulus was presented to the ear on the affected side. ABR latencies in the affected ear are markedly increased (Figures 12.4 and 12.5), and otoacoustic emissions are present since there is apparently no damage to the cochlea. If administered, the alternate binaural loudness-balance test will generally show either no recruitment or decruitment of loudness, and tone decay may be dramatic at all frequencies. Similarly, low SISI scores occur even when the test is modified by presenting the carrier tone at high sensation levels or by using large increments (e.g., 5 dB).

SPEECH AND HEARING CENTER
The University of Texas at Austin 78712
AUDIOMETRIC EXAMINATION

NAME: Last - First - Middle	SEX	AGE	DATE	EXAMINER	RELIABILITY	AUDIOMETER

AIR CONDUCTION

MASKING TYPE	RIGHT									LEFT								
	250	500	1000	1500	2000	3000	4000	6000	8000	250	500	1000	1500	2000	3000	4000	6000	8000
_NB_	O	5	10/10	5	5	10	5	5	5	10	15	15/15	20	30	35	50	55	60
																50*	55*	60*
EM Level in Opp. Ear																5	5	5

BONE CONDUCTION

MASKING TYPE	RIGHT						FOREHEAD						LEFT					
	250	500	1000	2000	3000	4000	250	500	1000	2000	3000	4000	250	500	1000	2000	3000	4000
_NB_							O	5	10	10	10	10	5	10	10	10	10	15
																30*	40*	50*
EM Level in Opp. Ear																35	35	40

		2 Frequency	3 Frequency		WEBER				2 Frequency	3 Frequency
	Pure Tone Average							Pure Tone Average		

SPEECH AUDIOMETRY

MASKING TYPE	RIGHT						LEFT					
	SRT 1	SRT 2	Recognition 1			Recognition 2	SRT 1	SRT 2	Recognition 1			Recognition 2
_WB_	5		1A List/SL 30	100 %		List/SL %	20		2A List/SL 30	60 %		List/SL %
EM Level in Opp. Ear										15		

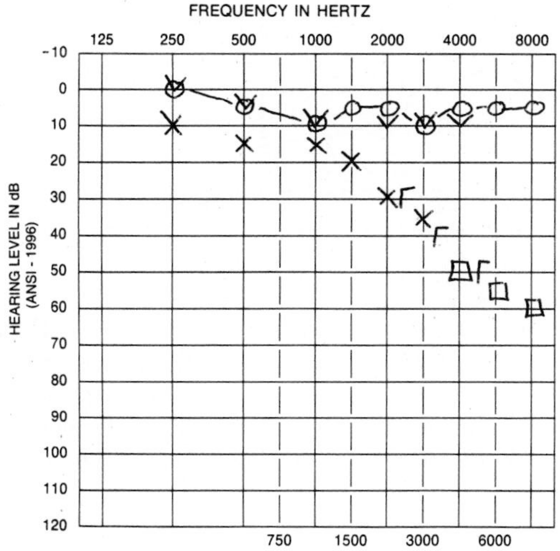

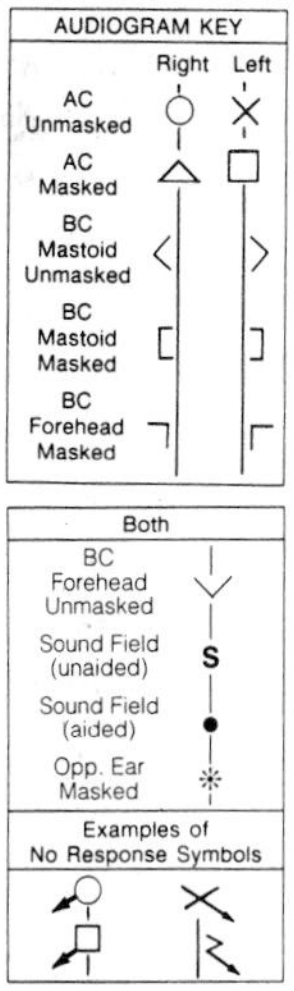

FIGURE 12.2   **Audiogram exemplifying a left acoustic neuroma. Although the hearing loss in the left ear is mild, word recognition is poor. Naturally, proper masking is essential in this case, especially for bone-conduction and word-recognition testing.**

SPEECH AND HEARING CENTER
The University of Texas at Austin 78712
IMMITTANCE

NAME: Last - First - Middle				SEX	AGE	DATE	EXAMINER		INSTRUMENT	

PRESSURE/COMPLIANCE FUNCTION

	– 400	– 350	– 300	– 250	– 200	– 150	– 100	– 50	0	+ 50	+ 100	+ 150	+ 200
Right					.44	.47	.53	.65	.85	.71	.57	.49	.46
Left					.66	.70	.73	.88	1.08	.91	.74	.70	.61

STATIC COMPLIANCE $C_x = C_2 - C_1$

RIGHT						LEFT					
.46	C_1	.85	C_2	.39	C_x	.61	C_1	1.08	C_2	.47	C_x

ACOUSTIC REFLEXES

	RIGHT				LEFT			
Frequency (Hz)	500	1000	2000	4000	500	1000	2000	4000
Ipsilateral (Probe same)		80	85			NR	NR	
Contralateral (Probe opposite)	75	75	80	80	100	105	NR	NR
Audiometric Threshold	5	10	5	5	10	15		
Reflex SL	70	65	75	75	90	90		
Decay Time (Seconds)	10+	10+			3	5		

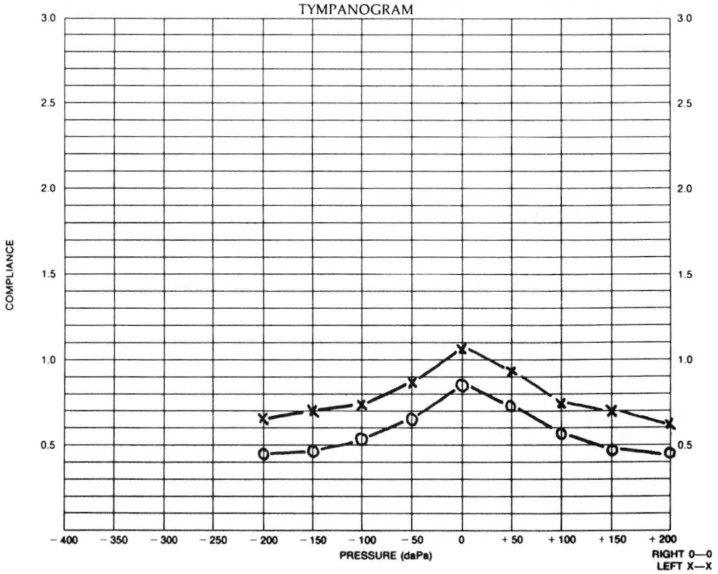

TYMPANOGRAM

FIGURE 12.3 Results on immittance measures for the theoretical patient illustrated in Figure 12.2. Tympanograms and static compliance are normal for both ears. The acoustic reflexes are normal when the tone is presented to the right (normal) ear. Reflex thresholds are elevated when tones are presented to the left ear (acoustic neuroma) in the low frequencies and absent for the higher frequencies. Reflex decay time is very rapid in the left ear in the low frequencies, with no decay in the right ear.

Valente and colleagues (1995) found that elevated or absent acoustic reflexes and abnormal findings on ABR testing were the best tests of correct diagnosis of acoustic neuromas. Josey (1987) reports the ABR has heightened test sensitivity to surgically confirmed lesions to 97 percent. The audiological test battery approach for acoustic neuromas is now often streamlined to pure tone and speech audiometry, acoustic reflex assessment, and ABR. A limitation of ABR testing presents itself in the

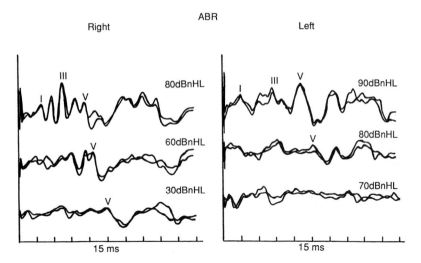

FIGURE 12.4   Results of auditory brainstem response testing on the patient with an VIIIth nerve hearing loss (acoustic neuroma) in the left ear (see Figure 12.2). See the latency-intensity functions for wave V in Figure 12.5.

presence of hearing poorer than 75 dB HL at 1000 to 4000 Hz (Josey, 1987). When the magnitude of hearing loss precludes ABR testing, the audiologist may need to employ more traditional, less sensitive, behavioral site-of-lesion tests.

Confirmation of acoustic neuroma is made through an interdisciplinary approach. Vestibular tests often show a number of abnormal signs, including spontaneous nystagmus with the eyes closed and generally decreased vestibular function on the affected side. An increase in the amount of protein in the cerebrospinal fluid is helpful in determining the presence of tumors. New advances in the specialty of medical imaging have vastly improved acoustic neuroma verification.

Medical Imaging

Remarkable technologies have been introduced to the science of medical imaging. The revolutionary development of **computed tomography (CT)** has permitted the viewing of numerous anatomical abnormalities in the body with a sensitivity unrivaled by previous techniques. In this procedure, often called *computerized axial tomography (CAT)*, an X-ray transmitter scans in a transverse plane (at right angles to the long axis) of the head or body, along a 180-degree arc, while an electronic detector simultaneously measures the intensity of the beam emerging from the other side of the patient. With the aid of a computer, the detector's information is converted to a picture, or "slice," of the patient. This technology has permitted the noninvasive detection of intracranial hemorrhages, tumors, and deformities with great sensitivity.

Magnetic resonance imaging (MRI) has become an exciting adjunct to CT scanning, using ionizing radiation to obtain images; MRI employs magnetic fields and radio waves to produce images in the different planes of the body. One of the most satisfying aspects of this technology is that the waves are believed to be virtually harmless. Furthermore, the technique is excellent for seeing many soft-tissue masses, such as acoustic neuromas, even when they are as small as just a few millimeters in diameter. An MRI scan of an acoustic neuroma is shown in Figure 12.6.

SPEECH AND HEARING CENTER
The University of Texas at Austin 78712

AUDITORY BRAINSTEM RESPONSE
(Adult Form)

NAME: Last · First · Middle	SEX	AGE	DATE	EXAMINER	RELIABILITY	INSTRUMENT

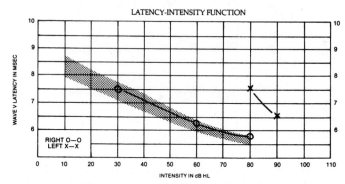

LATENCY-INTENSITY FUNCTION

RIGHT O—O
LEFT X—X

SHADED AREA REPRESENTS Normal Wave V Range for patients older than 16 mos. for 30 clicks per second.

	STIMULUS			WAVE LATENCY IN MSEC						
EAR	RATE	dB HL	FILTER	I	II	III	IV	V	VI	VII
R	13.1	80	150-1500	1.9		3.8		5.8		
L	13.1	90	150-1500	1.68		4.0		6.6		

SUMMARY OF RESULTS

INTERWAVE INTERVALS . . . . R __3.9__ L __4.92__

AMPLITUDE RATIO (V SAME OR > I) . . . . R _NORMAL_ L _NORMAL_

LATENCY CHANGE WITH INCREASED CLICK RATE . . . . R _____ L _____

INTERAURAL DIFFERENCES . . . . _____

ESTIMATED AIR CONDUCTION THRESHOLD IN dBHL (1-2 kHz) . . . . R _____ L _____

ESTIMATED BONE CONDUCTION THRESHOLD IN dB HL . . . . R _____ L _____

COMMENTS

_____

_____

_____

_____

_____

FIGURE 12.5   Latency intensity functions for wave V derived from the auditory brainstem response tracings shown in Figure 12.4, based on the patient with a unilateral retrocochlear hearing loss caused by an acoustic neuroma in the left ear (Figure 12.2). Wave V latencies are normal for the right ear and markedly increased for the left ear at all the sensation levels tested.

During head scans with both CT and MRI, the patient remains motionless while the head is scanned from within a large "doughnut" that surrounds it. Patients often find lying still on their backs difficult, and some, who suffer from different degrees of claustrophobia, become quite upset, even though the procedure is considered to be harmless. Often a chemical, such as gadolinium, is injected into the arm so that it can flow into the brain and serve as a contrast medium, allowing a mass to be

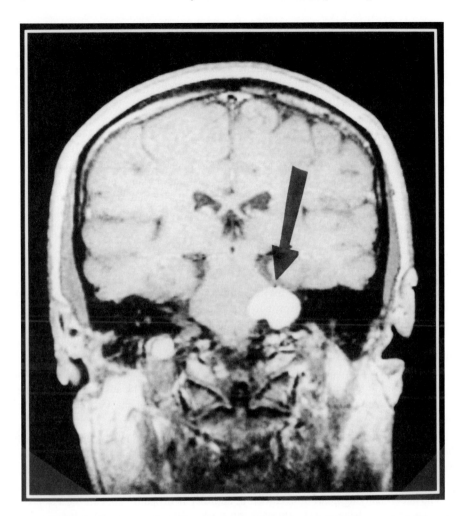

FIGURE 12.6   MRI scan showing a tumor in the left internal auditory canal. (Courtesy of MRI Center of Austin, Texas)

seen more clearly. The noise emitted by many imagers is so loud that many radiologists provide foam hearing protectors for their patients.

In a series of 100 patients with acoustic neuromas reported by Josey, Glasscock, and Musiek (1988), 93 had sufficient hearing to allow ABR testing, and 97 percent of that group showed abnormal ABR results reflecting the lesion. By contrast, 69 percent of the lesions were correctly identified by medical imaging alone. This result dramatizes the need to use both procedures in diagnosis.

An intriguing imaging procedure is now available that utilizes radioactive materials emitted from the body after injection. This procedure is called **positron emission tomography (PET)** and is considered safe, since the radioactivity levels decay very rapidly. PET is designed more to detect biochemical changes in the patient than anatomical changes, and it can be useful in the diagnosis of conditions like multiple sclerosis, Parkinson disease, stroke, schizophrenia, and even depression.

Telian and Kileny (1988) reported three case histories in which ABR, ENG, CT, and MRI at times suggested different problems. In other words, some of the tests resulted in both false positive and false negative results. Telian and Kileny also concluded that false normal ABR responses are more likely to occur when an acoustic tumor is in the cerebellopontine angle than when it is in the internal auditory canal.

Other Causes of VIIIth Nerve Hearing Loss

Because of their dramatic symptoms and the danger they pose to the life of the patient, acoustic neuromas come to the audiologist's mind first when VIIIth nerve signs appear. This is a safe and prudent attitude, but other conditions of the auditory nerve can produce identical audiological symptoms. These conditions include **acoustic neuritis** (inflammation of the vestibular or cochlear nerve) and **multiple sclerosis (MS).**

Auditory Neuropathy

Patients with **auditory neuropathy** may exhibit a mild to moderate sensorineural hearing loss with speech recognition difficulties disproportionate to the degree of measured hearing loss. These patients may also present with other peripheral neuropathies.

Patients with acoustic neuroma exhibit preservation of ABR wave I with an attenuation or delay of subsequent waves, unless the absence of all wave forms is reflected in the profound degree of hearing loss. In addition, these patients' neuromas will be evidenced on MRI. In contrast, patients with suspected auditory neuropathy may show all ABR waves to be absent when hearing thresholds may only be moderately impaired and no evidence of lesions of the VIIIth nerve or brainstem on MRI.

The type of VIIIth nerve lesion present in these patients is not clear. The abnormality may rest at the level of the inner hair cells, the juncture between the inner hair cells and the VIIIth nerve fibers, within the cell bodies of the auditory nerve or the nerve fibers themselves, or any combination of these.

The accompanying hearing loss seen in auditory neuropathy appears slowly progressive and does not benefit from hearing aids, although other rehabilitative efforts including speech reading and vibrotactile reproduction of speech signals (see Chapter 14) may be helpful. Physiological tests in conjunction with behavioral audiometrics aid in the differential diagnosis of auditory neuropathy. The expected findings in auditory neuropathy include absent or severely abnormal auditory brainstem potentials, including wave I in the presence of preserved otoacoustic emissions (Starr, Picton, Sininger, Hood, & Berlin, 1996).

Disorders of the Cochlear Nuclei

The cochlear nuclei represent the first of the relay stations in the central auditory nervous system and the last point at which entirely ipsilateral representation is maintained. Because the tonotopic layout of these nuclei allows for frequency analysis, lesions in these areas may produce clinical loss of hearing sensitivity. Beyond the cochlear nuclei, the stimulus presented to one ear is processed and transmitted along fibers on both sides of the brain.

Audiologists work under the assumption that lesions central to the cochlea will produce results specific to retrocochlear disorders on special diagnostic tests. Such results are usually observed with VIIIth nerve lesions but are not always the case in the cochlear nuclei. Carhart (1967) has pointed out that place and volley information, coded by the cochlea and transmitted by the auditory nerve, is processed separately in the cochlear nuclei. In certain situations in which the cochlear nuclei are damaged, a hearing loss will result, which means that site-of lesion tests must be performed at relatively high stimulation levels. In such cases special tests, such as the SISI and ABLB, may give rise to results that are similar to the results of tests performed on normal-hearing individuals at high sound-pressure levels. For patients with cochlear pathology, the sensation levels for these tests are low, but the sound-pressure levels are high.

There is often uncertainty about whether site-of-lesion test results in cases of damage to the cochlear nuclei will suggest a cochlear disorder, as in Méniére disease, or retrocochlear lesions, as in acoustic neuroma. The tests that are now available cannot completely solve this dilemma. Therefore, audiologists must proceed cautiously in cases of unilateral sensorineural hearing loss.

Causes of Cochlear Nuclei Disorders

Damage to the cochlear nuclei is difficult to diagnose with certainty without postmortem study. Lesions in the nuclei, like those in the auditory nerve, may result from disease, toxicity, irritation, pressure, or trauma.

Rh incompatibility was discussed briefly in Chapter 11 as a prenatal cause of cochlear hearing loss. Reports in the literature, such as by Blakely (1959) and Matkin (1965), show positive indications of cochlear pathology on site-of-lesion tests. Carhart (1967) poses a number of compelling arguments to suggest that hearing losses in Rh babies are caused by damage in the cochlear nuclei rather than in the cochlea, even though site-of-lesion tests may imply the opposite. Postmortem studies have shown deposits of bilirubin in the cochlea, as well as in different areas of the brain, including the cochlear nuclei. Goodhill (1950) coined the term *nuclear deafness* to describe the site of lesion in hearing-impaired children with cerebral palsy secondary to Rh incompatibility.

The term **kernicterus** has been used for some time to describe the condition characterized by bile deposits in the central nervous system. Kernicterus often results in degeneration of the nerve cells that come into contact with bile.

Disorders that interfere with or alter the blood supply to the cochlear nuclei may result in hearing loss. Such disorders, called *vascular accidents,* include the rupturing of blood vessels as well as clots that obstruct the arterial space. These clots may be either thromboses that form and remain in a specific area of the vessel, or embolisms that are formed by bits of debris that circulate through the system until they reach a narrow passageway through which they cannot pass. Either one may obstruct the blood vessel or cause it to burst. Arteries have also been known to rupture where aneurysms (dilations in the blood vessels) form, because aneurysms usually cause the walls to become stretched and thin. Cases of obstruction or rupture of blood vessels within the brain are called **cerebrovascular accidents (CVAs),** or strokes.

An increasingly common condition today is arteriosclerosis, or hardening of the arteries. In addition, the narrowing of the lumen within an artery may be associated with accumulations of fatty debris due to improper diet, insufficient exercise, or metabolic problems. When blood supply to critical nerve cells is diminished, the result is anoxia, which alters cell metabolism and may cause destruction of nerve tissue.

A number of congenital defects of the brain, including the central auditory pathways, have been described in the literature. These defects may be the result of birth trauma or agenesis of parts of the brain.

Pressure within the brainstem may also produce hearing loss. This pressure may be caused by tumors (either benign or malignant), by increased cerebrospinal fluid pressure produced secondary to trauma, or by direct insult to the head. Hemorrhage produced by vascular or other accidents may also cause pressure and damage.

Syphilis (lues) can produce damage anywhere in the auditory system, from the outer ear to the cortex. Cells are damaged or destroyed either by direct degeneration of the nerve units or, secondarily, by CVAs associated with the infection.

Degeneration of nerve fibers in the brain is expected with advancing age. Although presbycusis was listed as one of the causes of cochlear hearing loss, it has become accepted that with aging, changes occur virtually everywhere in the auditory system, including the brainstem. Diseases such as multiple sclerosis can produce degeneration of nerve fibers in younger people as well.

Disorders of the Higher Auditory Pathways

The types of disorders that affect the cochlear nuclei may also affect higher neural structures. Tumors, for example, are not limited to specific sites. Head injury, the major cause of death or serious brain damage among young people in the United States, can produce lesions in a variety of sites. Lesions may encompass large portions of the brain or be localized to small areas.

Factors influencing audiometric results include not only the sizes of the lesions but also their locations. Lesions of the temporal cortex, such as CVA or epilepsy, usually lead to abnormal results on special tests in the ear contralateral to the lesion. Lesions in the brainstem are not so predictable.

Jerger and Jerger (1975) point out that when a lesion is **extra-axial** (on the outside of the brainstem), audiometric symptoms appear on the same side of the head. Such patients often show considerable loss of sensitivity for pure tones, especially in the high frequencies. When the lesion is **intra-axial** (within the brainstem), central auditory tests may show either contralateral or bilateral effects. Often, hearing sensitivity for pure tones is normal or near normal at all frequencies.

Central Auditory Processing Disorders

The principal function of the central auditory system is found within its capacity to organize concurrent or sequential auditory input into definite patterns. The subsequent ability to comprehend and develop spoken language is primarily dependent upon the success of the central auditory system to process speech signals. Those with **central auditory processing disorders (CAPDs)** have difficulty in the interpretation of auditory information in the absence of a concomitant loss of hearing sensitivity. These processing difficulties are further compounded in the presence of surrounding auditory or sometimes even visual, distractions.

CAPDs occurring later in life, secondary to disorders such as CVAs, head trauma, brain tumor, or multiple sclerosis, have less chance of recovery than do CAPDs in the pediatric population. Because of the adaptive properties of the younger central nervous system, children have the advantage of compensatory development of other areas within the system. Auditory processing deficiencies secondary to CAPDs may result in lack of attention to auditory stimuli. This increases distractibility, decreases auditory discrimination and localization abilities, and makes comprehension of speech more difficult. Difficulty with auditory figure-ground differentiation, results in a decreased ability for selective attention. One cause for these deficiencies appears to be the decrease and fluctuation in the intensity of auditory input secondary to recurrent otitis media.

Minimal Auditory Deficiency Syndrome

The animal brain is characterized by an extremely well-organized system of representation for response to incoming signals. When there is deprivation of sensory input, such as to visual or auditory signals, marked changes may take place in the brain (Schwaber, 1992). The tendency of cells to become altered in order to conform to their environments is called **plasticity.** Neuroplasticity of structures in the brain may take place as a result of the sensory deprivation caused by either cochlear or conductive hearing losses.

The slight or mild hearing loss that is often associated with otitis media may go undetected in very young children. Even when it is correctly diagnosed, parents and physicians alike are relieved when symptoms abate and the child appears normal in all respects. Experts have recognized that even these transient and very mild conductive hearing losses may affect the development of skills essential to the learning of language. The term ascribed to this set of circumstances is the **minimal auditory deficiency syndrome (MADS).**

What may be happening in the young human brain has been demonstrated in the laboratory on experimental animals (e.g., Webster & Webster, 1977). Within 45 days, mice with conductive hearing loss surgically induced shortly after birth showed smaller neurons in the cochlear nuclei, superior olivary complex, and trapezoid body than did mice in the control group. Katz (1978) reported that the attenuation of sound may produce similar effects in children and contribute to the development of learning disabilities.

Concern over the relationship between language disorders and otitis media was demonstrated by Rentschler and Rupp (1984). These researchers found that 70 percent of a group of speech- and language-impaired children also had histories of hearing problems, and they suggested persistent monitoring of children with middle-ear disorders through tympanometric measures.

Although the population they studied was small, Gunnarson and Finitzo (1991) looked at a group of children with conductive hearing loss and the later effects on the electrophysiology of the brainstem. They concluded that there do appear to be effects of early transient hearing loss on auditory brainstem responses and that adequate sensory input to the central auditory nervous system is important to the brain during critical developmental periods.

The American Academy of Audiology (1992) issued a position paper on the guidelines for diagnosing and treating otitis media in children. Subsequent guidelines issued by the U.S. Public Health Service's Agency for Health Care Policy and Research outline recommended clinical diagnosis and treatment protocols for otitis media with effusion in young children (Stool, Berg, Berman, Carney, Cooley, Culpepper, Eavey, Feagans, Finitzo, & Friedman, 1994). Parties developing these guidelines are now convinced of a cause-and-effect relationship between early and recurrent otitis media and later communication disorders. There is no disagreement that the primary responsibility for treating otitis media lies within the medical domain; however, the diagnosis and management of subsequent hearing loss is the responsibility of the audiologist.

Although some controversy continues to exist, increasing numbers of professionals believe that children with repeated bouts of otitis media are at risk for the development of learning and communication disorders. It is not the extent of the hearing loss that is the precipitating factor, but rather the fluctuating nature of the disorder and the fact that differences in hearing sensitivity between the two ears of a child may result in abnormal development of auditory processing skills, which are dependent on binaural interactions in the brain. The American Academy of Audiology (1992) recommends the following:

1. *Identification.* This includes screening at-risk children, including those who develop otitis media before the age of six months, those who attend day-care centers, those with cleft palate or Down syndrome, and Native Americans. Screening should include the functions of the middle ear, hearing, and language development. Children who fail the screening should be referred for in-depth testing and possible remediation.
2. *Assessment.* Air- and bone-conduction audiometry for both ears should be carried out to determine the degree of hearing loss and the audiometric configuration. Speech audiometry, along with acoustic immittance tests and a battery of tests for central auditory disorders, should be administered when practicable. Referral to speech-language pathologists should be made on the basis of the outcome of these tests.
3. *Management.* Periodic audiometric follow-up should be completed, even when the child is asymptomatic. Hearing tests should be carried out at the beginning of every school year and at least once during the winter. Parents or caregivers should be kept apprised of hearing test results, and their concerns over their children's hearing status should be carefully heeded. Parents or caregivers should also be taught skills for dealing with their children during exacerbations of hearing loss, ways of recognizing the possible development of hearing loss, and systems for minimizing the disruption of classroom learning by attention to the learning environments of at-risk children.

Although it is recognized that not all children who suffer repeated bouts of otitis media will develop conditions that cause them to fall short of their genetic potential for learning, prudence demands that all persons who interact with these children should be alerted to the potential dangers.

Obscure Auditory Dysfunction

On occasion, patients present with complaints of decreased hearing abilities although subsequent routine audiometrics reveal normal peripheral hearing. These patients may be distressed over their difficulties in auditory functioning within social contexts, and concerned with potential deterioration in their hearing. In the absence of identifiable peripheral pathology or disconcerting unilateral symptoms, most of these patients are discharged with simple reassurance, leaving unanswered questions regarding the underlying problem. Patients following this scenario have been classified as having **obscure auditory dysfunction (OAD)** (Saunders & Haggard, 1989, 1993). Saunders and Haggard (1989) report OAD to be a multifactorial disorder that may incorporate linguistic, psychological, and auditory aspects.

Central Auditory Deafness

Cases of central deafness are extremely rare, occurring when both hemispheres of the brain are severely compromised. Although responses to behavioral audiometric tests may be absent, these patients typically have normal acoustic reflexes and ABRs. Such findings are usually secondary to vascular lesions of the middle cerebral artery or its branches.

Tests for Central Auditory Disorders

Lesions in the auditory nerve and cochlear nuclei produce obvious and dramatic hearing symptoms in the ear ipsilateral to the lesion. As stated earlier in this chapter, once the level of the olivary complex is reached, both sides of the brain are involved in the transmission of auditory information. Even large lesions in the brain may produce either no audiological symptoms or symptoms that are very subtle. For this reason, emphasis must be placed on developing tests that are specifically sensitive to lesions in the central auditory system, many of which are reviewed in this chapter.

For the most part, tests using pure tones have been unsuccessful in identifying central auditory lesions. Because pure-tone tests have been disappointing, much of the emphasis in diagnosing central auditory disorders has been placed on speech tests, many of which are available commercially.[2] As Keith (1981) points out, tests to evaluate these disorders in children share certain characteristics, including language-dependent administration and scoring. Tests that rely on speech stimuli must also be used with caution if the patient exhibits word recognition difficulties. Herein lies the *caveat*.

Performance-Intensity Function with PB Word Lists

Jerger and Jerger (1971) described the use of the *performance-intensity function for PB words* (PI-PB) as a method of screening for central auditory disorders. Patients with normal hearing sensitivity who show differences in the scores and shapes of the PI-PB curves may be suspected of central disorders. PB word lists are presented to the patient at a number of levels—for example, 10, 30, 70, and 90 dB above the SRT. The tests are scored and a graph may be drawn for each ear, showing the word recognition scores as a function of sensation level.

If a significant difference in scores occurs between ears (20 to 30 percent), it may be suspected that a central lesion is present on the side of the brain opposite the poorer score. Sometimes "rollover" of the curve occurs; that is, at some point scores begin to decrease as intensity increases (Figure 12.7). Rollover suggests a lesion on the side of the brain opposite the ear with the rollover or a lesion of the VIIIth nerve on the same side. PI-PB functions may not be helpful in detecting central lesions if a loss of hearing sensitivity is also present. A rollover ratio is derived by the following formula:

$$\text{Rollover ratio } (\%) = \frac{\text{PB Max} - \text{PB Min}}{\text{PB Max}}$$

PB Max is the highest score and PB Min the lowest score obtained at an intensity above that required for PB Max (Jerger & Jerger, 1971). Rollover ratios of .40 suggest cochlear lesions, whereas ratios of .45 or greater indicate an VIIIth nerve site. High rollover ratios are also seen in some elderly patients (Gang, 1976).

---

[2]Auditec of St. Louis (800-669-9065).

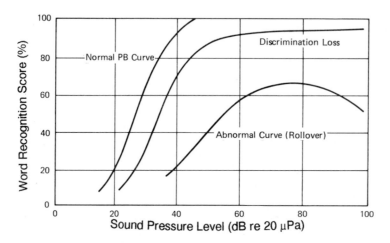

FIGURE 12.7 Typical performance-intensity functions for PB words showing the normal increase in word-recognition scores with increased intensity and the rollover (decreased discrimination beyond a certain level) evident in some ears contralateral to a central auditory disorder.

Two factors must be considered when determining rollover ratios. First, the procedure is not helpful if all word-recognition scores are low. Second, for the greatest accuracy, a number of levels must be tested. Establishing complete performance-intensity functions can be very time-consuming. However, when a central pathology is suspected, a comparison of performance of a high intensity speech recognition measure (90 dB HL, tolerance permitting) with that of the original speech recognition measure may be revealing. A decrease of 20 percent or more at the higher level can be considered an indication of central involvement. As this is a measure significantly above threshold, masking of the contralateral ear must usually be employed.

Filtered Speech Tests

Although standard tests for word recognition do not usually identify central lesions, distortion of the speech signal presented monaurally often results in reduced word recognition scores in the ear contralateral to a central lesion (Bocca & Calearo, 1963). This statement is true if the lesion does not impair the symbolization and memorization processes of the brain, which may result in much more demonstrable symptoms.

An early distorted speech measure utilized a low fidelity 1948 recording of the Harvard PB-50 word lists by Rush Hughes, a professional radio announcer. Goetzinger and Angell (1965) found that patients with suspected central auditory disorders had larger discrepancies between scores obtained with the Rush Hughes word list and other higher fidelity word lists than did those without central pathology.

Since that time, several methods have been used to distort the speech signal for central auditory tests. Speech has been periodically interrupted, masked, compressed in time, presented at low sensation levels, and filtered. Filtering some frequencies from the speech spectrum has become the most popular of these methods.

A signal may be passed through a filter that rejects the low frequencies and passes the highs (high-pass filter) or one that rejects the high frequencies and passes the lows (low-pass filter). A signal may also be processed through a filter that rejects both high and low frequencies above and below a prescribed range, so that only a band of frequencies is allowed through. This is called band-pass filtering and is usually described in terms of the range from the lowest to the highest frequencies passed.

Difficulty in recognizing filtered speech depends largely on the filter characteristics, such as whether the signal is high-pass, low-pass, or band-pass filtered; the cutoff frequency of the filter (the precise frequency above or below which the filtering takes place); and the filter rejection rate (usually expressed in decibels per octave). The steeper the rejection rate, the greater the distortion of the signal. Filtered speech tests may be performed monaurally or binaurally.

The classical work with monaurally filtered speech tests was done by Bocca, Calearo, and Cassinari (1954). These researchers used low-pass filtered speech, markedly attenuating frequencies above 800 Hz. Bocca (1967) has suggested that distorted sentence materials are superior to isolated words because they put greater stress on the brain's capacity for pattern recognition.

In temporal lobe lesions, word recognition may be much the same in both ears for unfiltered speech, but it may be markedly poorer in the ear contralateral to the lesion when filtered speech is used. Jerger (1960) found this to be true with low-pass filtered PB word lists in cases with lesions both in the brainstem and in the temporal lobe. Similar findings were observed in other temporal lobe lesions (Antonelli & Callearo, 1968; Hodgson, 1967; Lynn & Gilroy, 1977).

Filtered speech tests may also be carried out binaurally. Bocca (1955) found that combining a quiet undistorted signal to one ear with the same signal to the other ear, at a high level but distorted, yields surprising results when the central auditory pathways are intact. Discrimination for soft speech is naturally poor, as is discrimination for loud, distorted speech. When the two signals are presented simultaneously (soft to one ear, distorted to the other), a dramatic increase in the discrimination score is observed as the two signals are fused in the brain. No such summation of scores was observed by Jerger (1960) or Calearo (1957) in patients with temporal lobe disorders.

Band-pass Binaural Speech Audiometry

Matzker (1959) developed a test wherein different filtered portions of a speech signal are presented to each ear. Discrimination for either a low-frequency band passed signal alone or a high-frequency band-passed signal alone yields very poor speech intelligibility. If the brainstem is normal, the two signals are fused when presented simultaneously. Inability to demonstrate this binaural fusion suggests a lesion in the brainstem. Matzker's original materials were German PB words. A number of different filter setting have been used successfully in band-pass filtered speech audiometry (Table 12.1)

The test materials are fed from a CD or tape player to the two inputs of a stereo recorder. One channel is sent through a low-frequency band-pass filter, and the other channel is sent through a high-frequency band-pass filter. After the recording has been made, the two channels of the recorder can then feed the two channels of a speech audiometer.

One method for this test has been described by Smith and Resnick (1972). The low-frequency band of PB words is presented at 30 dB SL through one channel of a two-channel speech audiometer. The high-frequency band, controlled by the hearing-level dial of the second channel, is presented 10 dB above the level set for the low band. Three test conditions exist:

TABLE 12.1   Band-pass Filter Settings Used in Five Studies of Binaural Fusion

	Low-Frequency Band (Hertz)	High-Frequency Band (Hertz)
Matzker (1959)	500–800	1815–2500
Hayashi, Ohta, & Morimoto (1966)	300–600	1200–2400
Franklin (1969)	240–480	1020–2040
Smith & Resnick (1972)	360–890	1750–2200
Palva & Jokinen (1975)	420–720	1800–2400

1. Low band to the right ear, high band to the left ear (**dichotic**)
2. Low band to the left ear, high band to the right ear (dichotic)
3. Both bands to both ears (**diotic**)

The Smith and Resnick (1972) procedure with CNC words, which they call dichotic binaural fusion, has gained some clinical prominence. There appear to be no differences in the three scores in patients with normal hearing, cochlear lesions, or lesions of the temporal lobe. Patients with brainstem disorders show significant diotic-score enhancement over one or both of the dichotic scores.

The test designed by Palva and Jokinen (1975) also utilizes three test conditions with two narrow bands of filtered words. Each band alone, of course, yields very low discrimination scores. Results are obtained (1) with both bands in the right ear, (2) with both bands in the left ear, and (3) with the high band in the right ear and the low band in the left ear. Patients with disorders of the auditory cortex show poor scores on the monaural test in the ear contralateral to the lesions, although their dichotic scores are good. Patients with brainstem lesions show poor scores in any of the three conditions, especially the one involving binaural fusion.

Martin and Clark (1977) employed a comparison of diotic and dichotic presentations of the WIPI test to young children so that a picture-pointing procedure could be used as a screening test for children with auditory-processing disorders. They found that diotic presentation improved discrimination scores by 10 percent and that a control group did about as well on the more difficult dichotic task as on the diotic one. This procedure appears to have merit as a screening test for children who show normal hearing on standard audiometric procedures but whose histories suggest the possibility of central deficits. For those who fail the test, referral must be made for in-depth testing by language specialists.

Synthetic Sentence Identification Tests

The synthetic sentence identification (SSI) test, described in Chapter 5, may be used to identify lesions of the central auditory system. The sentences are made more difficult to identify by using a competing message, a recording of continuous discourse. This may be an *ipsilateral competing message (ICM),* which is presented to the test ear along with the synthetic sentences, or it may be a *contralateral competing message (CCM),* which is presented to the opposite ear. With the test materials (SSI) fixed at a given sensation level, the competing message may be varied in intensity so that a number of message-to-competition ratios (MCRs) are obtained (Jerger, 1973).

To perform the SSI-ICM test, a series of synthetic sentences is presented to one ear. The competing message is presented to the same earphone at a number of MCRs, beginning at +10 dB (the sentences 10 dB stronger than the competition) and increasing the intensity of the competition until the percentage of sentences identified correctly drops to 20 percent. The test is then repeated in the other ear.

According to Jerger (1973) normal-hearing persons will perform at the 100 percent level with an MCR of 0 dB, 80 percent with an MCR of –10 dB, 55 percent with an MCR of –20 dB, and 20 percent with an MCR of –30 dB (competing message 30 dB above the sentences). Patients with lesions of the brainstem show large differences in scores between the right and left ears on this test. With an increase in the level of the competing message, scores deteriorate more rapidly than normal when the test is performed in the ear contralateral to the lesion. For example, for a patient with a lesion of the left brainstem, SSI-ICM scores will be poorer in the right ear than in the left ear.

The SSI-CCM test is performed in precisely the same manner as the SSI-ICM, the only difference being that the competing message is presented to one ear and the sentences are presented to the opposite ear. The MCR is varied up to –40 dB.

Persons with normal hearing, and normal central auditory function, will perform very well on the SSI-CCM test, even at MCRs of –40 dB. The competition of the other ear seems to have little effect on the ability to understand the synthetic sentences. Patients with lesions of the temporal lobe perform well when the sentences are presented to the ear on the same side as the lesion while the competing message is presented to the other ear. When the sentences are presented to the ear on the unimpaired side and the competition is presented to the ear on the same side as the cortical lesion, deterioration of scores ensues. For example, in a left cortical lesion, SSI scores will be good with sentences in the left ear and competition in the right ear, but scores will be poor with sentences in the right ear and competition in the left ear. Jerger (1973) therefore believes that the use of ipsilateral and contralateral competing messages with the SSI not only reveals central disorders but actually separates lesions of the brainstem from those in the cortex.

Competing Sentence Tests

Building on work begun a decade earlier, Williford (1977) reported on the use of natural sentences in diagnosing central auditory disorders. The CST (Competing Sentence Test) is made up of natural sentences and, unlike the SSI procedure, uses an open-message set. To make the procedure useful, of course, a competing message is presented to the opposite ear.

The primary message is presented at a level 35 dB above the pure-tone average (PTA) while the competing message is presented at 50 dB above the PTA. Both sentences are the same length and on the same subject (e.g., time, food, weather, family). Fifteen sentences are used. The patient is told to repeat only the primary (softer) sentence. Because many brain-injured patients have difficulty in attending to soft stimuli or those under conditions of adverse message-to-competition ratios, modifications of the original method have been developed (Bergman, Hirsch, Solzi, & Mankowitz, 1987). Examples of the CST are included in the word list section under Forms in the literature section of the accompanying CD-ROM.

Patients with lesions of the temporal lobe show the greatest difficulty when the primary sentence is presented to the ear contralateral to the lesion. Simple versions of the procedure have been used successfully to identify children with learning disabilities. Children tend to improve on this test as they get older, which is not surprising because the central auditory nervous system probably continues to mature until about nine years of age.

Rapidly Alternating Speech Perception (RASP)

A test has been designed that rapidly alternates six- or seven-word sentences between the ears (Williford, 1977). The twenty sentences, presented at 50 dB above the SRT, are switched back and forth every 300 milliseconds. For the patient to understand and repeat the sentences, brainstem function must be normal because any segment presented to one ear alone is presumably too short to allow discrimination. The procedure is called the **Rapidly Alternating Speech Perception (RASP) test.**

The Dichotic Digits Test

Musiek (1983) describes a version of the **dichotic digits test** as being useful for diagnosing both brainstem and cortical disorders, although it may not be possible to tell one lesion site from the other on the basis of this test alone. Twenty sets of two-digit pairs are presented at 50 or 60 dB above the SRT. The digit 7 is omitted because it is the only one that has two syllables. The patient hears two successive pairs of two digits and is asked to repeat all four digits. The test can also be done with three-digit pairs but may result in low scores for some individuals because of short-term memory difficulties. For this reason, Mueller (1987a) believes that the two-digit pair test is probably better for detection of lesions in the central auditory nervous system.

The Staggered Spondaic Word (SSW) Test

Katz (1962, 1968) developed a test of dichotic listening that has undergone more standardization on English-speaking adults than most of the other tests for central auditory disorders and has been shown to differentiate between normal children and those with learning disabilities (Berrick, Shubow, Schultz, Freed, Fournier, & Hughes, 1984). The **Staggered Spondaic Word (SSW) test** is a measure of dichotic listening that utilizes spondees in a suprathreshold manner. Pairs of different spondaic words are presented to each ear, with some timing overlap for both ears. The first syllable of one spondee is presented to one ear; and, while the second syllable is presented, the first syllable of the other spondee is presented to the other ear. Then the second syllable of the second spondee is presented alone. This procedure is diagrammed as shown:

	Time $\longrightarrow$		
	1	2	3
Right Ear	OUT	SIDE	
Left Ear		IN	LAW

The words are recorded on two channels of a stereo tape for independent control by a two-channel speech audiometer. The items are presented so that the competing and noncompeting messages are reversed in terms of which ear is stimulated first. For example, the test may begin as: Right Noncompeting (RNC)–Right Competing (RC)–Left Noncompeting (LNC), followed by LNC–LC–RNC. The order of the ear receiving the first spondee is alternated throughout the test, which contains 40 items and takes about 20 minutes to complete.

The SSW test was designed to be performed at a level 50 dB above the SRT. If a PI-PB function has been determined, the SSW test may be delivered at the intensities in each ear at which PB Max was found. Using the PB Max intensity eliminates problems in word recognition posed by high-frequency peripheral hearing losses (Mueller, 1987b) or in patients with loudness tolerance problems.

During the SSW test, the patient is simply asked to repeat both spondees. Practice items are presented before the test is begun to ensure that the patient understands this unusual task. Because the SSW test is performed at relatively high sensation levels, if a hearing loss exists in one ear, no matter how mild, there is a chance that the better ear may, by contralateralization, aid in discriminating words presented to the poorer ear. Naturally, the very nature of this test precludes the use of masking, but insert receivers might be useful in increasing the interaural attenuation.

Scoring and interpreting the SSW test requires a special form, which is available commercially with the recording. Individual errors are summed first for each ear, both for competing and non-competing words. The total SSW score is the total number of errors obtained for both ears. Each monosyllable is given a weight of 2.5 percent, and the total of incorrect responses multiplied by 2.5 percent is subtracted from 100 percent to give the percentage of correct responses. To avoid penalizing the patient's SSW score for peripheral discrimination difficulties, the word recognition loss for PB words is credited to each ear by subtracting the percentage error for PB words from the percentage error on the SSW test for the same ear. Poor scores on the SSW test suggest a lesion in the higher brain centers on the side contralateral to the low-scoring ear. Although the SSW test is very popular, one lasting complaint concerns the amount of time needed to follow the complex scoring system. At least one computer program is now available for this purpose. Mueller (1987b) has suggested that diagnosis with the SSW test may be carried out simply by computing the score for each ear on the basis of the percentage of words identified correctly.

Masking-Level Difference

The phenomenon of binaural release from masking, or **masking-level difference (MLD),** has been known for some time (Hirsh, 1948). To determine the MLD, the binaural threshold is determined for a low-frequency tone presented in phase to the two ears in the presence of a binaural noise, also in phase. When the threshold is remeasured with the tones 180 degrees out of phase with the noise, a threshold improvement is found on the order of 10 to 15 dB. Abnormal MLDs in normal-hearing subjects strongly suggest a brainstem lesion (Noffsinger, Martinez, & Schaefer, 1985), but positive findings have also been observed in cases of acoustic neuroma, presbycusis, Méniére disease, and particularly multiple sclerosis (Mueller, 1987a). MLDs have also been measured using speech signals.

Although the effects of cochlear and cortical lesions on MLD are somewhat unpredictable, there is general agreement among researchers (e.g., Olsen & Noffsinger, 1976) that the release from masking is either absent or significantly less than normal in patients with lesions in the brainstem. If the clinician has access to a device capable of shifting the phase of the pure tone without affecting the phase of the noise, simply measuring several binaural pure-tone thresholds may provide additional insight into site of lesion. The procedure is complicated by any degree of peripheral hearing loss.

Time-Compressed Speech

With special recording devices it is possible to speed up the playback of speech stimuli without significantly creating the perception of higher vocal pitch. This **time-compressed speech** has been studied by using the words from the NU-6 lists. Central auditory lesions are best identified at 60 percent time compression (Kurdziel, Noffsinger, & Olsen, 1976). Kurdziel and colleagues found that in some brain lesions, time-compressed word recognition scores were poor in the ear contralateral to the lesion, whereas in other cases scores remained normal in both ears. There has not been much information in the recent literature on the use of time-compressed speech in cases of central auditory nervous system damage.

Screening Test for Auditory Processing Disorders

The **Screening Test for Auditory Processing Disorders (SCAN)**[3] was devised as a rapid procedure to detect auditory-processing difficulties in children aged 3 to 11, so that their risk factors may be determined and specific management strategies applied. Its standardization (Keith, 1986) appears to be more extensive than some of the other tests for central auditory disorders. The SCAN comprises three subtests: The filtered-word subtest contains two lists of 20 monosyllabic words that are low-pass filtered at 1000 Hz (rejection rate 32 dB/octave) and are presented by audiotape to one ear at a time. The auditory figure-ground subtest likewise contains two monosyllabic 20-word lists, presented to each ear in the presence of a background noise made up of a multitalker babble. A signal-to-noise ratio of +8 dB is used. The competing-word subtest comprises two lists of 25 monosyllabic words presented dichotically (one word introduced to each ear simultaneously). The child is instructed to repeat the word heard in the right ear followed by the word heard in the left ear. Comparisons to other tests for central auditory disorders suggest that the SCAN may be a useful procedure (Keith, Rudy, Donahue, & Katfamma, 1989).

In response to a need for well standardized central auditory tests for persons over 11 years of age, Keith (1994, 1995) modified the SCAN for use with older subjects. The SCAN-A is an upward extension of the SCAN designed for use with adolescents and adults with neurological disorders and learning disabilities.

Acoustic Reflex Test

Comparison of ipsilateral and contralateral acoustic reflexes can be of great value in determining the integrity of the crossover pathways in the trapezoid body of the brainstem. If, for example, a patient has normal hearing and normal ipsilateral acoustic reflexes in both ears, it is highly probable that the cochleas, the VIIth and VIIIth cranial nerves, and the middle-ear mechanisms are intact on both sides. If, in the same individual, the contralateral reflexes are absent, the most likely explanation is that damage exists within those crossover pathways (see Figures 6.7I and J).

Auditory Evoked Potentials

Auditory brainstem response audiometry has been useful in diagnosing central auditory disorders as long as any hearing loss in the two ears is essentially symmetrical and no more than a mild loss exists in either ear (Musiek, 1983). The presence of concomitant peripheral lesions may confound interpretation of ABR results if lesions are present in both the cochlea and the brainstem. Central lesions

---

[3]SCAN and SCAN-A available from The Psychological Corporation, Harcourt Brace Jovanovich. 1-800-228-0752.

will generally slow the conduction velocity of electrical impulses sent through the nerve fibers. Musiek suggests the following general observations:

Wave I (all waves) delay	Lesion in outer, middle, or inner ear
Wave I–III delay	Lesion in auditory nerve or lower brainstem
Wave III–V delay	Lesion in higher brainstem

In testing for lesions of the brainstem, it is useful to compare the latencies and intervals of waves I, III, and V as a function of increased click rates. Although the ABR results may provide important diagnostic information in testing for central auditory lesions, interpretation can be difficult when it is complicated by the absence of some waves, the influence of unusual audiometric configurations, and the patient's age and body temperature. The ABR is generally the most sensitive and specific test currently available for diagnosis of auditory brainstem lesions, although the use of the complete central test battery remains important (Chermak & Musiek, 1997).

The P300, or cognitive potential of the late auditory evoked response, is elicited by an "oddball" paradigm, whereby the subject tries to discriminate between a frequently occurring stimulus and a rarely occurring stimulus. For example, a 1000 Hz tone burst is presented 80 percent of the time, and a 2000 Hz tone burst is presented randomly 20 percent of the time. The subject is asked to count only the higher-pitched tones. The waveform elicited by the rare (2000 Hz) stimulus shows a large positive peak with a latency of approximately 300 milliseconds. Reduction in amplitude, or increase in the latencies of the P300, have been found in elderly individuals, those suffering from dementia, and head trauma patients. This procedure is thought to hold future promise as a diagnostic procedure for other disorders of the central auditory nervous system.

Otoacoustic Emissions

It has been emphasized in this book that otoacoustic emissions have come into their own as a powerful clinical tool, with a variety of applications. For example, Jerger, Ali, Fong, and Tseng (1992) reported on a patient with multiple sclerosis in whom it was possible to identify the source of the word-recognition difficulty she experienced in one ear as retrocochlear. The presence of distortion product otoacoustic emissions in this case suggested that at least the outer hair cells of the cochlea were functioning normally. The diagnosis of a more central lesion was confirmed by MRI of the brain. It is anticipated that further reports of this nature will be forthcoming. Cevette, Robinette, Carter, and Knops (1995) reported on the important contribution otoacoustic emissions can make to the diagnosis of multiple sclerosis.

Diagnostic Limitations

While administration of electrophysiologic tests is more costly than that of behavioral measures, behavioral tests are not always feasible as with patients with aphasia or central deafness. The sensitivity of testing for lesions of the auditory nerve and central auditory pathways increases when behavioral and electrophysiologic measures are combined. In addition, the audiologist's confidence in making a diagnosis of CAPD is heightened when abnormalities are found in both the behavioral and electrophysiologic domains (Chermak & Musiek, 1997).

There is much room for improvement in test design for CAPD given that tests currently available are largely drawn from methods developed for clinical and laboratory studies of physiology, neuroanatomy, and site of lesion (Harris, 1996). Of the commercially available tests for adult and pediatric CAPD, the SCAN and SCAN-A (Keith, 1986, 1995) appear to have the most complete development of normative data, yet both of these measures are designed as screening instruments. As Harris (1996) points out, it is ironic and unfortunate that tests with less comprehensive norms must then be used as follow-up approaches to confirm CAPD. The diagnosis of CAPD is best carried out through a team approach, capitalizing on the backgrounds of audiologists, speech-language pathologists, and educational psychologists.

Therapeutic Management

Patients with suspected lesions on the auditory nerve must be referred to a physician for medical and/or surgical management. Hearing loss, either preexisting or subsequent to medical intervention, may then be managed by the audiologist. These hearing losses may include the challenges of dramatically reduced word recognition or unilateral deafness.

From an audiological standpoint, adults with CAPD benefit from means of improving signal-to-noise ratios, as well as general communication guidelines provided to patients with peripheral hearing loss (Trychin, Clark, & Boone, 1986a, 1986b). Audiologists should be aware that older patients with presbycusic hearing loss may have central processing complications secondary to the aging process. Signal-to-noise enhancement and reduced speech rate can be beneficial for these individuals as well. Patients with OAD, as a group, do have difficulty understanding speech in noise. These patients benefit from recognition of the reality of their complaints, in spite of normal peripheral hearing, along with the provision of communication guidelines.

Many children with CAPD are placed within inappropriate therapy programs as their underlying disorder has not been identified. The child with CAPD may exhibit dysfluencies or hesitations in speech due to an inability to recall words or describe events. The misdiagnosis of these behaviors as stuttering can lead to incorrect intervention.

When a diagnosis of CAPD has been reached, controversy exists on the best remedial tack to be taken. Therapy programs designed for children are often based upon the deficiencies exhibited in language production. Some experts question, however, whether remediation of language processing deficits might better precede intervention for language production deficits. To this end, therapy is often directed toward improving auditory perceptual processing for such subskills as auditory attention, localization, figure-ground differentiation, discrimination, and sequencing.

In contrast, Northern and Downs (1991, p. 124) suggest that it may be wiser to attempt to identify the etiology of pediatric CAPD if we are to treat its symptoms more accurately. They reject a therapy program that is based upon the symptomatic treatment of auditory learning disorders, stating that this presupposes that the symptoms are the underlying cause of the exhibited language disorder, and that isolating and treating each symptom will remedy the language problem.

Classroom performance can be significantly affected by central auditory processing difficulties given the less than ideal signal-to-noise ratios in classrooms. Classroom management suggestions (Clark, 1980; Hall & Mueller, 1997) and classroom soundfield amplification (see Chapter 14) can be of benefit for children with CAPD.

Clearly the goal for both children and adults with CAPD is to attain improved listening ability and greater comprehension of spoken language. Toward this end, Chermak and Musiek (1997) outline a multifactored approach to remediation.

Summary

This chapter has dealt with the function and audiologic diagnosis of lesions of the auditory nerve and central auditory nervous system. Although considerable mystery continues to surround the central nervous system, nowhere is this mystery greater than in the higher auditory pathways. Impulses that pass from the cochlea are transmitted by the auditory nerve to the cochlear nuclei, which are waystations for transmission to higher centers and areas for complex frequency and temporal analysis. The cochlear nuclei also represent the highest centers at which the processing of neural stimuli represent auditory information obtained from just one ear. From the cochlear nuclei, auditory information is processed by the superior olivary complexes, the lateral lemnisci, the inferior colliculi, and the medial geniculate bodies. Impulses are finally transmitted to the cortex by the auditory radiations. Owing to the numerous decussations at higher centers, there is representation of each ear on both sides of the brain, with greater representation on the opposite side.

Caution should always be exercised when an audiologist attempts to determine the site of a lesion affecting the auditory system. A patient may, for example, have both a cochlear and a central disorder. Most auditory tests give results that reflect primarily the first lesion reached by the stimulus (the most peripheral lesion) but can be further complicated by the more central lesion. Ruling out one anatomical area of the auditory system should not result in a diagnosis of a lesion in a specific region elsewhere.

Behavioral tests for site of lesion may be positive in patients with lesions of the auditory nerve and cochlear nucleus. However, lesions in the higher centers produce more subtle symptoms and are often insensitive to many currently used tests. Special procedures have been devised for testing central disorders, but none has been demonstrated to be infallible. Much research is needed to improve techniques for detecting disorders in the central pathways and pinpointing the area of damage. There is little doubt that this is one of the most challenging areas for research in diagnostic audiology. Nearly 25 years ago, Williford (1977) lamented that audiology had only scratched the surface in its efforts to diagnose CAPD and that practical treatment programs were even less developed. Despite considerable progress to date, these are areas that still need much additional exploration.

STUDY QUESTIONS

1. Sketch from memory the auditory pathways arising from the cochlea. Label the different waystations, and specify, as far as you can, the functions of each.

2. Make a list of the possible causes of hearing disorders at each of the sites just named.

3. Draw an audiogram typical of an VIIIth nerve lesion. List the results of as many site-of-lesion tests as you can remember.

4. Why are lesions of the central auditory nervous system subtle and difficult to observe on standard audiometric tests?

5. List the tests that may be performed for central auditory lesions. Discuss the shortcomings of each test.

6. List the tests that can be done with evoked response audiometry and the areas of the auditory system assessed.

GLOSSARY

Acoustic neuritis Inflammatory or degenerative lesions of the auditory nerve.

Acoustic neuroma A tumor involving the nerve sheath of the auditory nerve.

Auditory nerve The VIIIth cranial nerve, which comprises auditory and vestibular branches, passing from the inner ear to the brainstem.

Auditory neuropathy A mild to moderate sensorineural hearing loss with speech recognition difficulties disproportionate to degree of loss. In contrast to acoustic neuroma, there is an unexpected absence of ABR wave forms and a normal MRI.

Auditory radiations A bundle of nerve fibers passing from the medial geniculate body to the temporal gyri of the cerebral cortex.

Central auditory processing disorders (CAPD) Impairment of the central auditory nervous system interfering with decoding of acoustic signals, including difficulties in sound localization and speech discrimination in noise.

Cerebellopontine angle (CPA) That area at the base of the brain at the junction of the cerebellum, medulla, and pons.

Cerebellum The lower part of the brain above the medulla and the pons. It is the seat of posture and integrated movements in the brain.

Cerebrovascular accident (CVA) A clot or hemorrhage of one of the arteries within the cerebrum; a stroke.

Commissure Nerve fibers connecting similar structures on both sides of the brain.

Computed tomography (CT) A procedure for imaging the inside of the body by representing portions of it as a series of sections. The many pictures taken are resolved by computer, and the amount of radiation to the patient is significantly less than with older procedures.

Decussation A crossing over, as of nerve fibers connecting both sides of the brain.

Dichotic Stimulation of both ears by different stimuli. This is usually accomplished with earphones and two channels of a CD or tape player.

Dichotic digits test A test for central auditory disorders performed by presenting two pairs of digits simultaneously to both ears.

Diotic Stimulation of both ears with stimuli that are approximately identical, as through a stethoscope.

Dorsal cochlear nucleus The smaller of two cochlear nuclei on each side of the brain; it receives the fibers of the cochlea on the ipsilateral side.

Extra-axial Outside the brainstem.

Heschl's gyrus See *Superior temporal gyrus*.

Inferior colliculus One of the central auditory pathways, found in the posterior portion of the midbrain.

Internal auditory canal A channel from the inner ear to the brainstem allowing passage of the auditory and vestibular branches of the VIIIth nerve, the VIIth nerve, and the internal auditory artery.

Insular Related to the insula, the central lobe of the cerebral hemisphere.

Intra-axial Inside the brainstem.

Kernicterus Deposits of bile pigment in the central nervous system, especially the basal ganglia. It is associated with erythroblastosis and the Rh factor.

Lateral lemniscus That portion of the auditory pathway running from the cochlear nuclei to the inferior colliculus and medial geniculate body.

Magnetic resonance imaging (MRI) A system of visualizing the inside of the body without the use of X rays. The body is placed in a magnetic field and bombarded with radio waves, some of which are re-emitted and resolved by computer, which allows for viewing soft tissues and various abnormalities.

Masking-level difference (MLD) The binaural threshold for a pure tone is lower when a binaural noise is 180 degrees out of phase than when the noise is in phase between the two ears.

Medial geniculate body The final subcortical auditory relay station, found in the thalamus on each side of the brain.

Medulla oblongata The lowest portion of the brain, connecting the pons with the spinal cord.

Minimal auditory deficiency syndrome (MADS) Changes in the size of neurons in the central auditory nervous system caused by conductive hearing loss in early life. The result is difficulty in language learning.

Multiple sclerosis (MS) A chronic disease showing hardening or demyelinization in different parts of the nervous system.

Neoplasm Any new or aberrant growth, as a tumor.

Neurofibromatosis (NF) The presence of tumors on the skin or along peripheral nerves; also called von Recklinghausen disease.

Obscure auditory dysfunction (OAD) Decreased hearing abilities, primarily in adverse listening conditions, in the absence of identifiable peripheral pathology.

Olivocochlear bundle (OCB) A grouping of nerve units in the brainstem that course to the cochlear nuclei and terminate in the cochleas. Efferent fibers from the OCB provide inhibitory connections to the auditory neurons.

Parietal lobe The division of each side of the cerebral cortex between the frontal and occipital lobes.

Plasticity The ability of cells, such as those in the auditory centers of the brain, to become altered in order to conform to their immediate environment.

Pons A bridge of fibers and neurons that connect the two sides of the brain at its base.

Positron emission tomography (PET) A medical imaging procedure that can indicate changes in the brain with a minimum of patient exposure to radioactivity. It is useful in identifying biochemical changes in the brain.

Rapidly Alternating Speech Perception (RASP) test A test for central auditory disorders in which sentences are rapidly switched from the left ear to the right ear. Normal brainstem function is required for discrimination.

Reticular formation Located in the brainstem, the reticular formation communicates with all areas of the brain and contains centers for inhibition and facilitation of afferent stimuli.

Screening Test for Auditory Processing Disorders (SCAN) A rapid test for central auditory processing disorders comprising three subtests: filtered words, auditory figure ground, and dichotic listening.

Staggered Spondaic Word (SSW) test A test for central auditory disorders utilizing the dichotic listening task of two spondaic words so that the second syllable presented to one ear is heard simultaneously with the first syllable presented to the other ear.

Superior olivary complex (SOC) One of the auditory relay stations in the midbrain, largely comprising units from the cochlear nuclei.

Superior temporal gyrus The convolution of the temporal lobe believed to be the seat of language comprehension of the auditory system.

Temporal lobe The part of the cerebral hemispheres usually associated with perception of sound. The auditory language areas are located in the temporal lobes.

Thalamus Located in the brain base, the thalamus sends projecting fibers to, and receives fibers from, all parts of the cortex.

Time-compressed speech A system of recording speech so that it is accelerated and therefore distorted, but the words remain discriminable.

Tonotopic Arranged anatomically according to best frequency of stimulation.

Trapezoid body Nerve fibers in the pons that connect the ventral cochlear nucleus on one side of the brain with the lateral lemniscus on the other side.

Ventral cochlear nucleus The larger of the two cochlear nuclei on each side of the brain; it receives the fibers of the cochlea on the ipsilateral side.

REFERENCES

American Academy of Audiology. (1992). Position Statement: Public meeting on clinical practice guidelines for the diagnosis and treatment of otitis media in children. *Audiology Today, 4,* 23–24.

Anderson, H., Barr, B., & Wedenberg, E. (1969). Intra-aural reflexes in retrocochlear lesions. In C. A. Hamberger & J. Wersall (Eds.), *Disorders of the skull base region* (pp. 49–55). New York: Wiley.

Antonelli, A., & Calearo, C. (1968). Further investigations on cortical deafness. *Acta Otolaryngologica* (Stockholm), *66,* 97–100.

Bergman, M., Hirsch, S., Solzi, P., & Mankowitz, Z. (1987). The threshold-of-interference test: A new test of interhemispheric suppression in brain injury. *Ear and Hearing, 8,* 147–150.

Berrick, J. M., Shubow, G. F., Schultz, M. C., Freed, H., Fournier, S. R., & Hughes, J. P. (1984). Auditory processing tests for children: Normative and clinical results on the SSW test. *Journal of Speech and Hearing Disorders, 49,* 318–325.

Blakely, R. W. (1959). Erythroblastosis and hearing loss: Responses of athetoids to tests of cochlear function. *Journal of Speech and Hearing Research, 2,* 5–15.

Bocca, E. (1955). Binaural hearing: Another approach. *Laryngoscope, 65,* 1164–1175.

———. (1967). Distorted speech tests. In A. B. Graham (Ed.), *Sensorineural hearing processes and disorders* (Henry Ford Hospital International Symposium). Boston: Little, Brown.

Bocca, E., & Calearo, C. (1963). Central hearing process. In J. Jerger (Ed.), *Modern developments in audiology* (pp. 337–370). New York: Academic Press.

Bocca, E., Calearo, C., & Cassinari, V. (1954). A new method for testing hearing in temporal lobe tumors: Preliminary report. *Acta Otolaryngologica* (Stockholm), *44,* 219–221.

Calearo, C. (1957). Binaural summation in lesions of the temporal lobe. *Acta Otolaryngologica* (Stockholm), *47,* 392–395.

Carhart, R. (1967). Audiologic tests: Questions and speculations. In F. McConnell & P. H. Ward (Eds.), *Deafness in childhood* (pp. 229–251). Nashville, TN: Vanderbilt University Press.

Chermak, G. D., & Musiek, F. E. (1997). *Central auditory processing disorders: New perspectives.* San Diego: Singular Publishing Group.

Clark, J. G. (1980). Central auditory dysfunction in school children: A compilation of management suggestions. *Speech, Language, and Hearing Services in Schools, 11,* 208–213.

Cevette, M. J., Robinette, M. S., Carter, J., & Knops, J. L. (1995). Otoacoustic emissions in sudden unilateral hearing loss associated with multiple sclerosis. *Journal of the American Academy of Audiology, 6,* 197–202.

Franklin, B. (1966). The effect on consonant discrimination of combining a low-frequency passband in one ear and a high-frequency passband in the other ear. *Journal of Auditory Research, 9,* 365–378.

Gang, R. P. (1976). The effects of age on the diagnostic utility of the rollover phenomenon. *Journal of Speech and Hearing Disorders, 41,* 63–69.

Goetzinger, C. P., & Angell, S. (1965). Audiological assessment in acoustic tumors and cortical lesions. *Eye, Ear, Nose and Throat Monthly, 44,* 39–49.

Goodhill, V. (1950). Nuclear deafness and the nerve-deaf child: The importance of the Rh factor. *Transactions of the American Academy of Ophthalmology and Otolaryngology, 54,* 671–687.

Gunnarson, A., & Finitzo, T. (1991). Conductive hearing loss during infancy: Effects on later auditory brain stem electrophysiology. *Journal of Speech and Hearing Research, 34,* 1207–1215.

Hall, J. W. & Mueller, H. G. (1997). *Audiologists' desk reference, Vol. I.* San Diego: Singular.

Harris, D. P. (1996). Central auditory processing disorders in children: Are we listening? In F. N. Martin & J. G. Clark (Eds.), *Hearing care for children* (pp. 161–179). Boston: Allyn & Bacon.

Hayashi, R., Ohta, F., & Morimoto, M. (1966). Binaural fusion test: A diagnostic approach to the central auditory disorders. *International Audiology, 5,* 133–135.

Hirsh, I. (1948). The influence of interaural phase on interaural summation and inhibition. *Journal of the Acoustical Society of America, 23,* 384–386.

Hodgson, W. (1967). Audiological report of a patient with left hemispherectomy. *Journal of Speech and Hearing Disorders, 32,* 39–45.

Jerger, J. (1960). Observations on auditory behavior in lesions of the central auditory pathways. *Archives of Otolaryngology* (Chicago), *71,* 797–806.

———. (1973). Diagnostic audiometry. In J. Jerger (Ed.), *Modern developments in audiology* (2nd ed., pp. 75–115). New York: Academic Press.

Jerger, J., Ali, A., Fong, K., & Tseng, E. (1992). Otoacoustic emissions, audiometric sensitivity loss, and speech understanding: A case study. *Journal of the American Academy of Audiology, 3,* 283–286.

Jerger, J., & Jerger, S. (1971). Diagnostic significance of PB word functions. *Archives of Otolaryngology, 93,* 573–580.

Jerger, J., Oliver, T. A., & Jenkins, H. (1987). Suprathreshold abnormalities of the stapedius reflex in acoustic tumors. *Ear and Hearing, 8,* 131–139.

Jerger, S., & Jerger, J. (1975). Extra- and intraaxial brain stem auditory disorders. *Audiology, 14,* 93–117.

Johnson, E. W. (1977). Auditory test results in 500 cases of acoustic neuroma. *Archives of Otolaryngology, 103,* 152–158.

Josey, A. F. (1987). Audiologic manifestations of tumors of the VIIIth nerve. *Ear & Hearing, 8,* 19S–21S.

Josey, A. F., Glasscock, M. E., & Musiek, F. E. (1988). Correlation of ABR and medical imaging in patients with cerebellopontine angle tumors. *The American Journal of Otology, 9* (Supplement), 12–16.

Katz, J. (1962). The use of staggered spondaic words for assessing the integrity of the central auditory nervous system. *Journal of Auditory Research, 2,* 327–337.

———. (1968). The SSW test: An interim report. *Journal of Speech and Hearing Disorders, 33,* 132–146.

———. (1978). The effects of conductive hearing loss on auditory function. *Asha, 20,* 879–886.

Keith, R. W. (1981). Tests of central auditory function. In R. J. Roeser & M. P. Downs (Eds.), *Auditory disorders in school children* (pp. 159–173). New York: Thieme-tratton.

———. (1986). *SCAN: A screening test for auditory processing disorders.* San Antonio: The Psychological Corporation, Harcourt Brace Jovanovich.

———. (1994). SCAN-A: *Test for auditory processing disorders in adolescents and adults.* San Antonio, TX: The Psychological Corporation, Harcourt Brace Jovanovich.

———. (1995). Development and standardization of SCAN-A: Test of auditory processing disorders in adolescents and adults. *Journal of the American Academy of Audiology, 7,* 286–292.

Keith, R. W., Rudy, J., Donahue, P. A., & Katfamma, B. (1989). Comparison of SCAN results with other auditory and language measures in a clinical population. *Ear and Hearing, 10,* 382–386.

Kurdziel, S., Noffsinger, D., & Olsen, W. (1976). Performance by cortical lesion patients on 40 and 60% time compressed materials. *Journal of the American Audiology Society, 2,* 3–7.

Lynn, G. E., & Gilroy, J. (1977). Evaluation of central auditory dysfunction in patients with neurological disorders. In R. W. Keith (Ed.), *Central auditory dysfunction* (pp. 177–222). New York: Grune & Stratton.

Martin, F. N., & Clark, J. G. (1977). Audiologic detection of auditory processing disorders in children. *Journal of the American Audiology Society, 3,* 140–146.

Matkin, N. D. (1965). *Audiological patterns characterizing hearing impairment due to Rh incompatibility.* Doctoral dissertation, Northwestern University, Evanston, IL.

Matzker, J. (1959). Two new methods for the assessment of central auditory functions in cases of brain disease. *Annals of Otology, Rhinology and Laryngology, 63,* 1185–1197.

Mueller, H. G. (1987a). An auditory test protocol for evaluation of neural trauma. *Seminars in Hearing, 8,* 223–238.

———. (1987b). The staggered spondaic word test: Practical use. *Seminars in Hearing, 8,* 267–277.

Musiek, F. E. (1983). The evaluation of brainstem disorders using ABR and central auditory tests. *Monographs in Contemporary Audiology, 4,* 1–24.

———. (1992). Neurotransmitters in the auditory system. *Audiology Today, 4,* 21.

Musiek, F. E., Gollegly, K. M., Kibbe, K. S., & Verkest, S. B. (1988). Current concepts on the use of ABR and auditory psychophysical tests in the evaluation of brain stem lesions. *The American Journal of Otology, 9,* 25–35.

NIH Consensus Statement. (1991). *Acoustic neuroma.* U.S. Department of Health and Human Services, NIH Consensus Development Conference, Bethesda, MD.

Noffsinger, D., Martinez, C., & Schaefer, A. (1985). Puretone techniques in evaluation of central auditory function. In J. Katz (Ed.), *Handbook of clinical audiology* (3rd ed., pp. 337–354). Baltimore: Williams & Wilkins.

Northern, J. L., & Downs, M. P. (1991). *Hearing in children.* Baltimore: Williams and Wilkins.

Olsen, W. O., & Noffsinger, D. (1976). Masking level differences for cochlear and brainstem lesions. *Annals of Otology, Rhinology and Laryngology, 85,* 820–825.

Palva, A., & Jokinen, K. (1975). The role of the binaural test in filtered speech audiometry. *Acta Otolaryngologica, 79,* 310–314.

Pool, J. I., Pava, A. A., & Greenfield, E. C. (1970). *Acoustic nerve tumors: Early diagnosis and treatment* (2nd ed.). Springfield, IL: Thomas.

Rasmussen, G. L. (1960). Efferent fibers of the cochlear nerve and cochlear nucleus. In G. I. Rasmussen & W. F. Windle (Eds.), *Neural mechanisms of the auditory and vestibular systems* (pp. 105–115). Springfield, IL: Thomas.

———. (1964). Anatomic relationships of the ascending and descending auditory systems. In W. S. Fields & B. R. Alford (Eds.), *Neurological aspects of auditory and vestibular disorders* (pp. 5–23). Springfield, IL: Thomas.

Rentschler, G. J., & Rupp, R. R. (1984). Conductive hearing loss: Cause for concern. *Hearing Instruments, 35,* 12–14.

Saunders, G. H., & Haggard, M. P. (1989). The clinical assessment of obscure auditory dysfunction - 1. Auditory and psychological factors. *Ear and Hearing, 10,* 200–208.

———. (1993). The influence of personality-related factors upon consultation for two different "marginal" organic pathologies with and without reports of auditory symptomatology. *Ear and Hearing, 14,* 242–248.

Schwaber, M. (1992). Neuroplasticity of the adult primate auditory cortex. *Audiology Today, 4,* 19–20.

Smith, B., & Resnick, D. (1972). An auditory test for assessing brain stem integrity: Preliminary report. *Laryngoscope, 82,* 414–424.

Starr, A., Picton, T. W., Sininger, Y., Hood, L., & Berlin, C. I. (1996). Auditory neuropathy. *Brain, 119,* 741–753.

Stool, S. E., Berg, A. O., Berman, S., Carney, C. J., Cooley, J. R., Culpepper, L., Eavey, R. D., Feagans, L. V., Finitzo, T., & Friedman, E. (1994, July). *Managing otitis media with effusion in young children: Quick reference guide for clinicians.* AHCPR Publication No. 94-0623. Rockville, MD: Agency for Health Care Policy and Research, U.S. Department of Health and Human Services.

Strasnick, B., Glasscock, M. E., Haynes, D., McMenomey, S. O., & Minor, L. B. (1994). The natural history of untreated acoustic neuromas. *Laryngoscope, 104,* 1115–1119.

Telian, S. A., & Kileny, P. R. (1988). Pitfalls in neurotologic diagnosis. *Ear and Hearing, 9,* 86–91.

Telian, S. A., Kileny, P. R., Niparko, J. K., Kemink, J. L., & Graham, M. D. (1989). Normal auditory brainstem response in patients with acoustic neuroma. *Laryngoscope, 99,* 10–14.

Trychin, S., Clark, J. G. & Boone, M. (1996a). Communication guidelines for people with hearing loss. In J. G. Clark & F. N. Martin (Eds.), *Effective counseling in audiology: Perspectives and practice* (pp. 275–276). Englewood Cliffs, NJ: Prentice Hall.

———. (1996b). Communication guidelines for speaking to people with hearing loss. In J. G. Clark & F. N. Martin (Eds.), *Effective counseling in audiology: Perspectives and practice* (pp. 273–274). Englewood Cliffs, NJ: Prentice Hall.

Valente, M., Peterein, J., Goebel, J. & Neely, J. G., (1995). Four cases of acoustic neuromas with normal hearing. *Journal of the American Academy of Audiology, 6,* 203–210.

Webster, D. B., & Webster, M. (1977). Neonatal sound deprivation affects brain stem auditory nuclei. *Archives of Otolaryngology, 103,* 392–396.

Williford, J. A. (1977). Differential diagnosis of central auditory dysfunction. *Audiology: An Audio Journal for Continuing Education, 2.*

SUGGESTED READINGS

Chermak, G. D., & Musiek, F. E. (1997). *Central auditory processing disorders: New perspectives.* San Diego: Singular.

Harris, D. P. (1996). Central auditory processing disorders in children: Are we listening? In F. N. Martin & J. G. Clark (Eds.), *Hearing care for children* (pp. 161–179). Boston: Allyn & Bacon.

Masters, M. G., Stecker, N. A., & Katz, J. (1998). *Central auditory processing disorders: Mostly management.* Boston: Allyn & Bacon.

Musiek, F., Baran, J., & Pinheiro, M. (1994). *Neuroaudiology, case studies.* San Diego: Singular.

Yost, W. A. (1993). *Fundamentals of hearing: An introduction* (3rd ed.). New York: Academic Press.

REVIEW TABLE 12.1　Audiological Symptoms of Retrocochlear Lesions

VIIIth Nerve and Cochlear Nucleus	Central Pathways
Negative SISI	Poor binaural fusion
Decruitment; no recruitment	Low SSI-ICM scores
Marked tone decay at all frequencies	Low SSI-CCM scores
Rapid acoustic reflex decay	Increased wave III-V interval
Elevated or absent acoustic reflexes	WRS for distorted speech poor in ear contralateral to lesion
Marked increase in ABR wave V latencies	
WRS for distorted speech poor in ear ipsilateral to lesion	

13 Nonorganic Hearing Loss

There are numbers of reasons why an individual might decide to fabricate or exaggerate a disability and many forms of expression for this decision. Law suits have been filed for compensation for low-back pain, memory loss, cognitive deficits, spinal cord injury, weakness, and, of course, hearing loss in addition to a host of litigious actions, many of which are related to claims for Worker's Compensation.

The past four chapters have discussed anatomical areas in the auditory system and hearing losses associated with lesions in each of these areas. The term **nonorganic hearing loss** describes an apparent loss of hearing, without an organic disorder, or with insufficient pathological evidence to explain the extent of the loss.

The source of patient referral, history of hearing loss, symptoms, and behavior both during and outside of hearing tests are factors to be considered before making a diagnosis of nonorganic hearing loss. Patients may exaggerate a hearing loss because they are incapable of more reliable behavior, because they are willfully fabricating or exaggerating a hearing disorder, or because they have some psychological disorder. Observation of the patient and special tests for nonorganic hearing loss often lead the audiologist to the proper resolution of the problem.

Chapter Objectives

This chapter should alert the reader to the problem of false or exaggerated hearing loss and some of the symptoms that make its presence known. The terms associated with this condition should be learned, as should the special tests that qualify and quantify it.

Terminology

Not all audiologists and other specialists concerned with hearing disorders use the term *nonorganic hearing loss*. Some prefer **pseudohypacusis,** which literally means "false hearing loss." Another popular term is **functional hearing loss.** The word *functional* is often used by physicians and psychologists to describe the symptoms of a condition that is not organic. Some audiologists use the term **psychogenic** (beginning in the mind) **hearing loss,** to describe a nonorganic problem the cause of which is psychological rather than deliberately feigned. An older term for psychogenic hearing loss is **hysterical deafness.**

In these days of heightened awareness about racist and sexist terminology, the word *hysterical* is an example of one whose precise meaning should be realized. Derived from the Greek, it means "uterus," since it was believed as far back as Hypocrites, the father of medicine, that such disorders were found only in women and were caused by sexual problems. In fact, it was claimed that the uterus literally moved from one part of the body to the other, creating a wide variety of nonorganic disorders. If the theory of the "wandering uterus" (Coleman, 1976) were true, the uterus would literally be found in the ear when nonorganic hearing loss is observed. Clinicians should select their terminology in sensitive ways.

One term probably used far too often is **malingering.** A malingerer is a deliberate falsifier of physical or psychological symptoms for some special gain. The slang military term *goldbrick* has been used to describe those persons who use the pretense of some disability to avoid undesired duty. Malingering is also frequently suspected in association with automobile and industrial accidents, when payment may be involved to compensate patients for damages. Many patients who are called malingerers actually have a hearing loss, but exaggerate its severity to increase their gains.

Although *nonorganic hearing loss* is the term used in this book, the reader should be aware of other terminology and should know that terms such as *nonorganic hearing loss, functional hearing loss,* and *pseudohypacusis* are general and do not suggest cause, as do the terms *malingering* and *psychogenesis.* There is no way to know for certain whether a patient with a nonorganic disorder is malingering, has a psychogenic problem, or suffers from some combination of the two. Unless the patient admits to lying, or the confirmed diagnosis of psychogenicity is made by a qualified psychologist or psychiatrist, audiologists should settle for more general terms.

Patients with Nonorganic Hearing Loss

Patients manifesting symptoms of nonorganic hearing loss may be of any age, sex, or socioeconomic background. It is probable that more adult males have been suspected of this disorder, because emphasis has been placed on eliminating its possibility among men applying to the Veterans Administration for compensation for hearing loss.

Most of the studies performed on patients with nonorganic hearing loss have been carried out on adult males because they have been "captive audiences," as in military studies. This leads one to wonder whether there are any age or gender differences in this respect, and the paucity of data along these lines regarding nonorganic hearing loss is not helpful. Some generalizations to nonorganic hearing loss may be made, however, from the literature on interpersonal communication.

Nonorganic hearing loss may be looked on as one form of *deception,* which can be defined as an intentional, conscious act. According to Burgoon, Buller, and Woodall (1989), in general, men find deceit more permissible than women. They further claim that when women lie it is usually to protect others, whereas men who lie tend to do so for more self-serving reasons. Because children's abilities to plan and execute deception successfully improve with age as they develop strategies for this purpose, we may assume that young children are less likely to feign a hearing loss successfully than adults or older children. There are reasons to believe that nonorganic hearing loss may be more common in children than has previously been thought, and that the dynamics that result in such behaviors may be much more deeply seated than has been supposed (Johnson, Weissman, & Klerman, 1992).

Ross (1964) has described the development of nonorganic hearing loss in children under some circumstances. Very often, children with normal hearing inadvertently fail screening tests performed in public schools. There are many reasons for failure to respond during a hearing test besides hearing loss: Equipment may malfunction, ambient room noise may produce threshold shifts, patients may have difficulty in following instructions, and so on. Children may find that as soon as school and parental attention focus on a possible hearing problem, they begin to enjoy a degree of gain in the form of favors, excuses for poor grades, and special attention. By the time some children are seen by hearing specialists, they may be committed to perpetuating the notion that they have hearing losses. Ross believes that public school referrals to audiologists or physicians should be made only after the individual responsible for the screening is fairly certain that a hearing loss is present.

There is probably a myriad of reasons why individuals might show nonorganic hearing loss. If a patient is, in fact, malingering or deliberately exaggerating an existing hearing loss, the motivation may be financial gain. Other reasons may simply be to gain attention, or to avoid performing some undesirable task. Because the underlying reasons are more difficult to understand, this problem has been considered a form of **conversion neurosis.** Whatever the dynamics of nonorganic hearing loss, they may be deeply enmeshed in the personality of the patient, and a cursory look at these dynamics in any single book must be recognized for its superficiality.

Signs of Nonorganic Hearing Loss

There are many signs that alert the audiologist to nonorganic hearing loss. These include the source of referral, the patient's history, behavior during the interview, and performance on routine hearing tests. Sometimes the symptoms of nonorganicity are so overt that they are easily recognized, even by nonprofessional personnel. At times the patient with nonorganic hearing loss is the comic caricature of a hard-of-hearing person, appearing to have no peripheral vision when approached in the waiting room, and so on. Other patients with nonorganic problems show no such easily recognized signs.

When a patient is referred to an audiologist with the specification that there is compensation involved, nonorganicity immediately becomes of prime concern. Such referrals may be made by the Veterans Administration, insurance companies, attorneys, or physicians. To be sure, only a small number of such patients show nonorganic behavior. The incidence of nonorganic hearing loss in this group, however, is bound to be higher than in the general population.

When a specific incident is cited as the cause of a hearing loss, and the patient stands to gain financially if hearing loss is proved, the audiologist's suspicion is likely to be raised. Often such patients' histories do not suggest nonorganicity, but it exists nevertheless. In many cases the manner in which information is volunteered by the patient is as revealing as the actual data. The audiologist should be alert for exaggerated hearing postures, extremely heavy and obvious reliance on lipreading, and so on.

Performance on Routine Hearing Tests

One of the first clues to nonorganic hearing loss is inconsistency on hearing tests. The test-retest reliability of most patients with organic hearing loss is usually quite good, with threshold differences rarely exceeding 5 dB. When audiologists find differences in pure-tone or speech thresholds that exceed this value, they must conclude that one or both of these measures is wrong. Sometimes, of course, the cause of such inconsistency is wandering attentiveness, and bringing the matter to the patient's attention solves the problem. In any case, the patient should be advised of the difficulty and increased cooperation should be solicited.

One of the most common symptoms of nonorganicity is incompatibility between the pure-tone average and the SRT. In audiograms that are generally flat, the agreement should be within 5 to 10 dB. If the audiometric configuration becomes irregular, as in sharply falling high-frequency hearing losses, the SRT may be closer to the two-frequency average, or even at or better than the best of the three speech frequencies. In older patients, or those suffering from abnormalities of the central auditory nervous system, the SRT is sometimes poorer than the pure-tone average. When the SRT is better than the pure-tone average, without an explanation such as audiometric configuration, nonorganicity is likely.

That the patient with nonorganic hearing loss often shows inconsistencies between thresholds for speech and pure tones is understandable. If, for example, a person were malingering, the objective would be to respond consistently to sounds above threshold, as if they were at threshold. Patients must therefore remember how loud a signal was the last time they heard it so that they can respond when the sound reaches that same level again. This is why test-retest differences are often so revealing. Some nonorganic patients have an uncanny ability to replicate their previous responses to speech or pure tones, but they fail in equating the loudness of the two. When spondees and pure tones are presented at the same intensities, the spondees appear louder, probably because the energy is spread over a range of frequencies.

Performance on other than threshold tests is sometimes helpful in detecting nonorganic hearing loss. The audiologist might wonder why a patient with a sensorineural hearing loss has excellent word-recognition scores. To be consistent on this test, the nonorganic patient may merely count the number of words and remember how many were deliberately missed.

Determination of acoustic reflex thresholds are discussed in Chapter 6, and the results of this test on different kinds of auditory lesions are described in Chapters 9, 10, 11, and 12. Except in cases of cochlear damage, the acoustic reflex threshold is expected to be at least 65 dB above the behavioral threshold. When the reflex threshold is less than 10 dB above the voluntary threshold, nonorganic hearing loss is a probability (Lamb & Peterson, 1967).

Another suggestion of nonorganicity comes from the apparent lack of cross-hearing in unilateral cases. Considerable attention is paid in Chapters 4 and 5 to contralateralization of pure tones and speech. When individuals feign a loss of hearing in one ear, without the knowledge of cross-hearing, they often give responses showing normal hearing in one ear and a profound (or total) loss in the other ear, exceeding the most extreme values of interaural attenuation (Figure 13.1A). A lack of cross-hearing is especially noticeable for bone conduction, where any interaural attenuation is negligible. In fact, a truly profound loss of hearing in one ear would appear as a conductive hearing loss; the air-conduction thresholds would be obtained from the nontest ear with about 55 dB lost to interaural attenuation, resulting in the appearance of a fairly flat air-conduction audiogram of about 55 dB HL, with bone conduction in the normal range (Figure 13.1B). The bone-conduction signals delivered to the poor ear would be heard in the better ear at normal levels (0 to 15 dB HL) since there is virtually no interaural attenuation for bone conduction. A true total unilateral loss is demonstrated audiometrically only with masking in the normal ear (note the masked symbols used in the audiogram in Figure 13.1C).

Many audiologists have noted a peculiar form of response from some nonorganic patients during SRT tests. Often these persons will repeat only half of each spondee at a number of intensities;

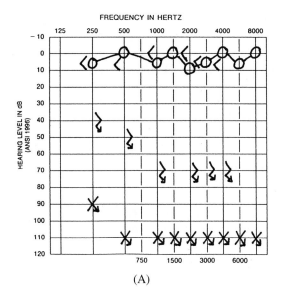

(A)

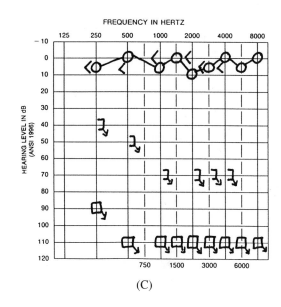

(C)

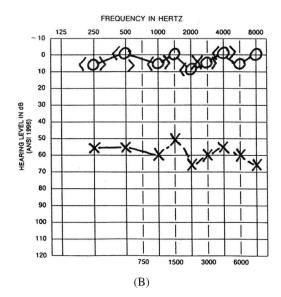

(B)

FIGURE 13.1 Theoretical test results showing normal hearing in the right ear and (A) a false total loss of hearing in the left ear (no evidence of cross hearing by air conduction or bone conduction); (B) a true total loss of hearing in the left ear showing tones cross-heard in the right ear, giving the appearance of a conductive hearing loss; and (C) a total loss of hearing in the left ear with proper masking in the right ear.

for example, *hot* (for *hot dog*) or *ball* (for *baseball*). Why this occurs has not been explained, but it has been reported fairly often.

Suspicion of nonorganic hearing loss is by no means proof. If it is suspected, it must be investigated further with great caution, using special diagnostic tests.

Tests for Nonorganic Hearing Loss

The primary purpose of special tests for nonorganic hearing loss is to provide information about the patient's hearing, even in cases in which cooperation is lacking. Behavioral tests for nonorganic hearing loss may be performed with pure tones or with speech. Some tests may be carried out with the usual diagnostic audiometer, and other tests require special equipment. Unfortunately, many of the tests are merely qualitative, that is, they produce evidence of nonorganicity, but do not reveal the threshold of hearing. Other tests are quantitative and reveal information about the patient's actual thresholds.

The Stenger Test

The **Stenger test** was designed for use with unilateral hearing losses. This test is based on the Stenger principle; that is, *when two tones of the same frequency are introduced simultaneously into both ears, only the louder tone will be perceived.* The test works best when there is a large difference (at least 25 dB) between the admitted thresholds of the two ears. The Stenger test may be carried out on a two-channel audiometer. A single pure-tone source may be split and controlled by two separate attenuators, or tones may be generated by two separate oscillators. If two oscillators are used, the tones must be locked in phase to avoid beats.

The thresholds of each ear for the desired frequencies are obtained first. Then, using one channel of the audiometer, a tone is introduced 10 dB above the threshold of the "better" ear. A response should always be obtained. A tone is then presented 10 dB below the threshold of the "poorer" ear. A response will be absent. There are two possible reasons why patients may not respond to the tone in their poorer ear. The first, obviously, is that they may not hear it. The second is that they may be unwilling, or psychologically unable, to respond to a tone that they do in fact hear. At this point, both tones are introduced simultaneously, 10 dB above the better-ear threshold reading and 10 dB below the poorer-ear threshold reading.

If patients fail to respond, it is because they hear the tone in the poorer ear, which they do not wish to admit. They will be unaware of the tone in the better ear, owing to the Stenger effect, and so will not respond at all. This is called a *positive Stenger*. If the patient responds when both ears are stimulated, this is called a *negative Stenger* and suggests the absence of nonorganicity, at least at the frequencies tested.

When positive results are found on the Stenger test, more quantitative information may be obtained. This is done by presenting the tone at 10 dB above the threshold for the better ear and at 0 dB HL in the poorer ear. With successive introductions, the level of the tone in the poorer ear is raised in 5 or 10 dB steps. The patient should always respond, because the 10 dB SL tone in the better ear provides clear audibility. If responses cease, the level of the tone in the poorer ear should be noted.

The lowest intensity that produces the Stenger effect is called the **minimum contralateral interference level.** This level may be within 20 dB of the actual threshold of patients with nonorganic hearing loss. Although some clinicians always perform the Stenger test by finding the minimum contralateral interference level, use of the screening procedure described first in this section, often saves considerable time when Stenger results are negative.

A negative result on the Stenger test is fairly conclusive evidence that there is no significant nonorganic component in the "poorer" ear. A positive Stenger tells the audiologist that the threshold results obtained in the poorer ear are inaccurate, but it does not reveal the true organic thresholds, although they may be approximated.

The Speech Stenger Test

Sometimes called the modified Stenger, the speech Stenger test may be carried out, using spondaic words, in exactly the same fashion as with pure tones. The principle is unchanged and requires that spondees be presented by a two-channel audiometer. The SRTs are obtained for each ear, using channel 1 for one ear and channel 2 for the other ear. Spondees are then presented 10 dB above the better-ear SRT, 10 dB below the level recorded as SRT of the poorer ear, and finally at these levels simultaneously.

Criteria for positive and negative on the speech and pure-tone Stenger tests are identical. Patients' failure to repeat words presented below the admitted threshold of the poorer ear suggests that they really do hear the words loudly enough to make them unaware that the words are presented above the threshold of the better ear at the same time.

Like the pure-tone Stenger test, the modified version often helps to identify the presence of nonorganic hearing loss but may not reveal the precise organic threshold of hearing. Positive results on this test, however, will encourage the audiologist to perform other tests to identify the true SRT. The speech Stenger test has the advantage over the pure-tone version in that there is no need for concern over the two tones beating. Determination of the minimum contralateral interference level for spondees may be made to help in estimating the SRT.

The Doerfler-Stewart Test

The **Doerfler-Stewart (D-S) test** is named for the audiologist and the engineer who devised it (Doerfler & Stewart, 1946). It is a confusion test that originally used spondaic words and **sawtooth noise;** later norms were collected so that white noise could be used. The test is performed binaurally and is contrived to confuse patients by presenting noise in their ears so that they lose their "loudness yardsticks" if their intentions are to respond consistently to the words above threshold as though they were at threshold.

The main problem with the D-S test is that, although it often indicates the presence of nonorganicity, it does not tell its extent, nor does it reveal the true SRT. The test is binaural and is therefore eliminated in unilateral cases. When speech discrimination scores are poor, either real or feigned, the patient may appear unable to repeat 100 percent of a list of spondees at any sensation level. This test is rarely performed today.

The Lombard Test

The **Lombard test** is based on the familiar phenomenon that people increase their vocal levels when they speak in a background of noise. If a noise is presented to the ears of speakers who do not hear the noise, they will of course, not change the loudness of their voices. If, however, the level of a person's voice goes up as noise is added, it is obvious that the noise is audible to that person.

The subject is positioned with air-conduction receivers over both ears and is asked to read or speak aloud. A neatly typed paragraph helps to avoid some difficulties professed during the performance of this kind of test. As the subject reads, a masking noise added to both ears is gradually increased in intensity. The examiner listens for increased vocal loudness. To help detect it, the subject may be asked to read into a microphone, which is fed into the VU meter of the audiometer being used. The gain on the VU meter may be adjusted so that the speaker's voice peaks around –5 VU. Any increases in the loudness of the reader's voice can then be observed visually as an increase in the value of the peaks on the VU meter.

If there is an increase in the loudness of the subject's voice, noted by observing the peaks on a VU meter, it can be said that the noise was at least loud enough to cause this voice reflex. No change in loudness might suggest that the noise was not heard or was not loud enough to cause the reflex. Surely a person with a 90 dB loss of hearing should not show a positive result on the Lombard test at 75 dB, and nonorganic hearing loss is immediately suspected in such a case. Beyond this, interpretation of the Lombard test must be made only in a general way.

As was implied, the Lombard test is not a strong test for nonorganic hearing loss. All attempts at finding normal values—that is, how many decibels above threshold a noise must be to cause the reflex—have failed. Some people begin to show some changes at 25 or 30 dB above threshold, and others may speak or read with noise at 100 dB SL in both ears with no noticeable changes in the loudness of their voices.

The Delayed-speech Feedback Test

People monitor the rate and loudness of their speech through a variety of feedback mechanisms, for example, tactile, proprioceptive, and, primarily, auditory feedback. After a phoneme is uttered, it is processed through the auditory system and the next phoneme is cued. Simultaneous feedback is essential for smooth articulation of speech sounds.

If a person's voice is recorded on magnetic tape, delayed 0.1 to 0.2 seconds, and played back, this **delayed auditory feedback (DAF)** causes subjects to alter their speech patterns, in some ways creating an effect similar to stuttering. Speakers may slow down, prolong some syllables, increase their loudness, or find it very difficult to speak at all. The creation of delayed feedback audiometry was inevitable as a test for nonorganic hearing loss, for surely a speaker's voice played back with a short delay can have no effect on speech production unless it is heard.

Subjects may be placed before a microphone, preferably in the patient room of a two-room audiometric suite. They wear a pair of air-conduction receivers. A prepared text that is easy to read and that can be completed in one-half to one minute is provided. The subjects are instructed to read the passage aloud and then to pause for a cue from the examiner, whereupon they read the passage aloud again, and so on. The first one or two readings should be allowed with no feedback, and the reading time should be recorded with a stopwatch. The VU meter of the audiometer should be adjusted so that the subject's word peaks average about –5 dB VU.

The delayed-speech portion of the test is begun after the preliminary steps. The test may be performed in both ears or one ear, with or without the nontest ear masked. The intensity of the signal is controlled by the attenuator of the audiometer and is first set at 0 dB HL. After each reading, the level is raised 10 dB until a positive result is seen. A positive result is defined as any change in the reading rate (sped up or slowed down by more than three to five seconds for a short passage), an increase in vocal intensity as seen on the VU meter (the Lombard effect), or obvious hesitations or prolongations on syllables or words.

In many ways, speech DAF is interpreted like the Lombard test. When changes occur in speaking rate, it must be assumed that subjects have heard their own voices and that this has had an effect on their monitoring systems. If this effect is noted at a low hearing level, it is assumed that hearing is probably normal or near normal, at least for the low and middle frequencies. Some speech changes have been observed as low as 10 dB above the SRT.

Some persons can tolerate delayed-speech feedback at very high sensation levels with no apparent breakdowns in their speech or voice patterns. Others are apparently much more susceptible to distraction by their own slightly delayed voices. As in so many tests, positive results on speech DAF are much more meaningful than negative results. When persons have difficulty reading or speaking under the DAF condition, this must mean that they have heard the signal at the level at which it was presented.

The Pure-tone Delayed Auditory Feedback Test

The principle of delayed auditory feedback has been applied to pure tones. Ruhm and Cooper (1964) devised a technique whereby subjects tap a pattern on a silent switch with their preferred index finger. The pattern may be two taps, pause, four taps, pause, two taps, and so on. The patient's arm is hidden from view. The forearm is placed down, so that tapping is done primarily with the finger. In this way the subjects are deprived, as much as possible, of visual, tactile, and auditory feedback of their tapping performance.

Patients are seated so that they cannot see the controls on the DAF apparatus. A two-room arrangement works well for this test. Patients are instructed on how to tap on the switch and are then asked to demonstrate this ability to the examiner. Earphones are placed over the ears and the test is begun.

The DAF device is designed so that if properly set, a brief tone (50 milliseconds) is presented to the subject's ear via an air-conduction earphone 200 milliseconds after each tap. The short delay from the tap on the key to the audibility of the tone causes subjects to modify their tapping behavior. Patients may change their tapping rates, increase their tapping pressure on the switch, or change the rhythm or the number of their taps (e.g., from a pattern of two and four to a pattern of one and three).

A tone of desired frequency is presented by means of the audiometer to which the DAF device is attached. The starting level should be 0 dB HL. Several tapping patterns are allowed between each increase in intensity, which is done in steps of 5 dB. The DAF threshold is the lowest level at which any alteration of tapping performance is noted. Responses may be monitored auditorily by the examiner, or a readout may be obtained on a graphic recorder that shows the tapping performance, including, in some cases, tapping pressure.

Ruhm and Cooper (1962) found that positive results on pure-tone DAF tests occur at sensation levels as low as 5 dB. The tone must be slightly above threshold for it to be audible 100 percent of the time. When positive results are seen, the examiner may infer that the patient's hearing threshold is no poorer than 10 dB below the DAF threshold.

Of all the tests described so far in this section, pure-tone DAF comes closest to doing what is necessary, identifying the patient's true organic threshold. Occasionally patients are seen who cannot or will not tap consistent patterns. In such cases the test cannot be performed.

Békésy Audiometry

At this time very few clinics perform Békésy audiometry (described briefly in Chapter 7) as a routine procedure (Martin, Champlin, & Chambers, 1998). It was used to identify nonorganic hearing loss when the pulsed-tone thresholds showed poorer hearing than the continuous-tone thresholds (called the Type V pattern) (Jerger & Herer, 1961), a phenomenon that was accentuated when the off-time of the signal was made longer (Hattler, 1970), when the intensity of the signal is decreased rather than increased (Chaiklin, 1990), or when some of these approaches are combined into a Békésy Ascending Descending Gap Evaluation (BADGE) (Hood, Campbell, & Hutton, 1964). This comparison of ascending and descending thresholds has also been described using a conventional audiometer (Cherry & Ventry, 1976; Harris, 1958; Thelin, 1997; Woodford, Harris, Marquette, Perry, & Barnhart, 1997). Schlauch, Arnce, Lindsay, Sanchez, and Doyle (1998) recommend an ascending procedure for SRT and a descending procedure for pure tones to identify nonorganic hearing loss.

The Varying Intensity Story Test

Another way of confusing a patient who may have a nonorganic hearing loss is to administer the **Varying Intensity Story Test (VIST)** (Martin, Champlin, & Marchbanks, 1998). The patient is asked to listen to a story in one ear, parts of which are presented above the admitted threshold and parts below this level. The story is delivered so rapidly that it is difficult for listeners to be certain what information was obtained that should and should not be admitted to. This test requires the use of a two-channel audiometer and a stereo tape player.

Patients are advised only that they will be told a story. The earphones are positioned over both ears, and one of the stories is played (see Figure 13.2). The hearing levels are set so that portions of the story are presented 10 dB above the admitted threshold and other portions 30 to 50 dB below this level. At the completion of the test the patient is given a short test. The story in Figure 13.2 has the advantage that the theme changes from a discussion of china (the dishes) to China (the country), when information presented at the softer level is included.

If the patient correctly answers any questions based on information presented below the admitted threshold, the conclusion must be drawn that hearing is no worse than the level at which that information was presented. This test can demonstrate graphically to patients, without otherwise discussing the situation, that if they are deliberately feigning or exaggerating a hearing loss, the examiner is aware of it.

Electrophysiological Tests

Nothing could be better suited to the testing of patients with nonorganic hearing loss than procedures that require no voluntary responses. By determining auditory thresholds in such a manner, the very lack of required cooperation would tend to discourage some patients from attempting to malinger. Some tests are available that can be administered with this objective in mind.

Acoustic Reflex Tests

An addition to the many uses already described for acoustic immittance meters is a method of estimating hearing sensitivity for patients who are unwilling or unable to cooperate. Following up on some earlier work on differential loudness summation, Jerger, Burney, Mauldin, and Crump (1974) developed what has come to be known as **Sensitivity Prediction from the Acoustic Reflex**

CHINA

PART I	PART II
PRESENTED ABOVE THRESHOLD	PRESENTED BELOW THRESHOLD

China,

despite overpopulation.

is well known for its delicate beauty

and its rugged terrain.

Many popular styles of

cooking originating in

china exist today. Patterns

of beautiful gardens

of flowers and geometric

landscaping

designs are equally common

in many modern Chinese cities.

Hand-painted scenes

of the natural beauty of China

can be found

in many museums

if one knows where to look.

Books about

China owned by your grandmother probably

contain much misinformation, because early 20th century China

is quite different from modern china. The computer age

has arrived and

changed the way complex designs are printed

on all types of textiles. A new age has dawned

on modern china.

FIGURE 13.2 Sample of a Varying Intensity Story Test.

(SPAR). Margolis (1993) has shown that with this procedure, hearing loss in excess of 30 dB can be detected with sensitivity and specificity greater than 90 percent.

The SPAR test is based on the fact that acoustic reflex thresholds get lower as the signal bandwidth gets wider. Stated differently, to elicit the reflex, a normal-hearing person will require greater intensity for a pure-tone than for a wide-band noise. The usual difference is about 25 dB. Patients with sensorineural hearing losses of mild to moderate degree show only a 10 to 20 dB difference, whereas patients with moderately severe losses show less than a 10 dB difference. Of course, patients with profound losses will show no acoustic reflex for either stimulus. To estimate the degree of hearing loss, the acoustic reflex thresholds (in dB SPL) at 500, 1000, and 2000 Hz are averaged and compared to the threshold for the broadband noise.

Electrodermal Audiometry

Electrodermal audiometry (EDA) combines Pavlovian conditioning with measurements of the psychogalvanic response. It has been known for some time that the skin serves as a conductor of electricity. By placing electrodes on the surface of the skin at two neighboring points, as at two adjacent fingertips, the electricity can be amplified and studied in terms of its electrical resistance.

Bordley and Hardy (1949) were the first to apply psychogalvanometry to audiometry. They reasoned that by pairing a tone with a small electric shock delivered by electrodes to the fingers of the hand opposite the pickup electrodes, the patient could be conditioned to respond to the tone. Because the shock always results in a drop in skin resistance, tones could be followed by shocks until the subject associated the two. This conditioning, similar to the conditioning of Pavlov's dogs, results in a drop in skin resistance following a tone, even if no shock is presented.

The days of EDA as a popular test have passed. This is partly true because the validity of the test is highly suspect in many cases. In addition, recent legislation protects individuals from being forced to receive noxious stimuli, such as electric shocks. Electrodermal audiometry has been called **objective audiometry.** Like other electrophysiological tests, it may be objective in the sense that patients do not play a voluntary role in stating when they hear a stimulus. Interpretation of responses, however, is a highly subjective matter.

Auditory Evoked Potentials (AEPs)

The use of AEP audiometry, described in Chapter 6, lends itself nicely to examining many difficult-to-test patients, especially those with suspected nonorganic hearing loss. Auditory brainstem response audiometry is increasing in popularity for this purpose, and often comes very close to predicting true audiometric thresholds in patients with nonorganic hearing loss. It must be remembered, however, that certain abnormal audiometric configurations yield ABR responses that erroneously suggest normal hearing (Glattke, 1983). Other electrophysiological tests, such as the auditory middle latency response, late evoked response, and electrocochleography, show promise for use with patients who demonstrate nonorganic behaviors. If performed early in the examination, a procedure like ABR may have a deterring effect on nonorganic behavior because patients should recognize early in the examination that the determination of hearing ability may be made without their active cooperation.

Otoacoustic Emissions (OAEs)

Transient evoked otoacoustic emissions (TEOAEs), also described in Chapter 6, may be of great value in the detection of nonorganic hearing loss (Musiek, Bornstein, & Rintelmann, 1995). Gollegly, Bornstein, and Musiek (1992) presented six cases in which voluntary thresholds were elevated but TEOAEs were normal. Gollegly (1994) concludes that TEOAEs can serve as a screening test for persons suspected of falsifying audiometric data, although if there is a possibility of a central disorder, ABR testing should also be done. When otoacoustic emissions are normal and retrocochlear pathology is ruled out, a reasonable conclusion to draw is that patients with elevated voluntary thresholds are manifesting nonorganic behaviors. Absence of OAEs does not mean that some exaggeration of auditory threshold is not taking place.

Other Confusion Tests

Often tests are administered that are designed to confuse patients suspected of nonorganic hearing loss, in hopes they will abandon this behavior. A series of tones may be introduced above and below the voluntary threshold, and the patient may be asked to count the tones and report the number that was heard (Ross, 1964). This becomes a problem for patients with nonorganic hearing loss, because they have to remember which tones they are willing to admit to hearing. The same procedure may be used to pulse the tones rapidly from one ear to the other in a unilateral case. The tones should be above the threshold of the "better" ear and below the admitted threshold of the "poorer" ear (Nagel, 1964).

The "yes-no" method described, by Frank (1976), is often useful in finding pure-tone thresholds for children. The child is instructed to say "yes" when a tone is heard and "no" when a tone is not heard. An ascending method is used. Many children falsifying test results will say "no" coincidentally with tonal presentation below their admitted thresholds. This method is easy and fast, and makes life simpler for the audiologist, when it works. Naturally, the more sophisticated patients are, the less likely they are to be tripped up by such an obvious subterfuge.

Nonorganic hearing loss may be identified by a standardized test for lipreading ability (Utley, 1946). The patient may be seated facing the examiner through the observation window separating the patient room from the control room. Lights in the patient room should be dimmed to eliminate glare. The patient wears the audiometer earphones and is given one form of the test with the intensity set well below admitted threshold, but above the level estimated as threshold by the audiologist. A different form of the test is given in identical fashion, but with the microphone switched off. Patients often do considerably better on the test when they hear, possibly because they are eager to prove they are good lipreaders.

Management of Patients with Nonorganic Hearing Loss

Creating an open confrontation with a patient demonstrating nonorganic hearing loss rarely results in improved test validity. After all, cooperation is hardly forthcoming in the presence of hostility. Clinicians may advise the patient that test inconsistencies exist, but they should try to shift the "blame" for this to their own shoulders, using such explanations as "Perhaps I didn't make it clear to you that you are to raise your hand even if the tone is very soft. You've been waiting until the tone is relatively loud before you've signaled. I'm sorry that I didn't make this clearer before, but let's try again." This provides patients with an honorable way out, which they often take.

As may be seen from the preceding section of this chapter, a number of tests for nonorganic hearing loss are at the disposal of the audiologist. In most cases, it is not difficult to uncover nonorganicity. Many tricks have been used. For example, audiologists may cover their mouths when speaking to patients who profess heavy reliance on lipreading. Patients may be given instructions through the audiometer below their admitted SRTs, such as "Remove the earphones; the test is over." Any movement of the hands toward the receivers tells the audiologist that the patient has heard the instruction and reacted before realizing that it was below the admitted threshold.

The greatest problem in dealing with patients with nonorganic hearing loss concerns the determination of the true threshold and how to manage these patients. If all patients with nonorganic hearing loss were liars, whose dishonesty was motivated by greed or laziness, perhaps the job would be easier. It is possible, however, that many patients with nonorganic hearing loss may be deeply troubled. As stated earlier, some hearing losses may be entirely feigned, others merely exaggerated, and still others produced on an unconscious level.

One of the temptations that all professional persons must avoid in working with disabled patients is that of making value judgments. Although we may be curious about the psychodynamics of a given situation, we cannot play psychiatrist with a patient suspected of having a psychogenic hearing loss. We also cannot play prosecutor, no matter how convinced we are that a patient is malingering. Malingering can be proved, without question, only if the patient admits to it.

When nonorganicity is demonstrated, it may be an unwise practice to draw the audiogram. Too many persons are prone to glancing at the red and blue symbols, with no study of the actual results and what they mean. When nonorganicity is suspected, it may be better to write "suspected nonorganic hearing loss" across the audiogram, to force anyone reading it to look more carefully at the report that should accompany the results of any hearing evaluation. In writing reports, audiologists should avoid the word *malingering,* but they should not hesitate to say *nonorganic hearing loss,* if they believe this to be the case. Referrals to psychiatrists or psychologists are sometimes indicated, but they should be made very carefully. Exactly how a patient should be advised of test results is an individual matter, and must be dictated by the experience of the audiologist.

Summary

Many patients seen in audiology clinics show symptoms of nonorganic hearing loss. They may be malingering, exaggerating hearing losses, or exhibiting psychogenic disorders. There may also be other reasons for test results to be inaccurate. The responsibility of the audiologist is to determine the true organic thresholds of hearing, even if this must be done with less than the full cooperation of the patient.

A number of tests can be performed when nonorganic hearing loss is suspected. Some of them merely confuse patients and provide evidence of nonorganicity; they might also convince the patients that they must be more cooperative. Other tests actually help determine auditory thresholds.

There is evidence (Martin & Monro, 1975; Martin & Shipp, 1982; Monro & Martin, 1977) that knowledge about the principles underlying some audiometric measures may assist the patient in "beating" some tests. Some procedures are more resistant to practice or sophistication than are others. Audiologists must consider these factors in working with patients demonstrating nonorganic hearing loss.

Audiologists have an obligation to serve the patient, even when the patient is uncooperative. The problems of writing reports and counseling are much greater with patients with nonorganic hearing loss than with those showing no evidence of this condition.

STUDY QUESTIONS

1. What are the first symptoms of nonorganic hearing loss that you might notice? How do they manifest during a test, and in a nontest situation?

2. Make a list of pure-tone tests for nonorganic hearing loss. Separate them into groups according to ease of performance, necessity for special equipment, identification of threshold, and so on.

3. Repeat question 2 for speech tests.

4. Consider the concepts of malingering, exaggeration, and psychogenicity as they relate to hearing loss.

5. What are the advantages and disadvantages of acoustic reflexes, ABR, and OAEs in the diagnosis of nonorganic hearing loss?

GLOSSARY

Conversion neurosis A Freudian concept by which emotional disorders become transferred into physical manifestations (e.g., hearing loss or blindness).

Delayed auditory feedback (DAF) The delay in time between a subject's creation of a sound (e.g., speech) and his or her hearing of that sound.

Doerfler-Stewart (D-S) test A binaural test for nonorganic hearing loss using spondaic words and a masking noise.

Electrodermal audiometry (EDA) A procedure for testing hearing using an auditory signal as a conditioned stimulus and an electric shock as an unconditioned stimulus.

Functional hearing loss See *Nonorganic hearing loss*.

Hysterical deafness An older term for *psychogenic hearing loss*.

Lombard test A test for nonorganic hearing loss based on the fact that speakers will increase the loudness of their speech when a loud noise interferes with their normal auditory monitoring.

Malingering The conscious, willful, and deliberate act of feigning or exaggerating a disability (such as hearing loss) for personal gain or exemption.

Minimum contralateral interference level On the Stenger test, the lowest intensity of a signal presented to the poor ear that causes the patient to stop responding to the signal that is above threshold in the better ear.

Nonorganic hearing loss The exaggerated elevation of auditory thresholds.

Objective audiometry Procedures for testing the hearing function that do not require behavioral responses.

Pseudohypacusis See *Nonorganic hearing loss*.

Psychogenic hearing loss A nonorganic hearing loss produced at the unconscious level, as by an anxiety state.

Sawtooth noise A noise made up of a fundamental frequency of 120 Hz, with equal amplitude at all harmonic frequencies. It was found on older speech audiometers.

Sensitivity Prediction from the Acoustic Reflex (SPAR) Prediction of approximate degree of hearing impairment based on the level of pure tones versus a broadband noise required to elicit the acoustic reflex.

Stenger test A test for unilateral nonorganic hearing loss based on the Stenger principle that states, "When two tones of the same frequency are introduced simultaneously into both ears only the louder one will be perceived."

Varying Intensity Story Test (VIST) Portions of a story are presented above the admitted "threshold" and portions below. If the patient remembers information presented below the admitted threshold, this is prima facie evidence that the hearing loss in that ear is exaggerated.

REFERENCES

Bordley, J. E., & Hardy, W. G. (1949). A study in objective audiometry with use of the psychogalvanic response. *Annals of Otology, 58,* 751–760.

Burgoon, J. D., Buller, D. B., & Woodall, W. G. (1989). *Nonverbal communication: The unspoken dialogue.* New York: Harper & Row.

Chaiklin, J. B. (1990). A descending LOT-Békésy screening test for functional hearing loss. *Journal of Speech and Hearing Disorders, 55,* 67–74.

Cherry, R., & Ventry, I. (1976). The ascending-descending gap: A tool for identifying a suprathreshold response. *Journal of Auditory Research, 16,* 281–187.

Coleman, J. C. (1976). *Abnormal psychology in modern life.* Glenville, IL: Scott Foresman.

Doerfler, L. G., & Stewart, K. (1946). Malingering and psychogenic deafness. *Journal of Speech Disorders, 11,* 181–186.

Frank, T. (1976). Yes-no test for nonorganic hearing loss. *Archives of Otolaryngology, 102,* 162–165.

Glattke, T. J. (1983). *Short-latency auditory evoked potentials. Fundamental bases and clinical applications.* Baltimore: University Park Press.

Gollegly, K. M. (1994). *Otoacoustic emissions and pseudohypacusis.* Poster Session presented at the Annual Convention of the American Speech-Language Hearing Association, New Orleans, LA.

Gollegly, K. M., Bornstein, S. P., & Musiek, F. E. (1992). *Otoacoustic emissions and pseudohypacusis.* Poster Session presented at the Annual Convention of the American Speech-Language-Hearing Association, San Antonio, TX.

Harris, D. A. (1958). A rapid and simple technique for the detection of nonorganic hearing loss. *Archives of Otolaryngology* (Chicago), *6X*, 758–760.

Hattler, K. W. (1970). Lengthened off-time: A self-recording screening device for nonorganicity. *Journal of Speech and Hearing Disorders, 35*, 113–122.

Hood, W. H., Campbell, R. A., & Hutton, C. L. (1964). An evaluation of the Békésy ascending descending gap. *Journal of Speech and Hearing Research, 7*, 123–132.

Jerger, J., Burney, P., Mauldin, L., & Crump, B. (1974). Predicting hearing loss from the acoustic reflex. *Journal of Speech and Hearing Disorders, 39*, 11–22.

Jerger, J., & Herer, G. (1961). An unexpected dividend in Békésy audiometry. *Journal of Speech and Hearing Disorders, 26*, 390–391.

Johnson, J., Weissman, M. M., & Klerman, G. L. (1992). Service utilization and social morbidity associated with depressive symptoms in the community. *Journal of the American Medical Association, 267*, 1478–1483.

Lamb, L. E., & Peterson, J. L. (1967). Middle ear reflex measurements in pseudohypacusis. *Journal of Speech and Hearing Disorders, 32*, 46–51.

Margolis, R. H. (1993). Detection of hearing impairment with the acoustic stapedius reflex. *Ear and Hearing, 14*, 3–10.

Martin, F. N., Champlin, C. A., & Chambers, J. (1998). Seventh survey of audiometric practices in the United States. *Journal of the American Academy of Audiology, 9*, 95–104.

Martin, F. N., Champlin, C. A., & Marchbanks, T. P. (1998). A varying intensity story test for simulated hearing loss. *American Journal of Audiology, 7*, 39–44.

Martin, F. N., & Monro, D. A. (1975). The effects of sophistication on Type V Békésy patterns in simulated hearing loss. *Journal of Speech and Hearing Disorders, 40*, 508–513.

Martin, F. N., & Shipp, D. B. (1982). The effects of sophistication on three threshold tests for subjects with simulated hearing loss. *Ear and Hearing, 3*, 34–36.

Monro, D. A., & Martin, F. N. (1977). The effects of sophistication on four tests for nonorganic hearing loss. *Journal of Speech and Hearing Disorders, 42*, 528–534.

Musiek, F. E., Bornstein, S. P. & Rintelmann, W. F. (1995). Transient evoked otoacoustic emissions and pseudohypacusis. *Journal of the American Academy of Audiology, 6*, 293–301.

Nagel, R. F. (1964). RRLJ: A new technique for the noncooperative patient. *Journal of Speech and Hearing Disorders, 29*, 492–493.

Ross, M. (1964). The variable intensity pulse count method (VIPCM) for the detection and measurement of the pure-tone threshold of children with functional hearing losses. *Journal of Speech and Hearing Disorders, 29*, 477–482.

Ruhm, H. B., & Cooper, W. A., Jr. (1962). Low sensation level effects of pure-tone delayed auditory feedback. *Journal of Speech and Hearing Research, 5*, 185–193.

———. (1964). Delayed feedback audiometry. *Journal of Speech and Hearing Disorders, 29*, 448–455.

Schlauch, R. S., Arnce, K. D., Lindsay, M. O., Sanchez, S., & Doyle, T. N. (1998), Identification of pseudohypacusis using speech recognition thresholds. *Ear and Hearing, 17*, 229–236.

Thelin, J. W. (1997). *Ascending-descending test for functional hearing loss*. Poster presented at the 1997 convention of the American Academy of Audiology, Ft. Lauderdale, FL.

Utley, J. (1946). A test of lipreading ability. *Journal of Speech and Hearing Disorders, 11*, 109–116.

Woodford, C. M., Harris, G., Marquette, M. L., Perry, L. & Barnhart, A. (1997). A screening test for pseudohypacusis. *The Hearing Journal, 4*, 23–26.

SUGGESTED READINGS

Martin, F. N. (1994). Pseudohypacusis. In J. Katz (Ed.), *Handbook of clinical audiology* (4th ed., pp. 553–567). Baltimore: Williams & Wilkins.

Rintelmann, W. F., & Schwan, S. A. (1991). Pseudohypacusis. In W. F. Rintelmann (Ed.), *Hearing assessment* (pp. 603–652). Boston: Allyn & Bacon.

REVIEW TABLE 13.1   Summary of Tests for Nonorganic Hearing Loss

| | Type of Signal | | | Type of Loss | | |
Name of Test	Pure Tone	Speech	Special Equipment Required	Unilateral	Bilateral	Estimates Threshold
ABR	X		X	X	X	X
Békésy audiometry	X		X	X	X	
Confusion tests	X	X		X	X	
Speech DAF		X	X	X	X	
Pure-tone DAF	X		X	X	X	
Doerfler-Stewart		X			X	
EDA	X	X	X	X	X	X
Lombard		X			X	
SPAR	X		X	X	X	X
Stenger	X	X		X		
TEOAE	X		X	X	X	
VIST		X	X	X		

PART IV

Management of Hearing Loss

The final part of this book is devoted to audiological management. Chapter 14 covers the subject of amplification/sensory systems and how they may be used to improve the communication of people with hearing loss. The closing chapter involves general patient treatment and is concerned with improving the lives of individuals with auditory disorders through specialized training and patient and family counseling.

14 Amplification/Sensory Systems

Amplification and sensory systems, either personal in the form of hearing aids or implants, or supplemental in the form of assistive devices such as television amplifiers, comprise a major component of management endeavors for the patient with hearing loss. When audiological rehabilitation is indicated, consideration should be given to amplification in the form of hearing aids. Although it is true that some patients cannot use or do not desire hearing aids, amplification should be considered for all patients with hearing impairment as part of a total rehabilitation program.

The task of the audiologist is to find the amplification/sensory system(s) most appropriate to the patient's needs and capabilities that will provide the greatest possible enhancement of speech understanding. This task becomes more challenging when working with very young children or individuals with multiple handicaps who cannot fully participate in the (re)habilitation process, those adult patients who deny the family's perceived need for rehabilitation, or the elderly whose declining mental and/or physical capabilities impede the rehabilitation process.

Chapter Objectives

This chapter provides an overview of the evolution of amplification systems, and the hearing aid styles and circuit options available at the opening of the twenty-first century. Considerations in the hearing aid selection and verification procedures for both children and adults are reviewed. Comprehensive management of hearing loss dictates that full consideration be given to assistive listening and alerting devices designed to augment the benefit derived through traditional amplification, or to bring awareness of auditory signals to those whose hearing cannot be otherwise assisted. Toward this end, the reader is presented with a review of the growing array of hearing assistance technologies for those with hearing loss.

Hearing Aid Development

Documentation of the historical development of devices to aid human hearing has been most fully chronicled by Berger (1988). The use of devices to collect and amplify sound for those with hearing loss may well be nearly as old as the human race. The earliest reference to sound collectors indicate that animal horns and sea shells were employed to gather sound waves and direct them into the external auditory canal. While many other devices were contrived through the years to collect and direct sound energy (Figure 14.1), it was not until the late nineteenth century that the first electronic hear-

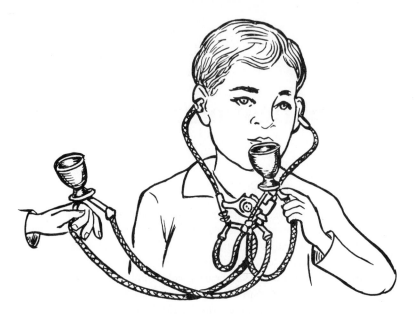

FIGURE 14.1   The Sexton Conversation Tube, an example of a sound collector for hearing enhancement. Presented by Samuel Sexton at the American Otological Society in July, 1885. (From Berger, K. W. (1984). *The Hearing Aid: Its Operation and Development.* **Livonia, MI: National Hearing Aid Society. Reproduced with permission from the International Hearing Society.)**

ing aid was produced (Berger, 1988). Because of size and weight, early electronic hearing aids often limited their users to the proximity of a table that could support the devices. Although some early carbon hearing aids could be body worn (Figure 14.2), it was nearly forty years after the development of electronic hearing aids before the **vacuum tube** allowed for any significant miniaturization. The vacuum tube also brought a significant increase in power and frequency bandwidth so that electronic amplification became feasible for a larger range of hearing losses than could be reached with the earlier carbon instruments.

The first **transistor,** developed by Bell Telephone Laboratories in 1947, was not initially useful in hearing aid design. However, an early refinement, the germanium junction transistor, found its first commercial use in hearing aids. Because of the junction transistor's smaller size and lower battery voltage requirements, significant miniaturization of hearing aids rapidly followed. As discussed by Berger (1988), earlier vacuum tube hearing aids had only gradually replaced the first carbon electronic hearing aids as their size, cost, and difficulties with the amplifier presented little competition to the carbon instruments. In contrast, transistor hearing aids completely replaced vacuum tube hearing aids within two to three years of their introduction in 1952.

Hearing aids have continued to evolve and improve through the use of **integrated circuits,** computer technology, and increased miniaturization. For years, audiologists have found hearing

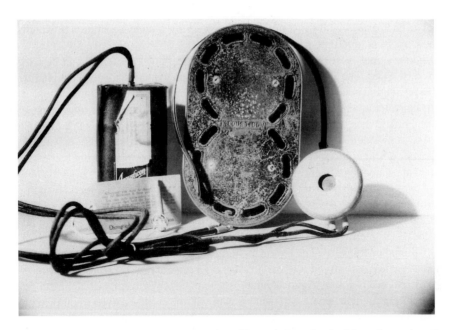

FIGURE 14.2   A complete carbon hearing aid consisting of a double carbon microphone for increased power, a receiver with headband and battery, circa 1910. (Photo courtesy of Dr. Irvin J. Gerling, Curator of the Kenneth W. Berger Hearing Aid Museum and Archives, Kent State University)

instrumentation to be the most rapidly developing and changing aspect of their clinical practice. The profession can look for this trend to continue.

Hearing Aid Circuit Overview

Hearing aids may be thought of as miniature, personalized, public address systems. Sounds that strike the microphone (input transducer) are amplified, transmitted electrically to a miniature loudspeaker (output transducer), and then into the patient's external ear canal. Some hearing aids utilize a bone-conduction vibrator that is held to the patient's mastoid by a metal headband like the bone-conductor vibrator of an audiometer. Power for the instruments is obtained from small batteries.

Hearing aids are signal processors: that is, they alter the signal input to improve it for the wearer. Traditionally, **analog hearing aids,** so called because the electrical signals generated are analogous to the sound that comes into the instrument, have involved technology much like the grooves of a phonograph record resemble the sound waves that were used when the record was cut (Pascoe, 1991). Analog technology involves modifying a continuous electrical signal. Completely **digital hearing aids** are relatively new to the selection of hearing aids available. Their purpose is to convert sound waves into numbers that are stored as binary digits (0s and 1s referred to as "bits"), the way a computer stores data. A digital instrument changes the continuous electrical signal by means of an analog-to-digital converter (A/D) into a series of many separate bits, which represent the frequency, intensity, and time patterns of the signal.

When a signal is in digital form, advanced processing operations can be carried out with lightning-fast speed. The altered signals are changed back to analog form by a digital-to-analog converter (D/A). Digital hearing aids are capable of providing improved clarity of signals and enhanced signal-to-noise ratios that are superior to those obtained with more traditional analog instruments. Digital technology has the potential to allow hearing aids to store sounds that enter the instrument and to separate wanted signals (those that will be used) from those that are unwanted (e.g., noise). Nevertheless, despite the superiority of digital instruments, they should not be perceived by clinicians, or represented to patients, as panaceas.

A "hybrid" hearing instrument allows for the digital shaping of the sound response of the hearing instrument, while the actual processing of the signal is through analog technology. These hearing instruments may be coupled to computers and programmed more precisely to an individual's hearing loss configuration and loudness tolerance levels than traditional hearing aids at a lesser cost than fully digital instruments. The hybrid technologies provide for models that allow separate amplifier characteristics to be stored into the hearing aid's memory, to be accessed by the wearer during different listening conditions. Such a feature is also possible with fully digital hearing aids.

In addition to the usual on-off switches and volume controls, even traditional analog hearing aids have internal and external adjustments to modify the amplification obtained in different frequency ranges, albeit not as precisely as their digital and hybrid counterparts. All hearing aids can be manufactured with **compression** circuitry to reduce loud sounds and keep them within the patient's dynamic range. Because patient loudness discomfort levels are not increased by the amount of sensorineural hearing loss, this circuitry is a valuable addition for those with loudness recruitment.

Some hearing aids also contain electromagnetic coils that, when switched into the circuit, bypass the microphone so that the user can hear more clearly over the telephone. These "T" switches have been used for improved telephone communication systems for many years, and today all corded telephones must be compatible with hearing aids (Beck, 1989). In addition to telephone use, T-switches allow access to a variety of assistive listening devices.

Characteristics of Hearing Aids

Hearing aids are usually described in terms of their electroacoustic properties, which include **output sound-pressure level (OSPL), acoustic gain, frequency response,** and **distortion.** Until the **Hearing Aid Industry Conference (HAIC)** (1961, 1975), these characteristics were loosely defined, which led to a number of misconceptions. The most recent specifications for hearing aids are published by the American National Standards Institute (ANSI, 1996). Measurements are made on an artificial ear with a 2 cm³ coupler to accommodate the earmold, the external receiver of the hearing aid, or to hold the plastic tubing that comes from the receiver. Although the 2 cm³ coupler measurement does not represent the hearing aid's function in a real ear, it does provide a standardized system for comparing different hearing aids. Most modern audiology clinics utilize a special hearing-aid test system (Figure 14.3) that contains a sound-treated enclosure for the hearing aid, a sweep-frequency audio oscillator and loudspeaker, and a microphone that picks up the signal after amplification by the hearing aid so that a curve can be printed out showing the characteristics of the signal

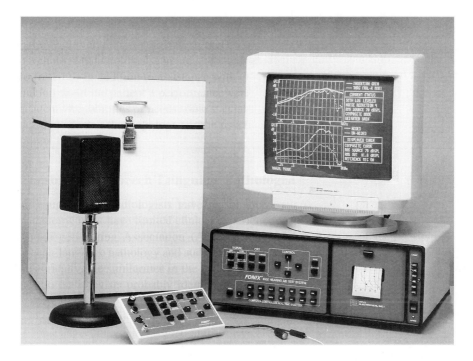

FIGURE 14.3 Hearing aid test system including sound chamber for 2 cc electroacoustic analysis of hearing instruments and probe-microphone measurements. (Courtesy of Frye Electronics)

after amplification. In most test boxes a graph is automatically drawn that shows the response of the hearing aid over a frequency range of 125 to 10,000 Hz.

Output Sound-Pressure Level (OSPL)

It is obvious that some control must be exercised by the manufacturer over the maximum sound pressure emitted from a hearing aid. If this pressure were unlimited, it could damage the wearer's hearing. The output sound-pressure level (OSPL), previously called the saturation sound-pressure level (SSPL), is the greatest sound pressure that can be produced by a hearing aid. The OSPL is considered one of the most important measurements and is usually made by using an input signal of 90 dB SPL with the hearing aid turned to full volume (OSPL90).

Acoustic Gain

The acoustic gain of a hearing aid is the difference, in decibels, between an input signal and an output signal. The gain (volume) control of the hearing aid is adjusted to its desired position, and a signal of 50 or 60 dB SPL is presented to the microphone. If the output SPL is 100 dB with an input of 60 dB SPL, the acoustic gain is 40 dB. **High-frequency average (HFA)** full-on gain is the average gain at 1000, 1600, and 2500 Hz when the volume control is turned as high as it can go. Although these measurements reflect maximum gain, they do not represent a true picture of the gain of the instrument on the patient, because hearing aids are rarely worn at full-volume settings. The ANSI standard is used for measuring acoustic gain below the aid's full-on position. This **reference test gain** allows for a more realistic appraisal of the way hearing aids might perform on a patient. The two main types of gain measured while the hearing aid is worn include **functional gain,** the measured difference between aided and unaided thresholds in the sound field, and **insertion gain,** the increase in sound-pressure level delivered by the hearing aid as measured at the tympanic membrane with a probe tube microphone.

Frequency Response

The range of frequencies that any sound system can amplify and transmit is limited. In the case of hearing aids, this range is restricted primarily by the transducers (microphone and receiver) and by the earmold configuration. Modern ear-level aids can provide wider frequency response ranges than their predecessors because of advances in technology. The frequency response of a hearing aid is determined by first measuring the reference test gain over a wide frequency range. Figure 14.4 shows a tracing from an in-the-ear hearing aid that provides maximum amplification in the 1500 to 6000 Hz range. To determine the frequency response, a line is drawn parallel with the baseline, which is 20 dB below a level showing the average gain at 1000, 1600, and 2500 Hz. The points of intersection of this line with the response curve may be considered the frequency range of the instrument.

Distortion

When a sound leaving a hearing aid differs in its frequency spectrum from the input signal, **frequency distortion** has taken place. **Amplitude distortion** refers to the differences in the relationships of the amplitudes of the input and output signals.

When sounds of one frequency are increased in amplitude, they may cause the electronic or mechanical portions of an amplifying system to be overstressed. This **harmonic distortion** can be expressed as the percentage of distortion of the input signal. The greater the distortion of a hearing aid, the poorer the quality of the amplified sounds of speech.

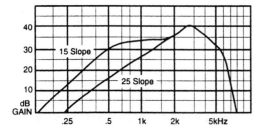

FIGURE 14.4   Frequency response characteristics of a typical in-the-ear hearing aid. Measurements were made with a 2-cm³ coupler and 60 dB input level.

Other Hearing-aid Parameters

Modern hearing-aid test equipment allows for a number of other checks to be made on the characteristics of hearing aids. Some of these checks include **equivalent input noise level,** battery drain, the performance of telephone induction coils, and the dynamic characteristics of circuitry, which alter the gain of the hearing aid as a function of the input signal (**automatic gain control**). Although definitions and descriptions are not presented here, the interested reader is encouraged to check the suggested reading list at the end of this chapter.

Binaural Amplification

A primary goal of any hearing aid fitting is to restore audition to as near normal a state as possible. As such, every attempt should be made to provide binaural hearing, assuming sufficient residual hearing and no contraindications presented by anatomical abnormalities. Research has documented patient comments that speech is clearer, louder, and less contaminated by background noise when two hearing aids are worn. In addition, localization of a sound source is usually enhanced with binaural hearing aids. The fact that evidence suggests a unilateral hearing aid fitting may result in auditory deprivation effects to the unaided ear (Gelfand & Silman, 1993) lends further credence to binaural hearing aid fittings. In a small percentage of cases, however, speech recognition is so poor in one ear that binaural aids decrease, rather than increase, the intelligibility of speech.

Types of Hearing Aids

Hearing aids come in a variety of shapes, sizes, colors, and types. Among the hearing aids available today are the traditional body-type, eyeglass, behind-the-ear, in-the-ear, in-the-canal, and completely in-the-canal instruments. Analog, analog/digital hybrid, and fully digital circuitry is available in even the smallest size hearing instruments.

Body-type Hearing Aids

Body-type hearing aids (Figure 14.5A) are usually reserved for patients with very profound hearing losses. They contain the microphone, amplifier, circuit modifiers, and battery compartment within a case that may be clipped to the wearer's clothing or worn in a pocket or a special pouch. A cord carries the electrical signals to a receiver, which is coupled to the patient's ear through a custom-fitted earmold (Figure 14.6). Body-type aids have several advantages: The controls are easy to adjust because they are relatively large, and the batteries often last longer than those for some types of aids. Battery compartments are large enough to allow easy access.

Problems with **acoustic feedback** are generally fewer with body-type hearing aids than with the other types. Acoustic feedback is a whistling sound that is the result of a cycle, when the amplified sounds leave the receiver and reach the microphone. Feedback is reduced by fabricating a tightly sealed earmold and by moving the receiver as far from the microphone as is practical.

Body-type instruments have several disadvantages, not the least of which is the cosmetic aspect. Despite attempts at public education, a stigma is often attached to hearing aids, and some

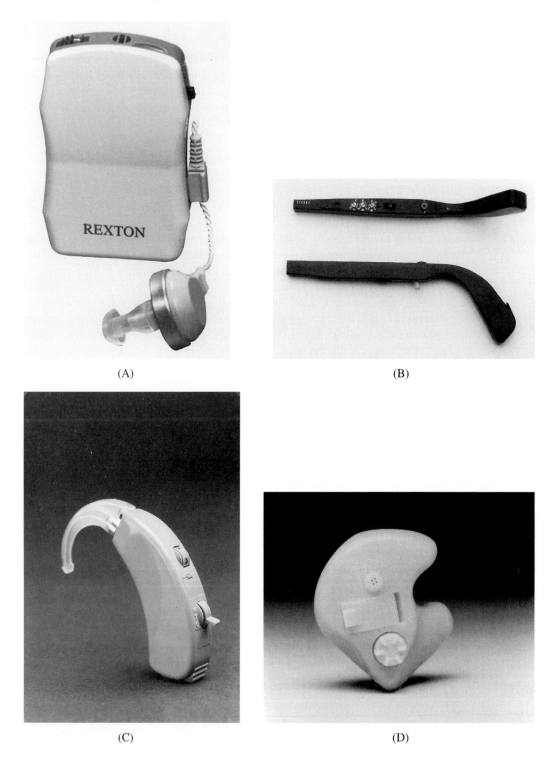

(A)

(B)

(C)

(D)

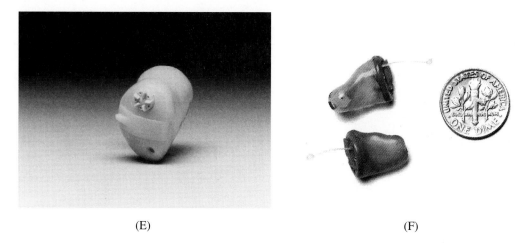

(E)   (F)

FIGURE 14.5   Six types of air conduction hearing aids showing: (A) body-type aid; (B) temple piece of eyeglass aid; (C) behind-the-ear (BTE) aid; (D) in-the-ear (ITE) aid; (E) in-the-canal (ITC) aid; and (F) completely in-the-canal (CIC) aid. (Courtesy of Rexton, Inc.)

people shun their use as a result. Not only are the cords considered unsightly, but they often break, causing the signal to be intermittent. In addition, when a body aid is worn under clothing, the rubbing of the microphone can cause a loud and disturbing noise. Because instruments are now available that can be worn on the ear and still provide the power previously found only in body-type instruments, the use of body aids has dropped sharply.

Eyeglass Hearing Aids

Hearing aids built into the temple bars of eyeglasses were among the first attempts at head-worn amplification following development of the transistor (Figure 14.5B). Patients who wear eyeglasses and hearing aids all the time used to prefer these instruments because they had less cumbersome hardware than body aids and were held in place more firmly than the large behind-the-ear aids that first appeared on the market. The once great popularity of eyeglass aids has diminished considerably in recent years, largely because of increased interest in in-the-ear hearing aids, and the dissatisfaction of having to wear two prostheses in one, creating practical problems when one needs repair or replacement.

Behind-the-ear (BTE) Hearing Aids

Hearing aids worn behind the ear (Figure 14.5C) and coupled via a hollow plastic elbow, or "ear hook," to a molded plastic insert (Figure 14.6) can be used by patients with mild to severe hearing losses. They allow for localization of sound, especially when a separate instrument is worn on each ear (binaural). Many patients report that it is easier to focus on a sound when they wear binaural ear-level instruments.

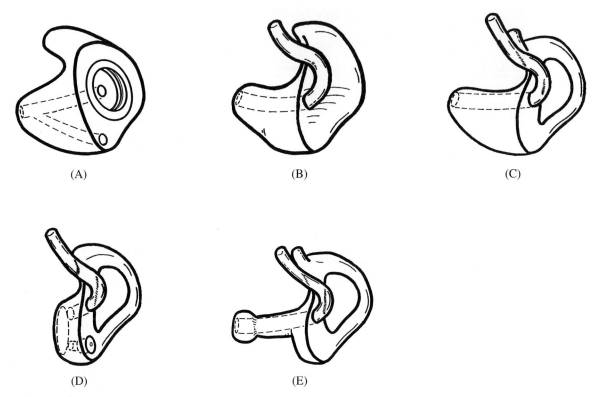

(A)   (B)   (C)

(D)   (E)

FIGURE 14.6   Five types of earmolds, showing: (A) receiver type for use with external transducer, vented to reduce low frequencies; (B) shell type for severe impairment; (C) skeleton (D) open-bore canal for enhanced high frequencies; (E) minimum contact mold for reduced occlusion effect. (Courtesy of Westone Laboratories)

Problems with clothing noise are eliminated with all head-worn hearing aids, as are difficulties with cords, because the receiver is built into the same case that houses the microphone and amplifier. The decreased size of the instrument makes adjustments of controls and insertion of batteries somewhat more difficult, especially for patients who are elderly or physically challenged. As the quality of BTE instruments improved and they became more powerful, their overall use increased. However, like their predecessors, they too are being overtaken in sales by the in-the-ear models.

In-the-ear (ITE) Hearing Aids

First developed in the late 1950s, instruments that are worn entirely in the concha and external auditory canal (Figure 14.5D) have been the most popular type for nearly twenty years. The circuitry is built into the earmold itself. Originally useful only for mild hearing losses, because of improved technology they can be used for hearing losses that range from mild to moderately severe.

In-the-canal (ITC) Hearing Aids

A major breakthrough in hearing aid design was the development of hearing instruments that fit entirely into the external auditory canal (Figure 14.5E), with only a slight protrusion into the concha. ITC aids are somewhat limited in power by their size, but they can be used by some patients with losses in the moderately severe range. This design takes advantage of the natural acoustic properties of the pinna, which are largely ignored by body, eyeglass, ITE, and BTE instruments. Improvements in the transducers allow for broader frequency response than was previously thought possible in a tiny instrument. The smaller size of the canal hearing aids makes them less useful than the ITE aids for some elderly patients.

Completely in-the-canal (CIC) Aids

The newest instrument available is the completely in-the-canal aid (Figure 14.5F), which is so tiny it is barely noticeable in many ears when it is inserted deep in the external auditory canal. Designed for mild or moderate hearing losses, the benefits of this instrument go beyond the obvious cosmetic appeal and include relatively easy use with telephones, lessening of wind-noise problems, increase of the usable gain of the instrument, and maximization of the contributions to hearing made by the pinna and the concha. What has come to be known as the "occlusion effect," the booming sound many hearing-aid wearers complain about when they speak, is often considerably lessened by CIC instruments (Mueller, 1994).

Because of the CIC's depth in the ear canal, the amplified sound is closer to the tympanic membrane and thus requires less gain and output than the other models. Such annoyances as weight and wind noise are lessened with this type of instrument. Even though the CIC is becoming a popular choice among potential hearing-aid users, the additional cost to the patient and the manual dexterity required to change the small batteries must be considered. In addition, as with many of the canal hearing aids, coupling to assistive listening devices is not possible.

CROS Aids

A patient with an unaidable unilateral hearing loss has a particular kind of listening difficulty, which can include trouble hearing soft speech from the "bad side." Little had been done in the way of amplification for such problems until Harford and Barry (1965) described a specially built instrument called **CROS (contralateral routing of offside signals).** In this configuration, the microphone is mounted on the side of the impaired ear, and the signal is sent to the amplifier, receiver, and plastic tube that are mounted on the side of the normal-hearing ear. The signal may be routed electrically through wires that are draped behind the head for BTE and ITE aids. The most popular method today is by way of FM transmitters and receivers, eliminating the need for wired connections. The signal presented to the canal of the "good" ear, either through a plastic tube or through a custom earmold, may contain an additional opening to allow unamplified sounds to enter the external ear canal normally. In this way patients hear from the "good" side in the usual fashion, but they also hear sounds from the "bad" side as they are amplified and led to the better ear.

The use of the CROS hearing instrument has expanded beyond its original intended use for unilateral hearing loss. It has been used both monaurally and binaurally (CRIS-CROS) for high-frequency losses and in other difficult cases in which traditional fitting results in acoustic feedback.

A **BiCROS** configuration allows for implementation of the traditional CROS principle, with the addition of amplification delivered directly to the better hearing ear when this ear also has some degree of hearing loss. Numerous variations of the CROS system are available for different types of hearing losses (Pollack, 1988).

Bone-conduction Hearing Aids

Bone-conduction hearing aids are selected for those patients with conductive hearing loss and otological conditions that preclude the use of air-conduction amplification (Figure 14.7). These conditions may include persistent or recurrent ear drainage, or hearing loss resulting from congenital ear canal or middle ear anomalies. The transducer is a vibrating receiver that is pressed firmly against the skin of the mastoid process. The transducer may be built within an eyeglass hearing aid, a post-auricular instrument worn with a headband, or coupled to a body-style hearing instrument. As vibration of the skull stimulates both cochleas from a single bone-conduction instrument, true binaural hearing, arising from timing and intensity differences of sounds reaching the two ears, is not attain-

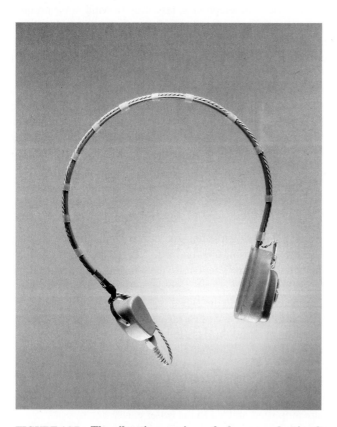

FIGURE 14.7   The vibrating receiver of a bone-conduction hearing aid sends sound waves to the cochlea through the bone conduction auditory pathways of the skull. (Courtesy of Starkey Laboratories)

able. The hearing aid industry indicates that between 0.2 and 0.3 percent of all hearing aids prescribed are bone-conduction hearing aids (Chasin, 1997).

Implantable Bone-conduction Devices

There are many people who suffer from conductive hearing losses for whom surgery either has failed to improve their hearing or is not an option. A number of these people have been helped in the past by bone-conduction hearing aids, but these devices are often found to be uncomfortable and/or unsightly. Some patients have shown preference for a relatively new option, involving a magnetic device that can be surgically implanted under the skin in the mastoid area. The procedure may be performed as outpatient surgery, using either local or general anesthesia. Several designs of such devices are now available (Figure 14.8) (Chasin, 1997, 1998).

For one design, a screw hole is prepared following a surgical incision in the mastoid, which is closed after the instrument is firmly screwed into place. After the incision has healed (about eight weeks), the patient is fitted with the induction device (which fits directly over the implant) and either an at-the-ear or body-worn, battery-powered processor. Patients report good sound quality, elimination of the acoustic feedback found with traditional hearing aids, and preference for this device over their previously worn hearing aids (Johnson, Meikle, Vernon, & Schleuning, 1988).

Naturally, since hearing stimulation is by bone conduction, patients must have significant air-bone gaps and reasonably good bone-conduction thresholds. DeChicchis, Bess, and Schwartz (1996) state that the bone-anchored hearing aid (BAHA) has proven effective for patients with bone-conduction pure-tone averages up to 45 dB HL. These investigators state that with the increased power of a connected body-style hearing instrument, the BAHA can be effective for patients with bone-conduction pure-tone averages up to 60 dB HL. Snik, Mylanus, and Cremers (1994) found that patients experienced better word recognition scores and improved subjective intelligibility when these devices were compared to previously worn traditional bone-conduction hearing aids. A follow-

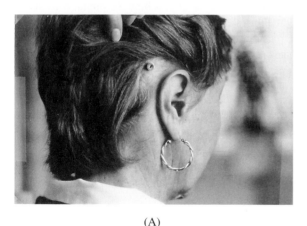
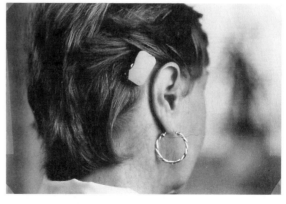

(A)   (B)

FIGURE 14.8   Bone-anchored hearing aid (BAHA): (A) The abutment is connected to a titanium screw threaded directly into the mastoid bone. (B) The BAHA attaches to the abutment allowing transmission of sound directly via the titanium screw. (Courtesy of Nobel Biocare USA, Inc.)

up study of 100 such devices (Tjellstron & Granstrom, 1994) revealed that 90 percent remained intact, while 5 percent became extracted because of trauma, and the other 5 percent became inoperative, but only after a number of years. Some patients experienced adverse skin reactions, but most of those were not considered serious. Time will reveal whether this procedure will become popular for individuals with conductive hearing loss.

Middle-ear Implants

A wide range of implantable hearing devices is being studied, both on humans and on experimental animals. The goal of implantable hearing aid research is the development of a totally implanted hearing device within the middle ear for moderate and severe sensorineural hearing loss (Dumon, Zennaro, Aran, & Bebear, 1995). The impetus behind the development of middle-ear implants is improved fidelity by driving the ossicles and/or cochlea directly without occlusion of the outer ear and reduction of acoustic feedback, because the energy is not transduced back to an acoustic signal. With the successful introduction of CIC hearing instruments, it is unlikely that middle-ear implants would be employed for cosmetic reasons alone. However, as these devices become perfected, a certain portion of those patients who are considered candidates for cochlear implants may instead be candidates for middle-ear implants (Chasin, 1997). There is no doubt that entirely new generations of such instruments will be forthcoming in the future and will be of great benefit for many patients.

Cochlear Implants

Several decades ago attempts were made to stimulate the cortex of the brain electrically to reproduce auditory sensations in people with hearing loss. These approaches were abandoned for a variety of technical reasons, but they led to the development of several systems for electrical stimulation of the cochlea. The **cochlear implant** (House, 1982) is a major step in the surgical implantation of instruments for patients with profound sensorineural hearing losses who are unable to use conventional amplification. The internal receiver, which is implanted under the skin behind the pinna, consists of wire electrodes and a tiny coil. Up to 22 active electrodes are placed 22 to 24 mm into the scala tympani within the cochlea. Ground electrodes are placed outside the bony labyrinth, often in the temporalis muscle (Figure 14.9). A small microphone is attached to an earhook and worn behind the ear. The microphone feeds electrical impulses to a speech processor, which codes the speech information to be transmitted to the electrode array. From the processor the signal goes to a transmitter, which converts it to magnetic impulses that are sent to the electrodes. An electrical signal is induced from the magnetic field in the cochlea and flows on to stimulate the auditory nerve (Figure 14.10).

Only a small number of adverse effects from cochlear implant surgery have been reported, and many of these have been corrected with revisions in the instruments and surgical procedures. Initially, only adults with profound hearing losses were provided with cochlear implants. A variety of tests had to be performed to ensure that the hearing losses were due to hair cell, rather than nerve cell damage. The hearing losses had to have been acquired after the development of speech and language, and the patients had to be free of physical or psychological conditions that might adversely affect adjustment. As the cochlear implant device was improved and diagnostic tests were expanded, candidacy for implantation grew to include children with profound congenital hearing losses.

Implant recipients are usually advised that they may not be able to discriminate among many of the sounds of speech. In spite of this, both objective and subjective outcome measures document the

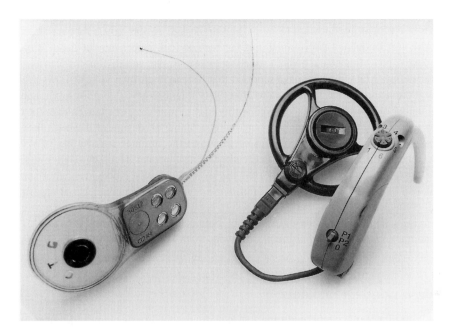

FIGURE 14.9 Example of an ear-level cochlear implant device showing its internal and external components. (Courtesy of Cochlear Corporation)

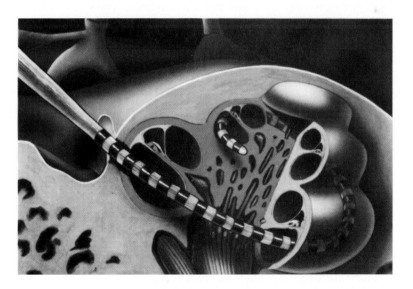

FIGURE 14.10 Implantation of a multielectrode array of a cochlear implant device. (Courtesy of Cochlear Corporation)

successes of cochlear implantation (Simons-McCandless & Parkin, 1997; Zwolan, Kileny, & Telian, 1997). Although frequency discrimination is far from perfect, voices may be heard at normal conversational levels, providing sound awareness and cues such as rate and rhythm that can assist the listener in speechreading. Many patients have reported that hearing their own voices allows them to monitor their vocal pitch and loudness much more effectively than was possible prior to implantation. A surprising number of patients report a marked ability to discriminate speech, even over the telephone.

As experience with cochlear implants increased and the design of the instruments improved, the number of physicians doing implant surgery and the number and variety of recipients have increased. The modern consensus is in agreement with Dorman, Hannley, Dankowski, Smith, and McCandless (1989), who concluded that the use of many channels provides better speech recognition than can be obtained with systems employing fewer channels. Because of reports in the news media, there is presently considerable interest in cochlear implants, and audiologists may be asked for information about them. It should always be pointed out that the cochlear implant is intended for those patients with hearing impairments so severe that they cannot be helped with other less invasive devices.

Auditory Brainstem Implants

Patients with bilateral acoustic neuroma that threaten either life or neurologic function are usually left with a loss of auditory function upon tumor removal. As they have no remaining cochlear nerve to stimulate, cochlear implantation provides no benefit. Advances in neuro-otology permit the cochlea and first order neurons to be bypassed, permitting direct stimulation of the cochlear nuclei.

Only patients with **neurofibromatosis type 2,** 90 percent of whom exhibit bilateral acoustic neuromas, are eligible for auditory brainstem implantation (ABI) under protocols set by the U.S. Food and Drug Administration (Hitselberger & Telischi, 1994). As with cochlear implantation, the implanted electrode is coupled through a transcutaneous magnetic connector to an external sound processor. While ABI creates an enhanced auditory awareness and improved speechreading performance, communication improvement is not as great as that obtained for cochlear implant recipients, regardless of the extent of auditory rehabilitation received following implantation.

Vibrotactile Instruments

Despite all attempts to take advantage of residual hearing through amplification, some patients simply cannot be helped by any of the devices just described. There is clear benefit to the use of instruments that amplify sound, not to augment hearing *per se,* but to provide tactile stimulation on the surface of the skin. An interest in such stimulation continues as, unlike cochlear implantation, **vibrotactile aids** are noninvasive and thereby pose less risk to young children than does surgery.

Vibrotactile aids (Figure 14.11) are designed on the principle that vibratory patterns can be generated on the skin that are directly related to the acoustic wave that strikes the microphone of the device. These instruments use microcomputers that assist in the perception of such cues as fundamental frequency and intonation. Small vibrators are worn on the chest, neck, wrist, or back of the hand and are connected by separate channels to the input unit, which can be worn in a carrying case or a pocket, much like a body-type hearing aid. The microphone may be built into the unit or clipped to the wearer's clothing. Noise-suppression circuitry helps to keep background sounds

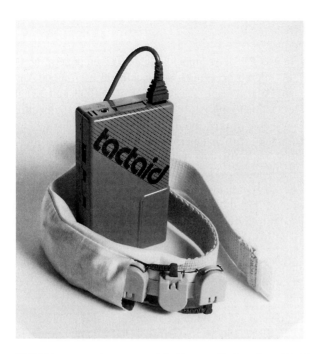

FIGURE 14.11   A commercial vibrotactile hearing aid. (Courtesy of Audiological Engineering Corporation)

from being picked up, and the wearer senses distinct vibratory patterns, which are unique to specific sounds.

An Australian vibrotactile device called the Tickle Talker was used on a small group of children in a total-communication training program (Galvin, Cowan, Sarant, Alcantara, Blamey, & Clark, 1991). It was found that the subjects could detect sound better with the tactile device than with hearing aids and that combining the two devices improved both hearing sensitivity and discrimination. Apparently the addition of the tactile device did not interfere in any way with the ability of the children to recognize manual signs.

The degree to which benefit is obtained from a vibrotactile instrument is largely determined by training and practice, although apparently instruments with different design specifications may provide differing amounts of information to enhance speechreading (Waldstein & Boothroyd, 1995). The greater the dedication to its use, the larger and more varied the number of speech sounds that can be perceived. With the proper use of vibrotactile aids, many patients may be able to increase their awareness of speech and environmental sounds, improve the rate and rhythm of their speech, augment speechreading, and possibly improve word-recognition skills.

To expect that vibrotactile aids will eventually replace traditional instruments for those with profound hearing loss is probably a mistake because the skin is less than an ideal receptor of vibratory information. It is advisable to explore traditional amplification thoroughly, especially with young children, before adopting a vibrotactile instrument.

Selecting Hearing-aid Candidates

In the past, general guidelines were used for determining whether a given patient should try hearing aids. Today audiologists often find such rules confining and lacking in usefulness. An old common rule was to recommend a hearing aid if the average hearing loss at 500, 1000, and 2000 Hz exceeded 30 dB in the better-hearing ear. Restriction to this kind of guideline ignores a number of critical factors, such as age, duration of hearing loss, speech-recognition ability, audiometric contour, intelligence, vocation, education, financial resources, and, perhaps most important of all, motivation to use hearing aids.

Before the era of modern middle-ear surgery, most patients wearing hearing aids had conductive hearing losses. Because these patients usually had good word-recognition ability and tolerance for loud sounds, many physicians encouraged them to try hearing aids. However, patients with sensorineural hearing losses were discouraged from wearing hearing instruments because of their difficulties with speech recognition and loudness tolerance. Complaints that the instruments merely amplified the distortion they heard, as well as problems with loudness recruitment, led many clinicians to conclude that patients with sensorineural hearing loss were often poor risks for amplification. It is unfortunate that this misperception lingers among many physicians, despite the numerous advances in hearing aid electronics.

With advances in middle-ear surgery, the number of people with conductive hearing loss wearing hearing instruments has decreased, and the number with sensorineural losses has increased. This is partly a result of improvements in the instruments and partly because of the influence of rehabilitative audiology. Selecting hearing aids for persons with sensorineural loss involves much more than simply scrutinizing the audiogram and making a recommendation. In many cases a trial period of several weeks with new hearing instruments can be a determining factor.

Selecting Hearing Aids for Adults

Carhart (1946) described a procedure for hearing-aid evaluation that was used for many years. This procedure included making measurements in the sound field using a number of different tests, performed both unaided and with a variety of different hearing aids. The differences between aided and unaided scores showed the amount of improvement provided by each aid. Measurements included the SRT, word-recognition scores in quiet and with background noise, most comfortable and uncomfortable loudness levels, range of comfortable loudness, and subjective estimates of clarity and quality. If four to six instruments were tested, the ideal one provided the lowest SRT, the highest word-recognition scores, a level of most comfortable loudness close to the level of normal conversation (60 to 70 dB SPL), and a broad range of comfortable loudness.

Opinions regarding the validity of these procedures has varied. Haug, Baccaro, and Guilford (1971) found them reliable and valid. Shore, Bilger, and Hirsh (1960) drew just the opposite conclusion. In addition to doubts about the replicability of sound-field speech audiometry with hearing aids, other problems presented themselves. Even if a selection was felt to be proper and a specific prescription was made for hearing aids, there was no guarantee that the instruments purchased would have the same characteristics as the ones recommended, even if they appeared identical in every way. There is strong evidence that the Carhart procedure and similar "comparative" methods are severely limited (Northern, 1992).

A more successful approach to hearing aid fittings is by prescription followed by some means of verifying the performance of the chosen circuit. A variety of prescription methods are currently employed by audiologists to match, as closely as possible, the acoustic characteristics of the earmold and hearing-aid configuration to the acoustic needs of the patient. Through venting and special earmold designs, for example, low-frequency energy can be deemphasized for patients with hearing losses that are primarily in the higher frequencies. Mid-frequency energy can be modified with acoustic dampers or filters in the tubing of the earmolds or ear hooks of the aids, and high-frequency energy can be enhanced with bell-shaped tubing and two earmold openings. Before the advent of this approach to acoustic modification, attempts at shaping the acoustic signals were limited to the use of electronic filters within the instruments.

Dissatisfaction with existing methods, improvements in hearing-aid design, and the ongoing desire to improve hearing health care have led to some interesting developments in recent years. Computer-based systems have been devised to simplify the various calculations required during hearing-aid selection procedures and to reduce potential errors when, for example, comparing gain at the tympanic membrane to gain in a hard-walled (e.g., 2 cm³) cavity, retrieving results from different instruments, or converting hearing-level values to sound-pressure levels (Kruger & Kruger, 1994). Hawkins (1992) has summarized the most commonly used prescriptive hearing-aid selection procedures.

Selecting Hearing Aids for Children

A child who is mature enough to perform behavioral hearing tests and is found to be in need of amplification may be tested by modifying certain adult selection procedures. The absence of receptive language skills, of course, usually precludes the use of speech audiometry in pediatric testing. Sometimes it is felt that a small child needs amplification even though no behavioral audiometric results have been obtained. Instruments selected for these children should be as electroacoustically flexible as possible so that modifications can be made as information is obtained about the child's hearing sensitivity. The high flexibility of programmable hearing instruments often makes these instruments an ideal choice for children. Many children, for whom a full hearing profile has not been determined, are enrolled in language-stimulation programs, where they should spend some time during each therapy session being conditioned to play audiometry. The earlier the age at which amplification through properly adjusted hearing aids can be provided, along with auditory training, the better the chances for development of normal language and intelligible speech and voice.

One of the obvious requirements in deriving maximum benefit from pediatric amplification is to get children to wear their hearing instruments. There are several reasons why some children are resistant. They may find their hearing aids physically uncomfortable, acoustically unpleasant, or cosmetically unappealing. Whereas vanity forces many adults to select the least conspicuous instrument, children are often attracted by those that are brightly colored and appealing. Allowing children to participate in the choice of the color of the instrument and earmold, whenever possible, makes them partners in the selection process, rather than passive participants. An additional advantage to a brightly colored device is the increased ease in finding it when it is dropped or lost, or in separating it from instruments worn by other children (DeConde, 1984). The dynamic nature of hearing instruments and the devices used to prescribe and fit them is such that the technology will probably be changed and updated on an almost constant basis for the foreseeable future. Science has truly come to the assistance of the hearing-aid user. Nevertheless, it is essential that patients themselves play active roles in the selection of their wearable hearing instruments.

Dispensing Hearing Aids

Until the late 1970s, the bylaws of ASHA did not allow its members to dispense hearing aids directly. Such sales were considered unethical because it was felt that the audiologist's objectivity might be compromised if any profit motive were injected into the selection process. The tide of this entire subject has turned. Not only are audiologists in many practice settings dispensing hearing aids directly to patients, but university training programs are preparing students for this practice.

Under proper conditions, direct dispensing of hearing aids appears to be an ideal procedure. The audiologist must be (1) aware of the characteristics and adjustments of the aids to be dispensed, (2) able to provide simple repairs, (3) capable of making and modifying earmolds, and (4) able to provide a total audiological rehabilitation program suited to each individual's needs. In addition, direct dispensing provides the unique opportunity for a patient to receive an entire rehabilitation program from one highly trained professional. Before embarking on a hearing-aid dispensing program, however, the audiologist must be aware of any pertinent state licensing laws. Many states now permit audiologists to dispense hearing aids without obtaining a second license through the hearing aid dispenser's licensing board.

When a patient deals directly with a nonaudiologist hearing-aid dispenser, direct guidance from an audiologist is absent. Patients may select dispensers arbitrarily, or they may be given lists of several dispensers. In this way patients can shop until they find an instrument that looks and sounds acceptable and is affordable. Of course, decisions are influenced to some extent by the dispenser's personality and sales expertise. Unfortunately, because some patients may suffer the confusion common to shoppers and may simply select hearing aids from the last dispenser they see, this is not a recommended procedure.

Occasionally audiologists practice within a location in which they do not dispense, and there are no dispensing audiologists in the community. If, after a patient's audiological assessment, an audiologist believes that hearing aids are indicated, a copy of the test results may be provided to the patient and contact made directly with a dispenser who is not an audiologist. Following selection of the instrument, the audiologist should see the patient again for an aided performance check to determine the efficacy of the hearing aids selected.

Some audiologists give their patients general kinds of prescriptions for hearing aids. These specifications might include whether both ears will be aided or, if not, the preferred ear; the type of aid; gain; OSPL90; frequency response; and so forth. In this way the dispenser fabricates an aid or selects from a stock of instruments and attempts to satisfy the needs of the patient within the confines of the recommendations.

Unless the patient returns to the audiologist after instruments have been obtained, there is no way to know whether the original recommendations have been followed by the hearing-aid dispenser, or whether the selected instruments are satisfactory. The audiologist and dispenser may discuss possible modifications of the original recommendations by telephone.

Regardless of how hearing aids are obtained, the audiologist must be prepared to assist patients who encounter difficulties with their instruments. Some common problems and solutions are summarized in Table 14.1. When there appears to be no simple correction for a malfunctioning instrument,

TABLE 14.1 Common Hearing Aid Problems and Their Solutions

Complaint	Explanation	Solution
Weak sound	Partial obstruction in earmold	Clean earmold
	Partial obstruction in tubing	Clean tubing
	Incorrect battery	Replace with proper battery
	Weak battery*	Replace with strong battery
Intermittent sound	Broken cord**	Replace cord
	Dirty battery contacts	Roll battery around in compartment or clean contacts with emery board or fine sandpaper
	Dirty controls	Move switches and controls through all positions to dislodge dirt Roll volume control several times through entire range Spray with contact cleaner
	Weak battery*	Replace with strong battery
No sound	Dead battery*	Replace with fresh battery
	Battery improperly inserted	Remove and replace battery
	Obstruction in earmold	Clean earmold
	Obstruction in tubing	Clean or replace tubing
	Twisted tubing	Untwist or replace tubing
	Broken cord**	Replace cord
	Broken receiver***	Replace receiver
	Set for telephone coil	Move to microphone position
	Improve use	Check owner's manual
Aid works but is noisy	Acoustic feedback	Check for tight-fitting mold Check for connection between mold and receiver Check for properly inserted mold Check for crack in tubing or ear hook Clear aid of clothing
	Clothing noise**	Use hearing-aid harness

*Use a battery tester that places a "load" on the battery.

**Body-type or CROS aid only.

***Body-type aid only.

factory repair may be required. The proper course can be guided by the audiologist, who must ascertain, among other things, that patients understand the terms of the new hearing aid's repair warranty.

Much of the stigma attached to wearing hearing aids was reduced by President Ronald Reagan's hearing-aid fitting in the early 1980s and President Bill Clinton's hearing-aid fitting in 1997. Because of this, along with the continued growth of the older segment of the population and the fact that more people than ever before can now be helped to hear better through corrective amplification, the number of hearing aids dispensed each year is increasing. Clearly, hearing aid dispensing is a role for which clinicians in training should be prepared.

Verifying Hearing Aid Performance

Audiologists have come to realize that despite the important measurements made in hard-walled 2 cm³ couplers, the "real ear" behaves quite differently. Amplified sound-pressure levels in the human ear are not accurately represented by the artificial cavity. This realization has encouraged the measurement of hearing-aid characteristics within the external auditory canal of the patient with tiny probe microphones (Figure 14.12). Such verification measurements reflect not only the acoustic characteristics of the hearing aid, but also the natural individual resonance of the ear itself and the interactions among these effects (Mueller, Hawkins, & Northern, 1992) .

When the earmold of a hearing aid is placed into the external ear canal, its first effect is to act like a plug, creating an additional hearing loss and altering the natural resonance of the ear. This is known as the **insertion loss.** Therefore, the first job of the hearing aid is to overcome the hearing loss it has created and the way the natural ear properties have been altered. For these reasons *in situ* (in position) measurements are extremely valuable in determining such important considerations as the real-ear unaided response, the real-ear aided response, and the insertion gain. With the advent of digitally programmable hearing aids, it is possible to use probe-tube measurements to tailor the response of the hearing instrument more closely to the sound-pressure needs of the individual.

Before the widespread clinical availability of probe-microphone measures of hearing-aid performance, sound-field tests with hearing instruments were common and are still used in some clinics today. If a child can be conditioned to take a pure-tone hearing test in the sound field, thresholds may be measured both with and without hearing aids at a number of different frequencies. The

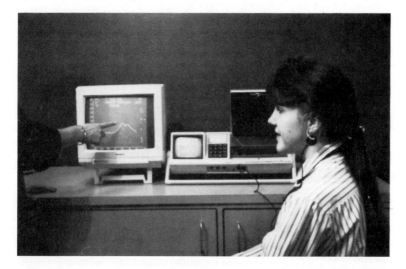

FIGURE 14.12   A probe tube microphone system for in situ measurement of hearing aid performance. (Courtesy of Starkey Texas)

improvements in thresholds obtained in the aided condition show the functional gain at different frequencies. If pure tones are used in the sound field, they should be either automatically pulsed on and off or warbled to avoid problems with interference patterns. A **warble tone** is one that is frequency modulated, that is, modified in frequency over time. A 1000 Hz tone warbled at 5 percent changes systematically in frequency from 950 to 1050 Hz.

The suitability of amplification cannot be judged solely on the basis of how closely aided thresholds approximate normal threshold levels. It is often impossible to reach normal threshold levels, or even a full audibility of the **speech spectrum** with some severe or profound hearing losses, because of the constraints of acoustic feedback and loudness tolerance levels associated with some hearing losses (Table 14.2).

Caution should be exercised in using sound-field measures given their poor test-retest reliability with children and the test's serious limitations (Clark, 1996). Probe-microphone measures of hearing-aid gain, in conjunction with speech audiometrics, are the recommended verification, because probe-microphone measures alone do not assess an individual's cognitive processing abilities. To prevent overamplification, a direct measurement of hearing-aid maximum output should also be obtained during hearing-aid verification (Hawkins, 1993).

It should be noted that verifying a hearing aid's ability to meet prescribed goals of amplification does not ensure a patient's favorable perception of benefit. Some formal means of validation that the patient's amplification needs have been addressed should be included within any hearing-aid fitting process. This may take the form of a pre- and post-fitting administration of a hearing handicap scale or other self-assessment measure.

TABLE 14.2 Aided Threshold Goals

Average Hearing Threshold[a] dB HL		+	Average Aided Real-ear Gain	=	Aided Threshold Goal[b] dB HL
Hearing Loss Descriptor[c]					
–10 –15	Normal hearing		NA		NA
16–25	Slight hearing loss		4–10		12–15
26–40	Mild hearing loss		10–20		16–20
41–55	Moderate hearing loss		20–30		21–25
56–70	Moderately severe loss		30–40		26–30
71–90	Severe hearing loss		40–45		31–45
91+	Profound hearing loss		46+		45–55

[a]Average 0.5, 1, and 2kHz re: ANSI-1989

[b]From Goodman (1965) as modified by Clark (1981)

[c]Goal based on sensorineural hearing impairment. Conductive and mixed hearing losses will tolerate more gain resulting in a lower threshold goal.

NA = not applicable

(From Clark, 1996)

Hearing Assistance Technologies

The inherent limitations of hearing aids often necessitate the use of a variety of technologies including various **assistive listening devices (ALDs)** and vibratory or visual alerting systems. One of the major disadvantages of wearable hearing aids is the environmental noise between the microphones of the hearing aids and the talker, which creates adverse signal-to-noise ratios and decreased speech intelligibility. The closer the talker is to the listener's hearing aids, the fewer the effects of intervening room noise. In addition, reverberation and other acoustic characteristics of any room may affect important parameters of sound waves as they travel through air. Getting talker and listener close together in space is often difficult in classrooms, as well as in a variety of other listening situations.

Older auditory training units were hard-wired, meaning that the microphone and amplifier were physically connected to receivers worn by the listeners. This configuration severely restricted the person speaking to proximity to the microphone and limited the person listening to a fixed location at the receivers. There are three types of assistive listening systems commonly used today that interface in a variety of ways with personal hearing aids, or small earphone receivers, for use in classrooms, theaters, hospitals, auditoriums, retirement facilities, libraries, and personal offices and homes. These systems utilize transmitters and receivers that allow freedom of movement for the talker and the listener.

In a frequency modulated (FM) system, the talker wears a small microphone, and signals are transmitted along a radio frequency (RF) carrier wave. Receivers worn by the listener allow the signal to be demodulated and delivered to the user in a variety of ways, including an induction loop that is worn around the neck. With a neck-worn induction loop fitting, the signal is then amplified for the user via the telecoils within the hearing aids. In lieu of the induction neck loop, a wire from the FM receiver unit permits coupling directly to the hearing aid. Both of these means of coupling the FM receiver to the hearing aids are rapidly being replaced by technological advances that have permitted the miniaturization of the FM receiver allowing the receivers themselves to be directly coupled to the hearing aids (Figure 14.13F).

Speech may also be delivered directly to hearing aids through infrared systems that utilize light frequencies invisible to the human eye to carry speech signals to a receiving unit worn by the listener. The receiving unit transduces the light signal into an auditory signal that may then be amplified to the desired level. The lack of any wires in the installation makes these systems easily installed, with the advantage of a lower cost than FM systems. Smaller infrared light systems may be used in the home for listening to television. Large area systems may be found in cinemas, theaters, and houses of worship.

A third system employs the same induction loop principal used with the neck loop described earlier. In this system, an electromagnetic field is created by a loop of wire around the room. As with the neck loop, the user receives the signal via the telecoils within the hearing aids. This system is the least expensive of the three, although some signal purity is sacrificed through electromagnetic coupling. Certainly different systems may be more appropriate for different purposes (Tyler & Schum, 1995).

In classrooms, FM technology can be coupled to sound-field speakers (Figures 14.14 and 14.15), providing greater acoustic accessibility of the teacher's instruction for all students in the room. Sound-field amplification must not be construed to be a replacement for a personal FM system. The former typically improves the classroom signal-to-noise ratio by 10 to 20 dB, the latter by as much as 20 to 30 dB. While some children's hearing losses require the greater signal-to-noise ratio

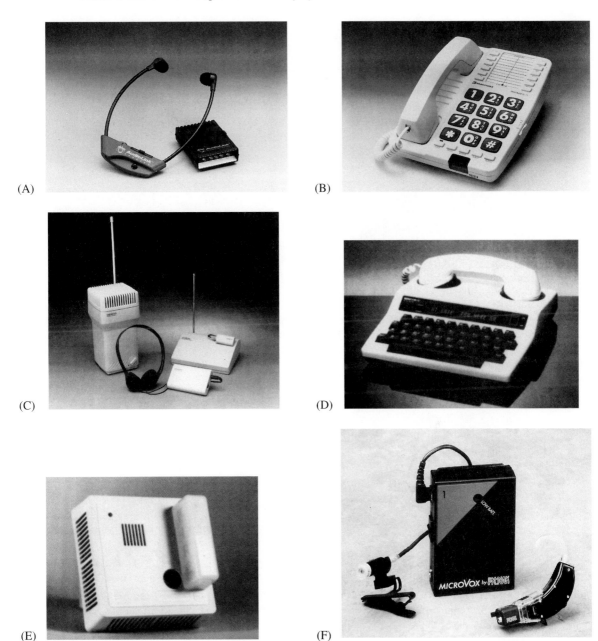

FIGURE 14.13 Examples of a few hearing assistance technologies for use by individuals with hearing impairment: (A) Audio-Link, an infrared system for transmission and reception of auditory signals through invisible light frequencies; (B) VCO telephone with built-in amplifier; (C) FM system, designed for home use, that includes a wireless remote speaker, or can be used with a headset for private listening; (D) Personal text telephone (TT) for a visual display of typed messages over the telephone lines (available with printer); (E) Smoke detector that both sounds a loud alarm and illuminates a powerful strobe light; (F) Phonak's Micro Link FM receiver plugs directly into the audio input jack of a BTE aid for reception of audio signals from a remote microphone. (Courtesy of Siemens Hearing Instruments, Inc., Phonak Hearing Instruments, and Ultratec, Inc.)

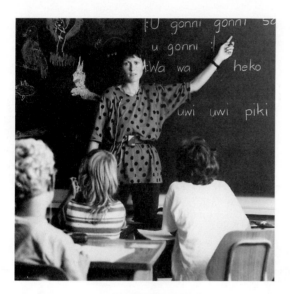

FIGURE 14.14   Classroom instruction is transmitted via FM technology from a teacher-worn microphone and transmitter to personal FM receivers (Figure 4.13F) or ceiling-mounted speakers (Figure 14.15). (Courtesy of Phonak Hearing Instruments)

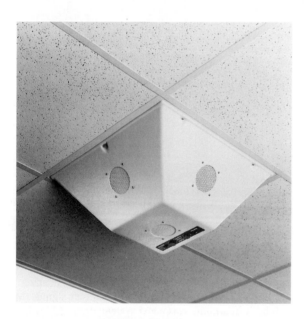

FIGURE 14.15   Significant enhancement of signal-to-noise ratios may be achieved through FM technology coupled to strategically placed ceiling mounted speakers. (Courtesy of Telex Communications, Inc.)

provided through a personal FM unit, sound-field FM technology has proven beneficial for children with fluctuating conductive hearing loss, unilateral hearing impairment, and slight, permanent, hearing loss (10 to 25 dB HL), as well as those with language, learning, attention, processing, or behavioral problems (Flexer, 1994).

A valuable addition to the array of assistive listening devices is the personal listening system, such as the pocket talker. Years ago hearing-aid manufacturers strove to increase the cosmetic appeal of hearing aids by making them as small as possible. Today there are many people with hearing impairment who are willing to use a device that is clearly visible and allows patients and those speaking with them easy access to a unit that is the size of a mini-audio cassette recorder, with large, easy-to-use controls. These devices are especially valuable in nursing homes, where looking after small hearing instruments can be a great inconvenience, and where patients often lack the fine motor control required of smaller units. An increasing number of physicians are learning of the pocket talker's value through audiologists. Confidential patient/physician dialogue is easily restored through these units for patients who have not yet been fitted with appropriate hearing aids.

Also included in the general category of hearing assistance technology are signaling or alerting units, which have been called "environmental adaptations" (Vaugn, Lightfoot, & Teter, 1988). The first of these devices amplified ringers of telephones and the transmitted talker's voice. Subsequently developed devices alert individuals through flashing lights or vibrations to the presence of emergency signals such as smoke or fire alarms; crying babies; or such mundane but important signals as timers, doorbells, and alarm clocks. Additional instruments to improve communication on the telephone include telecommunication devices for the deaf (TDDs) also known as text telephones (TTs). All television sets larger than 13-inch models sold after 1992 are equipped with telecaptioning decoders to allow printed text to be viewed on the screen. Modern technology and microcircuitry have created instruments that can markedly improve the quality of life for those with a hearing loss. Examples of several hearing assistance technologies may be found in Figure 14.13.

Summary

Devices designed to augment sound transmission to aid human hearing have evolved from simple sound collectors to instruments that employ some of today's most sophisticated miniature electronics. The styles and circuit options available are designed for both the hearing needs and cosmetic concerns of an ever-growing population of persons with hearing loss.

The audiologist's selection of appropriate amplification must always be followed by some means to verify that the performance received closely approximates the performance expected. Regardless of the style or whether a hearing instrument is designed with a simple analog circuit or advanced digital sound processing, the electroacoustic parameters of all hearing aids must meet certain standard specifications, and their performance should be monitored to ensure that adherence to standards is maintained.

The recommendation and fitting of appropriately selected hearing instruments is only one step within the complete hearing (re)habilitation services provided to patients. When the audiologist's (re)habilitative efforts with patients reveal the need for greater sound augmentation than hearing aids alone can provide, the appropriate recommendation and instruction for assistive listening/alerting devices should be given. To offer less than the full array of options available to those with hearing loss falls short of optimum patient care.

STUDY QUESTIONS

1. List and describe the electroacoustic characteristics of hearing aids.

2. What are the advantages and disadvantages of different types of hearing aids?

3. What measurements are made in hearing-aid evaluation and verification?

4. Why are speech audiometrics important in hearing-aid evaluation?

5. Briefly describe the differences among FM, infrared, and induction loop assistive devices.

6. List the basic components of a hearing aid and describe the purposes of each.

7. What is the difference between hybrid (digital/analog) hearing instruments and fully digital hearing instruments?

GLOSSARY

Acoustic feedback The whistling sound that is created when the signal leaving the receiver of a hearing aid leaks back into the microphone and is reamplified.

Acoustic gain The difference, in decibels, between the intensity of the input signal and the intensity of the output signal in a hearing aid.

Amplitude distortion The presence of frequencies in the output of an electroacoustic system that were not present at the input, resulting in a disproportional difference between the input and output waves.

Analog hearing aid An amplification system in which the electrical signal is analogous to the input acoustical signal in frequency, intensity, and temporal patterns.

Assistive listening devices (ALDs) Adjunct hearing instruments to improve signal-to-noise ratio. May include personal amplifiers, FM systems, TV listeners or telephone amplifiers.

Automatic gain control A special circuit within a hearing aid that prevents sounds from being overamplified for the impaired ear.

BiCROS hearing aid A modification of the CROS hearing aid (See *CROS*) in which there is one microphone on each side of the head, delivering signals to the better hearing ear when one ear is unaidable.

Cochlear implant A coil and series of electrodes surgically placed in the mastoid and inner ear. It is designed to provide sound to a patient with a profound hearing loss through a processor and external coil.

Compression A decrease in pressure. In a hearing aid, a method of limiting the amplification of louder sounds relative to weaker sounds.

CROS (contralateral routing of offside signals) A hearing aid originally developed for patients with unilateral hearing losses. The microphone is mounted on the side of the poorer ear, and the signal is routed to the better ear and presented by an "open" earmold.

Digital hearing aid An amplification system in which the input signal is stored, as by a computer, as sets of binary digits that represent the frequency, intensity, and temporal patterns of the input acoustical signal.

Distortion In a hearing aid, the result of an inexact copy of the input signal by the output signal. Distortion is usually caused by the microphone, speaker, and/or amplifier.

Equivalent input noise level The inherent noise level within a hearing aid with the input signal turned off and the hearing aid set at the reference test gain level.

Frequency distortion An inexact reproduction of the frequencies in a sound wave.

Frequency response The frequency range of amplification (as in a hearing aid), expressed in hertz, from the lowest to the highest frequency amplified.

Functional gain The difference in decibels between unaided and aided thresholds of hearing.

Harmonic distortion The distortion created when harmonic frequencies are generated in an amplification system; usually expressed in percentage of distortion.

Hearing Aid Industry Conference (HAIC) An organization of hearing-aid manufacturers that provides standardization of measurement and reporting on hearing-aid performance data.

High-frequency average (HFA) An ANSI hearing-aid specification expressed as the average SPL at 1000, 1600, and 2500 Hz.

Insertion gain The decibel difference between unaided and aided conditions as measured through a probe-tube microphone system. Commonly referred to as Real Ear Insertion Gain (REIG).

Insertion loss The additional loss of hearing created by placing a hearing aid, turned off, within the ear.

Integrated circuit An inseparable unification of several transistors and resistors on a small piece of silicon maintaining an electrical isolation of the circuit components.

Neurofibromatosis type 2 An hereditary disorder characterized by bilateral tumors along the cochleovestibular nerve; associated with hearing loss and other intracranial tumors.

Output sound-pressure level (OSPL) The newer term for maximum power output of a hearing aid; the highest sound-pressure level to leave the receiver of a hearing aid, regardless of the input level.

Reference test gain The acoustic gain of a hearing aid as measured in a hearing-aid test box. The gain control of the aid is set to amplify an input signal of 60 dB SPL to a level 17 dB below the OSPL90 value. The average values at 1000, 1600, and 2500 Hz determine the reference test gain.

Speech spectrum The overall level and frequency composition of the energy of everyday conversational speech.

Transistor An electronic device, with low power consumption and small space requirements, that amplifies electric current through the use of the semiconducting properties of an element such as silicon.

Vacuum tube A glass enclosure designed to regulate the flow of electric current.

Vibrotactile aids Devices that deliver amplified vibratory energy to the surface of the skin by special transducers. They are designed for patients whose hearing losses are so severe that assistance in speechreading cannot be obtained from traditional hearing aids.

Warble tone A tone that is frequency modulated within fixed limits around a set pure-tone frequency.

REFERENCES

American National Standards Institute (ANSI). (1996). *American National Standard for specification of hearing air characteristics.* ANSI S3.22-1987. New York: Author.

Beck, L. B. (1989, January-February). The "T" switch: Some tips for effective use. *Shhh,* 12–15.

Berger, K. W. (1988). History and development of hearing aids. In M. C. Pollack (Ed.), *Amplification for the hearing impaired* (3rd ed.; pp. 1–20). Orlando, FL: Grune & Stratton.

Carhart, R. (1946). Tests for selection of hearing aids. *Laryngoscope, 56,* 780–794.

Chasin, M. (1997). Current trends in implantable hearing aids. *Trends in Amplification, 2,* 84–107.

———. (1998). Implantable hearing aids. *The Hearing Review, 5*(2), 20–27.

Clark, J. G. (1981). Uses and abuses of hearing loss classification. *Asha, 23,* 493–500.

———. (1996). Pediatric amplification: Selection and verification. In F. N. Martin & J. G. Clark (Eds.), *Hearing care for children* (pp. 213–232). Boston: Allyn & Bacon.

De Chicchis, A. R., Bess, F. H., & Schwartz, D. M. (1996). Amplification selection for children with hearing impairment. In C. D. Bluestone, S. E. Stool, & M. A. Kenna (Eds.), *Pediatric otolaryngology, Volume 2* (3rd ed.; pp. 1632–1656). Philadelphia: W. B. Saunders.

De Conde, C. (1984). Children use colors to flaunt their new hearing aids. *Hearing Instruments, 35,* 22–26.

Dorman, M. F., Hannley, M. T., Dankowski, K., Smith, L., & McCandless, G. (1989). Word recognition by 50 patients fitted with the Symbion multichannel cochlear implant. *Ear and Hearing, 10,* 44–49.

Dumon, T., Zennaro, O., Aron, J. M., Bebear, J. P. (1995). Piezoelectric middle ear implant preserving the ossicular chain. In A. J. Mangiglia (Ed.), *Electronic implantation devices for partial hearing loss* (pp. 173–188). *The Otolaryngologic Clinics of North America*. Philadelphia: W. B. Saunders.

Flexer, C. (1994). *Facilitating hearing and listening in young children.* San Diego: Singular.

Galvin, K. L., Cowan, R. S. C., Sarant, J. Z., Alcantara, J. I., Blamey, P. J., & Clark, G. M. (1991). Use of a multichannel electrotactile speech processor by profoundly hearing-impaired children in a total communication environment. *Journal of the American Academy of Audiology, 2,* 214–225.

Gelfand, S. A., & Silman, S. (1993). Apparent auditory deprivation in children: Implications of monaural versus binaural amplification. *Journal of the American Academy of Audiology, 4,* 313–318.

Goodman, A. (1965). Reference zero levels for pure-tone audiometer. *Asha, 7,* 262–263.

Harford, E., & Barry, L. (1965). A rehabilitative approach to the problem of unilateral hearing impairment: The contralateral routing of signals (CROS). *Journal of Speech and Hearing Disorders, 30,* 121–138.

Haug, O., Baccaro, P., & Guilford, F. R. (1971). Differences in hearing aid performance. *Archives of Otolaryngology, 93,* 183–185.

Hawkins, D. B. (1992). Prescriptive approaches to selection of gain and frequency response. In H. Mueller, D. Hawkins, & J. Northern (Eds.), *Probe microphone measurements: Hearing aid selection and assessment* (pp. 91–112). San Diego: Singular.

———. (1993). Assessment of hearing aid maximum output. *American Journal of Audiology, 2,* 13–14.

Hearing Aid Industry Conference (HAIC). (1961). *Standard method of expressing hearing aid performance.* New York: Author.

———. (1975). *Standards for hearing aids.* New York: Author.

Hitselberger, W. E. & Telischi, F. F. (1994). Auditory brainstem implant. In D. E. Brackmann (Ed.), *Otologic surgery* (pp. 699–708). Philadelphia: W. B. Saunders.

House, W. F. (1982). Surgical considerations in cochlear implants. *Annals of Otology, Rhinology, and Laryngology, 91,* 15–20.

Johnson, R., Meikle, M., Vernon, J., & Schleuning, A. (1988). An implantable bone conduction hearing device. *American Journal of Otology, 9,* 93–100.

Kruger, B. A., & Kruger, F. M. (1994). Future trends in hearing aid fitting strategies: With a view towards 2020. In M. Valente (Ed.), *Strategies for selecting and verifying hearing aid fittings* (pp. 300–342). New York: Thieme Medical Publishers.

Mueller, H. G. (1994). CIC hearing aids: What is their impact on the occlusion effect? *The Hearing Journal, 47,* 29–35.

Mueller, H. G., Hawkins, D. B., & Northern, J. L. (1992). *Probe microphone measurements: Hearing aid selection and assessment.* San Diego: Singular.

Northern, J. L. (1992). Introduction to computerized probe-microphone real-ear measurements. In H. G. Mueller, D. B. Hawkins, & J. L. Northern (Eds.), *Probe microphone measurements: Hearing aid selection and assessment* (pp. 1–19). San Diego: Singular.

Pascoe, D. P. (1991). *Hearing aids: Who needs them?* St. Louis: Big Bend Books.

Pollack, M. C. (1988). Special applications of amplification. In M. C. Pollack (Ed.), *Amplification for the hearing impaired* (3rd ed.). Orlando, FL: Grune & Stratton.

Shore, I., Bilger, R. C., & Hirsh, I. J. (1960). Hearing aid evaluation: Reliability of repeated measurements. *Journal of Speech and Hearing Disorders, 25,* 152–170.

Simons-McCandless, M., & Parkin, J. (1997). Patient reported benefit and objective outcome data in adult cochlear implant patients. *Audiology Today, 9*(6), 27, 29, 31.

Snik, A. F. M, Mylanus, E. A. M., & Cremers, C. W. R. J. (1994). Speech recognition with the bone-anchored hearing aid determined objectively and subjectively. *Ear, Nose & Throat Journal, 73,* 115–117.

Tjellstron, A., & Granstrom, G. (1994). Long-term follow-up with the bone-anchored hearing aid: A review of the first 100 patients between 1977 and 1985. *Ear, Nose & Throat Journal, 73,* 112–114.

Tyler, R. S. & Schum, D. J. (1995). *Assistive devices for persons with hearing impairment.* Boston: Allyn & Bacon.

Vaugn, G. R., Lightfoot, R. K., & Teter, D. L. (1988). Assistive listening devices and systems (ALDS) enhance the lifestyles of hearing impaired persons. *American Journal of Otology, 9,* 101–106.

Waldstein, R. S., & Boothroyd, A. (1995). Comparison of two multichannel tactile devices as supplements to speechreading in a postlingually deafened adult. *Ear and Hearing, 16,* 198–208.

Zwolan, T. A., Kileny, P. R., & Telian, S. A. (1997). Self-report of cochlear implant use and satisfaction by prelingually deafened adults. *Ear and Hearing, 17,* 198–210.

SUGGESTED READINGS

Tyler, R. S. & Schum, D. J. (1995). *Assistive devices for persons with hearing impairment.* Boston: Allyn & Bacon.

Valente, M. (Ed.). (1996). *Hearing aids: Standards, options and limitations.* New York: Thieme Medical Publishers.

Valente, M. (Ed.). (1994). *Strategies for selecting and verifying hearing aid fittings.* New York: Thieme Medical Publishers.

15 Audiological (Re)Habilitation

Clinical audiologists have responsibilities that transcend diagnosis. When a medical condition causes, or contributes to, a patient's hearing problem, proper otological consultation must be sought. In the absence of medical treatment, or after its completion, the audiologist is the logical person to take charge of the patient's total audiological rehabilitation program. Also included among the audiologist's professional responsibilities are taking proper case histories, determining appropriate referrals upon completion of the examination, writing reports, and creating and maintaining liaisons with kindred professionals. If it is decided that hearing aids are indicated for a patient, the audiologist will select and fit the appropriate instruments and provide the needed orientation and follow-up care to ensure optimum efficiency in their use.

Of tremendous importance is the counseling session that should follow each audiological assessment, because what is said to the patient or family, and *how* it is said, can have great psychological impact. All the preceding materials in this book have led to what must be summarized briefly in the following pages. An understanding of normal and abnormal auditory functioning, together with diagnostic procedures, is without merit unless it culminates in activities that improve the lives of persons with hearing impairment.

Chapter Objectives

This chapter is designed to assist the reader in various aspects of patient management, such as taking histories, counseling, writing reports, cooperating with other professionals, and providing audiological rehabilitation. Less emphasis is placed on precise methodologies in this chapter than in previous chapters. The intention here is to give the reader a brief overview of a number of different aspects of audiology not previously detailed in this book.

Patient Histories

Proper documentation of a patient's history may be as important as the audiometric examination. The manner in which the history is recorded may follow one of several formats, ranging from informality to close adherence to a printed form. Some audiologists prefer to ask only questions that appear to relate to the patient's particular complaints and jot their remarks down informally. This approach requires much skill and experience and allows for possible omission of essential questions.

Some history forms are lengthy and contain more items than are essential for gathering data pertinent to a particular hearing problem. Short forms like those in Figures 15.1 and 15.2 have proven useful in the majority of cases. Although in some busy audiology centers case histories are recorded by ancillary personnel (technicians or clerks), or are mailed to the patient for completion before evaluation, it is best for the audiologist to ask the questions, or at least to review the questionnaire with the respondent.

Any case history form must provide space for a statement of the problem, including why the services of the audiologist were sought. It is helpful to know the patient's own attitude about the appointment. Knowing the reason for the visit to the clinic can provide powerful insight before the rest of the history has been completed, or the first test has been administered. Information about the duration and degree of hearing loss should be gleaned, along with family history of ear disease or hearing impairment, noise exposure, or trauma to the ear or head. Reports of vertigo, tinnitus, past surgery related to the ear, previous hearing tests, and so on are most important. History of experience with hearing aids is valuable. Developmental histories of children should be obtained along with any childhood illnesses or accidents, and any regressions in development associated with them.

The manner in which questions are answered may be revealing. Often a patient or caregiver hesitates in answering some questions, which may suggest that not too much credence should be given to the answers. This hesitancy sometimes reflects disagreement among family members. However, the fact that questions are answered rapidly and with apparent self-assurance does not, in itself, ensure validity. People who have repeatedly answered the same types of questions, perhaps posed by different specialists, become practiced at responding and may find themselves answering questions incorrectly with aplomb. The clinician should try to elicit objective responses as much as possible. Statements of a diagnostic nature, such as "I have Méniére disease" or "My child has a conductive hearing loss," should be investigated thoroughly, because they may represent the respondent's incorrect reflection of a previous diagnosis.

Referral to Other Specialists

Audiologists may refer their patients to other specialists for a variety of reasons. They may feel that additional help is needed for either diagnosis or treatment and require the talents of such professionals as otologists, speech-language pathologists, psychologists, or educators. In any case, a proper report should be sent to provide as much pertinent information as possible. It is mandatory that the patient or guardian sign a release form authorizing the audiologist to provide such information to interested parties. The form, properly filed, may prevent possible legal difficulties.

An audiogram, or other data obtained on hearing tests, should not be forwarded without qualifying remarks. The audiologist should not suppose that the recipient of test results will totally understand and interpret them correctly. At the other extreme, the audiologist should not include long, verbose reports conveying details of each and every test. Professional time is valuable and should not be occupied in reading unnecessary verbiage. In fact, it is probable that long reports are either not read at all or only scanned for the pertinent facts.

Each report must be written specifically for the type of specialist to whom it is sent. Audiologists should realize that reports sent about the same patient to an otologist and to a speech-language pathologist may differ greatly in the type of information included and in the manner in which statements are made. In addition, two otologists may differ in the type of information or degree of inter-

Clinic Number _____

THE UNIVERSITY OF TEXAS AT AUSTIN
Division of Communication Disorders

Pediatric Case History

Date _____

Patient's Name _____ Sex _____ D.O.B. _____
               Last   First   Middle

Age _____ Home Phone _____ Address _____

School _____ Grade _____ Teacher _____

Parents' Names _____

Referred by _____

Sex and Ages of Other Children _____

Pre–Birth
     Maternal Illness, Accident, Medication _____

     Rh Factor _____ Previous Miscarriages _____
     Length of Pregnancy _____

Birth
     Weight _____ Age of Mother _____ Cesarean _____
     Condition _____ Difficulty _____
     Jaundice, Anoxia, Cyanosis _____

Infancy and Childhood
     Seizures _____
     Motor Development _____
     Speech _____

     Illnesses, Accidents _____

     Familiar Hearing Loss _____
     Ear Infections and Surgery _____

     Drugs _____
     Nephritis, Mumps, Diabetes _____
     Other Problems _____

     Response to Sound _____

     Onset and Progression of Loss _____

     Previous Audiograms _____

     Hearing Aid: Ear _____ Type and Make _____
     Date and Place Bought _____
     Success with Aid _____
     Behavioral Problems _____

     School Progress _____
     Other Comments:

_____
Clinician

FIGURE 15.1 **Sample of a hearing history form for children.**

Clinic Number _____

THE UNIVERSITY OF TEXAS AT AUSTIN
Division of Communication Disorders

Adult Case History

Date _____

Patient's Name _____   Sex _____
                  Last   First   Middle

D.O.B. _____   Occupation _____

Address (City, State, Zip) _____
_____

Phone (Home) _____   (Office) _____
Referral Source _____
Family Physician_____

  I. Primary Complaint: _____
      _____

 II. Previous Hearing Evaluation: ( )Yes ( )No
     Where: _____   When: _____
     Remarks:_____
     _____

III. Hearing Loss
     Ear: ( )Right ( )Left ( )Both   Age of onset:_____
     Check if applicable: ( )Progressive ( )Fluctuant ( )Dysacusis ( )Paracusis willisii
               ( )Family History Who:_____
     Perceived handicap: _____
     Remarks: _____
     _____

 IV. Ear Infections: ( )Yes ( )No
     Ear: ( )Right ( )Left ( )Both   Age of onset:_____
     Check if applicable: ( )Drainage ( )Pain ( )Recurrent
     Treatment:_____
     Remarks:_____
     _____

  V. Ear Surgery: ( )Yes ( )No
     Ear: ( )Right ( )Left ( )Both   Date(s): _____
     Type(s) of surgery: _____
     Remarks:_____
     _____

 VI. Tinnitus: ( )Yes ( )No
     ( )Right ear ( )Left ear ( )Both ( )Non-localized ( )Constant ( )Fluctuant
     Describe:_____
     Irritation level: ( )mild ( )moderate ( )moderately severe ( )severe ( )Non-irritating

Adult Case History
Page 2

VII. Noise Exposure: ( )Yes ( )No
Type(s):__________
Duration:__________
Remarks:__________

VIII. Vertigo: ( )Yes ( )No
( )Positional ( )Rotary ( )light-headedness ( )Nausea
Treatment:__________
Remarks:__________

IX. Head Injuries: ( )Yes ( )No
Date(s): __________ Type(s):__________
( )Loss of consciousness ( )Affected hearing
Remarks:__________

X. Systemic Illnesses (Check those that apply)
( )Mumps ( )Measles ( )Diabetes ( )Renal ( )Infections ( )Circulatory
Other: __________

XI. Current Medications:
____

XII. Hearing Aids: ( )Worn in past ( )Currently worn ( )Never worn
Ear fit: ( )Right ( )Left ( )Binaural
Style: ( )BTE ( )ITE ( )ITC ( )CIC ( )Other Earmold (if applicable):__________
Make and Model: __________
Consistency of use:__________
Perceived benefit: __________
Remarks:__________

XIII. Audiologic Rehabilitation: ( )Yes ( )No
Remarks:__________

XIV. Comments__________

FIGURE 15.2 Sample of a form for recording an adult history of hearing loss and related conditions.

pretation they desire. As audiologists get to know particular referral sources, they develop an awareness of how reports should be written for each one. Some may require very formal documents,
whereas others will prefer informal synopses.

Briefly, the organization of a report sent to a professional person might be as follows:

- *First paragraph:* Identification of the patient (name, age, sex, short statement of history); the
  reason for referral.
- *Second paragraph:* Statement of the type and degree of hearing loss; reference to results that
  require special attention from the audiometric work sheets and tympanograms; interpretation
  of test results, where needed; implications for communication difficulties.
- *Third paragraph:* Specific recommendations, such as hearing aids; speech, language, or hearing therapy; return for follow-up; avoidance of noise exposure; and so on.

Audiology clinics and audiologists are often judged by the reports they send to other professional workers. Messy audiograms and poorly written or carelessly proofread reports may cause the
recipient to deduce that the audiological examination was also poorly done. Reports should be sent
out as quickly as possible after evaluations. Audiologists represent their clinics and their profession,
and good public relations may be as important to the proper management of the patient as good and
accurate testing, for one reflects the other.

Liaisons with Otolaryngologists

It is obvious that the audiologist is not the person to recommend or perform surgery or medical treatment. This is the duty of the physician, preferably an otologist in the case of ear disease. However,
most otologists are neither trained, nor interested, in the intricacies of diagnostic audiology, nor the
nonmedical aspects of audiological rehabilitation. Many cases of hearing loss have no medical
underpinnings, thereby necessitating no medical intervention. In other important, difficult, or con-
tradictory cases, however, consultation between the otologist and the audiologist is of great advantage to the patient. It is a mistake to think of the relationship between audiology and otology as one
in which the audiologist merely provides audiometric services for the use of the physician in a diagnosis. In such situations, the role of the audiologist may deteriorate to that of technician. The association between medicine and audiology should be a symbiotic one, a professional relationship that
leads to improved patient management.

In referring patients to a physician, audiologists should state in their reports the areas of concern and the reasons for referral. Recommendations for specific treatment should, of course, not be
made. If the patient has a disorder that appears partially or fully reversible (e.g., containing a conductive component caused by otitis media), the audiologist should reschedule the patient for testing
following medical attention to ascertain the degree of hearing improvement derived. After an air-
bone gap is closed, the sensorineural portion of a mixed loss may appear different from the pretreatment bone-conduction audiogram. A reevaluation of audiological rehabilitation needs may be
required in such cases.

Liaisons with Clinical Psychologists

Sometimes psychological consultation is required because the patient's problem is, at least partially,
complicated by an emotional disorder. The preprofessional training of most audiologists provides a

sufficient vocabulary of psychological terms, and association with psychological tests, to permit interpretation of a psychologist's report. As in referrals to physicians, when referring a patient to a psychologist, audiologists should state their particular concerns about the patient and their reasons for referral. In addition to assistance with emotional disorders, the psychologist can provide information about the patient's performance versus potential—for example, whether a child is reaching academic capabilities or needs some special help. At times, it is not until after consultation that it is decided whether the audiologist or the psychologist will become the central figure in the rehabilitation of the patient.

Liaisons with Speech-Language Pathologists

Although many audiologists have reasonably good academic backgrounds in speech-language pathology, most have limited clinical experience. A number of members of the American Speech-Language-Hearing Association (ASHA) hold the Certificates of Clinical Competence in both speech-language pathology and audiology, but many would not claim true competence in both areas. Historically, the similarities in the backgrounds and training in these two areas have been parallel, and so audiologists probably identify more closely with speech-language pathologists than with other specialists.

Often an audiologist will see patients because the speech-language pathologist wishes to know if some aspect of a communication disorder is related to a hearing problem, as well as the extent of this relationship. In the case of young, language-delayed children, the identification of a hearing disorder may play a large role in (re)habilitation. In such cases, collaboration between specialists can result in the proper planning of remediation. Some voice or articulation disorders are directly related to the inability to discriminate sounds or to hear in some frequency ranges.

Reports sent from audiologists to speech-language pathologists should be frank and direct. Audiologists should state their opinions regarding the type and extent of hearing impairment, and they should recommend referral to other specialists, such as otolaryngologists or psychologists, if indicated. The audiologist may state an opinion regarding the effects of hearing loss on a patient's speech, but should refrain from specific recommendations regarding therapy.

In working with some pediatric patients, an audiologist may have little more than a clinical hunch about the child's hearing. Phrases such as "hearing is adequate for speech," appear frequently in reports. In such cases, strong recommendations should be made so that follow-up testing is conducted at intervals until bilateral hearing sensitivity can be ascertained. Honest errors made by audiologists may not be caught until valuable time has been lost unless there is routine follow-up.

Liaisons with Teachers of Children with Hearing Impairments

Reports sent to teachers of children with hearing impairment are, in many respects, the same as those sent to speech-language pathologists. Events and developments of recent years have brought clinical audiologists and teachers closer together for the betterment of children with hearing disorders, largely because of the trend toward removing children from the self-contained environment of traditional schools for the deaf into mainstream education.

To permit children with hearing loss to compete with their hearing contemporaries, the combined efforts of the two specialties of clinical audiology and education of the "deaf" have come into closer harmony than ever before. This is largely true because of the emphasis now being placed by many educators on the use of residual hearing. As the barriers between the two groups break down, their formal educations include more overlapping course work. The harmony achieved can result in teamwork, with the children being the ultimate beneficiaries.

Teachers must learn to understand the implications of audiological management, and audiologists must learn to comprehend the difficulties in the day-to-day management of children in the classroom, especially when those children have impaired hearing. Items of mutual concern include hearing aids, classroom amplification systems, and implications of classroom acoustics. Audiologists' isolation from teachers of children with hearing impairment, and these teachers' reluctance to accept audiological intervention, will disappear as the interactions between these professions continue to increase.

Liaisons with Regular School Classroom Teachers

With the advent of Public Law 94-142, the Education for All Handicapped Children Act of 1975, an increasing number of children with hearing loss are being educated within regular classrooms by teachers with no formal preparation in the impact of, and remediation for, hearing impairment. The role of audiology in the delivery of appropriate education for these children, who were mainstreamed into the regular classroom, was a primary impetus for the development of educational audiology as a specialty area within audiology studies (Blair, 1996).

Educational audiology is still an underrepresented segment of the profession. Regular classroom teachers must usually rely on the information provided by the clinical audiologist in their efforts to meet the educational needs of mainstreamed children with hearing loss. When possible, direct consultation with a child's classroom teacher will go a long way toward helping the teacher, and the school, to address the hearing difficulties a child must endure, even following procurement of appropriate amplification. Reports, and/or consultations, should go beyond simple documentation of the hearing loss and amplification recommendations and must include specific implications of the hearing loss in concrete and functional terms. These may include such factors as the impact of background classroom noise, resultant fatigue from attempts at visual compensation for the hearing loss, and what high-frequency consonant sounds may still be missed even with amplification (Martin & Clark, 1996). Specific classroom management suggestions for children with hearing loss (Clark, 1996) are welcome additions to any communication with the regular classroom teacher.

Management of Adults with Hearing Impairments

The passage of Public Law 101-336, the Americans with Disabilities Act (1991), prohibits discrimination against persons with disabilities in such areas as transportation, state and local government, public accommodations, employment, and telecommunications. This law sprang from a grassroots movement and has had profound effects for individuals with hearing loss. It should be understood by audiologists, in addition to its technical implications, for in part it helps to reduce the negative images that are associated with physically and mentally challenged individuals, and it brings with it a new sensitivity to the feelings of those with hearing impairment. Audiologists are urged to consider the words they use in case management, for example, substituting *disability* for *handicap,* for a disabled person is only handicapped when faced with an insurmountable barrier. The person, and not the disability, should be emphasized as part of what has been called the "people first" movement; hence "person with a hearing loss" should replace "hearing-impaired person."

Adult patients requiring audiological management of their hearing problems are usually adventitiously impaired. Although some of these hearing losses are sudden, for example, the result of drug therapy or illness, most are gradual, almost insidious. It is important to separate the concepts of **hearing impairment,** an abnormality that is psychological, physiological, or anatomical (defined audiometrically), and **hearing disability,** which relates to individuals' inability to perform biologically and socially useful functions, from **hearing handicap,** the ways in which individuals are disadvantaged in fulfilling their desired roles (usually defined on self-assessment scales) (World Health Organization, 1980). The management of these patients has been termed aural rehabilitation, and more recently **audiological rehabilitation.**

The degree of handicap represented by the disability of a given hearing impairment can be highly individual and must be taken into account in rehabilitative planning. When labeling a disability based upon a given level of hearing impairment expressed in terms of the pure-tone average (PTA) (Table 4.1), it is important to remember that two- and three-frequency PTAs were designed to predict the threshold of speech, and as such, often misrepresent the impact of a given hearing loss. Although these averages are often used in assigning hearing disability labels, the prediction of speech thresholds and the assignment of disability labels are two quite different processes. A **variable pure-tone average (VPTA),** consisting of the poorest three frequencies of 500, 1000, 2000, and 4000 Hz, may serve better for the latter (Clark, 1981).

Audiological rehabilitation has changed in recent years for several reasons, including technological breakthroughs and cultural influences. Traditional rehabilitative techniques with adults, such as speechreading and auditory training, continue to be practiced, despite the fact that the data do not consistently prove these approaches to be effective. However, there is much that can be done to assist patients and their families in addressing the hearing problems that can become so intrusive in their lives.

While medical science has advanced in the treatment of diseases that cause hearing loss, similar advances have served to prolong life, with the result that for the first time in history, the population of the United States consists of more older people than younger people. Because hearing loss is the almost inevitable result of aging, the number of adults with acquired hearing loss is increasing. Audiologists must be prepared to meet this challenge.

Before an audiological rehabilitation program can begin, it is essential that the patient's hearing disability be assessed. It has been customary to base this assessment on objective audiometric data alone. The information provided earlier in this book is essential to patient management, but it does not supersede other information that may also be critical, such as the patient's own view of the disability, individual needs and preferences, socioeconomic status, education, vocation, and a host of other important considerations.

A number of attempts to assess the degree of hearing disability have been based both on audiometric data and on scales computed with the assistance of the patient. A review of hearing handicap scales is provided by Alpiner (1994). Although none of these methods is perfect, they assist the audiologist in compiling data about how the hearing impairment affects the central figure in the rehabilitation process. After all, it does little good to insist that a patient needs wearable amplification, when the patient minimizes the effects of the hearing loss and has no intention of using hearing aids.

The goal of adult audiological rehabilitation is always to make maximum use of residual hearing. Residual hearing is useful hearing, and it is not always easily discernible by looking at an audiogram, speech-recognition threshold, or word-recognition score. The patient's residual hearing is the difference, in decibels, between the auditory threshold and the uncomfortable loudness level. This is the dynamic range of hearing. The broader the dynamic range, the better candidate the patient is for hearing aids and audiological rehabilitation.

A number of decisions must be made after the hearing has been assessed. The decision on hearing aids must be made, and proper selection and orientation should be arranged. The nature of the orientation must be selected, that is, whether therapy should be done individually or in groups, who should constitute the specific group, what visual cues should be emphasized, how speech can be conserved, and so on. Rehabilitative efforts must be geared to the individual, whose curiosity and ability to comprehend should not be underestimated. The patient should be educated as fully as possible about hearing loss in general, and about the specific disability in particular. How the ear works and what has gone wrong, the effects of the loss on speech communication, implications for progression of the loss, the array of hearing assistance technologies available, and interactions with family and friends must all be discussed openly and honestly, with the patient in the presence of a close friend or family member, whenever possible.

Patients should be taught to maximize their communicative skills, in part by managing their environments. People should be encouraged to be in the same room with and facing others with whom they speak. Position in the room should be manipulated to take advantage of lighting. Room noise should be minimized during conversation, and assistive listening devices should be used when appropriate. Garstecki (1994) outlines a group audiological rehabilitation program that includes these topics within a three-week orientation. Ideally, at least some portion of audiological rehabilitation is performed in the audiology center in a group setting, but this is not always possible. In some cases the patient is homebound or in a facility for the elderly and cannot visit the clinic. Arrangements should be made to meet the needs of each patient whenever possible.

Many audiologists are more comfortable in the role of diagnostician than therapist. Modern audiology demands that the clinician be facile in both of these areas; and, indeed, it is within the latter that audiologists will find the greater autonomy. The reader is encouraged to explore the suggested readings at the end of this chapter for more information about managing hearing loss.

Counseling Adult Patients and Their Families

It has long been believed that one of the greatest responsibilities of the audiologist is to ensure that test results and diagnostic impressions are imparted adequately to patients and their families. Accurate test results are of paramount importance, but the tests serve merely as instruments to help clinicians give advice and counsel to patients and their families. Many people in our society have been conditioned to accept the recommendations of professionals without understanding the underlying reasons for them.

To many clinicians in all areas of human health care, the word *counseling* means telling patients what is wrong and what must be done about it. Counseling by audiologists must include much more. Audiological counseling is based on what Clark (1994) calls the "well-patient model," which is often valid because the majority of patients seen by audiologists are psychologically normal, but are trying to cope with the disruption a hearing loss has caused in their lives. Those occasional patients who face much deeper psychological difficulty may necessitate referral to a mental-health professional.

Expanding counseling beyond the mere transfer of information reflects a reconsideration of the counseling roles of audiologists that have been evident in recent years. Counseling should have a supportive base that helps patients and families to make practical changes in their lives that, in turn, will help them to develop a more positive approach to their own disabilities, the technological assistance available to them, and the residual communication difficulties that, for many, are inevitable (Clark, 1994).

The word *care* is one of the primary definitions of counseling, which is usually defined by health-care providers as a system of information transfer; that is, the counselor (audiologist, physician, hearing-aid dispenser) provides directions, which the client is expected to follow. This is no surprise since the word *client* comes from the Latin *cliens,* a follower, or one who bows or leans on another (as one's master) for protection. The alternative word *patient,* which is the one used in this book, is not much better since its root is in the Latin *patiens,* to suffer, that is, a person passively receiving care. It is little wonder then that the clinician may expect to operate from the position of strength, and the patient from one of subservience. Relationships between patients and their clinicians often come down to the exertion of control (Cassell, 1989), with the clinician exerting authority for what is believed to be in the best interest of the patient. Older, less educated patients seem to accept a more passive role than their younger, better educated counterparts (Haug & Lavin, 1983). However, the goal of the audiologist should be to help patients to achieve independence and to learn how to solve the problems associated with hearing loss, and the voice of clinical authority must often take a back seat.

Clark (1994) describes the differences between professional and nonprofessional counselors. He defines professional counselors as those who are specifically educated and trained in this area, including psychologists, social workers, and psychiatrists, although modern psychiatry appears to be turning away from a counseling profession to a neurochemical discipline. Nonprofessional counselors include those others who lack specific and advanced training in counseling, such as audiologists, speech-language pathologists, physicians, educators, clergy, attorneys, friends, and family. Psychotherapy is in the domain of the professional counselor. Understanding the differences between psychotherapeutic counseling and support counseling allows nonprofessional counselors to feel more comfortable within their counseling role. It is the audiologist's role in support counseling that is often slighted in patient care, and this role must be cultivated for the patient's benefit. Those who perform any counseling at all must know their strengths and limitations and must recognize the critical impact that their words and deeds can have on patients and their families.

To a large degree, the specific approach used, and the details included in counseling a patient or family, are determined by the audiologist's interests and professional experience. In the important area of content counseling it is helpful if the type and degree of loss are explained and the patient acquires a basic understanding of the audiogram. Results of speech audiometry and other special tests are often not well understood, but if some interest is shown in these tests, the results should be explained in as much detail as the patient desires, using the clearest terms possible with conscious avoidance of audiological jargon. What is surprising to many people is that initially many patients do not appear to show great interest in test results and want to go directly to the "bottom line," with questions about the need for hearing aids, progression of the loss, implications of the loss on general health, and so on. A sensible approach, after testing is completed, is simply to ask the patient what information is desired. If the patient is not prepared to listen, there is not much sense in pouring forth technical information. Since it is ideal for patients to be their own advocates, when they seem uncomfortable with the initial counseling session at least one follow-up should be scheduled. The counseling role of the audiologist cannot be overstressed, for there is evidence that much of what is explained by clinicians is not accurately retained, even by educated and intelligent patients (Martin, Krueger, & Bernstein, 1990).

In some cases it is necessary to avoid more than a perfunctory explanation of test results, for example, if there is a nonorganic component to a hearing loss or a potentially serious medical condition. On the one hand, an audiologist must not engage in discussions with patients of acoustic tumors and the like; this is the responsibility of the physician. On the other hand, if an audiologist suspects a condition for which a referral is made to an otologist, the patient will surely want to know the reason for the referral, and tact, diplomacy, and counseling skills are often tested under such conditions.

When discussing test results, the audiologist must create an atmosphere of calm professionalism, for this is often the basis for the patient's confidence in the clinician. Confidence is not determined by whether the audiologist wears a white coat or shows other outward postures of competence. Ordinarily, clinicians should not be separated from their patients by artificial barriers, like desks and tables. As the physical space between parties is decreased, the opportunities for trust and openness increase. The amount of time spent in counseling depends on the type of work setting and the motivation of the patient and audiologist. After an explanation of test results has been made, the audiologist should solicit questions from the patient and try to answer them in appropriate detail.

Often it is the unasked questions that audiologists must sense and answer. Patients, and their families, are frequently fearful of inquiring about the possible progression of hearing loss. Many older patients fear that it is only a matter of time before they will lose their hearing entirely. Although progression of hearing loss may or may not have been demonstrated by repeated hearing evaluations, it is possible for the audiologist to play a calming and reassuring role. It has been shown that progressive hearing loss in the elderly shows a concomitant progression of physical and psychosocial disorders, a situation to which the clinician must be sensitive. For every 10 dB increase in hearing loss there is a demonstrable increase in functional disability, such as problems with sleep, work, and alertness (Bess, Lichtenstein, Logan, Berger, & Nelson, 1989). Crandell (1998) found that the use of hearing aids may improve functional health status in elderly patients with sensorineural hearing loss due to decreases in the functional and psychosocial impacts of reduced communication.

Often elderly patients with hearing impairment are not referred to audiologists by other healthcare providers. It is not clear why this is the case, but it may be reasonable to assume that physicians, for example, simply expect hearing loss in their elderly patients as a normal consequence of aging, do not realize the extent to which many patients can be helped by counseling and amplification, or do not see hearing loss as a significant problem. In these matters the audiologist must educate not only the patient and the patient's family, but the medical community as well.

It has been known for some time that the diagnosis of hearing loss in children may be met with a number of emotional reactions, some of which may interfere with the very (re)habilitative measures that the audiologist intends. Many people have inferred that adults with acquired hearing loss do not suffer significant shock, disappointment, anger, sadness, or other emotions because they more or less expect the diagnosis they hear. Apparently, however, this is far from true in many cases, and adults may be much more emotionally fragile than had been supposed (Martin, Krall, & O'Neal, 1989). Assessing the emotional reaction of a patient to the news of a hearing loss often cannot be gauged accurately on the basis of a patient's affect, even by the most sensitive clinician (Martin, Barr, & Bernstein, 1992). As with parents, it is often difficult to distinguish those adults who receive what they perceive to be bad news about irreversible hearing loss in a matter-of-fact way from those for whom the same news is catastrophic.

It is almost always desirable to ask new patients to be accompanied to their hearing evaluations by someone significant to them, such as a spouse. Observing the tests, as well as the responses given, allows these individuals insights into the nature of the hearing disability that are difficult to comprehend when only explained. In all cases, it is the adult patient who should be addressed directly during post-evaluation counseling. Elderly people, as well as teenagers, resent being ignored or discussed as if they were not there. Assistive listening devices can be very useful in helping patients through the counseling process if they do not have their own hearing instruments (see Chapter 14).

Following the pronouncement that a hearing loss is probably irreversible, patients' emotional states may make it difficult for them to understand and process subsequently presented technical aspects of their hearing disorder and explanations of test results. At the same time, patients complain that they want to have much more information at the time of diagnosis than audiologists, physicians, and hearing-aid dispensers usually provide (Martin et al., 1989). A major complaint by patients is that they feel rushed while in the clinician's office. As stated earlier, one solution to this problem is to ask patients what they know about their problems and what they wish to be told. It should be emphasized that further counseling is available, and patients should be encouraged to call for more in-depth discussion of their hearing problems. After people have had a chance to compose themselves, they often think of many pertinent questions or details that they want explained. Many gaps can be filled in by providing printed materials or videotapes that can be viewed and reviewed at home.

Many adults find that support groups are of great assistance in dealing with their hearing loss. One such group is Self Help for Hard of Hearing People, Inc. (SHHH), which publishes its own consumer-oriented journal. Audiologists need to make referrals to support groups to supplement the (re)habilitation services they are providing their patients of all ages (see CD-ROM). What persons with hearing loss and their families are asking for is no more than they are entitled to: a concerned and compassionate clinician, who is willing to give sufficient time and express appropriate interest in what, to many people, is a profound and disturbing disability.

Hearing Therapy

A major task of the rehabilitative audiologist or therapist is to train the patient with hearing loss in the maximum use of residual hearing. In the past such intervention was referred to as auditory training—or more appropriately, auditory retraining—and often concentrated on a reeducation in listening for specific sounds. Professional attitudes on the value of auditory retraining vary. Although there is little evidence to prove that periods of professional training increase word-recognition scores, either with or without hearing aids, most audiologists are in favor of such programs. This is largely true as auditory retraining with adults has evolved to encompass instruction geared to enhanced recognition of and intervention for those variables within the environment, or poor speaker or listener habits, that impede successful communication (Trychin, 1994). This approach through **hearing therapy** classes has been shown to be more successful than a pure retraining in the perception of auditory signals. Such an approach is often integral to a more comprehensive delivery of audiological rehabilitation services and is endorsed by the primary consumer advocacy group for those with hearing loss as a recommended adjunct to hearing-aid fittings (Self Help for Heard of Hearing People, Inc., 1996). Hearing therapy classes are usually designed to be attended by the individual with hearing loss and a spouse, a close family member, or a friend.

The audiologist who recommends and fits the hearing aids may also serve as the audiological rehabilitation therapist, or for children, the latter may be a separate professional with a primary background in speech-language pathology or education of children with severe hearing loss. The vast majority of persons attending organized hearing therapy classes do so with the objective of improved use of their hearing aids. Unfortunately, even with the strongest attempts at intervention, some adult patients with sensorineural hearing losses cannot make the adjustment to hearing aids, or refuse to attempt to do so.

For both children and adults, hearing therapy may be given in groups or individually. Naturally, individual therapy allows for greater personal attention, but group work with adults has a psychotherapeutic value that cannot be underestimated. Many adults, particularly older people, become depressed over their hearing losses. They feel persecuted and alone. Although they may realize, on an intellectual level, that their problems are not unique, emotionally they feel quite isolated. The mere experience of being with people their own age and with similar problems may lift their spirits and aid in their rehabilitation. The opportunity for members of the group to share what has worked for them in their attempts to address their communication difficulties is beneficial to all group members. The educational and emotional values of therapy can only be approximated.

Speechreading Training with Adults

It is the mistaken concept among many laypersons, and among some professionals as well, that if hearing becomes impaired, it can be replaced by **lipreading,** in which the words of a speaker may be recognized by watching the lips. The term **speechreading** has replaced *lipreading,* because it is recognized that the visual perception of speech requires much more than attending to lip movements alone. Recognition of facial expressions, gestures, body movements, and so on, contributes to the perception of speech.

Many speech sounds are produced so that they may be recognized on the lips alone, at least in terms of their general manner and place of production. Some sounds, however, such as /p/, /m/, and /b/, are produced in such a way that they are difficult to differentiate from visual cues alone. Other sounds, such as /g/, /k/, and /h/, cannot be perceived visually at all.

Although much has been done to investigate the value of speechreading, and a number of methods are available to teach this skill to people with hearing loss, it is still a considerably misunderstood concept. It is a gross error to believe that speechreading alone can replace hearing in the complete understanding of spoken discourse. It is also an error to believe that more than about 50 percent of the sounds of speech may be perceived through speechreading alone.

For speechreading to be of maximum value to the patient, it should be taught in conjunction with the coping strategies addressed in hearing therapy, so that the combined effects of vision and residual hearing may be gained. When the two senses are used simultaneously, they interact synergistically; the combined effect on discrimination for speech is greater for watching and listening together than for either watching alone or listening alone.

Many people believe that speechreading is an art that requires an innate talent possessed more by some persons than by others. It is probably true that some people are more visually oriented than others. Some people do better on speechreading tests without training than do other people who have had a number of speechreading lessons.

The methods of teaching speechreading to adults vary considerably in their philosophy and implementation. Some include an analytic approach to the movements of the speaker's lips, whereas others are more synthetic. Computer-assisted training in speechreading has been used that implements videodisc technology. It is enough to say in this brief discussion that speechreading should be made as natural to the patient as possible, utilizing residual hearing through hearing aids if this is indicated.

Management of Children with Hearing Impairment

Although other conditions may contribute to delay the onset of normal language and speech, often hearing loss is the primary problem. Whether a hearing loss is present at birth or develops at some time afterward can make a profound difference in language acquisition. When it exists before the normal development of language, it is referred to as **prelinguistic hearing loss.** A hearing loss that begins after language concepts are formed is called **postlinguistic.** Naturally, the later in life a hearing loss begins, the better the chance to conserve the speech and language that a child has already learned through the hearing sense.

One obligation of the audiologist is to pursue medical reversal of a hearing loss as soon as that possibility presents itself. Determination of otologic or surgical treatment is based on medical decisions. Audiologists should make a medical referral immediately when otitis media or other infections are seen, or when there is any indication of a structural deviation that might involve the auditory system. If medical treatment of a hearing loss is impossible, or still leaves the child with some hearing loss, further audiological intervention is needed, including family counseling.

Counseling Parents and Families

Precisely how to convey to parents or caregivers the nature and extent of their children's hearing loss is not universally agreed upon. Many clinicians use a system of direct information transfer. That is, they present information, insofar as it is known, about a child's hearing loss. Often this includes descriptions of the audiogram, definitions of terms, and options for meeting the child's needs. The intent is to educate the caregivers to the point that they can best handle the child's hearing problems. Clinicians often do not realize that their choice of language, verbal and nonverbal, and even the amount of information provided, may have profound effects, both positive and negative, on the receiver of that information.

The reactions of parents to the realization that their child has a hearing impairment are not always the same. Whether externalized or internalized, it is safe to say that the effect is generally quite intense. As Moses (1979) points out, parents view their children as extensions of themselves, with hopes and dreams of perfection. When an imperfection is uncovered, the dreams become shattered. Because of its "invisibility," hearing impairment often does not appear to be a true disability, which makes the adjustment even more difficult for the parents.

Van Hecke (1994) reviewed the states through which many parents pass when they learn of their child's handicap. Initially, parents often go through a period of *denial* as a means of self-defense against very bad news. During this state it is frequently fruitless even to try to provide details of the diagnosis and recommendations for training, for parents are simply incapable of acceptance at this juncture.

As mourning over the loss of the perfect child continues, parents frequently express *anger* as they relinquish their feelings of denial. This anger may be transferred to loved ones, marital partners, audiologists, physicians, or God, leaving virtually no one invulnerable. Audiologists must be able to function as counselors and accept this anger, even if it is directed toward them. Objectivity at this point is crucial.

When anger has subsided, it is common for parents to go through a period of *guilt*. Parents who persist in seeking explanations for the cause of the hearing loss may be looking for a way out of the awful sense that they have somehow done this to their child or are being punished for some past sin. If the guilt is projected toward the other marital partner, the marriage can become shaky; divorce is not uncommon among parents of children with disabilities. Indeed, many parents never pass from the guilt state, with unfortunate consequences for children, who may become spoiled or overprotected or may never reach their full potential. Merely telling parents that they need not blame themselves is often fruitless, but the audiologist should try to avoid words or actions that promote guilt.

As parents cease reeling from the impact of the "bad news" about their child, they seek ways to maximize the child's potential. At this point they may be so overloaded with assignments, information, and advice (albeit well meaning) from professionals, family, and friends, that they believe they are inadequate for the job at hand. Subsequently, anxiety may increase, which must be dealt with before any form of intervention can become effective for the child.

Before parents can help their children, they must be helped themselves. They must be taught to cope with the challenge of parenting a child with a hearing impairment. They must learn to continue to give and to accept love and to include the entire family in normal activities, as well as in activities prescribed for the child with the hearing loss. The audiologist, as a sensitive and empathetic listener, must learn to see beyond the words to the feelings of family members. Therapy without personal concern may be useless.

Parents are often confused and disturbed by new and unusual terminology (Martin, 1994). Even the words used to describe the child's problems may be critical. For some time Luterman (1987), as well as others, has been concerned with the manner of giving information to parents. Martin, George, O'Neal, and Daly (1987) conducted a survey in the United States and learned that parents (or other caregivers) are often not receptive to detailed information immediately after they have learned that their child has an irreversible hearing loss. Respondents to this survey indicated that initial parental reactions include sorrow, shock, denial, fear, anger, helplessness, and blame. It takes varying and sometimes prolonged amounts of time for the diagnosis of hearing loss to be accepted. Acceptance of this diagnosis is often easier for parents and others if they have the opportunity to observe hearing tests as they are performed on their children.

When presenting diagnostic information that may be painful, audiologists must temper their enthusiasm for launching habilitative efforts with patience and understanding. Reliance on feedback from parents regarding their anxiety levels during counseling may be misleading. For example, what appears to be a lax or indifferent parental attitude may be a smokescreen for fear and bewilderment.

Sometimes caregivers opt for a plan of action that is not what the audiologist believes to be in a particular child's best interest. Because of their background and training, many audiologists believe that the first avenue followed should employ the aural/oral approach, maximizing residual hearing with amplification and encouraging communication through speech. A different decision by a parent may appear to be "wrong" to the clinician, but the clinician's opinion must be repressed.

The function of the audiologist should be to convey educational and habilitative options to the parents (Clark, 1983). These alternatives should be explained carefully, objectively, and without bias, so that the caregivers themselves can make informed decisions about the management of their child. Opportunities for further consultation with the clinician, as well as participation in parent support groups, should be provided at the earliest possible time. Audiological counseling should be viewed as a continuing process, and parents should feel that they can come to their audiologist/counselor when they need assistance. Grandparents and other close family members also experience sometimes devastating emotional response to the news of a child's hearing loss. A meeting with the audiologist or referral to appropriate support groups can be very beneficial to the child and family as they learn to cope with the changes they are confronting in their lives (Atkins, 1994).

One aspect of audiologist-caregiver interaction that must not be overlooked is the possible need for genetic counseling. Smith (1994) points out that this counseling should not merely provide medical and genetic information, but should also provide support for family members as they learn to deal with their child's hearing loss. The need to direct families to genetic counselors may be more than ethical, because failure to make such recommendations, when they are indicated, may place the clinician in legal jeopardy.

According to Smith (1994), families seek genetic counseling for a variety of reasons, once they realize that such services are available. They may be interested in the etiology or prognosis of their own or their children's hearing loss, or they may wish to decide whether to have children if there is a family history of hearing loss. They may have a child with a hearing loss and want to know the probabilities that a later child will have a similar condition. In some cases, if the parents have impaired hearing, they may look at the probability of having an offspring with a hearing loss as positive. It is not for the audiologist to decide what decisions should be made on the basis of genetic counseling, but rather to see that the family is aware of what is available and to know the team to whom the referral should be made. Such a team usually includes a geneticist (a medical doctor), a genetics counselor (usually holding a master's or doctoral degree), and others as needed.

It is natural for clinicians to present diagnostic information to the adults who have accompanied a child to the hearing evaluation. When children are old enough and have sufficient communication skills, they should be a part of the discussion. This serves to eliminate the resentment that many children feel when they have been excluded from discussions that relate directly to them. Naturally, when children are very young, severely hearing impaired, or multiply handicapped, it is the adults who should be addressed, but always with a mindful attitude about the child's feelings. When children are young and profoundly hearing impaired, it is their caregivers who must decide how the children are to be educated.

Auditory Training with Children

There are obvious differences in the approaches to patients with prelinguistic and postlinguistic hearing losses. Children who have suffered hearing loss from birth or early childhood cannot call on the memory of speech sounds, and so must begin training in special ways. Children with hearing impairment vary considerably in the enthusiasm with which they accept amplification. A great deal of the acceptance depends on the approach made by the family, audiologist, and therapist. The sudden presentation of loud and distorted sounds can be frightening to children. They may be confused and annoyed by the ear mold, or the hearing aids themselves. For the small child, there is no way for explanations to precede the wearing of hearing aids. Of course, the more readily the hearing aids are accepted, the sooner training can begin (see Figure 15.3). **Auditory training** programs for children may be quite comprehensive, and specific goals and objectives should be established

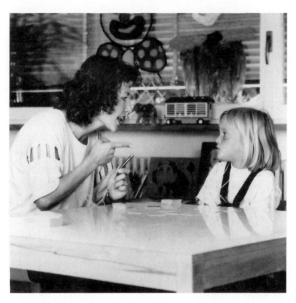

FIGURE 15.3   Direct auditory input enhances the signal-to-noise ratio during auditory training. (Courtesy of Phonak)

based on individual needs. There is no way to stress the importance of providing amplification to children, when indicated, at the earliest possible time. The notion that such action might be "too soon" is simply untrue.

Working with school-age children is often easier than working with younger children. The main problem, again, is the children's acceptance of their amplification devices. The approach can make a great and lasting difference in the children's attitudes toward amplification. The audiologist, therapist, and family should show enthusiasm for the project, but it is important that children not learn to use their hearing aids as instruments of punishment against their elders. Children have been known to pull hearing aids from their ears and throw them to the floor when they become angry with their parents.

Speechreading Training with Children

Speechreading for small children should begin early in life. They should be encouraged to watch the faces of their parents and others. Speech to these children should be slow, simple, and carefully articulated, without exaggeration of the movements of the face and mouth. The error committed by many parents is to mouth speech without voice, in the belief that the exaggerations will help the children speechread, and that voice is unnecessary since the children are "deaf." Using voice allows the production of the speech sounds to be more natural and, it is hoped, provides some auditory cues if the children's residual hearing has been tapped by amplification.

Educational Options

The precise modes of communication by which profoundly hard-of-hearing children should be educated continue to be debated. As mentioned earlier, many people believe that emphasis should be placed on speech, with amplification designed to take advantage of residual hearing. Strict adherents to this philosophy are often called *oralists;* they believe that since all children live in a world in which communication is accomplished through speech, their adjustment is best made by teaching them to speak so that they will "fit in" with the majority of others.

Other experts believe that manual communication, by signs and finger spelling, allows children with profound hearing losses to communicate more readily, so that communication skills can be learned more quickly, and specific subjects can be taught. Additionally, the *manualists* often believe that signing serves as a more useful communication system than speech for many children; their adjustment is made to the nonhearing world, where they will be accepted more completely.

According to Vernon and Mindel (1978), the greatest psychological danger to the child with a profound hearing loss is the inability of the parents, and the professional specialists with whom they deal, to understand the problems involved. Their belief is that the frequent failure of amplification, even with speechreading and auditory training, testifies to the need for the early use of manual communication. They feel that children's psychological and educational needs are not met by forcing them into artificial situations and insisting that they become something they are not—hearing persons. This belief that deafness need not be looked on as a handicap, but rather as a characteristic, is the philosophy of what has come to be called the "Deaf community." The term *Deaf* (with a capital D) should be used to denote those who identify themselves with Deaf culture, while the term *deaf* (small d) describes the hearing status of the individual (Woodward, 1972). From an audiological standpoint, "deaf" is reserved for description of individuals whose hearing loss is so profound that the auditory channel cannot be used as the primary channel for speech reception, or speech and language development.

Lane (1992) maintains that the Deaf community should not be regarded as disabled, but should be thought of as a "linguistic minority," with its own culture and language: American Sign Language. He speaks of the resentment of this group against the intrusion of the "audists" into the lives and educational decisions of deaf persons. This is a viewpoint that has become increasingly prevalent.

Lane (1987) also feels that the community of persons with severe to profound hearing losses is at odds with the professions that were designed to help it: "To achieve intellectual and emotional maturity at full participation in society most deaf children require an education conducted in their primary language, American Sign Language. . . ." Proponents of oral, or combined oral and manual approaches to teaching children with hearing impairments, may be just as adamant in their beliefs. Educational placement for children with hearing loss is an issue that is not easily resolved.

The Bureau of Education of the Handicapped was established in 1966, which in turn led to implementation of Public Law 94-142 in 1975, the Education for All Handicapped Children law. This law mandates **mainstreaming** children with disabilities whenever possible, their education to be carried out in the "least restrictive environment." Mainstreaming requires that children spend their entire school day in a regular classroom except for times specifically designed to receive support services related to their disability. More than half of the approximately 80,000 children with profound hearing losses in the United States were moved away from specialized schools, many of which began to close as a consequence (Lane, 1987). It is unfortunate that the least restrictive environment was interpreted as endorsing mainstreaming for *all* children. Restrictive environments may be more appropriately defined as settings that limit a child's classroom potential, and that the least restrictive environment is that environment most appropriate for the child (Ross, Brackett, & Maxon, 1991).

The Education of the Handicapped Act Amendments (P.L. 99-457) were enacted in 1986 to provide guidelines for offering assistance from birth to children with hearing loss and other disabilities. The purpose of this law, in addition to offering assistance and guidance to families with younger children, was to develop family-centered programs. P.L. 94-142 mandated the **individualized educational plan (IEP),** and P.L. 99-457 encouraged the **individualized family service plan (IFSP).** Early intervention services include audiometry, speech-language pathology, case management, family training, health services, nutrition, occupational therapy, physical therapy, psychological and social services, transportation, and more. The Individuals with Disabilities Education Act of 1990 (P.L. 101-476), and the Individuals with Disabilities Education Act Amendments of 1997 (P.L. 105-17), added legal clarification. All this legislation places educational audiology on a firm legal footing, although there is evidence that the enactment of laws does not necessarily translate into actual services for some of the children they are designed to assist (DeConde-Johnson, 1991). The laws do, however, provide for punitive action against noncompliant schools.

In all states, children who are suspected of having a hearing loss are entitled to free testing. The purpose, of course, is to identify, as early as possible, those children who require special assistance. In many states this is called "child find." Once the identification is made, audiological services should include appropriate professional referral, habilitative measures (auditory training, language stimulation, speechreading, **speech conservation**), counseling and guidance, and determination of specific amplification needs (Johnson, 1994).

The American Speech-Language-Hearing Association has detailed the responsibilities of the educational audiologist (ASHA, 1993). ASHA lists the effects a hearing loss has on the education of children as (1) a delay in the development of receptive and expressive communication skills, (2) a language deficit that reduces academic performance because of learning problems, (3) poor self-concept and social isolation resulting from communication difficulties, and (4) restriction of future vocational choices.

A variety of placement options may be available for the formal education of children with a hearing loss. These include privately and publicly funded institutions, residential and day schools, and public schools. Of all children in regular classrooms requiring special educational considerations, those with hearing impairment make up the largest groups (Flexer, Wray, & Ireland, 1989). Although classroom teachers have shown an interest in knowing more about their students with hearing loss, they admit that their present knowledge is inadequate for proper management (Martin, Bernstein, Daly, & Cody, 1988). In addition to educational management, teachers must have information about classroom acoustics, individually worn amplification devices, and systems to help improve the signal-to-noise ratios for children.

When children are mainstreamed, direct contact with the classroom teacher is the best way to see that their needs are met. If intervention is handled diplomatically, audiologists will find most teachers receptive and eager to learn how to help their students. Special help includes assigning preferential seating, providing maximum visual clues, encouraging the use of amplification, issuing written assignments when possible, and maintaining frequent contact with caregivers.

The ideal seat in the classroom is not necessarily right at the front near the teacher's desk. Each situation is different, but whenever possible light, especially from windows, should be at the child's back, so that glare and shadows are at a minimum. FM, or similar listening systems to enhance signal-to-noise ratios, should be used. When such systems are employed, an environmental microphone on the hearing aid should be used to pick up the voices of the other students in the class. The teacher should speak distinctly to the child, but should not overemphasize lip movements, which is a natural tendency when talking to any person with a hearing impairment. Shouting should be avoided, and the teacher should see that the hearing aids are in working order. Homework and other assignments should be printed on handouts, or written on the chalkboard, in addition to being explained orally. Sign-language interpreters, when used, should be welcome to the classroom, and their presence explained to the normal-hearing children.

It is axiomatic that any system of teaching children with hearing losses, in the classroom or speech and hearing clinic, will be most effective if it is complemented by a strong home program. Academic progress must be monitored with the parents on a more frequent basis than with normal-hearing students.

A parental decision to follow a certain course regarding a child's training may change, based on the reinforcement received for the efforts made, and on new information acquired. The responsibility of the pediatric audiologist is to remain as a source of information and support to families, to follow up the initial diagnosis with regular hearing evaluations, and to assist with hearing aids and other listening devices as needed. Insightful clinicians must develop skills that allow them to facilitate, rather than to direct, families in the series of decisions that are so critical to fulfill the potential of children with hearing impairments.

The reader may have noted that a scrupulous attempt has been made throughout this book to minimize the use of the word *deaf*. More than thirty years ago, Ross and Calvert (1967) pointed out that the "semantics of deafness" may have a profound effect on the ability of a family with a child with a hearing impairment to cope with the problems that arise. The lay public, and to a large extent the professional community, have polarized people into two groups, those who hear and those who do not. When people are labeled "deaf," it means to many that they cannot hear at all, and that they will remain mute. This can inhibit the use of residual hearing and the development of spoken language. Ross and Calvert state that ignoring the quantitative nature of hearing loss may affect the child's diagnosis, interaction with parents, educational placement and treatment, and expectations for achievement.

Brief descriptions follow of some of the more familiar teaching methods.

American Sign Language (ASL)

In American Sign Language, often called *Ameslan,* specific and often logical signs are created with the hands, which allows for faster communication than finger spelling. ASL is often thought to suffer from inaccuracies in English grammar and syntax, although it is not inaccurate when viewed as a language in its own right. ASL is considered by many educators to be a true language and is accepted by some colleges and universities as a means of satisfying the undergraduate foreign language requirement.

Auditory-Verbal Approach

Formerly referred to as unisensory or Acoupedics, the auditory-verbal philosophy is placed entirely on the use of audition and early amplification with hearing aids. This method stresses the auditory channel as the channel for the development of spoken receptive and expressive communication skills.

The Aural/Oral Method

Often called the multisensory or auditory-global approach, the aural/oral method attempts to tap the child's residual hearing through amplification and to employ auditory and speechreading (lipreading) training. The child's output is expected to be speech.

Cued Speech

Cued speech (Cornett, 1967) was devised to aid speechreading and speech development and employs eight formed handshapes in four positions, which are made close to the face of a speaker so they may supplement speechreading information. The cues assist in differentiating among sounds that appear to be the same on the lips (for example, /m/, /b/, and /p/). The child must simultaneously attend to both the speechreading and the cues, for the cues by themselves are meaningless.

Finger Spelling (Dactylology)

Finger spelling has been called "writing in the air" (Mayberry, 1978), because it is a system by which each letter of the alphabet is represented by a precise formation of the fingers of one hand; it allows users to spell out entire words, phrases, and sentences. Although finger spelling alone does not facilitate the development of language in children with significant hearing losses, it does preserve the rules of grammar and syntax, which are often compromised with some of the other systems. Figure 15.4 shows the manual alphabet.

Linguistics of Visual English (LOVE)

Linguistics of Visual English utilizes signs as in SEE 1 and SEE 2 but employs a slightly different written system, although it follows English word order. Finger spelling is used to show irregular tense use. LOVE is less commonly used than SEE 1 or SEE 2 (Mayberry, 1978).

Pidgin Sign English (PSE)

Pidgin Sign English is a combination of ASL and some of the elements of systems that use sign markers, such as SEE 1, SEE 2, and LOVE. According to Paul and Quigley (1987), PSE is probably the most popular form of sign communication used in classrooms in residential schools for the hearing impaired, because of problems associated with the consistent use of contrived signs in the other systems.

Rochester Method

Also known as visible speech, the Rochester Method was developed at the New York School for the Deaf. This method employs the simultaneous use of speech and fingerspelling in a "writing in air" technique superimposed on normal speech.

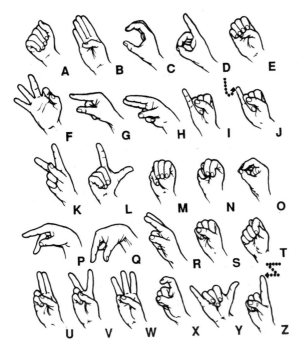

FIGURE 15.4 The manual alphabet.

Seeing Essential English (SEE 1)

Seeing Essential English primarily employs ASL, using word orders as they would appear in spoken or written English, with specific signs for some articles and verbs, and markers to help in identifying tense and number (Paul & Quigley, 1987). This system breaks down words into morphemes (e.g., *a-part-ment*). SEE 1 may allow a quicker grasp than ASL as a communication system for children, and may be faster to use.

Signed English (SE)

Signed English (Bornstein & Saulnier, 1973) is a manual system that follows the rules of English grammar. Finger spelling augments this system when no particular sign represents a word. SE takes ASL vocabulary and places it in English word order.

Signing Exact English (SEE 2)

Signing Exact English (Gustafson, Pfetzing, & Sawolkow, 1980) is similar to SEE 1 but is less rigid about following word order precisely in a sentence, which may account for its wide use (Paul & Quigley, 1987). This system breaks down words into morphemes that are individually accepted words (e.g., *cow-boy*).

Total Communication (TC)

Total communication is probably the most popular teaching system now employed for children with severe to profound hearing losses. It is accomplished by taking the best of the aural and sign systems, placing the emphasis on both to help the child to communicate. Proponents believe that language is learned more quickly and accurately through TC than by other methods, whereas critics maintain that it is unrealistic to expect some children to learn to listen, read lips, and follow signs at the same time.

Management of Tinnitus

Tinnitus has been mentioned several times in this book. Complaints of ear or head noises go back through recorded history and accompany, to some degree, almost every etiology of hearing loss. Many people experience tinnitus even though they have normal hearing, and a significant number suffer from severe, and near-debilitating tinnitus. While early measures of perceived tinnitus loudness suggested levels ranging from 1 to 20 dB SL (Graham & Newby, 1962), later measurement methods are more commensurate with the levels of tinnitus patients' distress, yielding values ranging from 8 to 50 dB SL (Goodwin, 1984). The prevalence of tinnitus in children may be greater than commonly realized, as children may be less likely to report these sounds unless questioned (Clark, 1984). Graham (1987) reported that more than 60 percent of surveyed children with hearing loss requiring amplification experienced some degree of tinnitus.

Although the origin of tinnitus has long been a source of debate among clinicians and researchers, recent investigation of cerebral blood flow suggests that the source of tinnitus may lie within auditory cortical regions of the brain rather than the cochlea itself (Lockwood, Salvi, Coad, Tosley, Wack, & Murphy, 1998). This would suggest that it may not be damage to the cochlea that gives rise to tinnitus, but rather aberrant changes within the central auditory pathways secondary to more peripheral impairment.

Figure 15.5 summarizes many of the contributors to the perception of tinnitus, which has been variously described by such adjectives as "ringing," "crickets," "roaring," "hissing," "clanging," "swishing," and a host of others. Tinnitus of a tonal quality, compared to "noise-type" tinnitus, is subjectively judged by patients as more annoying and is reported to occur more frequently (Press & Vernon, 1997). With the formation of the American Tinnitus Association (DeWeese & Vernon, 1975), consciousness has been raised on the subject, and professionals have learned to heed the complaints of tinnitus sufferers. Other than the use of masking sounds to cover up the tinnitus—for example, a clock radio or white noise generator at night, or hearing aids during the day—little help was available until about twenty years ago. Treatment has included drugs such as vitamins and vasodilators, such surgeries as labyrinthine or vestibular nerve destruction, nerve blocks, and cognitive therapy, all with varying results.

The wearable tinnitus masking unit has enjoyed some marginal popularity. Most such devices are similar to behind-the-ear and in-the-ear instruments (see Figure 14.6C and D) and are manufactured by some hearing-aid companies. The tinnitus masker, designed as a miniature masking unit, produces a band of noise that surrounds the frequency of the tinnitus. When no specific frequency or noise band is reported as characteristic of the tinnitus, a broadband signal may be used as the masker. With patience and gradual adjustments, a close match to a patient's tinnitus can be obtained.

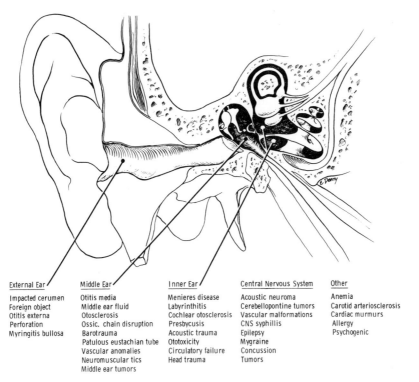

External Ear	Middle Ear	Inner Ear	Central Nervous System	Other
Impacted cerumen	Otitis media	Menieres disease	Acoustic neuroma	Anemia
Foreign object	Middle ear fluid	Labyrinthitis	Cerebellopontine tumors	Carotid arteriosclerosis
Otitis externa	Otosclerosis	Cochlear otosclerosis	Vascular malformations	Cardiac murmurs
Perforation	Ossic. chain disruption	Presbycusis	CNS syphillis	Allergy
Myringitis bullosa	Barotrauma	Acoustic trauma	Epilepsy	Psychogenic
	Patulous eustachian tube	Ototoxicity	Mygraine	
	Vascular anomalies	Circulatory failure	Concussion	
	Neuromuscular tics	Head trauma	Tumors	
	Middle ear tumors			

FIGURE 15.5   Possible contributors to the perception of tinnitus. (Courtesy of Dr. Ross Roeser)

Most patients have given disappointing reports on the effects of tinnitus maskers, but a few are extremely satisfied with the results. Some claim that not only is the tinnitus relieved by what they observe to be external sounds preferable to their own tinnitus, but also the tinnitus is temporarily absent after the masking device is removed. Although it is not completely understood, this effect may be explained by some residual inhibition in the auditory system. If a hearing loss is present, hearing aids with appropriate gain for the hearing loss often serve as effective tinnitus maskers.

The principles of biofeedback have also been applied for tinnitus relief. Biofeedback allows individuals to monitor their own physiological activity by attaching recording electrodes to special parts of the body; these permit the patient to observe and control the activity. Some patients have learned to monitor and suppress their tinnitus through biofeedback techniques.

Tinnitus Retraining Therapy (TRT) has been shown to provide patients with a means to habituate to the presence of their tinnitus (Jastreboff & Hazell, 1998). This therapy is based upon the observation that the auditory system's contribution to the annoyance of tinnitus may be secondary to that of the limbic (emotional) and the autonomic nervous systems. TRT requires a substantial amount of direct work with patients, but when done properly it yields a success rate for reducing tinnitus annoyance greater than 80 percent.

Some patients' complaints of tinnitus are much more dire than others with similar amounts of hearing loss, in whom one might predict a similar type and degree of tinnitus. Schechter, McDermott, and Fausti (1992) liken the affliction from tinnitus to experiences of pain. They suggest that, given a certain amount of neural activity stimulating the pain centers of the brains of two individuals, the experiences might be quite different, being modified by higher brain centers, and by such factors as mood, personality, and culture. They also suggest that the effects of tinnitus on any given individual's personal life may, at least in some cases, be influenced by that person's psychological state. Given the interactions between the often unknown physiological base of tinnitus, and the psychological reaction to it, the phenomenon of tinnitus continues to be perplexing.

Hyperacusis

Some patients with tinnitus report a decreased tolerance to loud sounds, and the majority of these report their **hyperacusis** to be equally disturbing as, or worse than, their tinnitus (Reich & Griest, 1991). Contrary to the common belief that hyperacusis represents an exceptionally acute sense of hearing, this disorder is more accurately described as a collapse of loudness tolerance. The threshold of loudness discomfort for the patient with hyperacusis is inversely related to frequency, with less loudness tolerance as frequency increases. The threshold of discomfort for these patients may be as low as 20 to 25 dB SL for low-frequency sounds (e.g., 250 Hz) declining to as little as 5 dB SL or less for sounds greater than 10,000 Hz (Vernon & Press, 1998). Hyperacusis is a separate phenomenon from recruitment, often considered to result from decreased inhibition within the central auditory system.

Those individuals with hyperacusis may react in a frightened or startled fashion to common sounds such as the telephone ringing or the noise of a vacuum cleaner. These persons may resort to the use of hearing protection to better endure their daily lives, although overprotection of the ears may actually cause a worsening of the condition. In addition to shunning protection of the ears from every day sounds, audiological rehabilitation has been successful with some with hyperacusis through a series of desensitization exercises over a protracted time (Vernon & Press, 1998).

Multicultural Considerations

Approximately one out of every three Americans is nonwhite, with Hispanics constituting the most rapidly growing of minority groups in the United States. The percentages of culturally and linguistically diverse groups among school-age children is nearly twice that in the general population (U.S. Bureau of the Census, 1990). Professionals have an obligation to become familiar with cultures apart from their own and to recognize the diversity existent within a given culture (Atkins, 1994). Variations within culturally acceptable family dynamics and cultural influences on outward interactions with those perceived to be in positions of authority can have a direct impact on acceptance and implementation of professional recommendations. In addition, language differences between audiologists and patients can directly influence both the evaluation and the subsequent counseling that is provided (Flores, Martin, & Champlin, 1996).

As described earlier, audiologists must remain cognizant of the views of those who align themselves within the culture of the Deaf community. Regardless of one's views on Deaf cultural issues, the Deaf community can serve as a valuable resource in hearing loss management for families and professionals alike.

Summary

Diagnosis of the type and degree of a patient's hearing loss is an essential beginning to audiological (re)habilitation. For proper management, the audiologist must become sophisticated in the intricacies of history taking. The importance of a proper professional relationship between the audiologist and the patient (or family) cannot be overstated. Advising and counseling sessions greatly affect the overall management of those with hearing impairment. Audiologists also must maintain good relationships with other professionals who may be involved in the rehabilitation of the patient. Proper relationships are strongly influenced by the exchanges among professionals, such as letters and reports.

Audiologists should be responsible for the total program of audiological rehabilitation of the adult patient with a hearing loss. They must make the determination of the need for special measures, such as speechreading, hearing therapy, auditory training, the acquisition of hearing aids, and tinnitus therapy or hyperacusis desensitization. If hearing aids are indicated, the audiologist will figure prominently in the selection procedure.

When working with children, audiologists must muster every resource at their disposal, including interactions with caregivers and other professionals in designing approaches that will maximize the human potential in every child with a hearing loss. To do less is a disservice to the children whose futures may be profoundly affected by professional decisions.

STUDY QUESTIONS

1. In what ways do the approaches to audiological rehabilitation differ for children and adults?

2. List the data you would include in a report sent to different specialists with a common interest in your patient. In what ways are the reports similar and dissimilar?

3. List the first five questions you would ask when recording a patient's history.

4. Design a case history form that might be suitable for (a) adult patients and (b) pediatric patients.

5. How may tinnitus and hyperacusis be treated?

6. How might acceptance of an acquired hearing loss be improved?

7. How would you approach the counseling of the parents of a child who has just been diagnosed with a hearing loss?

8. What are some of the topics that might be included in an adult hearing therapy class?

9. List the training and educational options for children with severe hearing impairments.

GLOSSARY

Audiological rehabilitation Treatment of those with adventitious hearing loss to improve communication through hearing aids, hearing therapy, speechreading, and counseling. Audiological *habilitation* of children may also include speech and language therapy, auditory training, and manual communication. Also known as aural rehabilitation.

Auditory training The training of the patient with a hearing loss in the optimum use of residual hearing.

Hearing disability An inability to perform socially useful functions due to hearing loss. A given disability may or may not present a handicap.

Hearing handicap The ways in which a hearing loss has a frustrating effect on individual roles or goals.

Hearing impairment Abnormality of structure or function that is physiological, psychological, or anatomical.

Hearing therapy An instruction, usually offered in groups, to enhance recognition of, and intervention for, those variables within the environment, or poor speaker or listener habits, that impede successful communication.

Hyperacusis A collapse of loudness tolerance with or without accompanying hearing loss.

Individualized Educational Plan (IEP) An annually updated, federally mandated plan for the education of children with handicaps.

Individualized Family Service Plan (IFSP) An annually updated, federally mandated plan for early intervention services for infants and toddlers with special needs and their families.

Lipreading See *Speechreading.*

Mainstreaming Integrating children with hearing impairments (or other disabilities) into the "least restrictive" educational setting. This often implies placement in a regular school classroom with special educational assistance, where necessary.

Postlinguistic hearing loss Hearing loss acquired by children after they have developed some language skills.

Prelinguistic hearing loss Hearing loss that is either congenital or acquired before language skills have been developed.

Speech conservation Therapy to maintain clear articulation when the auditory feedback for speech production has been hindered by postlinguistic hearing loss.

Speechreading The use of visual (primarily facial) cues to determine the words of a speaker.

Variable pure-tone average (VPTA) The average pure-tone threshold of the poorest three frequencies of 500, 1000, 2000, and 4000 Hz, used for the assignment of hearing loss impairment labels. Allows for a representation of hearing loss of either flat configuration or isolated primarily within either the lower or higher frequency range.

REFERENCES

Alpiner, J. G. (1994). Counseling geriatric patients and their families. In J. G. Clark & F. N. Martin (Eds.), *Effective counseling in audiology: Perspectives and practice* (pp. 278–309). Englewood Cliffs, NJ: Prentice Hall.

American Speech-Language-Hearing Association (ASHA). (1993). Guidelines for audiology services in the schools. *Asha, 35* (3) (Suppl.), 24–32.

Americans with Disabilities Act (ADA). (1991). United States Architectural and Transportation Barriers Compliance Board. Accessibility guidelines for buildings and facilities. *Federal Register, 56,* 144, 35455–35542.

Atkins, D. V. (1994). Counseling children with hearing loss and their families. In J. G. Clark & F. N. Martin (Eds.), *Effective counseling in audiology: Perspectives and practice* (pp. 116–146). Englewood Cliffs, NJ: Prentice Hall.

Bess, F. H., Lichtenstein, M. D., Logan, S. A., Burger, M. C., & Nelson, E. (1989). Hearing impairment as a determinant of function in the elderly. *Journal of the American Geriatrics Society, 37,* 123–128.

Blair, J. C. (1996). Educational audiology. In F. N. Martin & J. G. Clark (Eds.), *Hearing care for children* (pp. 316–334). Boston: Allyn & Bacon.

Bornstein, H., & Saulnier, K. (1973). Signed English: A brief follow-up to the first evaluations. *American Annals of the Deaf, 118,* 454–463.

Cassell, E. J. (1989). Making the subjective objective. In M. Stewart & D. Roter (Eds.), *Communicating with medical patients* (pp. 13–23). Newbury Park, CA: Sage.

Clark, J. G. (1981). Uses and abuses of hearing loss classification. *Asha, 23,* 493–500.

———. (1983). Beyond diagnosis: The professional's role in education consultation. *Hearing Journal, 36,* 20–25.

———. (1984). Tinnitus: An overview. In J. G. Clark & P. Yanick (Eds.), *Tinnitus and its management: A clinical text for audiologists* (pp. 3–14). Springfield, IL: Charles C Thomas.

———. (1994). Audiologist's counseling purview. In J. G. Clark & F. N. Martin (Eds.), *Effective counseling in audiology: Perspectives and practice* (pp. 1–17). Englewood Cliffs, NJ: Prentice Hall.

———. (1996). Guidelines for the classroom teacher: Appendix 9. In F. N. Martin & J. G. Clark (Eds.), *Hearing care for children* (pp. 359–360). Boston: Allyn & Bacon.

Cornett, R. O. (1967). Cued speech. *American Annals of the Deaf, 112,* 3–13.

Crandell, C. C. (1998). Hearing aids: Their effects on functional health status. *The Hearing Journal, 51,* 22–32.

DeConde-Johnson, C. (1991). The "state" of educational audiology: Survey results and goals for the future. *Educational Audiology Association Monograph, 2.*

DeWeese, D., & Vernon, J. (1975). The American Tinnitus Association. *Hearing Instruments, 18,* 19–25.

Education for All Handicapped Children Act of 1975. Public Law 94-142. U.S. Congress, 94th Congress, 1st Session, U.S. Code, section 1041-1456.

Education of the Handicapped Amendments. (1986, October). Public Law 99-457. *U.S. Statutes at Large, 100,* 1145–1176. Washington, DC: U.S. Government Printing Office.

Flexer, C., Wray, D., & Ireland, J. A. (1989). Preferential seating is *not* enough: Issues in classroom management of hearing-impaired students. *Language, Speech and Hearing Services in Schools, 20,* 11–21.

Flores, P., Martin, F. N., & Champlin, C. A. (1996). Providing audiological services to Spanish speakers. *American Journal of Audiology, 5,* 69–73.

Garstecki, D. C. (1994). Hearing aid acceptance in adults. In J. G. Clark & F. N. Martin (Eds.), *Effective counseling in audiology: Perspectives and practice* (pp. 210–246). Englewood Cliffs, NJ: Prentice Hall.

Goodwin, P. E. (1984). The tinnitus evaluation. In J. G. Clark and Yanick, P. (Eds.), *Tinnitus and its management: A clinical text for audiologists* (pp. 72–94). Springfield, IL: Charles C Thomas

Graham, J. (1987). Tinnitus in hearing-impaired children. In J. W. P. Hazel (Ed.), *Tinnitus* (pp. 131–143). Edinburgh: Churchill Livingston.

Graham, J. & Newby, H. (1962). Acoustical characteristics of tinnitus. *Archives of Otolaryngology, 75,* 162–167.

Gustafson, G., Pfetzing, D., & Sawolkow, E. (1980). *Signing Exact English: The 1980 edition.* Los Alamitos, CA: Modern Signs Press.

Haug, M., & Lavin, B. (1983). *Consumerism in medicine: Challenging physician authority.* Beverly Hills, CA: Sage.

Individuals with Disabilities Education Act of 1990 (IDEA). Public Law 101-476, U.S.C. 1400et seq.: *U.S. Statutes at Large, 104,* 1103–1151.

Individuals with Disabilities Education Amendments of 1997. Public Law 105-17, *U.S. Statutes at Large, 111,* 37–157.

Jastreboff, P. J., & Hazell, J. W. P. (1998). Treatment of tinnitus based on a neurophysiological model. In J. A. Vernon (Ed.), *Tinnitus: Treatment and relief* (pp. 201–217). Boston: Allyn & Bacon.

Johnson, C. D. (1994). Educational consultation: Talking with parents and school personnel. In J. G. Clark & F. N. Martin (Eds.), *Effective counseling in audiology: Principles and practice* (pp. 184–209). Englewood Cliffs, NJ: Prentice Hall.

Lane, H. (1987). Mainstreaming of deaf children—From bad to worse. *The Deaf American, 38,* 15.

———. (1992). *The mask of benevolence: Disabling the deaf community.* New York: Alfred A. Knopf.

Lockwood, A. H., Salvi, R. J., Coad, M. L., Tosley, M. S., Wack, D. S., & Murphy, B. W. (1998). The functional neuroanatomy of tinnitus: Evidence for limbic system links and neural plasticity. *Neurology, 50*(1), 114–122.

Luterman, D. M. (1987). Counseling parents of hearing-impaired children. In F. N. Martin (Ed.), *Hearing disorders in children* (pp. 303–319). Austin, TX: Pro-Ed.

Martin, F. N. (1994). Conveying diagnostic information. In J. G. Clark & F. N. Martin (Eds.), *Effective counseling in audiology: Principles and practice* (pp. 38–69). Englewood Cliffs, NJ: Prentice Hall.

Martin, F. N., Barr, M., & Bernstein, M. (1992). Professional attitudes regarding counseling of hearing-impaired adults. *American Journal of Otology, 13,* 279–287.

Martin, F. N., Bernstein, M. E., Daly, J. A., & Cody, J. P. (1988). Classroom teachers' knowledge of hearing disorders and attitudes about mainstreaming hard-of-hearing children. *Language, Speech and Hearing Services in Schools, 19,* 83–95.

Martin, F. N., & Clark, J. G. (1996). Behavioral hearing tests with children. In F. N. Martin & J. G. Clark (Eds.), *Hearing care for children* (pp. 115–134). Boston: Allyn & Bacon.

Martin, F. N., George, K., O'Neal, J., & Daly, J. (1987). Audiologists' and parents' attitudes regarding counseling of families of hearing impaired children. *Asha, 29,* 27–33.

Martin, F. N., Krall, L., & O'Neal, J. (1989).The diagnosis of acquired hearing loss: Patient reactions. *Asha, 31,* 47–50.

Martin, F. N., Krueger, J. S., & Bernstein, M. (1990). Diagnostic information transfer to hearing-impaired adults. *Tejas, 16,* 29–32.

Mayberry, R. T. (1978). Manual communication. In H. Davis & S. R. Silverman (Eds.), *Hearing and deafness* (4th ed., pp. 400–417). New York: Holt, Rinehart & Winston.

Moses, K. (1979). Parenting a hearing-impaired child. *Volta Review, 81,* 73–80.

Paul, P. V., & Quigley, S. P. (1987). Some effects of early hearing impairment on English language development. In F. N. Martin (Ed.), *Hearing disorders in children* (pp. 49–80). Austin, TX: Pro-Ed.

Press, L., & Vernon, J. (1997). Tinnitus in the elderly. *Hearing Health, 13*(6), 12–14, 20.

Reich, G., & Griest, S. (1991). *American Tinnitus Association hyperacousis survey.* Fourth International Tinnitus Seminar, Bordeaux, France.

Ross, M., Brackett, D., & Maxon, A. (1991). *Assessment and management of mainstreamed hearing-impaired children.* Austin: Pro Ed.

Ross, M., & Calvert, D. R. (1967). The semantics of deafness. *Volta Review, 69,* 644–649.

Self Help for Hard of Hearing People, Inc. (1996). Position statement on group hearing aid orientation programs. *SHHH, 3,* 29.

Schechter, M. A., McDermott, J. C., & Fausti, S. A. (1992). The incidence of psychological dysfunction in a group of patients fitted with tinnitus maskers. *Audiology Today, 4,* 34–35.

Smith, S. D. (1994). Genetic counseling. In J. G. Clark & F. N. Martin (Eds.), *Effective counseling in audiology: Perspectives and practice* (pp. 70–91). Englewood Cliffs, NJ: Prentice Hall.

Trychin, S. (1994). Helping people cope with hearing loss. In J. G. Clark & F. N. Martin (Eds.), *Effective counseling in audiology: Perspectives and practice* (pp. 247–277). Englewood Cliffs, NJ: Prentice Hall.

U.S. Bureau of the Census. (1990). *Statistical abstract of the United States: 1990* (110th ed.). Washington, DC: Government Printing Office.

Van Hecke, M. L. (1994). Emotional responses to hearing loss. In J. G. Clark & F. N. Martin (Eds.), *Effective counseling in audiology: Perspectives and practice* (pp. 92–115). Englewood Cliffs, NJ: Prentice Hall.

Vernon, J., & Press, L. (1998). Treatment for hyperacusis. In J. Vernon (Ed.), *Tinnitus: Treatment and relief* (pp. 223–227). Boston: Allyn & Bacon.

Vernon, M., & Mindel, E. (1978). Psychological and psychiatric aspects of profound hearing loss. In D. Rose (Ed.), *Audiological assessment* (pp. 99–145). Englewood Cliffs, NJ: Prentice-Hall.

Woodward, J. (1972). Implications of sociolinguistics research among the deaf. *Sign Language Studies, 1,* 1–7.

World Health Organization (WHO). (1980). *International classification of impairments, disabilities, and handicaps: A manual of classification relating to the consequences of disease* (pp. 25–43). Geneva: World Health Organization.

SUGGESTED READINGS

Alpiner, J. G., & McCarthy, P. A. (Eds.). (1993). *Rehabilitative audiology*. Baltimore: Williams & Wilkins.

Clark, J. G., & Martin, F. N. (Eds.). (1994). *Effective counseling in audiology: Perspectives and practice*. Englewood Cliffs, NJ: Prentice-Hall.

Hall, J. W., & Mueller, H. G. (1998). *Audiologists' desk reference, Vol. II: Audiologic management, rehabilitation, and terminology*. San Diego: Singular Publishing Group.

Hull, R. H. (Ed.). (1997). *Aural rehabilitation: Serving children and adults* (3rd ed.). San Diego: Singular Publishing Group.

Ross, M. (1997). A retrospective look at the future of aural rehabilitation. *Journal of the Academy of Rehabilitative Audiology, 30,* 11–28.

Sanders, D. A. (1993). *Management of hearing handicap: Infants to elderly* (3rd ed.). Englewood Cliffs, NJ: Prentice Hall.

AUTHOR INDEX

Page numbers in *italics* refer to the location of complete references.

SUBJECT INDEX

Page numbers in *italics* refer to the location of glossary definitions.

A

Academy of Dispensing Audiologists, 10
Academy of Rehabilitative Audiology, 10
Acoustic feedback, 395, *416*
Acoustic gain, 392, 393–394, *416*
Acoustic immittance, 151–159
Acoustic impedance, 151, *180*
Acoustic neurinoma, 341
Acoustic neuritis, 348, *364*
Acoustic neuroma, 341, *364*
Acoustic reflex, 152, 160–165, *180*
  arc, 160, *180*
  decay, 164, *180*
    test, 164, *180*
  screening of infants, 206
  threshold (ART), 160, *180*
Acoustic reflex tests, 360, 378–379
Acoustic trauma notch, 316, *329*
Acquired immune deficiency syndrome
    (AIDS), 311,
    329
Action potential (AP), 303, *329*
Active electrode, 168, *180*
Acute, 258, *287*
Aditus ad antrum, 251, *287*
Afferent, 303, *329*
Aided threshold goals, table, 411
Air conduction, 13, *22*, 74
  and bone conduction, relationship
    between, review table, 24
  measuring with pure-tone audiometer,
    48–49
  measuring with speech audiometer, 52
Air-bone gap (ABG), 92, *112*
Air-bone relationships, 96
Air-conduction audiometry, 81–89
Alexander Graham Bell Association for the
    Deaf, 10
All-or-none principle, 302
Allele, 308, *329*

Alternate Binaural Loudness Balance
    (ABLB), 186–187, *195*
Alternate Monaural Loudness Balance Test
    (AMLB), 186
American Academy of Audiology (AAA),
    9
American Auditory Society, 10
American National Standards Institute
    (ANSI), 42
American Speech and Hearing Association
    (ASHA), 9
American Speech Correction Association,
    9
American Standards Association (ASA),
    42
Amerslan. *see* American Sign Language
    (ASL)
Amplification/sensory systems, 389–418
  binaural amplification, 395
  characteristics of hearing aids, 392–395
    acoustic gain, 393–394
    distortion, 394
    frequency response, 394
    other parameters, 395
    output sound-pressure level (OSPL),
      393
  dispensing hearing aids, 408–410
  hearing aid circuit overview, 391–392
  hearing aid development, 389–391
  hearing aids, types of, 395–405
    auditory brainstem implants, 404
    behind-the-ear (BTE), 397–398
    body-type, 395–397
    bone-conduction, 400–401
    cochlear implants, 402–404
    completely in-the-canal (CIC), 399
    CROS, 399–400
    eyeglass, 397
    implantable bone-conduction,
      401–402

in-the-canal (ITC), 399
in-the-ear (ITE), 398
middle-ear implants, 402
vibrotactile instruments, 404–405
hearing assistance technologies,
    412–415
selecting hearing aids for adults,
    406–407
selecting hearing aids for children,
    407–408
selecting hearing-aid candidates, 406
verifying hearing-aid performance,
    410–411
Amplitude, 32, *65*
Amplitude distortion, 394, *416*
Ampulla, 294, *329*
Analog hearing aid, 391, *416*
Anechoic chamber, 63, *65*
Annulus, 235, *245*
Anotia, 237, *245*
Anoxia, 311, *329*
Aperiodic, 44, *65*
Apgar, Dr. Virginia, 201n
Apgar Test, 201, *224*
Artificial ear, 54, *65*
Artificial mastoid, 54, *65*
ASHA guidelines to audiologic screening
    of pediatric population, table, 221
Assistive listening device (ALD), 412, *416*
Athetosis, 309, *329*
Atresia, 238, *245*
Attenuation, 16, *22*
Audiogram, 84, *112*
Audiogram interpretation, 92–98
Audiological (re)habilitation, 419–448
  hyperacusis, 444
  management of adults with hearing
    impairments, 426–433
    counseling adult patients and their
      families, 428–431

455